LGBT-Parent Families

Abbie E. Goldberg • Katherine R. Allen
Editors

LGBT-Parent Families

Innovations in Research and Implications for Practice

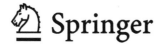

Editors
Abbie E. Goldberg
Department of Psychology
Clark University
Worcester, MA, USA

Katherine R. Allen
Department of Human Development
Virginia Polytechnic Institute
  and State University
Blacksburg, VA, USA

ISBN 978-1-4614-4555-5   ISBN 978-1-4614-4556-2 (eBook)
DOI 10.1007/978-1-4614-4556-2
Springer New York Heidelberg Dordrecht London

Library of Congress Control Number: 2012945937

Printed on acid-free paper

Springer is part of Springer Science+Business Media (www.springer.com)

LGBT-Parent Families: From Abnormal to Nearly Normative, and Ultimately Irrelevant

In 2003, I began teaching an undergraduate course titled "Sexual Diversity in Society" in what proved to be a turning point year for North American struggles for LGBT family rights. Gay rights plaintiffs in the USA and Canada scored a series of landmark court victories that year. State and provincial Supreme Courts in Massachusetts, Ontario, and British Columbia became the first in this hemisphere to judge bans on same-sex marriage unconstitutional, and in its historic ruling in the Lawrence v. Texas case, the USA Supreme Court reversed itself by overturning antisodomy laws. A scathing dissent by Justice Scalia correctly forecast the implications of this decision for the ultimate legalization of same-sex marriage.

I always begin my courses on sexual diversity by conducting an anonymous, informal survey about my students' sexual experiences, beliefs, attitudes, identities, and aspirations. Over the course of the past decade, I've noticed two intriguing, superficially contradictory, trends in the data produced by this decidedly unrepresentative sampling method. Unexpectedly, the number of women who label themselves lesbian has declined sharply, and the ranks of students claiming gay, or even straight, identities have been ebbing as well. Instead, students with nonconforming sexual or gender inclinations and practices, and women especially, have become more apt to describe themselves as "questioning, curious, undecided, or queer." Some refuse to define their sexuality at all.

This is not because my more recent cohorts of students are more fearful, reticent, or ashamed of their sexual desires than were their predecessors. They are not choosing to remain closeted due to internalized homophobia or a dread of social ostracism. On the contrary, like the public at large, my students express a steady rise in their acceptance of same-sex intimacy and in their level of support for same-sex marriage and parenthood. Indeed, virtually none of my students still considers heterosexuality to be prerequisite for forming families. Even those who proclaim the most dissident sexual and gender identities now seem to view their future entry into marriage and parenthood as social expectations that they variously embrace, defer, reject, or resist. No longer family outcasts, they are privileged members of the "post-closet" generation who do not feel obliged to define themselves or their family aspirations in terms of sexual identities.

The appearance of a handbook on LGBT-parent families similarly signals and advances the mainstreaming of a category of family that just a short time ago was utterly marginal, subversive, even illegal. As with same-sex marriage, what were once considered to be unacceptably queer forms of family have been moving rapidly from the realm of the clinically abnormal to that of the socially normative. Academic research has been intimately intertwined with the unexpectedly rapid normalization of at least lesbian- and gay-parent families. Court cases and legislative battles over bids for same-sex marriage, child custody rights, and access to foster care and adoption placements as well as to fertility and alternative reproductive services have relied heavily on the growing research literature on lesbian and gay parents and their children. Scholars working in this field, including yours truly, have been called to testify as experts in courtrooms and legislative hearings, and as public authorities and educators by the media and community institutions. Drawing on this mounting body of research, virtually all of the relevant major professional associations have weighed in, issuing a roster of reports and resolutions that affirm the effectiveness of lesbian and gay parents and formally support equal legal rights for them and their children. These include the *American Academy of Pediatrics, American Psychiatric Association, American Psychological Association, Canadian Psychological Association, American Psychoanalytic Association, American Academy of Child and Adolescent Psychiatry, National Association of Social Workers, Child Welfare League of America*, and the *North American Council on Adoptable Children*.

The publication of this handbook, like the launching of the *Journal of GLBT Family Studies* by the late Jerry Bigner in 2005, signals a coming of age, so to speak, of a subfield of research that gestated in the social movements for sexual and gender liberation and rights that generated its very subject matter. Both the journal and this substantial volume themselves serve as evidence of the astonishingly rapid growth, progress, and significance achieved by research in this field. They demonstrate that a formerly peripheral, somewhat suspect academic enterprise is now sufficiently mature and self-confident to undertake its own benchmarking self-assessments.

The impressively broad sweep of family forms, issues, and audiences addressed by this volume attests to this maturity. To date, the vast majority of research on LGBT-parent families actually treated only a narrow demographic band of families with parents who adopted the "L" word. In response to the weighty political context and uses of this research, during the first couple of decades, most researchers defensively compared lesbian-mother families to "normal" families with heterosexual parents, and their findings typically stressed the similarities in child outcomes. The earliest studies compared the families of lesbian and straight mothers who were raising children after a divorce from a heterosexual marriage. More recent studies typically focus on planned lesbian-parent families created via the use of donor sperm or legal adoption. Consequently, this volume opens with a series of useful overview chapters on these paths to lesbian motherhood that undertake a comprehensive, critical inventory of this most developed body of research.

However, Editors Abbie Goldberg and Katherine Allen know better than to sideline the families of the remaining constituents of the sexual minority alphabet. Ground-clearing, exploratory chapters included in this collection chart the more fledgling bodies of research on families with G, B, and T species of parents. The volume also boldly pushes the research goal posts by including chapters on important underrecognized subjects, such as LGBT grandparenthood, polyparenting, and the politically sensitive matter of the appearance of a "second generation"—children raised by LGBT parents who themselves develop LGBT identities.

Another sign of the maturity and confidence displayed by the editors and contributors to this handbook and by the subfield more broadly is their self-conscious awareness of ethnocentric limitations evident in most of the research that has been conducted to date. With rare exceptions, the LGBT-parent families that have been studied have been disproportionately composed of White, middle-class North Americans and West Europeans. Goldberg and Allen made a commendable effort to rectify this imbalance by including chapters that specifically treat the current state of research knowledge and ignorance about race, ethnic, and national diversity in patterns of LGBT-parent families. Likewise, most contributors to this volume adopt a unifying emphasis on an intersectional analysis of sexual, class, and racial-ethnic differences among families. Additionally, this book displays a keen sensitivity to understudied contextual factors that shape and constrain parenting practices, and children's experiences. Several chapters treat the impact of varied regional, occupational, and community environments on families with LGBT parents. Finally, the book assesses the status of research methods in the field and the implications of current knowledge for applied research, practice, and policy. Few readers of this volume will doubt that lesbian- and gay-parent families are well on their way to achieving normalization and that the more marginal ranks of transgender, bisexual, and polyamorous-parent families have embarked on the arduous struggle for recognition and respect.

In the end, however, the very existence of a specialized body of research on LGBT-parent families implies that there is something distinctive and important about them that merits explicit study. It implies that the families of lesbian, gay male, bisexual, and transgender parents share something important in common with one another that distinguishes them from those with heterosexual parents, and that all four categories are more like each other than any of them is like a family with straight parents. With one caveat, these presumptions are tendentious at best. The only undeniable factors that distinguish LGBT from straight-parent families are the social fact and the social effects of heteronormativity. What such families share is a need to cope with forms of prejudice, stigma, and discrimination that are rooted in aversion to the challenges to conventional gender and sexuality that their existence represents.

We are dealing here, in other words, with the effects of a distinction between a marked and unmarked category. Studies, books, and courses abound on African-American-parent families, but you're likely to search in vain for a course, study, or handbook assessing research on White-parent families. Research on working-class and poor families is marked, but rarely do we designate family research as about middle-class families. For similar reasons, we find no handbooks or courses on heterosexual-parent families. White, middle-class, heterosexual, married couple-parents are the taken for granted norm against which families composed of members of marked, and generally subordinate, categories are judged.

In the end, therefore, the ultimate fate of research on LGBT-parent families should be to help make its project anachronistic. Paradoxically, the research assessed and promoted here gestures optimistically toward a future where the sex and gender of parenthood has become a matter of social indifference. It helps us to imagine a world in which the very notion of studying LGBT-parent families might seem retro, quaint, and uninformed. Those comparatively privileged cohorts of students enrolling in my courses on sexual diversity, who already feel socially confident enough to resist sexual and gender badges, foreshadow such a future. Ironically, however, we still need much more careful research and practice of the sort presented in this book if we are ever to consign its very subject matter to the dustbin of history.

New York, NY, USA   Judith Stacey

Contents

Contributors

Katherine R. Allen, Ph.D. Department of Human Development, Virginia Polytechnic Institute and State University, Blacksburg, VA, USA

Mark Bartkiewicz, Ph.D. GLSEN (the Gay, Lesbian and Straight Education Network), New York, NY, USA

Dana Berkowitz, Ph.D. Department of Sociology and Program in Women's and Gender Studies, Louisiana State University, Baton Rouge, LA, USA

Henny Bos, Ph.D. Graduate School of Child Development and Education, College of Child Development and Education, Research Institute of Child Development and Education, University of Amsterdam, Amsterdam, The Netherlands

Amy Brainer, M.A. Department of Sociology, University of Illinois-Chicago, Harrison Street, Chicago, IL, USA

Eliza Byard, Ph.D. GLSEN (the Gay, Lesbian & Straight Education Network), New York, NY, USA

Cheryl Dobinson, M.A. Health Systems & Health Equity Research Group, Centre for Addiction & Mental Health, Toronto, ON, Canada

Jordan B. Downing, M.A. Department of Psychology, Clark University, Worcester, MA, USA

Rachel H. Farr, Ph.D. Department of Psychology, University of Massachusetts, Amherst, MA, USA

Christine A. Fruhauf, Ph.D. Department of Human Development & Family Studies, Colorado State University, Fort Collins, CO, USA

Jacqui Gabb, Ph.D. Department of Social Policy and Criminology, The Open University, Milton Keynes, UK

Abbie E. Goldberg, Ph.D. Department of Psychology, Clark University, Worcester, MA, USA

Peter Haydon, B.A. PolyVic, Melbourne, VIC, Australia

Stephen Hicks, Ph.D. School of Nursing, Midwifery, and Social Work, University of Salford, Salford, UK

Elizabeth Grace Holman, M.S., M.S.W. Department of Human and Community Development, University of Illinois at Urbana-Champaign, Urbana, IL, USA

Ann H. Huffman, Ph.D. Department of Psychology, W. A. Franke College of Business, Northern Arizona University, Flagstaff, AZ, USA

Anne Hunter, B.A. PolyVic, Melbourne, VIC, Australia

Eden B. King, Ph.D. Department of Psychology, George Mason University, Fairfax, VA, USA

Joseph Kosciw, Ph.D. GLSEN (the Gay, Lesbian and Straight Education Network), New York, NY, USA

Katherine Kuvalanka, Ph.D. Department of Family Studies and Social Work, Miami University, Oxford, OH, USA

Arlene Istar Lev, L.C.S.W-R., C.A.S.A.C. School of Social Welfare, and Choices Counseling and Consulting, University at Albany, Albany, NY, USA

Carien Lubbe, Ph.D. Department of Educational Psychology, University of Pretoria, Pretoria, South Africa

Nancy J. Mezey, Ph.D. Department of Political Science and Sociology, Monmouth University, West Long Branch, NJ, USA

Mignon R. Moore, Ph.D. Department of Sociology, University of California, Los Angeles, CA, USA

Joel A. Muraco, B.S. Norton School of Family and Consumer Sciences, University of Arizona, Tucson, AZ, USA

Nancy A. Orel, Ph.D., L.P.C. Gerontology Program, Department of Human Services, College of Health and Human Services, Bowling Green State University, Bowling Green, OH, USA

Ramona Faith Oswald, Ph.D. Department of Human and Community Development, University of Illinois at Urbana-Champaign, Urbana, IL, USA

Maria Pallotta-Chiarolli, Ph.D. Social Diversity in Health and Education School of Health and Social Development, Deakin University, Burwood, VIC, Australia

Charlotte J. Patterson, Ph.D. Department of Psychology, University of Virginia, Charlottesville, VA, USA

Chad I. Peddie, M.A. Human Resources Research Organization, Alexandria, VA, USA

Lori E. Ross, Ph.D. Department of Psychiatry, University of Toronto, Toronto, ON, Canada

Health Systems & Health Equity Research Group, Centre for Addiction & Mental Health, Toronto, ON, Canada

Stephen T. Russell, Ph.D. Norton School of Family and Consumer Sciences, University of Arizona, Tucson, AZ, USA

Aline G. Sayer, Ph.D. Department of Psychology, Center for Research on Families, University of Massachusetts, Amherst, MA, USA

Shannon L. Sennott, L.I.C.S.W. Translate Gender, Inc., Northampton, MA, USA

The Institute for Dialogic Practice, Northampton, MA, USA

Julie Shapiro, J.D. Fred T. Korematsu Center for Law and Equality, Seattle University School of Law, Seattle, WA, USA

JuliAnna Z. Smith, M.A. Department of Psychology, Center for Research on Families, University of Massachusetts, Amherst, MA, USA

Fiona Tasker, Ph.D. Department of Psychological Sciences, Birkbeck University of London, London, UK

Cynthia J. Telingator, M.D. Child and Adolescent Psychiatry, Cambridge Health Alliance, Harvard Medical School, Cambridge, MA, USA

Part I

Research: Overview Chapters

Lesbian and Gay Parenting Post-Heterosexual Divorce and Separation

Fiona Tasker

Pioneering Lesbian and Gay Parenting

Lesbian and gay parenting after a heterosexual relationship ends in separation or divorce was established as a field of research in the 1980s. Most of our knowledge about whether or not parental sexual orientation influences children's development is derived from studies of children raised by their lesbian mother and her new female partner after the child's mother and father separated. Lesbian and gay parenting post-heterosexual separation has not been a prominent topic in either published research or media headlines in recent years, as research interest has moved on to planned parenting by lesbians and gay men. Nevertheless, tantalizing questions of definition and fluidity both of sexuality and of parenting remain to be explored, and these are questions that speak to the heart of post-identity politics in a new era.

In reviewing the field I first contextualize lesbian and gay parenting post-heterosexual separation, noting difficulties of definition within our limited knowledge of the demographic profile of nonheterosexual parenting. Using U.S. Census data from 2000, Gates and Ost (2004) have estimated that about a quarter of same-gender

couples had children (under age 18 years) residing with them, with proportionately more children living in female couple-headed households than male couple-headed households. Gates (2008) has reasoned that a large proportion of these children were conceived in prior heterosexual relationships, as gay men and lesbians in same-gender couples who recorded previous heterosexual marriages were nearly twice as likely as those previously unmarried to have children. However, as Gates and Romero (2009) have explained, the U.S. Census did not ask a direct question about sexual identity, sexual behavior, or route to parenthood, and would have missed single lesbians or gay men or those with non-cohabiting partners. The Census used traditional definitions of the ending of a heterosexual marital relationship in divorce and the formation of stepfamily—thus confounding new partnership, co-residence, and stepparenting in presuming that a cohabiting same-gender partner would be involved in parenting and a non-cohabiting partner would not. Lesbian and gay parenting post-heterosexual separation does not necessarily fit traditional heterosexual patterns.

In the main body of this chapter I consider key published studies of lesbian and gay parenting post-heterosexual separation that have been undertaken, viewing them from a social constructionist position as situated within the sociohistorical context of various theoretical, legal, and social debates that have influenced the field. I have grouped the studies according to their thematic concerns: concerns about parental

F. Tasker, Ph.D. (✉)
Department of Psychological Sciences,
Birkbeck University of London, Malet Street,
Bloomsbury, London, WC1E 7HX, UK
e-mail: f.tasker@bbk.ac.uk

A.E. Goldberg and K.R. Allen (eds.), *LGBT-Parent Families: Innovations in Research and Implications for Practice*, DOI 10.1007/978-1-4614-4556-2_1, © Springer Science+Business Media New York 2013

separation or divorce and child well-being, hearing the voices of lesbian and gay parents, coming out, and acknowledging new partners. To highlight both theoretical perspectives and methodological aspects of the studies reviewed, I also have noted the academic discipline most associated with each thematic grouping as this too has contextualized the research.[1]

I conclude with a final section on new trends and future directions in which I consider an integrative perspective on the field, in particular drawing on the frameworks of life course theory (Bengtson & Allen, 1993; Elder, 1998), social constructionism (Gergen, 2009), and family systems theory (Broderick, 1993). These perspectives highlight (a) the importance of improving definition and measurement in quantitative research, (b) the need to contextualize lesbian and gay parenting by investigating intersectionality, and (c) the significance of queering the field and speaking the unspoken.

Where possible, I have prioritized studies that collect data from lesbian and gay parents themselves, and considered the often hidden perspectives of their same-gender partners, rather than dwelling on the more numerous studies on the perspectives and experiences of the children raised in these families. Children's perspectives are considered elsewhere in this volume (and see also Goldberg, 2010; Tasker & Patterson, 2007). Here I have aimed to direct attention to the diverse positions of lesbians and gay men engaged in parenting post-heterosexual separation or divorce.[2]

---

[1] In attempting to place the academic origins of particular studies I have undoubtedly simplified the complex multiple positions of scholars investigating lesbian and gay parenting. Nonetheless, discernable waves of research have ebbed and flowed upon particular theoretical and thematic currents navigated by investigators from particular academic disciplines.

[2] Post-heterosexual parenting takes place after the ending in separation or divorce of a heterosexual relationship in which children were conceived or adopted and the parent redefines their sexual orientation as nonheterosexual. In considering the published literature in the field I have focused on the position of lesbian and gay parents parenting post-heterosexual separation or divorce. Researchers in the field have sometimes noted the particular circumstances of their participants but most have not.

Concern About Parental Separation and Divorce: Influences from Child Psychology and Psychiatry

Clinicians working with children and their families were the first set of professionals to publish research on lesbian and gay parenting. Beginning in the 1970s and 1980s, papers by psychiatrists began to be published giving concise accounts of issues highlighted in case notes from individual sessions with lesbian mothers or gay fathers and their children. These papers tended to emphasize the difficulties children faced in lesbian- or gay-parent families post-heterosexual separation or divorce (Agbayewa, 1984; Weeks, Derdeyn, & Langman, 1975) or used psychoanalytic theory to examine children's psychosexual development (Javaid, 1983, 1993). Authors contextualized many of the issues encountered as similar to those faced by other children of separated or divorced heterosexual parents who had begun new sexual relationships. This work opened the door to later empirical work using control groups of children brought up by a single heterosexual parent after parental separation or divorce.

Initial studies of same-gender parenting were launched largely by developmental psychologists and child psychiatrists to empirically investigate pragmatic concerns raised by divorce settlements in the 1970s and 1980s restricting residence and visitation by lesbian mothers (e.g., Golombok, 2002). At this time observations were being made about the salience of father absence after parental divorce (e.g., Wallerstein & Kelly, 1980), and earlier conclusions regarding factors that constituted maternal deprivation were being reassessed (Rutter, 1981).

Studies also addressed theoretical questions on the influence of parenting on children's social development, testing out theories that emphasized the importance for children's development of having two resident parents of the opposite gender. Psychoanalytic theories emphasized the salience of the father's active presence in helping to resolve oedipal dilemmas for both sons and daughters (Socarides, 1978). Social learning theorists delineated not only the significance of same-gender role models for identity development but also the importance of both positive and negative reinforcement in shaping children's social behavior (Bandura, 1977). In contrast, social cognitive theories stressed the importance of the way children themselves organized knowledge about the world rather than parental influences per se (Martin & Halverson, 1981). These theories were evident in the studies as they focused attention on particular factors that might mediate the influence of lesbian parenting on children's developmental outcomes (Golombok & Tasker, 1994). Psychoanalytic theories drew attention to the amount of contact children had with their father subsequent to parental separation as moderating the influence of upbringing by a lesbian mother. Social learning theories indicated the significance of how the mother responded to her child's preferences related to gender and psychosexual development. Social cognitive theories highlighted children as active agents in their own social development and the salience of peer group norms rather than parental sources.

Beginning in the early 1980s, studies were published that examined the family relationships of children of separated or divorced lesbian mothers by comparing parent–child relationships in a group of lesbian-led families with a group of families headed by a single heterosexual mother. These studies carefully matched participants' characteristics between groups or statistically controlled for additional variables to rule out factors associated with the experience of parental separation or divorce. The most rigorous of these studies also used multiple measurements and independent reporters together with statistical techniques that calculated the probability of a finding being definitive beyond the particular sample that generated it (e.g., Golombok, Spencer, & Rutter, 1983; Green, Mandel, Hotvedt, Gray, & Smith, 1986).

Studies of this genre concentrated more on the parenting of the lesbian mother than on the parenting of her new same-gender partner and invariably concluded that lesbian mothers were just as warm, caring, and child-focused as heterosexual mothers (Golombok et al., 1983; Green et al., 1986;

Hoeffer, 1981; Kirkpatrick, Smith, & Roy, 1981; Lott-Whitehead & Tully, 1992; Mucklow & Phelan, 1979). Yet irrespective of this, lesbian mothers were more likely than heterosexual mothers to fear the loss of custody of their children (Lyons, 1983). The studies also concurred in finding that children raised by lesbian mothers after heterosexual separation or divorce were just as well adjusted as children raised in other post-divorce households. Specifically, these children showed no more evidence of psychological distress than population norms, generally had good relationships with their peers, displayed typical gender development patterns, and later most identified as heterosexual young adults (for reviews see Anderssen, Amlie, & Ytteroy, 2002; Tasker, 2005).

Knowledge of gay men's parenting has lagged behind knowledge of lesbian parenting post-heterosexual separation or divorce, perhaps in part because it has been difficult to recruit samples of gay men who had shared or full custody of their child after separating from the child's mother. Community surveys of gay fathers in the UK and USA confirmed that gay fathers and their new partners are more likely to have children visiting than they are to have children residing with them (Barrett & Tasker, 2001; Wyers, 1987). Further, unlike studies on lesbian motherhood, studies of gay fathers often have not included children as respondents and so have not systematically assessed developmental outcomes for children (Golombok & Tasker, 2010). Nevertheless, some studies have compared questionnaire data from nonresidential gay fathers and nonresidential heterosexual fathers. For example, Bigner and Jacobsen (1989a, 1989b, 1992) found that the divorced gay fathers they surveyed faced similar challenges to heterosexual divorced fathers in maintaining relationships with their children who lived apart from them. Compared with the heterosexual fathers surveyed, the gay fathers reported that they were more cautious in showing affection to their partner in front of their child, used a more child-centered approach to discipline, and set stricter limits on their child's behavior. One of the few studies to use questionnaire and interview data to compare 13 lesbian mother- and 10 gay father-headed families tentatively indicated that gay fathers reported less problematic relationships with their ex-spouse and were more likely to encourage their children to play with gender-typed toys than were lesbian mothers (Harris & Turner, 1985; Turner, Scadden, & Harris, 1990). At the same time, this study found that lesbian mothers tended to indicate more possible benefits to their children from their new family environment (Harris & Turner, 1985; Turner et al., 1990).

Hearing the Voices of Lesbian and Gay Parents: Activists and Feminists Critiquing the Frameworks of Debate

It is important not to neglect the invaluable perspective provided by lesbian mothers and gay fathers themselves on post-heterosexual separation or divorce families, who point to the diversity of family structures and unique advantages and challenges of living lesbian motherhood or gay fatherhood. Many of these voices were acknowledged by feminist activists and scholars and collected together in insightful anthologies. For example, the Boston Lesbian Psychologies Collective published reviews and research to highlight issues such as the diversity of women's sexual identities and experiences (Golden, 1987; Nichols, 1987) and vitally noted how motherhood, sexuality, ethnicity, and other cultural contexts intertwined (Espin, 1987; Hill, 1987). Other authors have stressed how children in these families, by seeing openly gay men and lesbians, would learn about the possibilities of nontraditional lives and appreciate diversity as positive rather than threatening, and so become more accepting of their own individual sexual behavior (Bigner, 1996; Riddle, 1978).

Increasing social tolerance and the push from the gay, lesbian, and feminist liberation movements, together with empirical findings from studies discussed in the previous section of this chapter, were influential in positively changing the context for legal decisions about custody and access post-heterosexual separation (Falk, 1989).

Nonetheless, in legal cases, particular research findings were highlighted that coincided with less accepting social attitudes toward nonheterosexual parenting. Legal cases and social debates in the USA were dominated by nexus test cases (Logue, 2002). Under nexus judgments, parental sexual orientation was considered irrelevant to child custody decisions unless a direct link could be made between the parents' sexual behavior and negative child outcomes. Nexus judgments not only considered particular child outcomes to be paramount, but also viewed these child outcomes in isolation from the context of familial and wider social, cultural, and historical systems that surrounded them. The criteria used in the "best interests of the child" debates focused attention on the child's individual developmental outcomes: That is, the child should not differ from population norms on well-being and peer relationships, lesbian or gay parenting should be equivalent to heterosexual parenting, and continued contact with the child's heterosexual opposite-gender parent should occur. Moreover, it was thought that the child's gender development should be prescribed by his or her biological sex, and that children should grow up to become heterosexual adults. Clarke, Ellis, Peel, and Riggs (2010) have argued that drawing the above distinctions between acceptable and unacceptable outcomes regulated the lives of many lesbian mothers, who felt compelled to present themselves as "good" mothers by downplaying their sexuality, providing male role models for their children, and remaining neutral about their child's sexual identity.

Several authors have contended that engaging with the best interests of the child debate constrained research in the field within the limitations of a liberal humanist agenda, anxious to promote justice by arguing from a "no difference" perspective on sexual orientation (Clarke, 2002; Malone & Cleary, 2002; Stacey & Biblarz, 2001). Confusing issues of justice and fair treatment with equal needs, and ignoring cultural or contextual differences, has been a problem in other research fields too, such as (dis)ability (Mulderrig, 2007) and cross-cultural counseling (Pedersen, 2003).

Certainly the research questions investigated in the first wave of studies were dominated by empirically investigating whether children brought up by lesbian mothers were disadvantaged; for example, most studies measured only the presence or absence of psychological distress (for a review see Tasker, 2005) with only two published studies measuring more positive indices such as self-esteem (Gershon, Tschann, & Jemerin, 1999; Huggins, 1989). Nevertheless this research opened up areas for further exploration; the two-tailed hypotheses used not only tested for disadvantage but also could suggest advantage. Further, in some studies, multivariate within-group analyses of lesbian- or gay-parented families revealed a more nuanced picture. For example, the studies by Huggins (1989) and Gershon et al. (1999) indicated evidence for a bimodal distribution of self-esteem scores in the small samples of adolescents from the post-heterosexual separated or divorced lesbian mother families they recruited. Namely, self-esteem scores were generally higher than control group scores for children who felt positively about their mother's lesbian identity (Huggins, 1989) and adolescents who perceived little stigma associated with having a lesbian mother (Gershon et al., 1999).

Coming Out: Sociologists and Psychotherapists Delineate Identity Pathways and Resources

In contrast to the controlled quasi-experimental studies focused on child outcome measures described previously, other empirical papers generally authored by those trained in sociology, psychotherapy, or social work focused on the lived experiences of lesbian mothers and gay fathers themselves. Authors described the motivations for forming and exiting heterosexual relationships and the process of coming out as lesbian, gay, or bisexual. Research in this tradition not only outlined the challenges experienced by lesbian and gay parents but also gave insight into the resources that parents drew upon and the resilience of family members.

These studies produced rich qualitative data outlining how women and men who identified as lesbian or gay had become parents through a heterosexual relationship. Findings from these investigations suggested that lesbian and gay parents often entered into a heterosexual relationship for a wide variety of reasons. Some women and men recalled earlier feelings of same-gender attraction, but in addition experienced intense interpersonal pressure to marry from an opposite-gender partner (Buntzly, 1993; Dunne, 2001) or their family of origin (Miller, 1979). Others felt the weight of societal expectations upon them to marry (Buntzly, 1993; Pearcey, 2005; Wyers, 1987) or desired the cultural status associated with marriage and parenthood (Bigner & Jacobsen, 1989a). Some reported thinking that a lesbian or gay identity was incompatible with parenthood or said they could not see a reflection of themselves in the negative stereotypes of lesbians or gay men they had encountered (Dunne, 2001). Several had hoped that marriage would move their sexual desires away from others of the same gender (Dunne, 2001; Ross, 1990; Wyers, 1987). Others had very little or no awareness of sexual interest in the same gender until after marriage (Bozett, 1981a; Coleman, 1990; Miller, 1979). Some cited more positive reasons for their heterosexual relationship, such as the desire to have children (Wyers, 1987) or a genuine affection for their partner (Coleman, 1990; Dunne, 2001; Miller, 1979; Ross, 1990; Wyers, 1987).

While authors such as Coleman (1990) have noted the absence of literature on bisexual and lesbian women "coming out" in heterosexual marriages, retrospective studies by sociologists Bozett (1981a, 1981b) and Miller (1978, 1979) have outlined the multifaceted identity careers of gay fathers. Miller (1978) suggested that fathers who were in the process of identifying as gay men increasingly found heterosexual marriage to be a difficult commitment to sustain; the turning point for many gay fathers often hinged on the development of an ongoing intimate relationship with another man. In Miller's terminology, men in this situation were at various stages in moving from seeing themselves as a *trade husband* (a man who opportunistically had sexual experiences with men), a *homosexual husband* (a man who had begun to acknowledge a nonheterosexual identity only to himself), a *gay husband* (a man who had acknowledged a gay identity to himself and to key others, including his wife), and a *faggot husband* (a man who had acknowledged his identity as an out gay father with pride and maintained an ongoing relationship with his children). Other authors have indicated that some opposite-gender couples in mixed orientation marriages may stay together many years, for instance by not responding to or avoiding external pressures to split up, enhancing the companionate nature of their own relationship, and finding kin and friends who will sustain their family rather than undermine it (Buxton, 2005).

A variety of experiences of coming out to their children were noted by the gay fathers in Benson, Silverstein, and Auerbach's (2005) qualitative study of 25 gay fathers. Some of the gay fathers described coming out as a transformative experience that increased honesty and closeness in their relationships generally. Other fathers decided not to disclose to their family because they worried about problems that disclosure might bring, or felt obligated to their wife or other family members not to tell on the marriage. Bozett (1981a) concluded that gay fathers experienced a fear of rejection in trying to conjoin both their identities as a separated or divorced father and as a gay man. Bozett argued that disclosure to others who affirmed both identities supported the gay father's own self-acceptance. Long-term individual psychotherapy with gay fathers has suggested that the emotional distress surrounding the coming out process can last for several years (Bigner, 1996).

Papers describing the resilience of lesbian-mother families and gay-father families also outlined the reasoning, strengths, and resources that family members drew upon. On the one hand, reports by Hall (1978) and Lewis (1980) on lesbian motherhood have suggested that some of the difficulties that children experienced in accepting their mother's new female partner were linked to resolving their feelings about the ending of their mother's and father's relationship. The 10 gay fathers interviewed by

Turner et al. (1990) also thought that any distress or problems their children had were more connected to parental separation or divorce than adjusting to having a gay parent. On the other hand, Lewis (1980) pointed out how some of the 21 children with lesbian mothers whom she interviewed did not feel ambivalent about their mother and in fact were proud of her for "standing up for what she believed" (p. 203) and permitting them also to break with conventional gender roles if they desired.

The issues faced by lesbian- or gay-parented families post-heterosexual separation or divorce were sometimes similar to those faced in families led by heterosexual parents post-separation or divorce, but also crucially different because of social stigma. Particular studies in the social work tradition gave insights into the fears expressed by adolescent sons and daughters that they would be judged and possibly rejected by their peers at school because of having a lesbian mother (Lewis, 1980; O'Connell, 1993) or a gay father (Bozett, 1987b). From her own experience running a psychotherapy clinic, Pennington (1987) highlighted that the most serious challenges faced by children and lesbian mothers were how to manage the heterosexism and homophobia they encountered in their daily lives at school, at work, and in their neighborhoods. Pennington stressed that the constraint and secrecy imposed by ignorance and prejudice outside the family could engender mistrust in family relationships.

Other authors have emphasized how isolating the experience of lesbian parenthood can be. Crawford (1987) found that lesbian mothers experienced separation from the social world of (presumed heterosexual) motherhood, while as mothers with children from heterosexual relationships their lesbian identity was sometimes doubted by lesbians without children. Other studies analyzing data from large community surveys of lesbian and bisexual women or gay men have found that parents who had children before identifying as lesbian, bisexual, or gay were significantly older than their peers when they first questioned their sexuality, had their first same-gender sexual experience, or first talked to someone about their sexual identity (Henehan, Rothblum, Solomon, & Balsam, 2007; Morris, Balsam, & Rothblum, 2002). Using the concept of a social clock highlighted by life course theorists (Bengtson & Allen, 1993), the findings of these studies suggest that adjustment to membership of a lesbian or gay community could be particularly challenging for lesbian mothers or gay fathers who had children before coming out, since they are going through developmental milestones "off-time" compared with lesbian or gay peers.

Acknowledging New Partners: Employing Stepfamily Dynamics to Investigate Parenting Post-Heterosexual Separation or Divorce

One unresolved issue that stood out in many early studies of lesbian and gay parenting post-heterosexual separation or divorce was the seeming absence of a same-gender partner; the lesbian or gay parent may be partnered but rarely did partners appear in studies focused on lesbian and gay parents. In part the specific research focus on children and biological parenting can be held culpable; nevertheless, this absence should be contextualized alongside more general societal pressures that have conspired to keep partners as "invisible members" of newly formed post-heterosexual divorce families. For instance, a household is more visibly headed by a lesbian or gay parent if a same-gender partner cohabits, and many jurisdictions placed residence or access restrictions on a lesbian or gay parent if the partner was present (Logue, 2002). Further, if a partner became involved in parenting, families faced a variety of issues to resolve: What roles would the partner take on in the family? And how would she or he be known—as a co-parent, a stepparent, or a special family "friend?" Authors also have come up against the problem of terminology; as Nelson (1996) has discussed, no term is problem free. In this review I have followed Nelson and used stepparent as the literal term to denote the married, cohabiting, or non-cohabiting partner of their biological parent.

Lesbian and Gay Stepparented Families: Archetypal Incomplete Institutions and Families of Choice?

Two theoretical advances in particular have inspired research on lesbian and gay stepparented families. First, Cherlin (1978) proposed the sociological concept of the incomplete institution to describe stepfamily relationships, and later identified stepfamily relationships, rising rates of cohabitation, and the advent of same-sex marriage and civil partnerships as key aspects in the weakening of social norms around marriage per se (Cherlin, 2004). Second, in her anthropological research on lesbians and gay men's conceptualization of family, Weston (1991) crucially expanded the concept of kinship networks to consider fluidity and meaning, not just biological and marital ties. Both theoretical concepts have been employed to investigate the internal and external social relationships of lesbian and gay stepparented families.

The stepfamily led by a same-gender couple has been described as an archetypical example of an incomplete institution (Erera & Fredricksen, 1999; Hall & Kitson, 2000; Hequembourg, 2004). As participants in an incomplete institution, same-gender stepfamily members encounter an absence of terminology for family relationships and the lack of legal or public acknowledgement of their family relationships. Conceptualizing the same-gender couple stepfamily as an example of an incomplete institution has highlighted the lack of definition and recognition surrounding same-gender stepfamily membership as a separate issue, distinct from, albeit connected with, prejudice against lesbian and gay parents. Crawford (1987) has described how the lack of language and cultural rites of passage can serve to work against and render invisible otherwise loving family relationships. Crawford further describes how invalidation can foster anxiety and insecurity leading to secrecy on the part of families. This invalidation and secrecy may in turn render the family being vulnerable to and unable to resist outside intrusion, for example, by ex-husbands or family of origin members feeling that they should have prior claim on the children. Finding terms to describe the relationship or role between a parent's new partner and the parent's child is complex. Ainslie and Feltey (1991) have described how no simple term described the variation in parenting roles that lesbian mothers ascribed to their partner and how partnership status often went unmarked or lacked recognition. While acknowledging the difficulties that absence of terminology presented, Ainslie and Feltey paradoxically noted that the absence of terminology also could free relationships from cultural assumptions, thus enabling these relationships to develop as family members deemed appropriate. Hequembourg's (2004) study also indicated that while lesbian-led stepfamilies can experience internal dynamics that have much in common with those reported within heterosexual stepfamilies, lesbian-led stepfamilies additionally encounter incomprehension and prejudice during their external interactions (e.g., with schools, the law) because their incompletely institutionalized position eluded recognition.

Ethnographic research by Weston (1991) detailing kinship networks first headlined the importance of nonbiological kin in "families we choose," emphasizing the importance of current partners, ex-partners, and those who are more than good friends in providing socioemotional, practical, and financial support for lesbians and gay men. Supportive networks, including family of choice as well as traditional kin, have been seen as particularly important for lesbian- and gay-parented families formed post-heterosexual separation, in dealing with the implications of both stigmatization and incomplete institutionalization. For example, Oswald (2002) has suggested two main family-supporting strategies employed in kin networks that center on lesbians and gay men: choosing supportive kin and selectively disclosing kin to others outside the family circle (intentionality); and using political action, such as changing surnames and legal deeds, to recognize kinship relationships (redefinition). Nevertheless two small qualitative studies that have explored kinship networks have yielded contradictory findings. Ainslie and Feltey (1991) highlighted

how lesbian feminist mothers parenting post-heterosexual separation described the importance of family of choice relationships that crucially helped out at critical points when usual household resources were stretched. In contrast, Gabb (2004), in her UK study of 13 post-heterosexual separation or divorce lesbian-led middle- and working-class families, reported that "'friends as family' neither represented the reality of their kinship networks nor was an ideal to which they aspired" (p. 169).

Same-Gender Stepparented Families: Similarities

Some authors have delineated the similarities of gay- and lesbian-led stepfamilies with stepfamilies led by heterosexual couples. Children in both types of stepfamilies have more of an emotional tie to their parent than their stepparent; they also tend to have a closer tie to their nonresident parent than their stepparent (Baptiste, 1987; Ganong & Coleman, 2004). Current-Juretschko and Bigner (2005) argued that the descriptions of stepfather roles and daily stepfamily life given by five gay stepparents living with their partner's biological children differed little from those provided by heterosexual stepfathers in other studies of stepfamily life.

Certainly there are structural similarities between same-gender couple and opposite-gender couple stepfamilies. First, the relational building block from which the stepfamily has taken shape is the relationship between parent and child that pre-dates that of parent and stepparent. Second, the stepfamily will have to consider the relationship of the parent's ex-partner to the child and manage the implications of this in family life. Third, separation and re-partnership have important implications for financial resources that go into maintaining a household; while some family members may gain resources as a result of household transitions most will lose, and some badly. Aspects of these three dynamics can be seen as having influence on stepfamily life in the studies detailed below. Nevertheless the particular implications of stepfamily dynamics depend on whether children are not resident or resident full or part-time and crucially are moderated by gender.

Other studies of gay fathers have highlighted the role that a new partnership can play in satisfaction with family life. For example, the British Gay and Bisexual Parenting Survey (GBPS) of 101 fathers, many of whom were parenting nonresident children from a previous heterosexual partnership, compared self-report ratings given by single gay fathers with ratings from gay fathers who had a male partner (Barrett & Tasker, 2001). This survey found that men with partners, particularly those who were cohabiting, rated themselves as more successful than single gay fathers at managing common household and parenting challenges. In another study of 48 families, the factor that was associated most with high levels of satisfaction with family life (as rated by gay fathers, male partners, and children) was the extent to which a new male partner had been integrated into family life (Crosbie-Burnett & Helmbrecht, 1993).

In contrast to the 23 post-heterosexual separation or divorce lesbian and gay parents in her sample, Lynch (2004a) reported that most of their lesbian and gay partners had not been involved in parenting prior to commencing that particular relationship; thus, how to be a stepparent to their new partner's child was a major question for them. Becoming a parent to a partner's child has been highlighted as a challenging issue faced by stepparents in other studies too, particularly in counterpoint to the issues faced by lesbian mothers in letting another "mother" her child (Ainslie & Feltey, 1991; Baptiste, 1987; Hall, 1978; Nelson, 1996).

Same-Gender Stepparented Families: Differences

While there are undoubtedly some similarities between same-gender and opposite-gender partnership stepfamilies in terms of stepfamily dynamics, there are important differences in terms of the legal recognition of the stepparent. Second-parent adoptions have been used in many states in the USA to give legal recognition to the stepparent's relationship with the child. However, second-parent adoption orders (which allow the stepparent to take parental responsibility for legal decisions for the child) are more commonly registered for resident heterosexual stepparents than lesbian or gay stepparents (Ganong & Coleman, 2004; Hequembourg & Farrell, 1999). Second-parent adoptions can be fraught with legal complications because state adoption laws generally require that the child's nonresident genetic parent has legally relinquished his or her parenthood before a second-parent adoption (as yet most jurisdictions refuse to allow a child having more than two legal parents and many require the stepparent to be married to the child's biological parent).

Studies by developmentalists have investigated how family life (including stepparent–child relationships) developed for children in lesbian parent-led families post-heterosexual separation or divorce. For example, most of the children in both groups of separated or divorced lesbian mothers and heterosexual mothers who were interviewed by Golombok and colleagues in the 1970s (Golombok et al., 1983) were reinterviewed in early adulthood, by which time over 80% of the mothers in both groups had cohabited with a new partner (Tasker & Golombok, 1995, 1997). Sons and daughters described a variety of different ways in which their mothers' female partners fit into family life in these lesbian stepparent families: sometimes female partners took on a major role in child care and were described as a second mother, while in other cases the young person described their mother's partner as more like a big sister, or an important family friend. The sons and daughters of lesbian mothers generally depicted their mother's female partner as integrating with existing family relationships rather than dividing them, whereas some of the young people with re-partnered heterosexual mothers regarded their stepfather with some hostility or resented him trying to take on a father's role. Perhaps women partnering with women with children from a prior heterosexual relationship "do stepparenting" differently than men partnering with women with children.

There are further crucial differences between same-gender and opposite-gender partnership stepfamilies in the degree of stigmatization that family members likely encounter. From his findings from a focus group study of six partnered lesbian mothers, Berger (1998a, 1998b) argued that lesbian stepfamilies are vulnerable to triple stigmatization (a) by mainstream society for identifying as lesbians, (b) for stepfamily membership, and (c) by the lesbian and gay community for being involved in parenting. Prejudice by nonparenting lesbians and gay men potentially could cause particular distress for lesbian and gay parents and their partners, because it creates distance between them and a source of community support.

Coming out as a same-gender couple-headed stepfamily can present an important challenge for parents and stepparents. Most of the 23 parents in Lynch's (2004b) study had gone simultaneously through the processes of self-identifying as lesbian or gay, coming out to others, dealing with stigma, separating from their spouses, and beginning stepfamily relationships. In the same study, many of the lesbian or gay partners described entry into stepfamily life as a second coming out process with different parameters and implications from their earlier disclosures because they had to make decisions as a family (Lynch, 2004a). Dealing with the possibility of their children experiencing prejudice from peers was of paramount importance in most lesbian and gay stepparenting families: Both parents and stepparents often held back disclosure to avoid prejudice despite the difficulties this posed for their couple relationship (Lynch & Murray, 2000). Changes in household composition post-heterosexual separation also may make a lesbian- or gay-parented family more visible and so more vulnerable to prejudice (Van Dam, 2004). Studies with gay fathers have pointed to the compromises that they made in exercising boundary control to compartmentalize their lives. For example, some of the 14 fathers interviewed by Bozett (1987a) described hiding any possible gay signifiers to avoid unwanted disclosure to their children's friends. The ongoing problem of social stigma and its impact on daily family life has been underscored by Robitaille and Saint-Jacques (2009) in their qualitative study of 11 sons' and daughters' experiences growing up in post-heterosexual separation or divorce lesbian and gay stepparented families.

Families led by lesbians or gay men where one or both of the same-gender partners had children from a previous heterosexual relationship seem to "do" family not only in different ways to heterosexual stepfamilies but also in different ways than same-gender couples who had or adopted children together (Perlesz et al., 2006). Planned gay or lesbian parenthood allows couples to plan and organize their parenting together in a process that often begins long before a child's arrival. Forming a same-gender relationship when a partner, or both partners, already have a child is complicated by preexisting family relationships including ex-partners and possibly extended family members; this complication may be particularly difficult if there has been a high level of conflict between ex-partners.

New Trends and Future Directions

At the beginning of the twenty-first century, a number of scholars have interrogated the field of lesbian and gay parenting. Some researchers have highlighted the importance of continuing to conduct outcome-based research, but also pointed to ways to develop the rigor of quantitative research (Goldberg, 2010; Tasker & Patterson, 2007). Other authors have suggested a more radical overhaul of the field to deploy social constructionist, queer theory, and psychoanalytic paradigms to consider the different social realities experienced by children growing up with LGBT parents (Biblarz & Stacey, 2010; Clarke et al., 2010; Malone & Cleary, 2002; Stacey & Biblarz, 2001). As I review below, these ideas all have exciting, and sometimes competing, implications for the field, some of which are already beginning to be taken up by researchers.

Improving Definition and Measurement in Quantitative Research

Over the last decade, there have been important steps in both sampling and measurement that have improved the quality of quantitative outcome based research (for reviews see Goldberg, 2010; Tasker & Patterson, 2007). Most empirical studies have sampled mainly White and middle-class self-selected samples of lesbian mothers. Thus, understanding of gay-father families, bisexual-parented families, and the impact of ethnicity and social class on LGB family life still lags far behind (Golombok & Tasker, 2010; Tasker & Patterson, 2007).

Recruiting lesbian-mother and gay-father families through national data sets has been a considerable step forward in our knowledge of the demographics of lesbian and gay parenting. Nevertheless, using national data sets may not necessarily address the issue of how representative those surveyed are of families with a lesbian or gay parent, since many such families slip through the net of traditional survey questions (see Chap. 22). In particular, the lack of clear criteria for defining lesbian or gay parenthood has presented a serious problem. While the sons and daughters of lesbian and gay parents have been extensively questioned about their sexual orientations, most studies have taken self-identification as a lesbian or gay parent to be the criterion for inclusion in the survey study group (Tasker & Patterson, 2007). The problem of self-identification is compounded further as many of the comparative studies reviewed above also relied on the presumption that none of the members of the heterosexual parent comparison groups had ever experienced same-gender attractions or relationships. The reluctance of epidemiological researchers to ask the general public questions about sexual orientation has meant that recent research studies benefiting from nationally representative samples have had to compromise on specificity and rely instead on extensive data checking to deduce that children in the study group were indeed being raised in a lesbian-led

family (Wainright & Patterson, 2006; Wainright, Russell, & Patterson, 2004).

Another issue of sampling definition is ensuring that researchers routinely collect adequate data on different pathways to parenthood. Regrettably, there are no methods of distinguishing between planned or post-heterosexual separation or divorced lesbian- or gay-parented families in the Add Health data set used by Wainright et al. (2004) and Wainright and Patterson (2006). Small-sample qualitative studies that can detail route to parenthood and family relationships have raised intriguing questions in the field, but these studies may produce contradictory findings. For example, earlier in this chapter I noted differences between the findings reported by Ainslie and Feltey (1991) and Gabb (2004) with regard to the importance of family of choice kinship networks between couples parenting in post-heterosexual separation lesbian-led stepfamilies. Without properly controlled quantitative comparison studies it is not possible to ascertain the strength of different associations in the data and discover whether or not findings constitute a predictable, or indeed a general, pattern.

Measurement reliability, validity, and comparability across different studies have also remained an issue for quantitative studies, and how to pool findings across studies has been a challenge for meta-analytic and narrative reviews alike (Crowl, Ahn, & Baker, 2008; Tasker & Patterson, 2007). Further, only a few studies gather and compare data from multiple family members, use independent observers blind to family type, and collect prospective data to attempt to discern causal pathways (Tasker, 2005). New models of association both between and within different types of families await to be discerned in future quantitative research employing rigorous measurement standards.

Deconstructing and Contextualizing Lesbian and Gay Parenting

Social constructionist ideas have emphasized the crucial importance of considering the particular intersections of demographic characteristics, to take into account the complexities of cultural context in creating a diversity of subject positions and subjective experiences. Sexuality has been underinvestigated in gender studies and class analysis (Taylor, 2011) while studies of race and ethnicity have considered mostly men who are presumed to be heterosexual (Glenn, 2000). While queer theoretical approaches have placed diversity and fluidity in the foreground, they have often sidelined the gender- and class-based materiality of sexuality (Jackson, 2011). These complex intersections challenge us to move beyond additive accounting of advantage versus disadvantage to consider group-, process-, and system-centered understandings of interactions (Choo & Ferree, 2010).

Future research should take into account the complex intersections of gender, sexuality, (dis) abilities, racial or ethnic differences, and routes to parenthood in creating particular patterns of parenting in families led by LGBT parents. U.S. census data have revealed that African-American and Hispanic women and men in same-gender couples are, respectively, two and three times more likely than White Americans to be bringing up children (Gates, 2008) yet samples recruited to research same-sex parenting have not reflected these proportions (see Chap. 9). Without representative sampling we do not know the cultural parameters of parenting. For example, previous research on lesbian couples who had planned lesbian parenthood together found that women aspired to and attained a feminism-inspired egalitarian division of child care and household labor (Patterson, 1995; Sullivan, 2004). However, this pattern may be particular to the mainly White, middle-class couples engaged in planned lesbian parenthood. Moore (2008) used a mixed methods approach to collect data on household decision making of Black lesbian couples where one partner was the mother of a child from a previous heterosexual relationship. Both partners contributed financially to the household; however, biological mothers earned less than their partner, did more of the household work, and exercised more authority over bringing up the children and family finances. Lesbian mothers mainly attributed their authority to their feelings of responsibility for their children and the importance of preserving their economic independence; both of these positions could be linked to African-American women's cultural heritage. Nonetheless findings from Hare and Richards's (1993) and Gabb's (2004) qualitative studies have indicated that this pattern may also pertain to White lesbian mothers parenting post-heterosexual separation where the custodial lesbian mother's relationship remained central to her child's life in contrast to the more peripheral role played by her partner in parenting.

An exciting new crossover into the field has been from clinicians bringing formulations derived from social constructionism and systemic practice with families into research on lesbian and gay parenting (Tasker & Malley, 2012). For example, previous authors had considered coming out as a step toward authenticity for the gay or lesbian parent (e.g., Dunne, 1987). In contrast, Lynch and Murray (2000), working from a family systems perspective, point out that coming out decisions raise other considerations for lesbian and gay parents bringing up children from previous heterosexual relationships as they consider the multiple systems that contextualize their lives. Lynch and Murray crucially viewed coming out not as an individual parental decision but a fluid family process centered around the child's needs and adapted to circumstances. Other researchers have considered multiple systemic perspectives in qualitative analyses of individual interviews with young adult sons and daughters of separated or divorced gay fathers to explore how young persons' awareness of their father's sexual identity has been contextualized by the ending of their mother and father's marriage and their awareness of their father's same-gender partnerships. Young adults' own tales of coming out to others about their father were influenced both by variations in their feelings about their father and consideration of the potential responses of different audiences (Tasker, Barrett, & De Simone, 2010).

Perlesz et al. (2006) have drawn on a systemic perspective, together with social constructionist ideas regarding the ability of language to empower and disempower (Shotter, 1993), in their work. They interviewed members of 25 different lesbian-led family networks to explore the complexities of coming out issues for children, lesbian couples, and extended family members. For example, Brown and Perlesz (2007) counted 45 different terms used to describe the lesbian parent who has not given birth to some or all of her children—depending on the term used and linguistic context, her parenting role was either placed in the foreground, sidelined, or disappeared.

Queering the Field and Speaking the Unspoken

Other authors have made intriguing links between queer theory and Lacanian psychoanalytic thinking to argue that the exclusionary binary of gay/lesbian versus heterosexual paralyzes research on lesbian-led families, such that if the family is deemed to be "acceptable" then sexual signifiers are absented (Malone & Cleary, 2002). Malone and Cleary (2002) suggested that researchers "carefully scrutinize the meanings of families as well as the unconscious and psychological dimensions of the family as a vehicle for intergenerational perpetuation" (p. 273). Without this scrutiny, lesbian-led families appear to fulfill the fantasy of the perfect, equal, companionate couple with no differences in power, living an ideal that is only seen to be troubled by homophobia. Malone and Cleary have argued that other power differentials exist, for example, a power differential between an established identity of motherhood and the otherness that challenges it. It is this power differential that may be particularly pertinent to same-gender couple stepfamilies formed after post-heterosexual separation when the child's relationship with the parent pre-dates the partnership and previously heterosexual styled parenting is challenged by the arrival of new expectations.

One example of work that has been enlivened by new paradigms of social constructionism and queer theory has been scholarship that examines the implications of queer parenting for queering the gender and sexual development of their children. Studies have suggested that some adult offspring engaged in a more open-minded consideration of their own psychosexual development, while others reported current or previous worries that their own or a partner's sexual identity might unpredictably change (Goldberg, 2007; Tasker & Golombok, 1997). Both types of stance may be seen at present as querying, but not necessarily queering (Lev, 2010), while some offspring of lesbian or gay parents have intentionally embraced a queer perspective on their own lives (Kuvalanka & Goldberg, 2009) the majority identify as heterosexual (Goldberg, 2007; Tasker & Golombok, 1997).

Interesting questions remain as to how parental sexual orientation may link into children's psychosexual development. First, the large majority of adult sons and daughters studied to date spent at least some of their childhood growing up in the matrimonial home with two ostensibly heterosexual parents before either their mother and/or father began to identify as lesbian or gay. Perhaps we see a particular linkage between the lesbian or gay parent's transitioned sexual identification and their children's questioning, which may or may not be manifest in the psychosexual developmental pathways of children brought up within planned gay or lesbian-led families.

Second, many members of the first wave of out lesbian mothers identified their sexual identity through their engagement with the feminist movements of the 1970s and 1980s. Studies intentionally sampled feminist lesbian mothers (e.g., Ainslie & Feltey, 1991) or had a noticeable group of participants who clearly identified with feminist ideas (e.g., Harris & Turner, 1985; Hoeffer, 1981). For example, some of the lesbian mothers in Hoeffer's (1981) study clearly avoided promoting gender stereotypes in their nominations of the toys they preferred for their children; however, no differences were evident in the gender-typical behavior and toy choices of the children of lesbian mothers and the comparison group of children of heterosexual single mothers. Perhaps any influences from the attitudes conveyed by feminist mothers remain latent until adolescence or adulthood when associations emerge in a more open-minded consideration of psychosexual development particularly among daughters (Tasker & Golombok, 1997).

Queer theory may provide a particularly useful lens through which to explore how lesbian and gay parents who came out of (or indeed remained in) opposite-gender relationships critique and position their own sexuality. As noted earlier, researchers have not specifically explored parental self-identification of sexual orientation yet studies have suggested a wide variety of different paths to heterosexual parenthood among lesbian and gay parents who had children prior to coming out. The heterosexual relationships recorded in studies to date seem to encompass a vast range of very different experiences from exploitative or abusive encounters, an enjoyable sampling of an opposite-gender relationship, or a long-term committed relationship that partners leave and grieve. Other fields of research have pointed to the particular fluidity of women's sexual identification (Diamond, 2008; Kitzinger & Wilkinson, 1995; Peplau & Garnets, 2000). What difference does transitioned sexual orientation make to parenting? Research is yet to explore this question specifically with LGBT parents themselves.

Conclusion

On the one hand, much of our knowledge of LGBT parenting is based on studies of lesbian and gay parents who had their children in previous heterosexual relationships. On the other hand, our knowledge of same-gender parenting post-separation or divorce remains partial with few studies addressing gay fatherhood, limited consideration of research questions other than those focused on developmental outcomes for children, and little investigation of the intersection of parental sexual orientation with cultural variation and the plurality of identity positions that LGBT parents may occupy over time. The research field awaits consideration of how transitioned lesbian and gay parenting post-heterosexual separation or divorce may differ from parenting planned by LGBT parents. Future research studies will need to conceptualize diversity and fluidity in parental sexual orientation and consider contextual variation in parenthood utilizing a variety of different theoretical frameworks and research methodologies to collect quantitative and qualitative data.

Acknowledgments The author would like to thank Abbie Goldberg and Katherine Allen for their editorial comments, enthusiasm, and patience.

References

Agbayewa, M. O. (1984). Fathers in the newer family forms: Male or female? *Canadian Journal of Psychiatry, 29*, 402–405.

Ainslie, J., & Feltey, K. M. (1991). Definitions and dynamics of motherhood and family in lesbian communities. *Marriage & Family Review, 17*, 63–85. doi:10.1300/J002v17n01_05

Anderssen, N., Amlie, C., & Ytteroy, E. A. (2002). Outcomes for children with lesbian or gay parents: A review of studies from 1978 to 2000. *Scandinavian Journal of Psychology, 43*, 335–351. doi:10.1111/1467-9450.00302

Bandura, A. (1977). *Social learning theory*. Englewood Cliffs, NJ: Prentice Hall.

Baptiste, D. A. (1987). The gay and lesbian stepparent family. In F. W. Bozett (Ed.), *Gay and lesbian parents* (pp. 112–137). New York, NY: Praeger.

Barrett, H., & Tasker, F. (2001). Growing up with a gay parent: Views of 101 gay fathers on their sons' and daughters' experiences. *Educational and Child Psychology, 18*, 62–77.

Bengtson, V. L., & Allen, K. R. (1993). The life course perspective applied to families over time. In P. G. Boss, W. J. Doherty, R. LaRossa, W. R. Schumm, & S. K. Steinmetz (Eds.), *Sourcebook of family theories and methods: A contextual approach* (pp. 469–499). New York, NY: Plenum Press.

Benson, A. L., Silverstein, L. B., & Auerbach, C. F. (2005). From the margins to the center: Gay fathers reconstruct the fathering role. *Journal of GLBT Family Studies, 1*(3), 1–29. doi:10.1300/J461v01n03_01

Berger, R. (1998a). Gay stepfamilies: A triple-stigmatized group. *Families in Society, 81*, 504–516. doi:10.1300/J087v29n03_06

Berger, R. (1998b). *Stepfamilies: A multi-dimensional perspective*. New York, NY: Haworth Press.

Biblarz, T. J., & Stacey, J. (2010). How does the gender of parents matter? *Journal of Marriage and Family, 72*, 3–22. doi:10.1111/j.1741-3737.2009.00678.x

Bigner, J. J. (1996). Working with gay fathers: Developmental, post-divorce parenting, and therapeutic issues. In J. Laird & R. J. Green (Eds.), *Lesbians and gays in couples and families: A handbook for therapists* (pp. 370–403). San Francisco, CA: Jossey-Bass.

Bigner, J. J., & Jacobsen, R. B. (1989a). The value of children to gay and heterosexual fathers. In F. W. Bozett

(Ed.), *Homosexuality and the family* (pp. 163–172). New York, NY: Harrington Park Press.

Bigner, J. J., & Jacobsen, R. B. (1989b). Parenting behaviors of homosexual and heterosexual fathers. In F. W. Bozett (Ed.), *Homosexuality and the family* (pp. 173–186). New York, NY: Harrington Park Press.

Bigner, J. J., & Jacobsen, R. B. (1992). Adult responses to child behavior and attitudes toward fathering: Gay and nongay fathers. *Journal of Homosexuality, 23*, 99–112.

Bozett, F. W. (1981a). Gay fathers: Evolution of the gay-father identity. *American Journal of Orthopsychiatry, 51*, 552–559. doi:10.1111/j.1939-0025.1981.tb01404.x

Bozett, F. W. (1981b). Gay fathers: Identity conflict resolution through integrative sanctioning. *Alternative Lifestyles, 4*, 90–107. doi:10.1007/BF01082090

Bozett, F. W. (1987a). Gay fathers. In F. W. Bozett (Ed.), *Gay and lesbian parents* (pp. 3–22). New York, NY: Praeger.

Bozett, F. W. (1987b). Children of gay fathers. In F. W. Bozett (Ed.), *Gay and lesbian parents* (pp. 39–57). New York, NY: Praeger.

Broderick, C. B. (1993). *Understanding family process: Basics of family systems theory*. London, UK: Sage.

Brown, R., & Perlesz, A. (2007). Not the "other" mother: How language constructs lesbian co-parenting relationships. *Journal GLBT Family Studies, 3*, 352–403. doi:10.1300/J461v03n02_10

Buntzly, G. (1993). Gay fathers in straight marriages. *Journal of Homosexuality, 24*(3/4), 107–114.

Buxton, A. P. (2005). A family matter: When a spouse comes out as gay, lesbian, or bisexual. *Journal GLBT Family Studies, 1*(2), 49–70. doi:10.1300/J461v01n02_04

Cherlin, A. (1978). Remarriage as an incomplete institution. *American Journal of Sociology, 84*, 634–650. doi:10.1086/226830

Cherlin, A. (2004). The deinstitutionalization of American marriage. *Journal of Marriage and Family, 66*, 848–861. doi:10.1111/j.0022-2445.2004.00058.x

Choo, H. Y., & Ferree, M. M. (2010). Practicing intersectionality in sociological research: A critical analysis of inclusions, interactions, and institutions in the study of inequalities. *Sociological Theory, 28*, 129–149. doi:10.1111/j.1467-9558.2010.01370.x

Clarke, V. (2002). Sameness and difference in research on lesbian parenting. *Journal of Community & Applied Social Psychology, 12*, 210–222. doi:10.1002/casp.673

Clarke, V., Ellis, S. J., Peel, E., & Riggs, D. W. (2010). *Lesbian, gay, bisexual, trans & queer psychology: An introduction*. Cambridge, UK: Cambridge University Press.

Coleman, E. (1990). The married lesbian. In F. W. Bozett & M. B. Sussman (Eds.), *Homosexuality and family relations* (pp. 119–135). New York, NY: Harrington Park Press.

Crawford, S. (1987). Lesbian families: Psychosocial stress and the family-building process. In Boston Lesbian

Psychologies Collective (Ed.), *Lesbian psychologies: Explorations and challenges* (pp. 195–214). Chicago, IL: University of Illinois.

Crosbie-Burnett, M., & Helmbrecht, L. (1993). A descriptive empirical study of gay male stepfamilies. *Family Relations, 42*, 256–262. doi:10.2307/585554

Crowl, A. L., Ahn, S., & Baker, J. (2008). A meta-analysis of developmental outcomes for children of same-sex and heterosexual parents. *Journal of GLBT Family Studies, 4*, 385–407. doi:10.1080/15504280802177615

Current-Juretschko, L., & Bigner, J. J. (2005). An exploratory investigation of gay stepfathers' perceptions of their role. *Journal of GLBT Family Studies, 1*(4), 1–20. doi:10.1300/J461v01n04_01

Diamond, L. M. (2008). Female bisexuality from adolescence to adulthood: Results from a 10-year longitudinal study. *Developmental Psychology, 44*, 5–14. doi:10.1037/0012-1649.44.1.5

Dunne, E. J. (1987). Helping gay fathers come out to their children. *Journal of Homosexuality, 14*, 213–222.

Dunne, G. A. (2001). The lady vanishes? Reflections on the experiences of married and divorced non-heterosexual fathers. *Sociological Research Online, 6*(3). doi:10.5153/sro.636.

Elder, G. H., Jr. (1998). The life course as developmental theory. *Child Development, 69*, 1–12. doi:10.2307/1132065

Erera, P. I., & Fredricksen, K. (1999). Lesbian stepfamilies: A unique family structure. *Families in Society, 80*, 263–270.

Espin, O. M. (1987). Issues of identity in the psychology of Latina lesbians. In Boston Lesbian Psychologies Collective (Ed.), *Lesbian psychologies: Explorations and challenges* (pp. 35–55). Chicago, IL: University of Illinois.

Falk, P. J. (1989). Lesbian mothers: Psychosocial assumptions in family law. *American Psychologist, 44*, 941–947. doi:10.1037//0003-066X.44.6.941

Gabb, J. (2004). Critical differentials: Querying the incongruities within research on lesbian parent families. *Sexualities, 7*, 167–182. doi:10.1177/1363460704042162

Ganong, L. H., & Coleman, M. C. (2004). *Stepfamily relationships: Development, dynamics, and interventions*. New York, NY: Kluwer.

Gates, G. (2008). Diversity among same-sex couples and their children. In S. Coontz (Ed.), *American families: A multicultural reader* (pp. 394–399). New York, NY: Routledge.

Gates, G. J., & Ost, J. (2004). *The gay and lesbian atlas*. Washington, DC: Urban Institute.

Gates, G. J., & Romero, A. P. (2009). Parenting by gay men and lesbians: Beyond the current research. In H. E. Peters & C. M. Kamp Dush (Eds.), *Marriage and family: Perspectives and complexities* (pp. 227–243). New York, NY: Columbia University Press.

Gergen, K. J. (2009). *An invitation to social construction* (2nd ed.). London, UK: Sage.

Gershon, T. D., Tschann, J. M., & Jemerin, J. M. (1999). Stigmatization, self-esteem, and coping among the adolescent children of lesbian mothers. *Journal of Adolescent Health, 24*, 437–445. doi:10.1016/S1054-139X(98)00154-2

Glenn, E. N. (2000). The social construction and institutionalization of gender and race: An integrative framework. In M. M. Ferree, J. Lorber, & B. B. Hess (Eds.), *Revisioning gender* (pp. 3–43). Oxford, UK: AltaMira Press.

Goldberg, A. E. (2007). (How) does it make a difference? Perspectives of adults with lesbian, gay, and bisexual parents. *American Journal of Orthopsychiatry, 77*, 550–562. doi:10.1037/0002-9432.77.4.550

Goldberg, A. E. (2010). *Lesbian and gay parents and their children: Research on the family life cycle.* Washington, DC: American Psychological Association Books. doi:10.1037/12055-001

Golden, C. (1987). Diversity and variability in women's sexual identities. In Boston Lesbian Psychologies Collective (Ed.), *Lesbian psychologies: Explorations and challenges* (pp. 18–34). Chicago, IL: University of Illinois.

Golombok, S. (2002). Why I study … lesbian mothers. *The Psychologist, 15*, 562–563.

Golombok, S., Spencer, A., & Rutter, M. (1983). Children in lesbian and single-parent households: Psychosexual and psychiatric appraisal. *Journal of Child Psychology and Psychiatry, 24*, 551–572.

Golombok, S., & Tasker, F. (1994). Children in lesbian and gay families: Theories and evidence. *Annual Review of Sex Research, 5*, 73–100.

Golombok, S., & Tasker, F. (2010). Gay fathers. In M. E. Lamb (Ed.), *Role of the father in child development* (5th ed., pp. 319–340). New York: Wiley.

Green, R., Mandel, J. B., Hotvedt, M. E., Gray, J., & Smith, L. (1986). Lesbian mothers and their children: A comparison with solo parent heterosexual mothers and their children. *Archives of Sexual Behavior, 7*, 175–181. doi:10.1007/BF01542224

Hall, M. (1978). Lesbian families: Cultural and clinical issues. *Social Work, 23*, 380–385.

Hall, K. J., & Kitson, G. C. (2000). Lesbian stepfamilies: An even more "incomplete institution". *Journal of Lesbian Studies, 4*, 31–47. doi:10.1300/J155v04n03_02

Hare, J., & Richards, L. (1993). Children raised by lesbian couples: Does context of birth affect father and partner involvement? *Family Relations, 42*, 249–255. doi:10.2307/585553

Harris, M. B., & Turner, P. H. (1985). Gay and lesbian parents. *Journal of Homosexuality, 12*, 101–113.

Henehan, D., Rothblum, E. D., Solomon, S. E., & Balsam, K. F. (2007). Social and demographic characteristics of gay, lesbian, and heterosexual adults with and without children. *Journal GLBT Family Studies, 3*, 35–79. doi:10.1300/J461v03n02_03

Hequembourg, A. (2004). Unscripted motherhood: Lesbian mothers negotiating incompletely institutionalized family relationships. *Journal of Social and Personal Relationships, 21*, 739–762. doi:10.1177/0265407504047834

Hequembourg, A. L., & Farrell, M. P. (1999). Lesbian motherhood: Negotiating marginal-mainstream identities. *Gender and Society, 13*, 540–557. doi:10.1177/089124399013004007

Hill, M. (1987). Child rearing attitudes of black lesbian mothers. In The Boston Lesbian Psychologies Collective (Ed.), *Lesbian psychologies: Explorations and challenges* (pp. 215–226). Chicago, IL: University of Illinois Press.

Hoeffer, B. (1981). Children's acquisition of sex-role behavior in lesbian-mother families. *American Journal of Orthopsychiatry, 5*, 536–544. doi:10.1111/j.1939-0025.1981.tb01402.x

Huggins, S. L. (1989). A comparative study of self-esteem of adolescent children of divorced lesbian mothers and divorced heterosexual mothers. In F. Bozett (Ed.), *Homosexuality and the family* (pp. 123–135). New York, NY: Harrington Park Press.

Jackson, S. (2011). Heterosexual hierarchies: A commentary on class and sexuality. *Sexualities, 14*, 12–20. doi:10.1177/1363460710390572

Javaid, G. A. (1983). The sexual development of the adolescent daughter of a homosexual mother. *Journal of the American Academy of Child Psychiatry, 22*, 196–201. doi:10.1016/S0002-7138(09)62336-0

Javaid, G. A. (1993). The children of homosexual and heterosexual single mothers. *Child Psychiatry and Human Development, 23*, 235–248. doi:10.1007/BF00707677

Kirkpatrick, M., Smith, C., & Roy, R. (1981). Lesbian mothers and their children: A comparative survey. *American Journal of Orthopsychiatry, 51*, 545–551. doi:10.1111/j.1939-0025.1981.tb01403.x.

Kitzinger, C., & Wilkinson, S. (1995). Transitions from heterosexuality to lesbianism: The discursive production of lesbian identities. *Developmental Psychology, 31*, 95–104. doi:10.1037//0012-1649.31.1.95

Kuvalanka, K., & Goldberg, A. E. (2009). Second generation voices: Queer youth with lesbian/bisexual mothers. *Journal of Youth and Adolescence, 38*, 904–919. doi:10.1007/s10964-008-9327-2

Lev, A. I. (2010). How queer! - The development of gender identity and sexual orientation in LGBTQ-headed families. *Family Process, 49*, 268–290.

Lewis, K. G. (1980). Children of lesbians: Their point of view. *Social Work, 25*, 198–203.

Logue, P. M. (2002). The rights of lesbian and gay parents and their children. *Journal of the American Academy of Matrimonial Lawyers, 18*, 95–129.

Lott-Whitehead, L., & Tully, C. (1992). The family of lesbian mothers. *Smith College Studies in Social Work, 63*, 265–280.

Lynch, J. M. (2004a). Becoming a stepparent in gay/lesbian stepfamilies: Integrating identities. *Journal of Homosexuality, 48*(2), 45–60.

Lynch, J. M. (2004b). The identity transformation of biological parents in lesbian/gay stepfamilies. *Journal* of *Homosexuality*, *47*(2), 91–107. doi:10.1300/J082v47n02_06

Lynch, J. M., & Murray, K. (2000). For the love of the children: The coming out process for lesbian and gay parents and stepparents. *Journal of Homosexuality*, *39*(1), 1–24. doi:10.1300/J082v39n01_01

Lyons, T. A. (1983). Lesbian mother's custody fear. *Women and Therapy*, *2*, 231–240. doi:10.1300/J015v02n02_23

Malone, K., & Cleary, R. (2002). (De)sexing the family. *Feminist Theory*, *3*, 271–293. doi:10.1177/146470002762492006

Martin, C. L., & Halverson, C. (1981). A schematic processing model of sex typing and stereotyping in children. *Child Development*, *52*, 1119–1134. doi:10.2307/1129498

Miller, B. (1978). Adult sexual resocialization: Adjustments toward a stigmatized identity. *Alternative Lifestyles*, *1*, 207–234. doi:10.1007/BF01082077

Miller, B. (1979). Gay fathers and their children. *The Family Coordinator*, *28*, 544–552. doi:10.2307/583517

Moore, M. R. (2008). Gendered power relations among women: A study of household decision making in black, lesbian stepfamilies. *American Sociological Review*, *73*, 335–356. doi:10.1177/000312240807300208

Morris, J. F., Balsam, K. F., & Rothblum, E. D. (2002). Lesbian and bisexual mothers and nonmothers: Demographics and the coming-out process. *Journal of Family Psychology*, *16*, 144–156. doi:10.1037//0893-3200.16.2.144

Mucklow, B. M., & Phelan, G. K. (1979). Lesbian and traditional mothers' responses child behavior and self-concept. *Psychological Reports*, *44*, 880–882. doi:10.2466/pr0.1979.44.3.880

Mulderrig, J. (2007). *Equality and human rights: Key concepts and issues*. Edinburgh, Scotland: University of Edinburgh. Working paper available at http://eprints.lancs.ac.uk/1274

Nelson, F. (1996). *Lesbian motherhood: An exploration of Canadian lesbian families*. Toronto, ON: University of Toronto Press.

Nichols, M. (1987). Lesbian sexuality: Issues and developing theory. In The Boston Lesbian Psychologies Collective (Ed.), *Lesbian psychologies: Explorations and challenges* (pp. 97–125). Chicago, IL: University of Illinois.

O'Connell, A. (1993). Voices from the heart: The developmental impact of a mother's lesbianism on her adolescent children. *Smith College Studies in Social Work*, *63*, 281–299.

Oswald, R. F. (2002). Resilience within the family networks of lesbians and gay men: Intentionality and redefinition. *Journal of Marriage and Family*, *64*, 374–383. doi:10.1111/j.1741-3737.2002.00374.x

Patterson, C. J. (1995). Families of the lesbian baby boom: Parents' division of labor and children's adjustment. *Developmental Psychology*, *31*, 115–123. doi:10.1037//0012-1649.31.1.115

Pearcey, M. (2005). Gay and bisexual married men's attitudes and experiences: Homophobia, reasons for marriage, and self-identity. *Journal of GLBT Family Studies*, *1*(4), 21–42. doi:10.1300/J461v01n04_02

Pedersen, P. B. (2003). Culturally biased assumptions in counseling psychology. *The Counseling Psychologist*, *31*, 396–403. doi:10.1177/0011000003031004002

Pennington, S. B. (1987). Children of lesbian mothers. In F. W. Bozett (Ed.), *Gay and lesbian parents* (pp. 58–74). New York, NY: Praeger.

Peplau, L. A., & Garnets, L. D. (2000). A new paradigm for understanding women's sexuality and sexual orientation. *Journal of Social Issues*, *56*, 330–350. doi:10.1111/0022-4537.00169

Perlesz, A., Brown, R., Lindsay, J., McNair, R., de Vaus, D., & Pitts, M. (2006). Families in transition: Parents, children and grandparents in lesbian families give meaning to 'doing family'. *Journal of Family Therapy*, *28*, 175–199.

Perlesz, A., Brown, R., McNair, R., Lindsay, J., Pitts, M., & de Vaus, D. (2006). Lesbian family disclosure: Authenticity and safety within private and public domains. *Lesbian and Gay Psychology Review*, *7*, 54–65.

Riddle, D. I. (1978). Relating to children: Gays as role models. *Journal of Social Issues*, *34*, 38–58. doi:10.1111/j.1540-4560.1978.tb02613.x

Robitaille, C., & Saint-Jacques, M.-C. (2009). Social stigma and the situation of young people in lesbian and gay stepfamilies. *Journal of Homosexuality*, *56*, 421–442. doi:10.1080/00918360902821429

Ross, M. W. (1990). Married homosexual men: Prevalence and background. In F. W. Bozett & M. B. Sussman (Eds.), *Homosexuality and family relations* (pp. 35–57). New York, NY: Harrington Park Press.

Rutter, M. (1981). *Maternal deprivation reassessed*. London, UK: Penguin.

Shotter, J. (1993). *Conversational realities: Constructing life through language*. London, UK: Sage.

Socarides, C. W. (1978). *Homosexuality*. New York: Aronson.

Stacey, J., & Biblarz, T. (2001). (How) does the sexual orientation of parents matter? *American Sociological Review*, *66*, 159–183. doi:10.2307/2657413

Sullivan, M. (2004). *The family of woman: Lesbian mothers, their children, and the undoing of gender*. Los Angeles, CA: University of California Press.

Tasker, F. (2005). Lesbian mothers, gay fathers and their children: A review. *Journal of Developmental and Behavioral Pediatrics*, *26*, 224–240. doi:10.1097/00004703-200506000-00012

Tasker, F., Barrett, H., & De Simone, F. (2010). "Coming out tales": Adult sons and daughters' feelings about their gay father's sexual identity. *Australian and New Zealand Journal of Family Therapy*, *31*, 326–337. doi:10.1375/anft.31.4.326

Tasker, F., & Golombok, S. (1995). Adults raised as children in lesbian families. *American Journal of Orthopsychiatry*, *65*, 203–215. doi:10.1037/h0079615

Tasker, F. L., & Golombok, S. (1997). *Growing up in a lesbian family: Effects on child development*. New York, NY: Guilford Press.

Tasker, F., & Malley, M. (2012). Working with LGBT parents. In J. J. Bigner & J. L. Wetchler (Eds.), *Handbook of LGBT-affirmative couple and family therapy*. New York, NY: Routledge.

Tasker, F., & Patterson, C. J. (2007). Research on lesbian and gay parenting: Retrospect and prospect. *Journal of GLBT Family Studies, 3*, 9–34. doi:10.1300/J461v03n02_02

Taylor, Y. (2011). Sexualities and class. *Sexualities, 14*, 3–11. doi:10.1177/1363460710390559

Turner, P. H., Scadden, L., & Harris, M. B. (1990). Parenting in gay and lesbian families. *Journal of Gay and Lesbian Psychotherapy, 1*, 55–66. doi:10.1080/19359705.1990.9962145

Van Dam, M. A. A. (2004). Mothers in two types of lesbian families: Stigma experiences, supports, and burdens. *Journal of Family Nursing, 10*, 450–484. doi:10.1177/1074840704270120

Wainright, J. L., & Patterson, C. J. (2006). Delinquency, victimization, and substance use among adolescents with female same-sex parents. *Journal of Family Psychology, 20*, 526–530. doi:10.1037/0893-3200.20.3.526

Wainright, J. L., Russell, S. T., & Patterson, C. J. (2004). Psychosocial adjustment, school outcomes and romantic relationships of adolescents with same-sex parents. *Child Development, 75*, 1886–1898. doi:10.1111/j.1467-8624.2004.00823.x

Wallerstein, J. S., & Kelly, J. B. (1980). Effects of divorce on the visiting father-child relationship. *The American Journal of Psychiatry, 137*, 1534–1539.

Weeks, R. B., Derdeyn, A. P., & Langman, M. (1975). Two cases of children of homosexuals. *Child Psychiatry and Human Development, 6*, 26–32. doi:10.1007/BF01434429

Weston, K. (1991). *Families we choose: Lesbians, gays, kinship*. New York, NY: Columbia University Press.

Wyers, N. L. (1987). Homosexuality in the family: Lesbian and gay spouses. *Social Work, 32*, 143–148.

Lesbian-Mother Families Formed Through Donor Insemination

2

Henny Bos

For decades, theory and research on family functioning focused on two-parent families consisting of a father and a mother. Over the past 30 years, however, the concept of what makes a "family" has changed. Some children now grow up in "patchwork" or "blended" families; namely, families headed by two parents, one of whom has a child or children from a previous relationship. Other children grow up in "planned" lesbian-parent families; that is, families headed by two lesbian mothers who decided to have children together through adoption, foster care, or donor insemination. These lesbian mothers and their children differ from lesbian mothers whose children were born into previous heterosexual relationships. A child who was born into a previous heterosexual relationship of the mother before she identified herself as a lesbian will have experienced the mother's divorce and coming-out process, and this transition might influence the child's psychological well-being. Many other variations in family structures, or combinations of the above-mentioned family types, are possible; for example, a situation where two lesbian women have a relationship and a child has been born into that relationship, but both mothers also have a child or children from a previous heterosexual relationship or marriage (Chap 1). This chapter, however, focuses only on lesbian-mother families in which all children were conceived through donor insemination (planned lesbian-mother families).

Since the 1980s, assisted reproductive technologies have made it possible for lesbians with the economic means to access sperm banks and thus become parents. As a result, planned lesbian-mother families are now an integral part of the social structure of many Western countries (Parke, 2004). For example, at the time of the 2000 United States Census, one third of female-partnered households contained children (Simmons & O'Connell, 2003). In 2002 there were an estimated 21,000 female cohabiting couples in the Netherlands, and almost 15% of these couples had children younger than 18 years old; in 2009, there were 25,000 female cohabiting couples in the Netherlands, of which 20% had children younger than 18 years old (Bos & van Gelderen, 2010; Steenhof & Harmsen, 2003). It is unclear, however, whether these children were born into lesbian relationships.

It is expected that the number of children born into lesbian relationships and raised by two lesbian mothers will continue to increase. In 2001, a Kaiser Family Foundation survey of 405 randomly selected, self-identified lesbians in the USA found that almost half (49%) of those who

H. Bos, Ph.D. (✉)
Graduate School of Child Development and Education,
College of Child Development and Education,
Research Institute of Child Development and Education,
University of Amsterdam, P.O. Box 94208,
1090 GE Amsterdam, The Netherlands
e-mail: H.M.W.Bos@uva.nl

A.E. Goldberg and K.R. Allen (eds.), *LGBT-Parent Families: Innovations in Research and Implications for Practice*, DOI 10.1007/978-1-4614-4556-2_2, © Springer Science+Business Media New York 2013

were not already parents indicated that they would like to have children of their own in the future. A recent study in the Netherlands found that among 1,101 lesbian and bisexual women between aged 16 and 25, 60% of the women wanted to become parents in the future (Van Bergen & van Lisdonk, 2010).

The right and fitness of lesbians to parent is widely disputed in the media and in the legal and policy arena. Opponents of lesbian parenting claim that the children of lesbian parents are at risk of developing a variety of behavior problems, because they are raised in fatherless households, lack a biological tie with one of the mothers, and might be teased by their peers because their mothers are lesbian (for an analyses of the arguments of opponents, see Clarke, 2001). To deflect these concerns, advocates of same-sex marriage and lesbian parenthood rely on the few studies that have been conducted on planned lesbian-mother families. These advocates emphasize that in these studies no evidence was found for the proposition that the traditional, nuclear mother–father family is the ideal environment in which to raise children (Rosky, 2009).

In the present literature review I distinguish among three types of foci in studies on planned lesbian-mother families; namely, questions that focus on (a) a comparison between planned lesbian-mother families and two-parent heterosexual families on family characteristics, parenting, and child outcomes; (b) differences and/ or similarities between biological mothers (or "birthmothers") and nonbiological mothers (or "co-mothers" or "social mothers") on such aspects as motives to become a mother, parenting, and division of labor; and (c) the diversity within planned lesbian-mother families (in areas such as experiences of stigmatization and donor status) and the consequences of this diversity on parenting and child outcomes. These three research areas are grounded in different theoretical backgrounds. I then present an overview of the most important findings of each category of research. Finally, I describe some scientific limitations of the summarized studies as well as challenges of future research.

Planned Lesbian-Mother Families Compared with Two-Parent Heterosexual Parent Families

Early studies, in particular, on planned lesbian-mother families were often aimed at establishing whether lesbians can be good parents, whether they should be granted legal parenthood, and whether they should have access to assisted reproductive technologies (e.g., Kirkpatrick, Smith & Roy, 1981; Mucklow & Phelan, 1979). The emphasis was originally on proving the normality of planned lesbian-mother families and the children who grow up in them (for overviews, see Clarke, 2008; Sandfort, 2000; Stacey & Biblarz, 2001). To inform family policy and regulations on assisted reproduction, it continues to be important to compare parents and children in planned lesbian-mother families and two-parent heterosexual-parent families. It is also important to continue this research focus to further theoretical understanding of the influence of family structure (same-sex vs. opposite-sex parents) and family processes (parent–child relationships, relationships between parents) on child development. The association between family structure and outcomes for children can be complex, with family structure often playing a less important role in children's psychological development than the quality of the family relationships (Parke, 2004).

The results of studies that compare planned lesbian-mother families and two-parent heterosexual-parent families are presented below. These studies tended to focus on three main areas (a) family characteristics, (b) parenting, and (c) the development of offspring.

Family Characteristics

Age of Mother and Desire and Motivation to Have Children

In a Dutch study of 100 planned lesbian-mother families and 100 heterosexual two-parent families (with children between 4 and 8 years old), Bos, van Balen, and van den Boom (2003) found that both biological and co-mothers in planned lesbian-mother families were, on average, older than heterosexual parents. This age difference might be related to several issues: Lesbian women start to think about having children at an older age than heterosexual women; they have to make several decisions regarding the conception (e.g., deciding on donors), which takes time; and it takes longer to get pregnant through donor insemination than by natural conception (Botchan et al., 2001).

In Bos et al.'s (2003) study, participants were also asked about their motives to become a parent. The lesbian biological mothers and co-mothers differed from heterosexual mothers and fathers in that they spent more time thinking about their motives for having children. This difference might be because lesbians more carefully weigh the pros and cons of having children, or because their process to parenthood is comparable to that of infertile heterosexual couples, whereby they possess an enhanced awareness of the importance of parenthood in one's life. However, lesbian parents and heterosexual parents seem to rank their parenthood motives rather similarly: Both reported feelings of affection and happiness in relation to having children, and the expectation that parenthood will provide life fulfillment, as their most important motives for having children (Bos et al., 2003).

Division of Family Tasks

How parents in lesbian-mother families and heterosexual two-parent families divide their time between family tasks (household tasks and childcare) and work tends to be measured in two ways. For example, Chan, Brooks, Raboy, and Patterson (1998) studied 30 lesbian couples and 16 heterosexual couples in the USA and asked each parent to complete a questionnaire, the "Who Does What" measure; Cowan & Cowan, 1988), indicating whether she/he or her/his partner carried out a specific tasks. In the earlier mentioned Dutch study by Bos, van Balen, and van den Boom (2007), the division of household tasks and childcare was evaluated by means of a structured diary record of activities. This diary was

completed by both parents in the 100 lesbian-mother families and both parents in the 100 heterosexual two-parent families (Bos et al., 2007). The findings of these studies were similar and did not differ as a function of approach to measuring the division of labor. Lesbian-parent families with young children were likely to share family tasks to a greater degree than heterosexual two-parent families. Perhaps the absence of gender polarization in lesbian-mother families leads to more equal burden sharing, which might explain findings that lesbian mothers are more satisfied with their partners as co-parents compared to heterosexual parents (Bos et al., 2007). Analysis of diary data also revealed that lesbian biological mothers and co-mothers spent similar amounts of time on employment outside the home, in contrast to heterosexual two-parent families (fathers spent much more time at their work outside the home than their partners did) (Bos et al., 2007). It might be that lesbian partners understand each other's career opportunities and challenges better than partners in a heterosexual relationship (see also Dunne, 1998).

Parental Justification

Bos et al. (2007) also examined whether Dutch lesbian mothers feel more pressure to demonstrate to people in their environment that they are good parents. A significant difference in this feeling, which can be described as "parental justification," was found only between lesbian co-mothers and heterosexual fathers: Lesbian co-mothers felt more pressured to justify the quality of their parenthood than heterosexual fathers. According to the authors, this finding might be explained by the co-mother's absence of a biological tie with the children, which drives them to do their utmost to be "good moms." Like adoptive parents, lesbian social mothers may face difficulties in developing an adequate sense of acting as full parents (Grotevant & Kohler, 1999). It is also likely that lesbian social mothers feel pressured to be visible as mothers (e.g., Nekkebroeck & Brewaeys, 2002), because they think that their position is different from that of biological parents, whether lesbian or heterosexual.

Parenting

Parental Stress

In their study of Dutch lesbian-mother families with young children, Bos, van Balen, Sandfort, and van den Boom (2004) found that lesbian mothers' experience of parental stress was comparable to that of heterosexual parents. These findings are congruent with other studies carried out in other countries which found that lesbian mothers do not differ from heterosexual mothers in two-parent families on parental stress (Shechner, Slone, Meir, & Kalish, 2010). Shechner et al. (2010), for example, examined maternal stress in 30 lesbian two-mother families, 30 heterosexual two-parent families, and 30 single-mother families (all with children between 4 and 8 years old). This study—which was carried out in Israel—found that single heterosexual mothers reported higher levels of stress than lesbian mothers and two-parent heterosexual mothers, and the lesbian mothers' stress scores did not differ from the heterosexual mothers in two-parent families. Patterson (2001) administered the Symptom Checklist (SCL-90; Derogatis, 1983) which addresses a variety of psychological and somatic symptoms, to 66 lesbian mothers (with children between 4 and 9 years old), and compared the mothers' scores with the norms of a female nonpatient sample (Derogatis, 1983). In this study, too, no significant differences between groups were found on any of the SCL-90 measured psychological or somatic symptoms.

Parenting Styles

Studies carried out in the UK, the USA, the Netherlands, and Belgium have shown that based on parent self-report data in lesbian-mother families with young children, the co-mothers had higher levels of emotional involvement, parental concern, and parenting awareness skills than fathers in heterosexual two-parent families (Bos et al., 2007; Bos, van Balen, & van den Boom, 2004; Brewaeys, Ponjaert, van Hall, & Golombok, 1997; Flaks, Ficher, Masterpasqua, & Joseph, 1995; Golombok, Tasker, & Murray, 1997). In Bos et al.'s (2007) Dutch study of 100 lesbian-mother families and 100 heterosexual two-parent families, data were also gathered by means of observations of the parent relationship during a home visit. During this visit, parent and child were videotaped performing two instructional tasks, which were later scored by two different trained raters. It was found that the co-mothers differed from the fathers in that they showed lower levels of limit setting during the parent–child interaction (Bos et al., 2007). These differences were not found between lesbian biological mothers and heterosexual mothers. These differences may be due to gender: Women are supposed to be more expressive, nurturant, and sensitive, while men more often exhibit instrumental competence (such as disciplining) (Lamb, 1999).

Golombok et al. (2003) examined, by means of standardized interviews, the quality of parent–child relationships of a community sample of 7-year-old children in 39 lesbian-mother families (20 headed by a single mother and 19 by a lesbian couple), 74 two-parent heterosexual families, and 60 families headed by single heterosexual mothers. When lesbian-mother families were compared with the two-parent heterosexual families, a significant difference was found for emotional involvement, with fathers scoring higher than co-mothers. According to the authors, this difference might have to do with the fact that although the children involved in this study were also born into lesbian relationships, a substantial number of the lesbian co-mothers were stepmothers, who were not actively involved in the decision to have a child and did not raise the child from birth. Another significant difference found in this study was that the frequency of smacking was greater among the fathers than among the co-mothers; this difference is an important finding because smacking is associated with aggressive behavior in children (Eamon, 2001).

In a longitudinal study in the UK, the researchers compared 20 families headed by lesbian mothers (11 couples and 9 single mothers) and 27 families headed by single heterosexual mothers with 36 two-parent heterosexual families, at the time the offspring reached adolescence (Golombok & Badger, 2010). They found that the mothers in the lesbian-mother families and in the single heterosexual-mother families were more emotionally involved with their adolescents than mothers in traditional father–mother families. Lesbian mothers and single heterosexual mothers also showed lower levels of separation anxiety than mothers in the two-parent heterosexual families. Although no differences were found between the lesbian mothers and the single heterosexual mothers on these aspects, they did not differ on disciplinary techniques and conflicts: The lesbian mothers showed higher levels of these characteristics than the single mothers.

Thus, empirical studies reveal a consensus that there are some differences between lesbian and heterosexual parents: Lesbian mothers are more committed as parents, spend more time caring for their children, and report higher levels of emotional involvement with their children. The question is whether this more competent and involved parenting is reflected in the children's development.

Offspring Development

Psychosocial Development

Research on children and adolescents in planned lesbian-mother families has mainly focused on their psychological adjustment and peer relationships. In general, growing evidence suggests that there are no differences between young children raised in lesbian-parent families and those raised in two-parent heterosexual families with regard to problem behavior and well-being (Bos et al., 2007; Bos & van Balen, 2008; Brewaeys, Ponjaert-Kristoffersen, van Steirteghem, & Devroey, 1993; Flaks et al., 1995; Patterson, 1994; Steckel, 1987). Thus, the higher levels of positive parenting found among lesbian-parent families do not generally translate into more positive child outcomes. In this respect, the findings of various studies support the ideas of Roberts and Strayer (1987) concerning a leveling-off effect (i.e., a sigmoid curve) of involved parenting.

There are, however, some exceptions to the above-mentioned findings. In the U.S. National Longitudinal Lesbian Family Study (U.S. NLLFS), for example, the mean score of the thirty-eight 10-year-old girls in lesbian-mother

families on externalizing problem behavior (as measured by the Child Behavioral Checklist, or CBCL; Achenbach, 1991; Achenbach & Rescorla, 2001) was significantly lower than that of an age-matched control group of girls in heterosexual two-parent families (Gartrell, Deck, Rodas, Peyser, & Banks, 2005). For this publication of the U.S. NLLFS, CBCL norms were used as the comparison group (Achenbach, 1991; Achenbach & Rescorla, 2001). In their longitudinal study in the UK, Golombok et al. (1997) found that when the offspring of the planned lesbian mothers were 6 years old, they rated themselves less cognitively and physically competent than did their counterparts in father-present families. At the age of 9, however, there were no significant differences on psychological adjustment between the two groups (MacCallum & Golombok, 2004).

Vanfraussen, Ponjaert-Kristoffersen, and Brewaeys (2002) also found a significant difference in their study in Belgium: Although the 24 children in lesbian-parent families were not more frequently teased than the 24 children in heterosexual two-parent families about such matters as clothes or physical appearance, family-related incidents of teasing were mentioned only by children from lesbian-parent families. Vanfraussen et al. (2002) also gathered data on the children's well-being through reports from teachers, parents, and children. Teachers reported more attention problem behavior by children from lesbian-mother families than by children from mother–father families. However, based on the reports from mothers and the children themselves, no significant differences on the children's problem behavior were found. An explanation for this discrepancy might be that teachers' evaluations are based on a different setting from that of mothers and children.

The above-mentioned studies on the psychological development of children were all based on convenience samples: The planned lesbian-mother families were recruited with the help of gay and lesbian organizations, through friendship networks, through hospital fertility departments, and sometimes through a combination of these methods. However, several studies used a different recruitment strategy. Golombok et al. (2003)

extracted household composition data from the U.K. Avon Longitudinal Study of Parents and Children data set; they used this information to identify households headed by two women and compared them with two-parent heterosexual families. They found no differences in the psychological well-being of young children in the two types of households.

A similar strategy was used by Wainright and colleagues (Wainright & Patterson, 2006, 2008; Wainright, Russell, & Patterson, 2004), who used the U.S. National Longitudinal Study of Adolescent Health (Add Health) data set to identify households headed by two mothers. They could identify 44 families headed by two mothers, and each of them was matched with an adolescent of the Add Health data set who was reared in a two-parent heterosexual family. They found no differences in substance use, relationships with peers, and progress through school between adolescents in households headed by two women and those in two-parent heterosexual families.

The results of two other studies on adolescents are also available. Gartrell and Bos (2010) found that at the age of 17 years, the U.S. NLLFS offspring (39 boys and 39 girls) demonstrated higher levels of social, school/academic, and total competence than gender-matched normative samples of American teenagers (49 girls and 44 boys), indicating the healthy psychological adjustment of the U.S. NLLFS offspring. Although the authors showed that the U.S. NLLFS sample and the comparison sample are similar in socioeconomic status, they were neither matched on nor did the authors control for race/ethnicity or region of residence. This matching, however, was done in another U.S. NLLFS publication about substance use (Goldberg, Bos & Gartrell, 2011). For this study, the researchers used the Monitoring the Future (MTF) data as a comparison group, and by using a 1:1 match procedure on gender, age, race/ethnicity, and parental education, they randomly selected seventy-eight 17-year-old adolescents from the MTF data set. Compared to the matched adolescents, U.S. NLLFS adolescents with same-sex parents were not more likely to report heavy substance use (Goldberg et al., 2011). Second, the above-mentioned U.K. longitudinal study by

Golombok and Badger (2010) found that at the age of 19, adolescents born into lesbian-mother families showed lower levels of anxiety, depression, hostility, and problematic alcohol use, and higher levels of self-esteem, than adolescents in traditional father–mother families. According to Bos and van Balen (2010), the positive findings regarding adolescents in planned lesbian-parent families may be partly explained by the mothers' commitment to and involvement in the rearing of their offspring, or by other aspects regarding the quality of the relationships within the family (e.g., having a supportive partner).

Gender Role, Sexual Questioning, and Sexual Behavior

Other frequently studied aspects of the development of children in planned lesbian-parent families are the children's gender roles and sexual behavior. MacCallum and Golombok (2004) studied 25 lesbian-mother families, 38 families headed by a single heterosexual mother, and 38 two-parent heterosexual families in the UK and found that boys in lesbian or single-mother families showed more feminine personality traits than boys in two-parent heterosexual families. However, other studies that focused on children's aspirations to traditionally masculine or feminine occupations and activities (and which were also carried out in Western countries) did not find differences between children in lesbian-parent families and those in two-parent heterosexual families (Brewaeys et al., 1997; Fulcher, Sutfin, & Patterson, 2008; Golombok et al., 2003).

Bos and Sandfort (2010) studied the gender development of the offspring of lesbian mothers in the Netherlands from a multidimensional perspective by focusing on five issues (a) gender typicality (the degree to which children felt that they were typical members of their gender category), (b) gender contentedness (the degree to which children felt happy with their assigned gender), (c) pressure to conform (the degree to which children felt pressure from parents and peers to conform to gender stereotypes), (d) intergroup bias (the degree to which children felt that their gender was superior to the other gender), and (e) children's anticipation of future heterosexual romantic involvement. The authors found that when the offspring of the parents were between 8 and 12 years old, the 63 children in the lesbian-parent families felt less parental pressure to conform to gender stereotypes, were less likely to experience their own gender as superior (intergroup bias), and were more likely to question future heterosexual romantic involvement than the 68 children in the two-parent heterosexual families. An explanation for these findings might be that lesbian mothers have more liberal attitudes than heterosexual parents toward their children's gender-related behavior (Fulcher et al., 2008). That children in lesbian-mother families are less sure about future heterosexual romantic involvement might be because they grow up in a family environment that is more tolerant toward homoerotic relationships.

The above-mentioned findings are all based on studies of children. The three studies that were conducted on adolescents also included questions about sexual and romantic behavior, and sexual orientation. The longitudinal U.K. study by Golombok and colleagues (2010) found that as young adults (mean age 19), individuals with lesbian mothers were more likely to have started dating than those from heterosexual-parent families. However, the U.S. NLLFS found that the 17-year-old offspring of lesbian mothers were significantly older at the time of their first heterosexual contact compared to an age- and gender-matched comparison group from the National Survey of Family Growth (Gartrell, Bos, & Goldberg 2010). A study using Add Health data, on the other hand, revealed no significant differences in heterosexual intercourse or romantic relationships between young adults with lesbian mothers and young adults with heterosexual parents (Wainright et al., 2004). In all three studies, almost all the children of the lesbian mothers identified themselves as heterosexual. However, the daughters of U.S. NLLFS lesbian mothers were significantly more likely to have had same-sex sexual contact (Gartrell et al., 2010), which might be because this type of family environment makes it more comfortable for adolescent girls with same-sex attractions to explore intimate relationships with

their peers (Biblarz & Stacey, 2010; Stacey & Biblarz, 2001).

Comparison Between Biological Mothers and Nonbiological Mothers in Planned Lesbian-Mother Families

In studies that compare biological and nonbiological mothers in planned lesbian-parent families, there are three main topics of interest (a) the pregnancy decision-making process and the desire and motivation to have children, (b) the division of tasks, and (c) parenting. Interest in the differences and similarities between biological and nonbiological mothers is linked to the role and position of the mothers who did not bear a child, especially because these mothers are living in a societal context in which the biological relatedness of the parents is perceived as very important. In addition, for nonbiological mothers in planned lesbian-mother families, in many countries there is also the issue of the lack of legitimacy under the law (Waaldijk, 2009a, 2009b, 2009c). As a consequence, nonbiological mothers might feel excluded in their role as parents by institutions. In addition to experiencing greater feelings of exclusion, nonbiological mothers might experience lack of recognition, entitlement, and security in their parental role.

Pregnancy Decision-Making Process, and Desire and Motivation to Have Children

Several studies have examined the decision-making process concerning which of the partners in lesbian couples will conceive and bear the children. Goldberg (2006), for example, interviewed 29 American lesbian couples about their decision regarding who would try to get pregnant and the reasons behind this decision. The most frequently mentioned reason was the biological mother's desire to experience pregnancy and childbirth; for some, it was also important to have a genetic connection with the child (Goldberg, 2006).

However, many couples had other reasons. For example, one reason was age: the older partner was chosen because it could have been her last chance to become pregnant, or the younger partner was chosen because they both thought that the age of the older partner might make it difficult for her to conceive. Another reason was employment situation: The partner with the most flexible job was chosen to conceive. Chabot and Ames (2004) interviewed 10 American lesbian couples (age of the children was between 3 months and 8 years) and also observed these couples during support group meetings for lesbian parents. Similar results were found on how the couples decided who would carry the child as in the above-mentioned study of Goldberg (2006).

Women in lesbian couples can theoretically have each partner carry a child. Studies, however, have shown that few couples make the decision to do this. For example, a study of 95 lesbian couples who were undergoing artificial donor insemination (AID) treatment at a infertility clinic in Belgium found that only 14% of the couples wanted both partners to become pregnant—first the older and then the younger partner (Baetens, Camus, & Devroey, 2003). A study of 100 Dutch lesbian couples who already had one or more children (with the oldest child between 4 and 8 years old) found that in only a minority (33%) of cases had both mothers given birth to a child (Bos et al., 2003). While in Baetens et al.'s (2003) study it was the oldest partner who had been the first to try to get pregnant, in Bos et al.'s (2003) study there was no significant age difference between the two would-be parents.

In Bos et al.'s (2003) study, the authors also compared the mothers who did get pregnant with those who did not. They found that the former group had spent more time on thinking about why they wanted to become mothers, stated more frequently that they had had to "give up almost everything" to get pregnant, and more frequently reported "parenthood as a life fulfillment" as a motive for seeking parenthood. Indeed, it would be interesting to examine the extent to which gender identity (i.e., the extent to which women use stereotyped feminine or masculine personal-

ity traits to describe themselves) is a predictor of the desire to experience pregnancy and childbirth. For a heterosexual woman in a Western society, being a mother is still considered evidence of her femininity (Ulrich & Weatherall, 2000), and it would be interesting to look at how this perception is related to a lesbian woman's desire to become a mother or to give birth in a lesbian relationship.

Division of Tasks

Several studies have found that the biological lesbian mothers were more involved in childcare than their partners, that the nonbiological lesbian mothers spent more time working outside the home, and that the mothers shared the housework relatively equally (Bos et al., 2007; Goldberg & Perry-Jenkins, 2007; Patterson, 2002; Short, 2007). Several other studies, however, found an equal division of both unpaid and paid work between the partners in planned lesbian-mother families. For example, Chan et al. (1998) studied 30 American lesbian-parent families and 16 heterosexual-parent families and found that same-sex couples shared childcare, housework, and employment fairly equally whereas heterosexual couples did not. These results are similar to findings from the third and fourth wave of the U.S. NLLFS (the children were then 4 and 10 years old, respectively); namely, in most families in which the mothers were still together, biological mother and nonbiological mother shared child rearing relatively equally (Gartrell et al., 1999, 2000).

Based on theses inconsistent findings, one could conclude that there is a great deal of variability in the labor arrangements within lesbian couples (Goldberg, 2010). A next step is to investigate the differences between the planned lesbian-parent families that do have an equal division of labor and those that do not, and to gain more information (via in-depth interviews) about whether this division is based on a conscious decision. In the families in which this division is a conscious decision, it would be interesting to examine what factors (e.g., stereotyped feminine or masculine personality traits, career opportunities, age, or socioeconomic status) are related to such decision.

Parenting

Only a few studies have examined whether there are differences in parenting styles and parenting behavior between partners in planned lesbian-mother families. When such a comparison is made, the unit of analyses is the biological tie (or its absence) with the child(ren). Goldberg, Downing, and Sauck (2008) asked the lesbian mothers whom they interviewed whether they observed in their children a preference for the biological or the nonbiological mother. Many of the women mentioned that as infants their children had preferred the birth mother, but that over the years this preference had faded such that at the time of the interviews, the children (who were then 3.5 years old) had no preference. According to the mothers, the initial preference of the child was related to the pregnancy and the experience of breastfeeding during the first months. Notably, some nonbiological mothers were jealous of these experiences of their partners. Gartrell et al. (1999) also found that lesbian co-mothers of 2-year-old children reported feelings of jealousy related to their partners' bonding with the child (see also Gartrell, Peyser, & Bos, 2011).

One of the publications emanating from the Dutch study by Bos et al., (2007) compared biological and nonbiological mothers in the 100 planned lesbian-mother families with respect to parenting styles and parental behavior. No differences were found between the partners on most of the variables: They did not differ significantly on emotional involvement, parental concern, power assertion, induction (all measured with questionnaires), supportive presence, or respect for the child's autonomy (all measured with observations of child–parent interactions). However, lesbian biological mothers scored higher on limit setting on the child's behavior during the observed parent–child interactions.

Diversity Within Planned Lesbian-Mother Families

The focus of the third set of studies is on diversity among planned lesbian-mother families and the potential effects of such diversity on child rearing and children. Three aspects of diversity within planned lesbian-mother studies that have been studied are (a) donor status (known or as yet unknown donor), (b) absence of male role figures, and (c) the mothers' and the offspring's experiences of stigmatization. The focus on diversity within lesbian-parent families represents a relatively new type of inquiry in studies of lesbian-mother families.

Questions regarding why mothers use known or as yet unknown donors, and what the choice means for the mothers and their offspring, should be placed in a broader discussion in which some authors have theorized that the absence of information about their donors may affect the offspring's identity and psychological development, especially during the vulnerable period of adolescence (for an overview see Hunfeld, Passchier, Bolt, & Buijsen, 2004). Interest in the role of male involvement in these families is based on theories and ideas about gender identification, and how the absence of a traditional father or father figure may affect children. Interest in the experience and role of stigmatization in lesbian-mother families should be understood in terms of perspectives emphasizing the role of personal, family, and community resources in reducing the negative impact of homophobia on the offspring's psychological development (Van Gelderen, Gartrell, Bos, & Hermanns, 2009).

Donor Status

Many fertility clinics in the USA offer couples the option of using either the sperm of a donor who will remain permanently anonymous (unknown donor) or that of a donor who may be met by the offspring when she or he reaches the age of 18 (identity-release donor) (Scheib, Riordan, & Rubin, 2005). In her US study of 29 pregnant lesbians and their partners, Goldberg (2006) found that 59% of the women wanted to have an unknown donor, and the main reason for this preference was that they wanted to raise their children without interference from a third party. Touroni and Coyle (2002), who interviewed nine lesbian couples in the UK, found that six of them made the decision for a known donor, and a reason that they gave for this was they believed that children have the right to know their genetic origins and/or to form relationships with their donors early in life. Gartrell et al. (1996) found that among the lesbian women in their study who preferred a known donor, many did this because they worried that children conceived by unknown donors might experience psychological and identity problems during adolescence or later in life.

There are few data on what it means for offspring to have known or unknown donors. In Belgium, Vanfraussen, Pontjaert-Kristoffersen, and Brewaeys (2003a, 2003b) asked 24 children (mean age = 10 years old) with lesbian mothers whether, if it were possible, they would want to have more information about their donors. Nearly 50% of the children answered "yes," and they were especially curious about their donors' physical features and personalities. Scheib et al. (2005) found that for adolescents conceived by identity-release donors and raised in lesbian-mother families, the most frequently mentioned questions were "What's he like?," "What does he look like?," "What's his family like?," and "Is he like me?" The Belgian study also assessed whether the children who wanted to know more about their donors differed in self-esteem or emotional and behavioral functioning from their counterparts who did not share this curiosity. No significant differences were found on self-esteem or emotional and behavioral functioning between the group of children who wanted to learn more about their donors and those who did not have this curiosity (Vanfraussen et al., 2003a, 2003b).

At the time of the first U.S. NLLFS data collection, the mothers-to-be were either pregnant or inseminating, and the donor preferences were almost equally divided between permanently anonymous and identity-release donors (Gartrell et al., 1996). In the fifth wave of the U.S. NLLFS, nearly 23% of the adolescents with unknown donors stated that they wished they knew their donors, while 67% of those who would have the option to meet their donors when they turned 18 planned to do so. Unfortunately, the U.S. NLLFS adolescents were not asked why they intended to contact their donors, nor what they hoped to experience by meeting them.

The U.S. NLLFS also gathered data on the offspring's problem behavior by means of parental reports using the CBCL (Achenbach & Rescorla, 2001). This data collection by means of the parental reports of the CBCL was done in the fourth and fifth waves (when the children were 10 and 17 years old, respectively), which made it possible to assess the role of donor status regarding the offspring's problem behavior over time. The authors (Bos & Gartrell, 2010a) found only a few differences between the offspring when they were 10 and when they were 17 years old: That is, when they were 17 years old, their scores on social problems and aggressive behavior were lower, and their scores on thought problems and rule-breaking behavior were higher, than when they were 10 (Bos & Gartrell, 2010a). For all findings, no differences were found between adolescents with known donors and those with as yet unknown donors. These findings are important, because lesbian women are often uncertain about the long-term consequences of donor selection and the well-being of their offspring, and these findings indicate that donor type has no bearing on the development of the psychological well-being of the offspring of lesbian mothers over a 7-year period from childhood through adolescence.

Male Role Models

Little research has focused on lesbian mothers' ideas about male involvement in the lives of their offspring, and no studies have looked at what it means for children and adolescents growing up in lesbian-mother families with or without male role models. The U.S. NLLFS found that when the mothers were pregnant or undergoing the process of insemination, 76% stated that they hoped to provide their children with positive male role models (often described as "good, loving men") (Gartrell et al., 1996), and by the time the children were 10 years old, half of the families had incorporated male role models into these children's lives (Gartrell et al., 2005).

Goldberg and Allen (2007) interviewed 30 lesbian couples in the USA, during the pregnancy and when the children were 3 months old and found that more than two-thirds of the women were highly conscious of the fact that their children would grow up in the absence of a male figure; they believed this might have negative consequences for their offspring's psychological well-being. Many of them, in turn, had already made plans to find such men. According to the authors, as well as Clarke and Kitzinger (2005), this awareness and anticipation may be a response to the cultural anxieties about the necessity of male role models in the development of children.

All of the above studies evaluated what mothers reported about male role figures in the lives of their offspring, and on what these mothers thought the presence or absence of such figures might mean for the development of their children. The influence of male role figures on the offspring's gender role development and psychological adjustment has not yet been studied.

Stigmatization

Mothers' Experiences of Stigmatization

The U.S. NLLFS found that while pregnant or undergoing the process of insemination, most mothers saw raising a child in a heterosexist and homophobic society as a challenge they would have to deal with in the future (Gartrell et al., 1996). Experiences of stigmatization and rejection were assessed in the Dutch longitudinal study by Bos et al. (2004). The 200 mothers (100 couples) were asked about such experiences when the children were between 4 and 8 years old. The authors developed a scale to measure the mothers' perceived experiences of rejection.

This instrument included 7 forms of rejections related to being a lesbian mother. Lesbian mothers were asked to indicate how frequent ($1 = never$, $2 = sometimes$, $3 = regularly$) each form of rejection had occurred in the previous year (Bos et al., 2004). The forms of rejection that were most frequently reported (i.e., the mothers answered that they sometimes or regularly experienced it) were "Other people asking me annoying questions related to my lifestyle" (reported by 68% and 72% of the biological mothers and the co-mothers, respectively) and "Other people gossiping about me" (27.3% and 32.7% of the biological and the co-mothers, respectively). Less frequently reported experiences were disapproving comments (13% and 12.1% of the biological and the co-mothers, respectively) and being excluded (12% and 9.1% of the biological and the co-mothers, respectively). The 7 items formed a reliable scale, and based on this scale the authors calculated the associations between rejection and the extent to which the mothers reported parental stress (parental burden), the need to demonstrate to others that they are good parents (parental justification), and feelings of not being able to handle their children (feeling incompetent as a parent). The results show that higher levels of rejection were associated with more experiences of parental stress, feeling a greater need to justify the quality of the parent–child relationship, and feeling less competent as a parent (Bos, van Balen, Sandfort et al., 2004).

It should be mentioned that the study from which these data are drawn was conducted in the Netherlands, which has a relatively positive climate regarding lesbian and gay people and same-sex marriage (Sandfort, McGaskey, & Bos, 2008). The level of stigmatization may therefore be more pronounced in other Western countries. Shapiro, Peterson, and Stewart (2009) also showed that differences in sociolegal context (namely countries in which same-sex marriage is possible compared to countries in which it is not) can influence the experience of lesbian parenthood: They found that lesbian mothers in Canada reported fewer worries about discrimination than lesbian mothers in the USA.

Children's and Adolescents' Experiences of Stigmatization

In the follow-up of the above-mentioned study that was carried out in the Netherlands, the children (who were now between 8 and 12 years old) were asked about their experiences of rejection (Bos & van Balen, 2008). Sixty percent of the children in the lesbian-mother families reported that peers made jokes about them because they had lesbian mothers. Other frequently reported negative forms of rejection were: annoying questions about the parents' sexual orientation (56.7%), abusive language related to the mothers' sexual orientation (45.2%), peers gossiping about the lesbian mothers (30.6%), and exclusion by peers because of their family situation (26.2%).

Here, differences in sociolegal context between countries are also important. In the fourth wave of the U.S. NLLFS, Gartrell et al. (2005) measured experiences with homophobia among the children by asking them: "Did other kids ever say mean things to you about your mom(s) being a lesbian?" Almost 38% of the 41 boys and 46% of the 38 girls answered "yes" on this question. Responding to exactly the same question to children in Dutch planned lesbian families, 14.7% of the 36 boys and 22.2% of the 38 girls answered "yes." In the last wave of the U.S. NLLFS data collection (when the offspring were 17 years old), 35.9% of the boys and 46.2% of the girls reported experiences of homophobic stigmatization.

Although studies that compared the children of lesbian and heterosexual parents showed that having same-sex parents is not in itself a risk factor (e.g., Bos et al., 2007; Golombok et al., 2003), both the Dutch longitudinal study and the U.S. NLLFS found that when children are confronted with their peers' disapproval of their lesbian mothers' sexual orientation, they lose self-confidence and exhibit more behavioral problems (Bos & van Balen, 2008; Bos, van Balen, Sandfort et al., 2004; Gartrell et al., 2005). However, among the children who reported being stigmatized, three groups exhibited greater resilience: namely, children who attended schools that had lesbian/gay awareness on their curricula; children whose mothers

described themselves as active members of the lesbian community; and children who had frequent contact with other offspring of same-sex parents (Bos, Gartrell, van Balen, Peyser, & Sandfort, 2008; Bos & van Balen, 2008). In the fifth wave of the U.S. NLLFS it was found that among the adolescent offspring of lesbian mothers, stigmatization was associated with more problem behavior, but that having close, positive relationships with their mothers mitigated this negative influence (Bos & Gartrell, 2010b). Bos and Gartrell (2010b) hypothesized that family conversations about possible future homophobic stigmatization reduces the negative impact of these experiences on the well-being of the offspring; however, in the data on the 17-year-old offspring of the U.S. NLLFS, no evidence was found to support this hypothesis (Bos & Gartrell, 2010b).

Limitations and Challenges

There are several limitations of the comparison studies and of the studies that focus solely on planned lesbian-parent families and the mechanisms within these families. First, most studies collected data by means of semi-structured interviews with parents or self-administered questionnaires completed by parents. It might be that results based on parental reports are biased because the mothers want to demonstrate that they are good parents. Gathering data on the parent–child relationship and the offspring's psychological adjustment from such sources as teacher reports or observations of parent–child interactions (which some studies already do) might counter the degree to which self-report bias is a limitation.

Second, there is the issue of the representativeness of the samples used in the studies, and the generalization of the findings. Most studies on planned lesbian-mother families used comparatively small samples, and respondents were recruited via such sources as organizations of lesbian and gay parents. As a consequence they are not representative, which has consequences for the generalizability of the findings (Tasker, 2010).

It should also be noted that most studies on planned lesbian-mother families are carried out among upper-middle-class, highly educated, urban-dwelling, White lesbian parents (Clarke, 2008; Gabb, 2004). This limitation means that there is an absence of class-based analysis, which also has consequences for the representativeness of the samples and the findings.

A practical solution to these issues of representativeness is to apply large, general sample frames, and to screen for households headed by two women (Sandfort, 2000). However, such a solution would be very costly. An alternative is to include some identifying questions about the family structure, genetic relationship between parents and offspring, and sexual orientation in general population studies set up by other researchers on topics that are related to the field of parenting or child development (Tasker, 2010). This strategy might also make it possible to get more diversity in SES and race in the samples of planned lesbian-mother families.

The above-mentioned strategy was used in two studies (Golombok et al., 2003; Wainright et al., 2004; Wainright & Patterson, 2007, 2008). However, in the data sets the researchers used there were only questions about the structure of the families in which the children and adolescents were living, and the parents' sexual orientation was not specified. Therefore the analyses may be confounded by the inclusion of women who live together but do not identify as lesbian (Gartrell & Bos, 2010).

It is also a limitation that in most studies, planned lesbian-mother families are compared with two-parent heterosexual families (e.g., Bos et al., 2007). In such a design, however, issues related to unraveling the influence of gender, a genetic link, and minority status remain unresolved. Researchers should therefore initiate other designs. A comparison, for example, between planned lesbian-families, two-parent heterosexual families, gay-father families and/or gay-father and lesbian-mother families in which the mother became a parent after her coming out and is sharing the child-rearing task, might help to tease apart the relative influences of gender, genetic link, and minority status on child rearing and child development.

Another limitation is that most of the previous studies on planned lesbian mother families used a cross-sectional design; thus, one has to be cautious in ascribing causal directions to the associations that were found (e.g., between experiences of stigmatization and the offspring's psychological adjustment). There are several studies in which data are gathered in several waves (e.g., Bos et al., 2007; Bos & Sandfort, 2010; Gartrell et al., 1996; Golombok et al., 1997; Golombok & Badger, 2010). However, the instruments that were used were different across phases, and as a consequence it was not possible to examine the psychological well-being of the offspring from a longitudinal perspective. Longitudinal studies, for example, on the long-term consequences of stigmatization and resilience are needed.

Conclusion

Most existing studies on planned lesbian-mother families made a comparison between planned lesbian-mother families and heterosexual two-parent families with the aim of gathering more information on whether lesbian women could be "good" parents. These comparative studies of the significance of the "critical ingredients" of child rearing and family processes are important, to gather more information about what they do and how they contribute to the healthy development of children's well-being. However, as a consequence of the tremendous diversity within the lesbian community, recent research has increasingly focused on diversity within lesbian-mother families and the effects of family variation on parenting and child outcomes. There has been a trend toward investigating new kinds of research questions that are more centered on the mechanisms within lesbian-parent families, instead of comparing them with heterosexual two-parent families. For example, these studies focus on differences and similarities in parenting between biological and nonbiological mothers, and on how lesbian mothers deal with circumstances in which they differ from heterosexual parents.

To evaluate the psychological development of offspring in planned lesbian-mother families, it is important to consider the sociolegal context and cultural climate in which the families live (Bos, Gartrell, Peyser, & van Balen, 2008; Shapiro et al., 2009; Tasker, 2010). The comparison study of the U.S. NLLFS data and those of a Dutch study (Bos, Gartrell, van Balen et al., 2008) indicates that cross-national differences in the acceptance of homosexuality and same-sex parenthood have consequences for the well-being of children in lesbian-mother families, with greater acceptance of lesbian and gay people and same-sex parenting associated with less problem behavior among the children. Future research should compare the experiences of parents and their offspring in multiple countries that have different levels of official recognition of lesbian couples.

References

Achenbach, T. M. (1991). *Manual for the child behavior checklist and revised child behavior profile*. Burlington, VT: University of Vermont Department of Psychiatry.

Achenbach, T. M., & Rescorla, L. A. (2001). *Manual for ASEBA school-age forms and profiles*. Burlington, VT: University of Vermont, Research Center for Children, Youth, and Families.

Baetens, P., Camus, M., & Devroey, P. (2003). Counseling lesbian couples: Request for donor insemination on social grounds. *Reproductive BioMedicine Online, 6*, 75–83. doi:10.1016/S1472-6483(10)62059-7

Biblarz, T. J., & Stacey, J. (2010). How does the gender of the parents matter? *Journal of Marriage and Family, 72*, 3–22. doi:10.1111/j.1741-3737.2009.00678.x

Bos, H. M. W., & Gartrell, N. (2010a). Adolescents of the US National Longitudinal Lesbian Family Study: The impact if having a known or an unknown donor on the stability of psychological adjustment. *Human Reproduction, 26*, 630–637. doi:10.1093/humrep/deq359

Bos, H. M. W., & Gartrell, N. (2010b). Adolescents of the US National Longitudinal Lesbian Family Study: Can family characteristics counteract the negative effects of stigmatization? *Family Process, 49*, 559–572.

Bos, H. M. W., Gartrell, N. K., Peyser, H., & van Balen, F. (2008). The US National Longitudinal Lesbian Family Study: Homophobia, psychological adjustment, and protective factors. *Journal of Lesbian Studies, 12*, 455–471. doi:10.1080/10894160802278630

Bos, H. M. W., Gartrell, K., van Balen, F., Peyser, H., & Sandfort, Th. G. M. (2008). Children in planned lesbian families: A cross-cultural comparison between the USA and the Netherlands. *American Journal of Orthopsychiatry, 78*, 211–219. doi:10.1037/a0012711

Bos, H. M. W., & Sandfort, Th. (2010). Children's gender identity in lesbian and heterosexual two-parent families. *Sex Roles, 62*, 114–126. doi:10.1007/s11199-009-9704-7

Bos, H. M. W., & van Balen, F. (2008). Children in planned lesbian families: Stigmatisation, psychological adjustment and protective factors. *Culture, Health, & Sexualities, 10*, 221–236. doi:10.1080/13691050701601702

Bos, H. M. W., & van Balen, F. (2010). Children of the new reproductive technologies: Social and genetic parenthood. *Patient Education and Counseling, 81*, 429–435. doi:10.1016/j.pec.2010.09.012

Bos, H. M. W., van Balen, F., Sandfort, Th. G. M., & van den Boom, D. C. (2004). Minority stress, experience of parenthood, and child adjustment in lesbian families. *Journal of Reproductive and Infant Psychology, 22*, 291–305. doi:10.1080/02646830412331298299

Bos, H. M. W., van Balen, F., & van den Boom, D. C. (2003). Planned lesbian families: Their desire and motivation to have a child. *Human Reproduction, 18*, 2216–2224. doi:10.1093/humrep/deg427

Bos, H. M. W., van Balen, F., & van den Boom, D. C. (2004). Experience of parenthood, couple relationship, social support, and child rearing goals in planned lesbian families. *Journal of Child Psychology and Psychiatry, 45*, 755–764. doi:10.1111/j.1469-610.2004.00269.x

Bos, H. M. W., van Balen, F., & van den Boom, D. C. (2007). Child adjustment and parenting in planned lesbian-parent families. *American Journal of Orthopsychiatry, 77*, 38–48. doi:10.1037/0002-9432.77.1.38

Bos, H. M. W., & van Gelderen, L. (2010). Homo en lesbisch ouderschap in Nederland. In S. Keuzenkamp (Ed.), *Steeds gewoner, nooit gewoon. Acceptatie van homoseksualiteit in Nederland* (pp. 104–118). The Hague, The Netherlands: Sociaal en Cultureel Planbureau.

Botchan, A., Hauser, R., Gamzu, R., Yogev, L., Paz, G., & Yavetz, H. (2001). Results of 6139 artificial insemination cycles with donor spermatozoa. *Human Reproduction, 16*, 2298–2304. doi:10.1093/humrep/16.11.2298

Brewaeys, A., Ponjaert, I., van Hall, E. V., & Golombok, S. (1997). Donor insemination: Child development & family functioning in lesbian mother families with 4 to 8 year old children. *Human Reproduction, 12*, 1349–1359. doi:10.1093/humrep/deh581

Brewaeys, A., Ponjaert-Kristoffersen, I., van Steirteghem, A. C., & Devroey, P. (1993). Children from anonymous donors: An inquiry into homosexual and heterosexual parents' attitudes. *Journal of Psychosomatic Obstetrics and Gynaecology, 14*, 23–35.

Chabot, J. M., & Ames, B. D. (2004). "It wasn't let's get pregnant and go do it": Decision-making in lesbian couples planning motherhood via donor insemination. *Family Relations, 53*, 348–356. doi:10.1111/j.0197-6664.2004.00041.x

Chan, R. W., Brooks, R. C., Raboy, B., & Patterson, C. J. (1998). Division of labor among lesbian and heterosexual parents: Associations with children's adjustment. *Journal of Family Psychology, 12*, 402–419. doi:10.1037/0893-3200.12.3.402

Clarke, V. (2001). What about the children? Arguments against lesbian and gay parenting. *Women's Studies International Forum, 24*, 555–570. doi:10.1016/S0277-5395(01)00193-5

Clarke, V. (2008). From outsiders to motherhood to reinventing the family: Constructions of lesbian parenting in the psychological literature – 1886–2006. *Women's Studies International Forum, 31*, 118–128. doi:10.1016/j.wsif.2008.03.004

Clarke, V., & Kitzinger, C. (2005). 'We're not living on planet lesbian': Constructions of male role models in debates about lesbian families. *Sexualities, 8*, 137–152. doi:10.1177/1363460705050851

Cowan, C. P., & Cowan, P. A. (1988). Who does what when partners become parents: Implications for men, women and marriage. *Marriage and Family Review, 12*, 105–131.

Derogatis, L. R. (1983). *SCL-90-R administration, scoring, and procedures manual.* Towson, MD: Clinical Psychometric Research.

Dunne, G. A. (1998). Pioneers behind our own front doors: New models for the organization of work in domestic partnerships. *Work, Employment, and Society, 12*, 273–296. doi:10.1177/0950017098122004

Eamon, M. K. (2001). Antecedents and socioemotional consequences of physical punishment on children in two-parent families. *Child Abuse and Neglect, 25*, 787–802. doi:10.1016/S0145-2134(01)00239-3

Flaks, D. K., Ficher, I., Masterpasqua, F., & Joseph, G. (1995). Lesbian choosing motherhood: A comparative study of lesbian and heterosexual parents and their children. *Developmental Psychology, 31*, 105–114. doi:10.1037/0012-1649.31.1.105

Fulcher, M., Sutfin, E. L., & Patterson, C. (2008). Individual differences in gender development: Associations with parental sexual orientation, attitudes, and division of labor. *Sex Roles, 58*, 330–341. doi:10.1007/s11199-007-9348-4

Gabb, J. (2004). Critical differentials: Querying the contrarieties between research on lesbian parent families. *Sexualities, 7*, 171–187. doi:10.1177/1363460704042162

Gartrell, N., Banks, A., Hamilton, J., Reed, N., Bishop, H., & Rodas, C. (1999). The national lesbian family study: 2. Interviews with mothers of toddlers. *American Journal of Orthopsychiatry, 69*, 362–369. doi:10.1037/h0080410

Gartrell, N., Banks, A., Reed, N., Hamilton, J., Rodas, C., & Deck, A. (2000). The national lesbian family study: 3. Interviews with mothers of five-year-olds. *American Journal of Orthopsychiatry, 70*, 542–548. doi:10.1037/h0087823

Gartrell, N., & Bos, H. M. W. (2010). The US National Longitudinal Lesbian Family Study: Psychological adjustment of 17-year-old adolescents. *Pediatrics, 126*, 1–9. doi:10.1542/peds.2010-1807

Gartrell, N., Bos, H. M. W., & Goldberg, N. (2010). Adolescents of the US National Longitudinal Lesbian Family Study: Sexual orientation, sexual behavior, sexual risk exposure. *Archives of Sexual Behavior, 40*(6), 1199–1209. doi:10.1007/s10508-010-9692-2 (online since November 6, 2010)

Gartrell, N., Deck, A., Rodas, C., Peyser, H., & Banks, A. (2005). The national lesbian family study: 4. Interviews with the 10-year-old children. *American Journal of Orthopsychiatry, 75*, 518–524. doi:10.1037/0002-9432.75.4.518

Gartrell, N., Hamilton, J., Banks, A., Mosbacher, D., Reed, N., Sparks, C. H., & Bishop, H. (1996). The national lesbian family study: 1. Interviews with prospective mothers. *American Journal of Orthopsychiatry, 66*, 272–281. doi:10.1037/h0080178

Gartrell, N., Peyser, H., & Bos, H. (2011). Planned lesbian families: A review of the U.S. National Longitudinal Lesbian Family Study. In D. M. Brodzinsky & A. Pertman (Eds.), *Adoption by lesbian and gay men* (pp. 112–129). Oxford, NY: Oxford University Press.

Goldberg, A. E. (2006). The transition to parenthood for lesbian couples. *Journal of GLBT Family Studies, 2*, 13–42. doi:10.1300/J461v02n01_02

Goldberg, A. E. (2010). *Lesbian and gay parents and their children: Research on the family life cycle.* Washington, DC: American Psychological Association.

Goldberg, A. E., & Allen, K. R. (2007). Lesbian mothers' ideas and intentions about male involvement across the transition to parenthood. *Journal of Marriage and Family, 69*, 352–365. doi:10.1111/j.1741-3737.2007.00370.x

Goldberg, A. E., Downing, J. B., & Sauck, C. C. (2008). Perceptions of children's parental preferences in lesbian two-mother households. *Journal of Marriage and Family, 70*, 419–434. doi:10.1111/j.1741-3737.2008.00491.x

Goldberg, A. E., & Perry-Jenkins, M. (2007). The division of labor and perceptions of parental roles: Lesbian couples across the transition to parenthood. *Journal of Social and Personal Relationships, 24*, 297–318. doi:10.1177/0265407507075415

Goldberg, N., Bos, H. M. W., & Gartrell, N. (2011). Substance use by adolescents of the US National Longitudinal Lesbian Family Study. *Journal of Health Psychology.* doi:10.1177/1359105311403522

Golombok, S., & Badger, S. (2010). Children raised in mother-headed families from infancy: A follow-up of children of lesbian and heterosexual mothers, at early adulthood. *Human Reproduction, 25*, 150–157. doi:10.1093/humrep/dep345

Golombok, S., Perry, B., Burston, A., Murray, C., Mooney-Somers, J., Stevens, M., & Golding, J. (2003). Children with lesbian parents: A community study. *Developmental Psychology, 39*, 20–33. doi:10.1037/0012-1649.39.1.20

Golombok, S., Tasker, F. L., & Murray, C. (1997). Children raised in fatherless families from infancy: Family relationships and the socio-emotional development of children of lesbian and single heterosexual mothers. *Journal of Child Psychology and Psychiatry, 38*, 783–791. doi:10.1111/j.1469-7610.1997.tb01596.x

Grotevant, H. D., & Kohler, J. K. (1999). Adoptive families. In M. E. Lamb (Ed.), *Parenting and child development in 'nontraditional families'* (pp. 161–190). Mahwah, NJ: Lawrence Erlbaum Associates.

Hunfeld, J. A. M., Passchier, J., Bolt, L. L. E., & Buijsen, M. A. J. M. (2004). Protect child from being born: Arguments against IVF from heads of the 13 licensed Dutch fertility centres, ethical and legal perspectives. *Journal of Reproductive and Infant Psychology, 22*, 279–289. doi:10.1080/02646830412331298341

Kaiser, H. J., & Foundation, F. (2001). *Inside-out: A report on the experiences of lesbians, gays, and bisexuals in America and the public's views on issues and policies related to sexual orientation*. Menlo Park, CA: The Henry J. Kaiser Family Foundation.

Kirkpatrick, M., Smith, C., & Roy, P. (1981). Lesbian mothers and their children: A comparative survey. *American Journal of Orthopsychiatry, 51*, 545–551. doi:10.1111/j.1939-0025.1981.tb01403.x

Lamb, M. E. (1999). Parental behavior, family processes, and child development in non-traditional and traditionally understudied families. In M. E. Lamb (Ed.), *Parenting and child development in 'non-traditional families'* (pp. 1–14). Mahwah, NJ: Lawrence Erlbaum Associates.

MacCallum, F., & Golombok, S. (2004). Children raised in fatherless families from infancy: A follow-up of children of lesbian and single heterosexual mothers at early adolescence. *Journal of Child Psychology and Psychiatry, 45*, 1407–1419. doi:10.1111/j.1469-7610.2004.00324.x

Mucklow, J. F., & Phelan, G. (1979). Lesbian and traditional mother's responses to child behavior and self-concept. *Psychological Report, 44*, 880–882.

Nekkebroeck, J., & Brewaeys, A. (2002). Lesbische moeders en heteroseksuele ouders, hun rol bekeken vanuit het kindperspectief [Lesbian mothers and heterosexual parents, parenting roles identified from the child's perspective]. *Tijdschrift voor Seksuologie, 26*, 125–130.

Parke, R. D. (2004). Development in the family. *Annual Review of Psychology, 55*, 365–399. doi:10.1146/annurev.psych.55.090902.141528

Patterson, C. J. (1994). Children of the lesbian baby boom: Behavioral adjustment, self-concepts, and sex-role identity. In B. Greene & G. Herek (Eds.), *Contemporary perspectives on lesbian and gay psychology: Theory, research and application* (pp. 156–175). Beverly Hills, CA: Sage.

Patterson, C. J. (2001). Families of the lesbian baby boom: Maternal mental health and child adjustment. *Journal of Gay and Lesbian Psychotherapy, 4*, 91–107. doi:10.1300/J236v04n03_07

Patterson, C. J. (2002). Children of lesbian and gay parents: Research, law, and policy. In B. L. Bottoms, M. Bull Kovera, & B. D. McAuliff (Eds.), *Children, social science, and the law* (pp. 176–199). Cambridge, MA: Cambridge University Press.

Roberts, W. L., & Strayer, J. (1987). Parents' responses to the emotional distress of their children: Relations with children's competence. *Developmental Psychology, 23*, 415–422. doi:10.1037/0012-1649.23.3.415

Rosky, C. J. (2009). Like father, like son: Homosexuality, parenthood, and the gender of homophobia. *Yale Journal of Law and Feminism, 20*, 256–355.

Sandfort, Th. G. M. (2000). Homosexuality, psychology, and gay and lesbian studies. In Th. G. M. Sandfort, J. Schuyf, J. W. Duyvendak, & J. Weeks (Eds.), *Lesbian and gay studies. An introductory, interdisciplinary approach* (pp. 14–45). London, England: Sage.

Sandfort, Th. G. M., McGaskey, J., & Bos, H. M. W. (2008, July). *Cultural and structural determinants of acceptance of homosexuality: A cross-national comparison*. Paper presented at the International Congress of Psychology, Berlin, Germany.

Scheib, J. E., Riordan, M., & Rubin, S. (2005). Adolescents with open-identity sperm donors: Reports from 12–17 year olds. *Human Reproduction, 20*, 239–252. doi:10.1093/humrep/deh581

Shapiro, D. N., Peterson, C., & Stewart, A. J. (2009). Legal and social contexts and mental health among lesbian and heterosexual mothers. *Journal of Family Psychology, 23*, 255–262. doi:doi:10.1037/a0014973

Shechner, T., Slone, M., Meir, Y., & Kalish, Y. (2010). Relations between social support and psychological and parental distress for lesbian, single heterosexual by choice, and two-parent heterosexual mothers. *American Journal of Orthopsychiatry, 80*, 283–292. doi:10.1111/j.1939-0025.2010.01031.x

Short, L. (2007). Lesbian mothers living well in the context of heterosexism and discrimination: Resources, strategies, and legislative changes. *Feminism & Psychology, 13*, 106–126. doi:10.1177/0959353507072912

Simmons, T., & O'Connell, M. (2003). *Married-couple and unmarried-partner households: 2000*. Retrieved from http://www.census.gov/prod/2003pubs/censr-5.pdf

Stacey, J., & Biblarz, T. (2001). (How) does the sexual orientation of parents matter? *American Sociological Review, 66*, 159–183.

Steckel, A. (1987). Psychosocial development of children of lesbian mothers. Gay and lesbian parents. In F. Bozett (Ed.), *Homosexuality and family relations* (pp. 23–36). New York, NY: Harrington Park Press.

Steenhof, L., & Harmsen, C. (2003, June/July). *Same-sex couples in the Netherlands*. Paper presented at the Workshop on Comparative Research, Rome, Italy.

Tasker, F. (2010). Same-sex parenting and child development: Reviewing the contribution of parental gender. *Journal of Marriage and Family, 72*, 35–40. doi:10.1111/j.1741-3737.2009.00681.x

Touroni, E., & Coyle, A. (2002). Decision-making in planned lesbian parenting: An interpretative phenomenological analysis. *Journal of Community and Applied Social Psychology, 12*, 194–209. doi:10.1002/casp.672

Ulrich, M., & Weatherall, A. (2000). Motherhood and infertility. Viewing motherhood through the lens of infertility. *Feminism and Psychology, 10*, 323–336. doi:10.1177/ 0959353500010003003

Van Bergen, D., & van Lisdonk, J. (2010). Psychisch welbevinden en zelfacceptatie van homojongeren [Psychological well-being and self acceptation of gay and lesbian youth]. In S. Keuzenkamp (Ed.), *Steeds gewoner, nooit gewoon. Acceptatie van homoseksualiteit in Nederland* (pp. 174–196). Den Haag, the Netherlands: Sociaal en Cultureel Planbureau.

Van Gelderen, L., Gartrell, N., Bos, H. M. W., & Hermanns, J. (2009). Stigmatization and resilience in adolescent children of lesbian mothers. *Journal of GLBT Family Studies, 5*, 268–279. doi:10.1080/1550 4280903035761

Vanfraussen, K., Ponjaert-Kristoffersen, I., & Brewaeys, A. (2002). What does it mean for youngsters to grow up in a lesbian family created by means of donor insemination? *Journal of Reproductive and Infant Psychology, 20*, 237–252. doi:10.1080/0264683021000033165

Vanfraussen, K., Pontjaert-Kristoffersen, I., & Brewaeys, A. (2003a). Family functioning in lesbian families created by donor insemination. *American Journal of Orthopsychiatry, 73*, 78–90. doi:10.1037/0002-9432.73.1.78

Vanfraussen, K., Pontjaert-Kristoffersen, I., & Brewaeys, A. (2003b). Why do children want to know more about the donor? The experience of youngsters raised in lesbian families. *Journal of Psychosomatic Obstetrics and Gynecology, 24*, 31–38.

Waaldijk, C. (2009a). *Legal recognition of homosexual orientation in the countries of the world. A chronological overview with footnotes.* Los Angeles, CA: The Williams Institute.

Waaldijk, C. (2009b). Overview of forms of joint legal parenting available to same-sex couples in European countries. *Droit et Société, 72*, 383–385.

Waaldijk, C. (2009c). Same-sex partnership, international protection. In R. Wolfrum (Ed.), *Max Planck encyclopedia of public international law* (pp. 1–9). Oxford, NY: Oxford University Press.

Wainright, J. L., & Patterson, C. J. (2006). Delinquency, victimization, and substance use among adolescents with female same-sex parents. *Journal of Family Psychology, 20*, 526–530. doi:10.1037/0893-3200.20.3.526

Wainright, J. L., & Patterson, C. J. (2008). Peer relations among adolescents with female same-sex parents. *Developmental Psychology, 44*, 117–126. doi:10.1037/0012-1649.44.1.117

Wainright, J. L., Russell, S. T., & Patterson, C. J. (2004). Psychosocial adjustment, school outcomes, and romantic relationships of adolescents with same-sex parents. *Child Development, 75*, 1886–1898. doi:10.1111/j.1467-8624.2004.00823.x

Lesbian and Gay Adoptive Parents and Their Children

3

Rachel H. Farr and Charlotte J. Patterson

Many lesbian and gay adults have adopted children in the USA and in other parts of the world (Gates, Badgett, Macomber, & Chambers, 2007; Patterson & Tornello, 2011). According to data from national surveys, lesbian and gay adults are raising 4% of all adopted children in the USA (Gates et al., 2007), and many other lesbian and gay adults express a desire to become parents (Gates et al., 2007; Riskind & Patterson, 2010). Despite the fact that adoptive families headed by lesbian and gay parents exist, there is continued controversy surrounding the adoption of children by lesbian and gay adults (Patterson, 2009). Adoption of children by lesbian and gay adults is regulated by a complex array of laws and policies, and these often vary from one jurisdiction to another. The resulting patchwork of law and policy creates challenges for adoptive families with lesbian and gay parents and for all those who work with them. Until recently, there has been little empirical research that can specifically inform decision making on this topic. Within the last decade, a growing body of research on the adoption of children by lesbian and gay parents has begun to address questions that have been at the center of public controversies.

In this chapter, we review research on lesbian and gay adoptive parents and their children in the context of an interdisciplinary framework. Studies of lesbian and gay adoptive parenting have emerged primarily from the fields of developmental and clinical psychology, but research from social work, family studies, demography, sociology, public policy, law, and economics is also relevant. In the context of research on adoption, and controversies about lesbian and gay adoptive parents, we provide an overview of recent research in this area. We consider work describing the pathways to adoption for lesbian and gay adults, and we summarize findings on their experiences in the adoption process. We also review research on psychosocial and adjustment outcomes for children, parents, and families when lesbian and gay parents adopt children. Throughout the chapter, similarities among lesbian, gay, and heterosexual adoptive parent families are discussed, such as those regarding outcomes for children adopted by lesbian, gay, and heterosexual parents. Ways in which lesbian and gay adoptive parents may differ from heterosexual adoptive parents are also noted, such as their reasons for adopting children. Finally, we offer recommendations for future research and practice.

R.H. Farr, Ph.D. (✉)
Department of Psychology, University of Massachusetts Amherst, 623 Tobin Hall, Amherst, MA 01003, USA
e-mail: rfarr@psych.umass.edu

C.J. Patterson, Ph.D.
Department of Psychology, University of Virginia, P. O. Box 400400 Gilmer Hall, Charlottesville, VA 22904, USA
e-mail: cjp@virginia.edu

A.E. Goldberg and K.R. Allen (eds.), *LGBT-Parent Families: Innovations in Research and Implications for Practice*, DOI 10.1007/978-1-4614-4556-2_3, © Springer Science+Business Media New York 2013

Research on Adoptive Families

One context for understanding issues facing lesbian and gay adoptive parents and their children is the body of research on adoption. A large literature explores adoptive family dynamics and psychosocial outcomes of adopted children, with samples predominantly comprising heterosexual couples and parents and their adopted children (Brodzinsky & Palacios, 2005; Javier, Baden, Biafora, & Comacho-Gingerich, 2007; Palacios & Brodzinsky, 2010; Wrobel, Hendrickson, & Grotevant, 2006; Wrobel & Neil, 2009). From the late 1950s through the 1990s, much of the research on adoption focused on outcomes for adopted children (Palacios & Brodzinsky, 2010). Over the last two decades, however, research has also expanded to include consideration of many different adoption-related issues, such as openness in adoption (Grotevant et al., 2007) outcomes for members of birth families (Henney, Ayers-Lopez, McRoy & Grotevant, 2007), transracial adoption (Burrow & Finley, 2004), and communication within families about adoption issues (Wrobel, Kohler, Grotevant, & McRoy, 2003).

Research regarding outcomes of children who have been adopted has indicated that, relative to their non-adopted peers (i.e., children remaining with their biological families), adopted children are at risk for some negative outcomes (Palacios & Brodzinsky, 2010), prominent among which are behavior problems. Children who experience institutionalization before being adopted appear to be particularly at risk for later problems. For example, Gunnar, Van Dulmen, and The International Adoption Project Team (2007) assessed child behavioral adjustment using the Child Behavior Checklist (CBCL) with 1,948 internationally adopted children. Those children who had experienced institutionalization for longer periods ($n=899$) had greater behavior problems than those who had experienced shorter or no periods of institutionalization ($n=1,038$). Other research has indicated that children adopted through foster care often fare worse in terms of behavioral and adjustment outcomes than do children adopted through private domestic

agencies or international agencies (Howard, Smith, & Ryan, 2004; Vandivere & McKlindon, 2010). Simmel, Barth, and Brooks (2007) found that youth adopted from foster care ($n=293$) exhibited higher rates of behavior problems than did adopted nonfoster care youth ($n=312$), as reported by adoptive parents on the Behavioral Problems Index. Both groups, however, had greater behavioral difficulties than those in the general population.

Negative outcomes do not, however, characterize adoptive children across the board. For instance, Juffer and Van IJzendoorn's (2007) meta-analysis of 88 studies comparing 10,997 children who were adopted internationally, domestically, and/or transracially with 33,862 children who were not adopted revealed no significant differences in children's self-esteem as a function of adoption. In addition, adopted children had higher self-esteem than their non-adopted, institutionalized peers. In a meta-analysis of studies examining the IQ and school performance of 17,767 adopted children, van IJzendoorn, Juffer, and Poelhuis (2005) found no significant differences in IQ between adopted and non-adopted children. School performance and language of adopted children, however, lagged behind the performances of their non-adopted peers. In contrast, adopted children scored higher on IQ tests and performed better in school than did children who remained in institutional care. Overall, adoption appears to be an effective intervention for children who face certain kinds of adversity early in life.

In an effort to reconcile differences in results among studies of children's outcomes, researchers have examined the role of a number of mediating factors, such as pre-adoptive life circumstances (Grotevant et al., 2006), adoptive family environments (Whitten & Weaver, 2010), the interaction of pre-adoptive factors and adoptive family environments (Ji, Brooks, Barth, & Kim, 2010), family relationships and interactions (Rueter, Keyes, Iacono, & McGue, 2009), communication about adoption (Grotevant, Rueter, Von Korff, & Gonzalez, 2012), awareness of adoption and adoptive identity (Grotevant, Dunbar, Kohler, & Esau, 2007; Juffer, 2006), the role of open adoption (Von Korff, Grotevant, & McRoy, 2006), and the role of appraisal in adoption (Storsbergen, Juffer, van Son, & van Hart, 2010). As in other types of families, the quality of family relationships, parenting, and interactions have been found to be significantly associated with child outcomes and family functioning (Lansford, Ceballo, Abbey, & Stewart, 2001; Rueter et al., 2009).

Most of the research on adoptive families to date has focused on families with heterosexual parents. More recently, research including lesbian and gay adoptive parents (and lesbian and gay prospective adoptive parents) has been conducted. Outcomes of children adopted by lesbian and gay parents have been considered, as well as a number of other facets of adoptive family dynamics in adoptive families headed by lesbian and gay parents. In this chapter, research findings about lesbian and gay adoptive parents and their children are compared with the broader literature about adoptive families wherever possible. We use a developmental and family systems perspective as well as an ecological systems approach to consider the experiences of lesbian- and gay-parent adoptive families in the context of broader social structure issues. The emergence of studies about adoptive families with lesbian and gay parents seems to have been motivated, in part, by controversy surrounding the adoption of children by lesbian and gay parents, and it is to this topic that we turn next.

Controversy Surrounding Lesbian and Gay Parent Adoption

The adoption of children by lesbian and gay adults has been a controversial issue in the USA and in many places around the world. Questions have been raised about the suitability of lesbian and gay parents as role models for children. Critics contend that a heterosexual mother and father are necessary for children's optimal development. Such questions and concerns have impacted policy and law regarding adoption by lesbian and gay adults. Indeed, adoptions of minor children by openly lesbian and gay

individuals and couples are permitted by law in some places and not in others. For example, in the USA, some jurisdictions (e.g., Mississippi and Utah) ban adoption by same-sex couples (Patterson, 2009). For many years, Florida law barred lesbian and gay individuals or couples from becoming adoptive parents. In 2010, however, the courts ruled that this law was unconstitutional, and overturned the ban (Miller, 2010). Many states (e.g., California, Massachusetts, Connecticut) prohibit discrimination on the basis of sexual orientation in matters of adoption and have laws that expressly permit the adoption of children by same-sex couples (Kaye & Kuvalanka, 2006). As a result, lesbian and gay adults have completed stranger adoptions[1] in a number of states, including California, Maryland, Ohio, and the District of Columbia (Patterson, 2009). Second-parent adoptions have been permitted in 26 states and the District of Columbia. Four states (Colorado, Nebraska, Ohio, and Wisconsin), however, have rejected second-parent adoptions by lesbian and gay adults (Patterson, 2009). Around the world, there is also considerable variation in law and policy in this regard. In Spain, Sweden, Canada, the Netherlands, and the UK, lesbian and gay adults are permitted to adopt children, but in Italy, Germany, and France, this is not permitted (LaRenzie, 2010). In the USA and in other countries, religious and political leaders have clashed repeatedly about whether the law should allow openly lesbian and gay adults to adopt minor children (LaRenzie, 2010; Miller, 2010). Controversy surrounding the adoption of children by lesbian and gay persons has contributed, in part, to research addressing questions about outcomes for children adopted

---

[1] Stranger adoptions describe situations in which biological parents are unwilling or unable to take care of a child. A stranger adoption is completed when a court dissolves the legal bonds between the child and his/her biological parents and establishes new legal ties between the child and his/her adoptive parents. In second-parent adoptions, legal parenting status is created for a second parent without terminating the rights or responsibilities of the first legal parent. In families headed by same-sex couples, second-parent adoptions create for the child the possibility of having two legally recognized parents (Patterson, 2009).

by lesbian and gay parents, the capabilities of lesbian and gay adults as parents, and overall family processes and dynamics in adoptive families with lesbian and gay parents. We next turn to discussing this research.

Research on Lesbian- and Gay-Parent Adoptive Families

In this section, we discuss the research on how lesbian and gay adults become adoptive parents, their strengths and challenges, their transition to adoptive parenthood, and outcomes of such adoptions for children, parents, and parenting couples. As will become clear, many lesbian and gay adults are becoming adoptive parents today. In some respects, they have experiences that are very like those of other adoptive parents, but lesbian and gay adoptive parents also face some issues that are specific to their circumstances.

Adoption as a Pathway to Parenthood

National survey data, together with findings from other research, suggest that lesbian and gay adoptive parents share a number of demographic characteristics with heterosexual adoptive parents (Gates et al., 2007). Like heterosexual adoptive parents, lesbian and gay adoptive parents are often older, well educated, affluent, and predominantly White (Brodzinsky & Pinderhughes, 2002; Erich, Leung, & Kindle, 2005; Farr, Forssell, & Patterson, 2010a; Gates et al., 2007; Goldberg, 2009a; Ryan, Pearlmutter, & Groza, 2004). It is important to note that these demographic factors are generally characteristic of known cases of legally recognized adoption. The demographic profile of families formed through more informal methods, such as kinship adoption, may be different.

Lesbian, gay, and heterosexual adults who adopt children may be motivated to do so for many similar reasons, but lesbian and gay adults may also adopt children for reasons that are distinct from those of heterosexual adults (Mallon, 2000). For example, in Farr and Patterson's (2009)

study of 106 adoptive families (29 lesbian, 27 gay, and 50 heterosexual couples), virtually all couples reported that they "wanted to have children" as a reason for pursuing adoption, regardless of parental sexual orientation. On the other hand, there were differences in expressed motivations for adoption as a function of family type. The vast majority of heterosexual couples reported "challenges with infertility" as a motivation for adopting children, but fewer than half of same-sex couples reported this as a reason for choosing to adopt. Many more same-sex than opposite-sex couples reported that they "did not have a strong desire for biological children." Similarly, Goldberg, Downing, and Richardson (2009) found that among a sample of 30 lesbian and 30 heterosexual adoptive couples, lesbian couples were less likely than heterosexual couples to report a commitment to biological parenthood. Goldberg and Smith (2008) reported that compared with heterosexual couples ($n = 39$), lesbian couples ($n = 36$) were less likely to try to conceive and also less likely to pursue fertility treatments. Many investigators have reported that heterosexual adoptive parents often described adoption as a "second choice" pathway to parenthood, chosen only after struggles with infertility convinced them that biological parenthood was not a realistic option (e.g., Mallon, 2007; Turner, 1999). Thus, unlike heterosexual couples, lesbian and gay adoptive parents may be more likely to have chosen adoption as their first choice as a route to parenthood. Indeed, Tyebjee (2003) found that lesbian and gay adults demonstrated greater openness to adopting children than did heterosexual adults. As such, lesbian and gay adults have sometimes been described as "preferential adopters" (Brodzinsky & Pinderhughes, 2002).

Another way that lesbian and gay adoptive parents may differ from heterosexual adoptive parents is in their willingness to adopt across racial lines, that is, to adopt a child from a racial or ethnic background different than their own. Among pre-adoptive couples, lesbian couples have been found to be more open than heterosexual couples to transracial adoption (Goldberg, 2009a; Goldberg & Smith, 2009a). Lesbian and gay adoptive couples have also been found to be more likely than heterosexual adoptive couples to have completed a transracial adoption (Farr & Patterson, 2009). Indeed, some heterosexual couples have been found to prefer same-race adoptions (Brodzinsky & Pinderhughes, 2002).

One reason that lesbian and gay couples may be more willing to adopt transracially is that same-sex couples are more likely than heterosexual couples to be interracial (Rosenfeld & Kim, 2005), and, in turn, interracial couples are more willing than same-race couples to complete transracial adoptions (Farr & Patterson, 2009). Also, some researchers have described racial integration as a characteristic of urban lesbian and gay communities (e.g., Stacey, 2006). For lesbian and gay parents in these communities, greater contact with racial minority groups may increase levels of comfort in interracial interactions (Emerson, Kimbro, & Yancey, 2002), and this could be a factor in their greater openness to transracial adoption. Because they are often less committed than heterosexual couples to achieving biological parenthood, same-sex couples may also be more open than heterosexual couples to transracial adoptions (Farr & Patterson, 2009; Goldberg et al., 2009).

Another way that lesbian and gay adoptive couples may be different than heterosexual adoptive couples is in terms of gender preferences in adoption. Goldberg (2009b) studied 47 lesbian, 31 gay, and 56 heterosexual couples who were actively seeking to adopt, and reported that, while heterosexual men were unlikely to express a gender preference, gay men often preferred to adopt boys. Lesbian participants who expressed a preference, generally preferred to adopt girls, as did the heterosexual women in the sample. Thus, only about half of participants overall expressed gender preferences, but among those who expressed preferences, all except the gay male participants preferred to adopt girls. These findings are consistent with earlier research regarding the preferences for child gender of both heterosexual adoptive couples and lesbian couples using donor insemination (Gartrell et al., 1996; Herrmann-Green & Gehring, 2007; Jones, 2008).

Why were these gender preferences observed? Lesbian and gay adoptive parents in Goldberg's (2009b) study often explained their preferences for child gender by reference to concerns about gender socialization and heterosexism. For example, some participants felt uncertain about parenting a child of a gender different than their own. It is possible that lesbian and gay couples, being made up of two parents of the same gender, may feel inadequate to parent a child of a different gender. Heterosexual couples, on the other hand, may feel equally "equipped" to parent a child of either gender since one parent of each gender is represented in the parenting couple. In this case, at least one partner in the couple may feel prepared for and knowledgeable about gender-specific socialization. Aside from this study, however, little is known about why lesbian and gay pre-adoptive parents expressed this feeling more often than did heterosexual pre-adoptive parents.

In choosing adoption as a route to parenthood, the child's race and gender are two concerns, but there are many other issues to consider as well. Indeed, gay men have been found to consider children's likely age, race, health, and a host of other factors in selecting their particular route to adoption (Downing, Richardson, Kinkler, & Goldberg, 2009). As adoptions may be domestic or international, may be accomplished through public or private agencies, may involve adoption of infants or children, and may involve open as well as closed arrangements, much remains to be learned about varied pathways to adoptive parenthood among lesbian and gay adults, and about factors related to these variations. Each variation comes with its own challenges, and research is only beginning to examine the relevant issues (Brodzinsky & Pinderhughes, 2002; Howard et al., 2004).

Challenges and Strengths of Adoptive Lesbian and Gay Parents

Although all prospective adoptive parents progress through a series of steps in adopting their child—including an application process, training and workshops for prospective parents, and a home study[2] (Brodzinsky & Pinderhughes, 2002)—lesbian and gay parents often face additional challenges. As mentioned earlier, lesbian and gay adults are not permitted to adopt children in all jurisdictions in the USA or elsewhere (Kaye & Kuvalanka, 2006; Ryan et al., 2004). Moreover, not all adoption agencies and/or adoption workers are open to working with lesbian and gay prospective parents. Brodzinsky, Patterson, and Vaziri (2002) found that among a sample of 369 public and private adoption agencies throughout the USA (i.e., in 45 states and the District of Columbia), 63% of reporting agencies had accepted applications from openly lesbian and gay prospective adoptive parents and 37% had placed children with openly lesbian and gay parents. A majority of public agencies and Jewish-affiliated private adoption agencies reported placing children with lesbian and gay parents, while only a minority of Catholic- and Protestant-affiliated agencies reported having done this. Among adoption social workers, Ryan (2000) found that homophobic attitudes were related to lesser likelihood of placing a child with lesbian and gay parents. Also, 14% of the 80 social workers in this study reported that their state prohibited adoptions by lesbian and gay adults, even when this was not the case. Thus, lesbian and gay adults face a number of institutional and attitudinal barriers in the adoption process.

In reports of the adoption journeys of lesbian and gay adults, the experience of discrimination from adoption agencies and workers is a recurring theme (Downs & James, 2006; Mallon, 2007; Matthews & Cramer, 2006). For example, Brooks and Goldberg (2001) conducted focus groups with 11 current and prospective lesbian and gay adoptive parents. The researchers found that lesbian and gay parents reported encountering more obstacles than did heterosexual foster and adoptive parents. Such obstacles included mistaken or harmful beliefs about lesbian and gay parenting, heterosexist attitudes, and a lack of formal policies and practices in working with sexual minority clients. Downs and James (2006) also reported that among a sample of 60 lesbian, gay, and bisexual adults, a majority faced discrimination in working with the child welfare system. Since more studies have included lesbian adoptive mothers than gay adoptive fathers, several studies have indicated that lesbian adoptive mothers have experienced various barriers and forms of bias in the adoption process (Goldberg, Downing, & Sauck, 2007; Ryan & Whitlock, 2007).

In a study of gay men seeking to adopt ($n = 32$), Downing et al. (2009) found that some men reported experiencing discrimination on the basis of gender as well as sexual orientation. Indeed, gay men seeking to adopt may face many barriers as a result of being both male and gay; for example, men may be seen by some adoption workers as not competent to parent infants or very young children (see also Gianino, 2008; Lobaugh, Clements, Averill, & Olguin, 2006; Schacher, Auerbach, & Silverstein, 2005). In addition to facing discrimination during all phases of the adoption process, Brown, Smalling, Groza, and Ryan (2009) found that lesbian and gay adoptive parents ($n = 182$) also reported feeling that they had few role models to guide them through this process. Also, some lesbian, gay, and bisexual foster and adoptive parents have noted the lack of acceptance they felt from other foster parents (Downs & James, 2006). Societal resistance to lesbian and gay parenting is commonplace in the form of homophobia, stereotyping, and discrimination (Downs & James, 2006). Lesbian and gay parents have reported experiencing discrimination and significant barriers to becoming adoptive parents not only in the USA but also in Canada (Ross et al., 2008; Ross, Epstein, Anderson, & Eady, 2009), Australia (Riggs, 2006), and the UK (Hicks, 2006).

At the same time, lesbian and gay individuals and couples may offer special strengths as adoptive parents. Farr and Patterson (in press)

---

[2] A home study is the in-depth evaluation that any prospective adoptive parent must complete in the USA as a requirement of the adoption process. It is intended as a way to educate and support parents throughout the adoption process and also to evaluate their fitness as potential parents (Brodzinsky & Pinderhughes, 2002).

found that, among 104 adoptive couples from a larger study (i.e., Farr et al., 2010a), lesbian and gay couples were more likely than heterosexual couples to report sharing the duties of parenthood in an equal fashion. Moreover, among same-sex couples, this shared parenting was associated with greater couple relationship adjustment and greater perceived parenting competence (Farr 2011). With regard to family interaction, lesbian mothers were more supportive of one another in observations of triadic (i.e., parent/parent/child) interaction than were heterosexual or gay parents. Among all family types, more supportive interaction was associated with positive adjustment for young adopted children in this sample (Farr & Patterson, in press).

Goldberg, Kinkler, and Hines (2011) reported that among couples who had recently adopted a child, lesbian ($n=45$) and gay adoptive couples ($n=30$) were less likely to internalize adoption stigma (e.g., feeling that being an adoptive parent is inferior to being a biological parent) than were heterosexual adoptive couples ($n=51$). Those parents who reported lower internalization of stigma also reported fewer depressive symptoms. Thus, it appears that lesbian and gay adoptive parents may be less likely than heterosexual adoptive parents to suffer from depressive symptoms related to the internalization of adoption stigma. Overall, lesbian and gay adoptive parents have been found to display some positive characteristics that may benefit their children.

Many adoptive and foster parents report satisfaction in being parents (Downs & James, 2006; Goldberg et al., 2007; Ryan & Whitlock, 2007). For example, in Schacher et al.'s (2005) qualitative study of 21 gay adoptive fathers, many participants described how they had grown closer with members of their families of origin as a result of becoming parents, and others expressed pride in their roles as fathers. In other studies, many adoptive parents have reported that they enjoyed being a role model for other lesbian, gay, and/or adoptive parents, that they received more support than they had expected from members of their families of origin after adopting, and that they felt satisfied with their experience of adoption (Brown et al., 2009; Ryan & Whitlock, 2007).

The Transition to Adoptive Parenthood

Regardless of parental sexual orientation, the transition to parenthood brings both joys and challenges. After the arrival of a first child, which can be marked by stress and compromised mental and physical health as well as by happiness and excitement, parents experience a period of adjustment (e.g., Cowan & Cowan, 1988). For those adopting children, the transition to parenthood involves a rigorous screening process by adoption professionals and a variable waiting time for placement of a child (Brodzinsky & Pinderhughes, 2002). In a systematic review of the literature, McKay, Ross, and Goldberg (2010) reported that rates of distress appear to be lower among adoptive parents as compared with biological parents, but post-adoption depressive symptoms are not uncommon. Post-adoption services appear to be helpful for some families (McKay et al. 2010). In one of the few studies comparing 52 biological parenting couples and 52 adoptive parenting couples across the transition to parenthood, adoptive parents demonstrated levels of psychological adjustment that were similar to those of biological parents (Levy-Shiff, Bar & Har-Even, 1990).

The transition to adoptive parenthood has been studied most carefully among heterosexual couples, but several studies have also examined this life transition among lesbian and gay adoptive couples. Consistent with the general literature on the transition to parenthood, Goldberg, Smith, and Kashy (2010) found that, among 44 lesbian, 30 gay, and 51 heterosexual adoptive couples, relationship quality declined across the transition to parenthood for all couple types. Women reported the greatest declines in love, and those in relationships with women (i.e., both heterosexual and lesbian partners) reported the greatest ambivalence. In another study of the same sample, Goldberg and Smith (2009b) found that all parents reported increases in perceived parenting skill across the transition to parenthood. Relational conflict and expectations of completing more childcare were related to smaller increases in perceived parenting skill.

In a study examining factors affecting lesbian and gay adoptive couples across the transition to parenthood, Goldberg and Smith (2011) found that greater perceived social support and better relationship quality were associated with more favorable mental health, as would be expected on the basis of findings from the general adoption literature. Sexual minority parents who had higher levels of internalized homophobia and who lived in areas with unfavorable legal climates with regard to adoption by lesbian and gay parents experienced the greatest increases in anxiety and depression across the transition to parenthood. In another study that retrospectively examined the transition to parenthood for gay male adoptive couples, Gianino (2008) conducted qualitative analyses of interviews with eight gay male couples. Participants discussed reactions of extended family and friends, coping with feelings of isolation, and the difficulties of dealing with (in)visibility, disclosure, and discrimination. The adoptive gay fathers in this sample also noted the pride they felt in their families, the ways in which they had taken on nontraditional parenting roles, and the greater feelings of intimacy and relationship permanence they experienced.

Child Outcomes

In controversies surrounding the adoption of children by lesbian and gay parents, debate has often centered on children's development. Questions have been raised by opponents of lesbian and gay adoptions about whether lesbian and gay adults can provide children with adequate parenting, appropriate role models, and effective socialization, particularly in the areas of gender development and sexual identity. The overall research on sexual orientation and parenting has been informative here (Patterson, 2009); children of lesbian and gay parents in general appear to be developing in ways that are very like their peers with heterosexual parents (Biblarz & Stacey, 2010; Goldberg, 2010; Tasker & Patterson, 2007). Until recently, however, little of this research focused specifically on outcomes among adoptive families.

There have, however, been some studies examining child development specifically in adoptive families with lesbian and gay parents, and the findings are consistent with those of the broader literature. We review research on children's outcomes in families with adoptive lesbian and gay and parents in three areas: child behavior and conduct, parent–child relationships, and gender development. We also review research on outcomes in transracial adoption. Next, we summarize results of research on parenting and outcomes for adoptive parents and for the whole adoptive family system. Finally, we provide an overview of research on factors beyond parental sexual orientation that affect parenting, family functioning, and children's outcomes. Considered as a group, the results of these studies show that parental sexual orientation is not a strong predictor of children's outcomes. Rather, other factors, such as prevailing laws and policies in a family's environment, may be quite important.

Behavioral adjustment has been a topic of great interest in studies of child outcomes in adoptive families with lesbian and gay parents. Erich et al. (2005) found no significant differences in child outcomes as a function of parental sexual orientation among a sample of 47 lesbian- and gay-parent adoptive families and 25 heterosexual-parent adoptive families with children ranging in age from infancy to adolescence. In Ryan's (2007) study of 94 adoptive families with lesbian and gay parents, children's scores on measures assessing socioemotional development were normative or above population averages. In a study of 155 adoptive families with lesbian or gay parents, and 1,004 adoptive families with heterosexual parents that included a wide age range of children (1.5–18 years old), Averett, Nalavany, and Ryan (2009) found that assessments of adopted children's behavior problems were unrelated to parental sexual orientation, even after controlling for child age, child sex, and family income. In a sample of 93 girls (averaging five and a half years old) adopted from China by single heterosexual mothers, lesbian couples, or heterosexual couples, Tan and Baggerly (2009) reported no significant differences in behavioral adjustment as a function of family type. Farr et al.

(2010a) studied behavioral adjustment among preschool-aged children adopted at birth by lesbian, gay, or heterosexual couples in 106 adoptive families. Both parents and teachers described these children as having relatively few behavior problems; there were no significant differences in this regard among children in the three groups. Thus, it appears that children adopted by lesbian and gay parents are developing well, with behavioral adjustment on par with that of children adopted by heterosexual parents.

In one study specifically targeting adopted adolescents of lesbian and gay parents, adolescents' disclosure practices were examined, with particular attention to issues related to having been adopted by lesbian or gay parents. Using qualitative interview data from 14 racially diverse adopted children ranging in age from 13 to 20 years old, Gianino, Goldberg, and Lewis (2009) explored how adolescents disclose their adoptive status and parental sexual orientation within friendship networks and school environments. With regard to having lesbian and gay parents, the results revealed that adolescents engage in a wide variety of strategies, ranging from not disclosing to anyone to telling others openly. Several participants noted that they had felt "forced" to disclose by virtue of their visibility as a transracial adoptive family with same-sex parents, and many indicated their apprehension in "coming out" about their families. Overall, adolescents indicated that they had received positive reactions and responses from others about their adoptive status. Gianino et al. (2009) suggested that parental preparation for dealing with issues surrounding their child's adoption, racism, and heterosexism and homophobia may have helped children in negotiating the disclosure process.

Two studies have been conducted to date that have examined the qualities of parent–child relationships in adoptive families with lesbian and gay parents. In a qualitative study of 15 lesbian couples who had adopted children, Bennett (2003) found that all parents reported that their children had strong emotional bonds with both of their mothers. However, parents' reports also suggested that children showed a primary bond with one mother in 12 of the 15 families, despite shared parenting and equal division of childcare between the two mothers. In a study of 210 adopted adolescents with 154 lesbian, gay, or heterosexual parents, Erich, Kanenberg, Case, Allen, and Bogdanos (2009) found that qualities of parent–adolescent relationships were not associated with parental sexual orientation, according to reports from both adoptive parents and adolescents. Thus, available data suggest that the qualities of adolescents' relationships with their adoptive parents have thus far been reported to be unrelated to parental sexual orientation.

Children's gender development in adoptive families with lesbian, gay, and heterosexual adoptive parents has been assessed in two studies involving the same sample of 106 adoptive families (Farr, Doss & Patterson, 2011; Farr et al., 2010a). Farr et al. (2010a) reported no significant differences in parents' reports of preschoolers' gender development as a function of parental sexual orientation. Boys and girls showed characteristics and preferences for toys and activities typical of their gender, and they did not differ as a function of having two mothers, two fathers, or one mother and one father. The results from observational data on children's play were consistent with those from parents' reports (Farr et al., 2011). Observations revealed that boys preferred to play with "boy-typical" toys and girls preferred to play with "girl-typical" toys. No significant differences as a function of parental sexual orientation were found in the numbers or types of toys that parents offered their children. Lastly, children were rated as appearing gender typical in their dress, regardless of family type (Farr et al., 2011). Thus, adopted children in this sample enacted typical gender role behavior at early ages, regardless of whether they were reared by lesbian, gay, or heterosexual parents.

Outcomes for children adopted transracially by lesbian, gay, and heterosexual parents were also examined among the sample of 106 adoptive families previously mentioned (Farr & Patterson, 2009). Results showed that children's behavioral adjustment did not vary with transracial adoptive status. Regardless of whether they had been adopted inracially or transracially, children were described by parents and teachers (or outside caregivers) as being well adjusted and as having relatively few behavior problems. A significant qualification to this finding, however, was the relatively young age of the children in this study. It would be helpful to follow such a sample into adolescence to explore the ways in which transracial adoptions unfold over time.

In short, from the existing literature, children adopted by lesbian, gay, and heterosexual parents have been found to demonstrate healthy adjustment and typical development in a number of domains. Across different types of adoption, different family structures, and different stages of development, children with adoptive lesbian and gay parents appear to fare as well as do those with adoptive heterosexual parents. Still, much remains to be learned.

Parent, Couple, and Family Outcomes

A handful of studies of adoptive families with lesbian and gay parents have examined outcomes for parents and for couples, as well as for overall family functioning. Goldberg and Smith (2011) reported relatively few depressive symptoms overall among lesbian and gay adoptive parents. An earlier report based on the same sample had also revealed that, among lesbian and heterosexual couples waiting to adopt children, there were no differences in overall well-being as a function of parental sexual orientation (Goldberg & Smith, 2008). With regard to parenting, Ryan (2007) found that lesbian and gay adoptive parents ($n=94$) scored in the normative or above average range on a measure assessing parenting ability. In a study focusing on the parenting experiences of gay adoptive fathers, Tornello, Farr, and Patterson (2011) found that participants ($n=231$) reported levels of parenting stress that were well within the normative range. Farr et al. (2010a) found that lesbian, gay, and heterosexual adoptive parents in their sample of 106 adoptive families reported relatively little parenting stress, with no significant differences by family type. Similarly, lesbian, gay, and heterosexual adoptive parents in this study were found to use effective parenting techniques, with no significant differences as a

function of parental sexual orientation. In observational data on family interaction among families in this same sample, lesbian, gay, and heterosexual adoptive parents were found to be relatively warm and accepting with their children overall; regardless of sexual orientation, mothers tended to be warmer with their children than did fathers (Farr, 2011).

In terms of couple relationships among lesbian and gay adoptive parents, Goldberg and Smith (2009b) found that lesbian ($n=47$) and gay adoptive couples ($n=56$) in their sample reported relatively low levels of relationship conflict. Farr et al. (2010a) also found that among their sample of 106 adoptive couples, adoptive parents reported high average levels of couple relationship adjustment. There were no significant differences among lesbian, gay, and heterosexual parents in this regard. A majority of couples reported long-term relationships with their partners or spouses, in which they reported considerable feelings of security and high relationship satisfaction (Farr, Forssell, & Patterson, 2010b). Lesbian and gay adoptive couples in this sample also reported overall satisfaction with current divisions of childcare labor, which participants generally described as being shared by both parents in the couple (Farr & Patterson, in press).

Consistent with findings from the broader literature, quality of parenting and of parent–child relationships appear to have more influence than parental sexual orientation on outcomes for parents and children. In their study of 106 families headed by lesbian, gay, and heterosexual adoptive couples, Farr et al. (2010a) found that qualities of family interactions were more strongly associated with child outcomes than was family structure. Across all family types, positive parenting and more harmonious couple relationships were significantly associated with parents' reports of fewer child behavior problems (Farr et al., 2010a). Using the same sample, Farr and Patterson (in press) found that quality of coparenting interaction was significantly related to children's behavioral adjustment, such that more supportive and less undermining behavior between parents was associated with fewer child behavior problems. Among Ryan's (2007) sample of 94 lesbian and gay adoptive parents, results showed that parents' positive perceptions of their own parenting as well as of the parent–child relationship were significantly associated with parents' perceptions of their children as having more strengths. Erich et al. (2009), in their study of 210 adopted adolescents and 154 parents, also reported that qualities of adolescents' relationships with their lesbian, gay, or heterosexual adoptive parents were associated with adolescents' reported life satisfaction, parents' reported relationship satisfaction with their child, and with the number of prior placements the adolescent had experienced, but were unrelated to parental sexual orientation.

With regard to family-level variables, Erich et al. (2005) found no significant differences in overall family functioning among adoptive families headed by lesbian, gay, and heterosexual parents. Rather, they reported that family functioning was associated with demographic variables, such as children's grade level and parents' prior experience with fostering children. In Leung, Erich, and Kanenberg's (2005) study of adoptive families with special needs children, better family functioning was more likely to occur in cases where adoptions involved younger, nondisabled children but was unrelated to parental sexual orientation. Farr (2011) found that, among adoptive families headed by lesbian, gay, and heterosexual couples with young children, observations of family interaction revealed high levels of family cohesion. Families headed by lesbian mothers were, however, significantly more cohesive than were the other family types. Thus, only one association between parental sexual orientation and overall family functioning has been identified to date, and it favored the families of lesbian mothers. Further study will be needed before firm conclusions can be drawn about associations between parental sexual orientation and family functioning among adoptive families.

Summary, Conclusions, and Future Directions

In this final section, we first summarize the overall findings of research to date and consider what conclusions may be justified on the basis of current

findings on adoptive families with lesbian and gay parents. We also suggest directions for further research and practice.

Summary of the Research Findings

In sum, research on lesbian and gay adoptive parents and their children has grown markedly in the last several years. In the USA, many lesbian and gay adults are adoptive parents, and many more wish to adopt children. Some of the reasons that lesbian and gay adults adopt children, as well as some of the experiences of lesbian and gay adoptive parents, are similar to, and some are different from, those of heterosexual adoptive parents. In recent studies, lesbian and gay adults have reported experiencing discrimination and facing many obstacles in becoming adoptive parents. At the same time, having overcome obstacles to parenthood, lesbian and gay adoptive parents appear to be as capable and effective as are heterosexual adults in their roles as adoptive parents. Children adopted by lesbian and gay parents have been found to develop in ways that are similar to development among children adopted by heterosexual parents. Regardless of parental sexual orientation, quality of parenting and quality of family relationships are significantly associated with adopted children's adjustment. Thus, as in other types of families, it is family processes, rather than family structure, that matter more to child outcomes and to overall family functioning among adoptive families.

Directions for Research, Policy, and Practice

While existing research on adoption by lesbian and gay parents is informative, work in this area has only recently begun, and there are many directions for further study. These include exploration of new topic areas of interest and expansion of the kinds of methodological strategies that are used to study adoptive families with lesbian and gay parents. Research in this area can yield information that will further our understanding of general developmental processes. It may also be useful in informing policy, practice, and law related to adoptions by lesbian and gay adults. In this section, we touch briefly on each of these ideas.

Future research on adoptive families with lesbian and gay parents would benefit from fuller consideration of the contexts of adoptive family life. These might include social, economic, and legal aspects of family environments. Research might consider the importance of characteristics of proximal aspects of family environments (e.g., social contacts that families encounter in their daily lives) as well as characteristics of more distal aspects of family environments (e.g., regional, state, and national laws and policies). Federal, state and local law may affect the choices that adoptive lesbian and gay parents can make for their families, and their daily interactions with neighbors, coworkers, and friends are also likely to exert important influences on their experiences. Inasmuch as laws, policies, and attitudes vary considerably across jurisdictions, both in the USA and in other countries, and inasmuch as change in this area is more the rule than the exception today, the impact of environments on the adoptive families of lesbian and gay parents is a rich and important topic for further study.

Adoption is a complex topic, and different issues arise in public versus private adoptions, domestic versus international adoptions, and in adoptions of infants versus adoptions of children or adolescents. Similarly, transracial adoptions bring with them issues that are not always posed by same-race adoptions, such as considerations of racial and ethnic socialization, identity, and diversity in one's community. The gender of adopted children may also emerge as an issue of special interest, especially for same-sex couples, as some existing research suggests that lesbian and gay adults may have particular preferences about child gender in adopting. Future research in this area could be strengthened by consideration of the variations among different types of adoptions.

Another valuable direction for future research would be to devote more attention to family processes and dynamics, as well as to family outcomes.

What are the special family dynamics, if any, that are associated with same-sex parenting couples, and how do these affect children, for better or for worse? What are the important ways in which lesbian and gay adoptive parents may be similar to and different from one another, and what does this mean for children? How, in short, are changing family configurations related to family interactions and relationships?

The voices of adoptive children themselves also need to be heard. How do children and youth understand the difficulties and the opportunities of their lives as adoptive offspring of lesbian or gay parents? How do children and youth see their experiences as having been linked with (or unaffected by) the contextual factors and varied family configurations discussed above? Greater attention to the views of adoptive children and youth growing up with lesbian and gay parents seems likely to broaden understanding in this area.

Greater integration across fields of adoption study would also be beneficial in providing a more comprehensive understanding of adoptive families with lesbian or gay parents. Scholarship in fields as diverse as law, economics, demography, family science, social work, sociology, and psychology is already contributing to understanding in this area. Further integration of work in these diverse fields might contribute to construction of a more comprehensive understanding of adoptive families with lesbian or gay parents. For example, empirical research is needed to document the social and economic consequences of changing adoption laws and policies.

From a methodological standpoint, use of more diverse research strategies seems likely to be fruitful. Much of the empirical work to date has relied on self-report data. Studies based on observations of actual behavior of both parents and children, as Farr and Patterson (in press) and Farr et al. (2011) used, have the potential to make strong contributions to this literature. Similarly, the effort to gather data from sources that are outside the families under study (e.g., from teachers, neighbors, or peers) also seems to be an important methodological direction for scholars to consider. Much existing work has used either quantitative or qualitative approaches to research, but mixed-methods approaches that embrace both quantitative and qualitative approaches to data collection could enrich our understanding. Many samples of lesbian and gay adoptive parents in the existing literature are predominantly White and well educated. More diverse samples could make valuable contributions, as the experiences of racial minority adoptive parents likely differ from those of White adoptive parents. Low-income adoptive parents, who may be likely to adopt children through public versus private adoption (or to foster children for long periods of time without legally adopting them), would also be expected to differ in their experiences from the more affluent adoptive parents who have been included in most studies to date. Furthermore, the few existing studies of lesbian and gay adoptive parents have generally not included bisexual or transgender parents. More inclusive samples of sexual and gender minority adoptive parents would contribute to our understanding of the experiences of diverse adoptive family systems. The majority of research to date has been cross-sectional in nature; longitudinal studies of adoptive families could also be pursued and might yield fresh insights about child development, parenting, and family functioning over time.

With regard to policy implications of research on lesbian- and gay-parented adoptive families, a number of directions can be identified. First and foremost, the results of research in this area should be used to inform law, policy, and practice. Many children in the USA alone await placement with permanent families. More than 500,000 children are in the child welfare system and more than 100,000 children are currently waiting to be adopted (U.S. Department of Health & Human Services, 2010). Compounding the challenge of finding permanent families for waiting children is a perceived dearth of prospective adoptive parents (Ryan et al., 2004). If adoption agencies were to recruit more prospective parents from lesbian and gay communities, many additional children might find permanent homes. Based on the findings of research to date, one would expect this to benefit such children in many ways. At the time of this writing, several states in the USA, such as Arizona,

are considering policies that would limit adoption to opposite-sex married couples (Center for Arizona Policy, 2011). If such a policy were to be adopted in Arizona, this would mean that otherwise qualified lesbian or gay prospective adoptive parents would be prohibited from adopting children in that state. Research findings to date clearly do not provide support for any such prohibition. Indeed, the existing evidence suggests that a prohibition of this kind would be detrimental to the welfare of children waiting for placement into permanent homes.

How do prohibitions on the adoption of children by lesbian and gay adults affect the likelihood of placement of children waiting to be adopted? Kaye and Kuvalanka (2006) compared placement rates of children from foster care in states with laws that prohibit adoptions by openly lesbian and gay adults with placement rates in states that permit such adoptions. They found that, in states where adoption laws prohibit adoptions by openly lesbian and gay adults, more children remained in foster care. In contrast, states that permitted lesbian and gay adults to adopt children had proportionately fewer children in foster care. Indeed, if lesbian and gay adults were permitted to adopt children in every jurisdiction within the USA, Gates et al. (2007) estimated that between 9,000 and 14,000 children could be removed from foster care and placed in permanent homes each year. If so, the results of research to date suggest that children would benefit.

To support lesbian and gay adults seeking to adopt children, a number of organizations have begun programs related to adoption issues. For example, the Human Rights Campaign (HRC) has implemented the "All Children—All Families" program (Human Rights Campaign, 2011). This initiative seeks to assist adoption agencies and child welfare professionals in their efforts to recruit prospective adoptive parents from lesbian and gay communities, work successfully with them, and in so doing, place more children into permanent homes (Human Rights Campaign, 2011). This initiative also serves as an educational resource for lesbian and gay adults who may be considering adoption as a pathway to parenthood.

Conclusion

In conclusion, the adoption of children by lesbian and gay parents is a growing reality in the USA and in at least some other parts of the world. Empirical research on adoptive families with lesbian and gay parents has begun to address some questions about how children adopted by lesbian and gay parents fare. While lesbian and gay individuals may face a number of challenges in becoming adoptive parents, lesbian- and gay-parent families formed through adoption appear to experience generally positive outcomes. Much remains to be learned, however, especially about the diversity among lesbian and gay adoptive parents and their children, and about the ways in which their lives are shaped by characteristics of the environments in which they live.

References

Averett, P., Nalavany, B., & Ryan, S. (2009). An evaluation of gay/lesbian and heterosexual adoption. *Adoption Quarterly, 12*, 129–151. doi:10.1080/10926750903313278

Bennett, S. (2003). Is there a primary mom? Parental perceptions of attachment bond hierarchies within lesbian adoptive families. *Child and Adolescent Social Work Journal, 20*, 159–173. doi:10.1023/A:1023653727818

Biblarz, T. J., & Stacey, J. (2010). How does the gender of parents matter? *Journal of Marriage and Family, 72*, 3–22. doi:10.1111/j.1741-3737.2009.00678.x.

Brodzinsky, D. M., & Palacios, J. (2005). *Psychological issues in adoption: Theory, research and practice.* Westport, CT: Greenwood.

Brodzinsky, D. M., Patterson, C. J., & Vaziri, M. (2002). Adoption agency perspectives on lesbian and gay prospective parents: A national study. *Adoption Quarterly, 1*, 43–60. doi:10.1300/J145v05n03_02

Brodzinsky, D. M., & Pinderhughes, E. (2002). Parenting and child development in adoptive families. In M. Bornstein (Ed.), *Handbook of parenting* (2nd ed., pp. 279–312). Mahwah, NJ: Lawrence Erlbaum Associates.

Brooks, D., & Goldberg, S. (2001). Gay and lesbian adoptive and foster care placements: Can they meet the needs of waiting children? *Social Work, 46*, 147–157.

Brown, S., Smalling, S., Groza, V., & Ryan, S. (2009). The experiences of gay men and lesbians in becoming and being adoptive parents. *Adoption Quarterly, 12*, 226–246. doi:10.1080/10926750903313294

Burrow, A. L., & Finley, G. E. (2004). Transracial, same-race adoptions, and the need for multiple measures of adolescent adjustment. *American Journal of Orthopsychiatry, 74*, 577–583. doi:10.1037/0002-9432.74.4.577

Center for Arizona Policy. (2011, January). *Family issue fact sheet: SB 1188 – Adoption; Marital Preference.* Phoenix: Center for Arizona Policy.

Cowan, P. A., & Cowan, C. P. (1988). Changes in marriage during the transition to parenthood: Must we blame the baby? In G. Y. Michaels & W. A. Goldberg (Eds.), *The transition to parenthood: Current theory and research* (pp. 114–154). New York: Cambridge University Press.

Downing, J., Richardson, H., Kinkler, L., & Goldberg, A. (2009). Making the decision: Factors influencing gay men's choice of an adoption path. *Adoption Quarterly, 12*, 247–271. doi:10.1080/10926750903313310

Downs, A. C., & James, S. E. (2006). Gay, lesbian, and bisexual foster parents: Strengths and challenges for the child welfare system. *Child Welfare, 85*, 281–298.

Emerson, M. O., Kimbro, R. T., & Yancey, G. (2002). Contact theory extended: The effects of prior racial contact on current social ties. *Social Science Quarterly, 83*, 741–765. doi:10.1111/1540-6237.00112

Erich, S., Kanenberg, H., Case, K., Allen, T., & Bogdanos, T. (2009). An empirical analysis of factors affecting adolescent attachment in adoptive families with homosexual and straight parents. *Children and Youth Services Review, 31*(3), 398–404. doi:10.1016/j.childyouth.2008.09.004

Erich, S., Leung, P., & Kindle, P. (2005). A comparative analysis of adoptive family functioning with gay, lesbian and heterosexual parents and their children. *Journal of GLBT Family Studies, 1*, 43–60. doi:10.1300/J461v01n04_03

Farr, R. H. (2011). *Coparenting among lesbian, gay, and heterosexual adoptive couples: Associations with couple relationships and child outcomes.* Available from ProQuest Dissertations and Theses database (UMI No. 3448525). doi:10.1037/12328-006

Farr, R. H., Doss, K. M., & Patterson, C. J. (2011). *Gender conformity among lesbian, gay, and heterosexual parents and their adoptive children.* Unpublished manuscript, University of Virginia, Virginia

Farr, R. H., Forssell, S. L., & Patterson, C. J. (2010a). Parenting and child development in adoptive families: Does parental sexual orientation matter? *Applied Developmental Science, 14*, 164–178. doi:10.1080/10888691.2010.500958

Farr, R. H., Forssell, S. L., & Patterson, C. J. (2010b). Lesbian, gay, and heterosexual adoptive parents: Couple and relationship issues. *Journal of GLBT Family Studies, 6*, 199–213. doi:10.1080/15504281003705436

Farr, R. H., & Patterson, C. J. (2009). Transracial adoption by lesbian, gay, and heterosexual parents: Who completes transracial adoptions and with what results? *Adoption Quarterly, 12*, 187–204. doi:10.1080/10926750903313328

Farr, R. H., & Patterson, C. J. (in press) Coparenting among lesbian, gay, and heterosexual couples: Association with adopted children's outcomes. *Child Development*

Gartrell, N., Hamilton, J., Banks, A., Mosbacher, D., Reed, N., Sparks, C. H., et al. (1996). The National Lesbian Family Study: 1. Interviews with prospective mothers. *American Journal of Orthopsychiatry, 66*, 272–281. doi:10.1037/h0080178

Gates, G. J., Badgett, M. V. L., Macomber, J. E., & Chambers, K. (2007). *Adoption and foster care by gay and lesbian parents in the United States*. Los Angeles: UCLA School of Law Williams Institute.

Gianino, M. (2008). Adaptation and transformation: The transition to adoptive parenthood for gay male couples. *Journal of GLBT Family Studies, 4*, 205–243. doi:10.1080/15504280802096872

Gianino, M., Goldberg, A., & Lewis, T. (2009). Disclosure practices among adopted youth with gay and lesbian parents. *Adoption Quarterly, 12*, 205–228. doi:10.1080/10926750903313344

Goldberg, A. E. (2009a). Lesbian and heterosexual pre-adoptive couples' openness to transracial adoption. *American Journal of Orthopsychiatry, 79*, 103–117. doi:10.1037/a0015354

Goldberg, A. E. (2009b). Heterosexual, lesbian, and gay preadoptive parents' preferences about child gender. *Sex Roles, 61*, 55–71. doi:10.1007/s11199-009-9598-4

Goldberg, A. E. (2010). *Lesbian and gay parents and their children: Research on the family life cycle*. Washington, DC: American Psychological Association.

Goldberg, A. E., Downing, J. B., & Richardson, H. B. (2009). The transition from infertility to adoption: Perceptions of lesbian and heterosexual preadoptive couples. *Journal of Social and Personal Relationships, 26*, 938–963. doi:10.1177/0265407509345652

Goldberg, A. E., Downing, J. B., & Sauck, C. C. (2007). Choices, challenges, and tensions: Perspectives of lesbian prospective adoptive parents. *Adoption Quarterly, 10*(2), 33–64. doi:10.1300/J145v10n02

Goldberg, A. E., Kinkler, L. A., & Hines, D. A. (2011). Perception and internalization of adoption stigma among gay, lesbian, and heterosexual adoptive parents. *Journal of GLBT Family Studies, 7*, 132–154. doi:10.1080/1550428X.2011.537554

Goldberg, A. E., & Smith, J. Z. (2008). Social support and psychological well-being in lesbian and heterosexual preadoptive couples. *Family Relations, 57*, 281–294. doi:10.1111/j.1741-3729.2008.00500.x

Goldberg, A. E., & Smith, J. Z. (2009a). Predicting non-African American lesbian and heterosexual preadoptive couples' openness to adopting an African American child. *Family Relations, 58*, 346–360. doi:10.1111/j.1741-3729.2009.00557.x

Goldberg, A. E., & Smith, J. Z. (2009b). Perceived parenting skill across the transition to adoptive parenthood among lesbian, gay, and heterosexual couples. *Journal of Family Psychology, 23*, 861–870. doi:10.1037/a0017009

Goldberg, A. E., & Smith, J. Z. (2011). Stigma, social context, and mental health: Lesbian and gay couples across the transition to adoptive parenthood. *Journal of Counseling Psychology, 58*, 139–150. doi:10.1037/a0021684

Goldberg, A. E., Smith, J. E., & Kashy, D.A. (2010). Pre-adoptive factors predicting lesdian, gay, and heterosexual couples relationship quality across the transition to adoptive parenthood. *Journal of Family Psychology, 24*, 221–232. doi: 10.1037/a0019615

Grotevant, H. D., Dunbar, N., Kohler, J. K., & Esau, A. L. (2007). Adoptive identity: How contexts within and beyond the family shape developmental pathways. In R. A. Javier, A. L. Baden, R. A. Biafora, & A. Comacho-Gingerich (Eds.), *Handbook of adoption* (pp. 77–89). Thousand Oaks, CA: Sage.

Grotevant, H. D., Rueter, M., Von Korff, L., & Gonzalez, C. (2012). Post-adoption contact, adoption communicative openness, and satisfaction with contact as predictors of externalizing behavior in adolescence and emerging adulthood. *Journal of Child Psychology and Psychiatry, 52*, 529–536. doi:10.1111/j.1469-7610.2010.02330.x

Grotevant, H. D., van Dulmen, M. H., Dunbar, N., Nelson-Christinedaughter, J., Christensen, M., Fan, X., et al. (2006). Antisocial behavior of adoptees and nonadoptees: Prediction from early history and adolescent relationships. *Journal of Research on Adolescence, 16*, 105–131. doi:10.1111/j.1532-7795.2006.00124.x

Grotevant, H. D., Wrobel, G. M., Von Korff, L., Skinner, B., Newell, J., Friese, S., et al. (2007). Many faces of openness in adoption: Perspectives of adopted adolescents and their parents. *Adoption Quarterly, 10*, 79–101. doi:10.1080/10926750802163204

Gunnar, M. R., Van Dulmen, M. H. M., & The International Adoption Project Team. (2007). Behavior problems in postinstitutionalized internationally adopted children. *Development and Psychopathology, 19*, 129–148. doi:10.1017/S0954579407070071

Henney, S. M., Ayers-Lopez, S., McRoy, R. G., & Grotevant, H. D. (2007). Evolution and resolution: Birthmothers' experience of grief and loss at different levels of adoption openness. *Journal of Social and Personal Relationships, 24*, 875–889. doi:10.1177/0265407507084188

Herrmann-Green, L. K., & Gehring, T. M. (2007). The German lesbian family study: Planning for parenthood via donor insemination. *Journal of GLBT Family Studies, 3*, 351–395. doi:10.1300/J461v03n04_02

Hicks, S. (2006). Maternal men – perverts and deviants? Making sense of gay men as foster carers and adopters. *Journal of GLBT Family Studies, 2*, 93–114. doi:10.1300/J461v02n01_05

Howard, J. A., Smith, S. L., & Ryan, S. (2004). A comparative study of child welfare adoptions with other types of adopted children and birth children. *Adoption Quarterly, 7*, 1–30. doi:10.1300/J145v07n03_01

Human Rights Campaign. (2011). *All children – all families*. Retrieved from http://www.hrc.org/issues/parenting/adoptions/12111.html

Javier, R. A., Baden, A. L., Biafora, R. A., & Comacho-Gingerich, A. (Eds.). (2007). *Handbook of adoption*. Thousand Oaks, CA: Sage.

Ji, J., Brooks, D., Barth, R. P., & Kim, H. (2010). Beyond preadoptive risk: The impact of adoptive family environment on adopted youth's psychosocial adjustment. *American Journal of Orthopsychiatry, 80*, 432–442. doi:10.1111/j.1939-0025.2010.01046.x

Jones, J. (2008). Adoption experiences of women and men and demand for children to adopt by women 18–44 years of age in the United States, 2002. *Vital and Health Statistics 23, 27*, 1–36.

Juffer, F. (2006). Children's awareness of adoption and their problem behavior in families with 7-year-old internationally adopted children. *Adoption Quarterly, 9*, 1–22. doi:10.1300/J145v09n02_01

Juffer, F., & Van IJzendoorn, M. H. (2007). Adoptees do not lack self-esteem: A meta-analysis of studies on self-esteem of transracial, international and domestic adoptees. *Psychological Bulletin, 133*, 1067–1083. doi:10.1037/0033-2909.133.6.1047

Kaye, S., & Kuvalanka, K. (2006). State gay adoption laws and permanency for foster youth. *Maryland Family Policy Impact Seminar*. Retrieved http://www.hhp.umd.edu/FMST/_docsContribute/GayadoptionbriefFINAL0806.pdf

Lansford, J. E., Ceballo, R., Abbey, A., & Stewart, A. J. (2001). Does family structure matter? A comparison of stepfather, and stepmother households. *Journal of Marriage and Family, 63*, 840–851. doi:10.1111/j.1741-3737.2001.00840.x

LaRenzie, A. (2010). *Laws of gay adoption*. Retrieved from http://www.ehow.com/about_5434538_laws-gay-adoption.html

Leung, P., Erich, S., & Kanenberg, H. (2005). A comparison of family functioning in gay/lesbian, heterosexual and special needs adoptions. *Children and Youth Services Review, 27*, 1031–1044. doi:10.1016/j.childyouth.2004.12.030

Levy-Shiff, R., Bar, O., & Har-Even, D. (1990). Psychological adjustment of adoptive parents- to-be. *American Journal of Orthopsychiatry, 60*, 258–267. doi:10.1037/h0079165

Lobaugh, E. R., Clements, P. T., Averill, J. B., & Olguin, D. L. (2006). Gay-male couples who adopt: Challenging historical and contemporary social trends toward becoming a family. *Perspectives in Pediatric Care, 42*, 184–195. doi:10.1111/j.1744-6163.2006.00081.x

Mallon, G. P. (2000). Gay men and lesbians as adoptive parents. *Journal of Gay and Lesbian Social Services, 11*, 1–22. doi:10.1300/J041v11n04_01

Mallon, G. P. (2007). Assessing lesbian and gay prospective foster and adoptive families: A focus on the home study process. *Child Welfare, 86*, 67–86.

Matthews, J. D., & Cramer, E. P. (2006). Envisaging the adoption process to strengthen gay- and lesbian-headed families: Recommendations for adoption professionals. *Child Welfare, 85*, 317–340.

McKay, K., Ross, L. E., & Goldberg, A. E. (2010). Adaptation to parenthood during the post-adoption period: A review of the literature. *Adoption Quarterly, 13*, 125–144. doi:10.1080/10926755.2010.481040

Miller, C. M. (2010). Appeals court: Florida ban on adoption by gays unconstitutional. *Miami Herald*. Retrieved from http://www.tampabay.com/news/courts/civil/appeal-court-florida-ban-on-gay-adoption-unconstitutional/1123284

Palacios, J., & Brodzinsky, D. (2010). Review: Adoption research: Trends, topics, outcomes. *International Journal of Behavioral Development, 34*, 270–284. doi:10.1177/0165025410362837

Patterson, C. J. (2009). Children of lesbian and gay parents: Psychology, law, and policy. *American Psychologist, 64*, 727–736. doi:10.1037/0003-066X.64.8.727

Patterson, C. J., & Tornello, S. L. (2011). Gay fathers' pathways to parenthood: International perspectives. *Zeitschrift für Familienforschung (Journal of Family Research), 7*, 103–116.

Riggs, D. (2006). Developmentalism and the rhetoric of best interests of the child: Challenging heteronormative constructions of families and parenting in foster care. *Journal of GLBT Family Studies, 2*, 57–71. doi:10.1300/J461v02n02_03

Riskind, R. G., & Patterson, C. J. (2010). Parenting intentions and desires among childless lesbian, gay, and heterosexual individuals. *Journal of Family Psychology, 24*, 78–81. doi:10.1037/a0017941

Rosenfeld, M., & Kim, B. (2005). The independence of young adults and the rise of interracial and same-sex unions. *American Sociological Review, 70*, 541–562. doi:10.1177/000312240507000401

Ross, L. E., Epstein, R., Anderson, S., & Eady, A. (2009). Policy, practice, and personal narratives: Experiences of LGBTQ people with adoption in Ontario, Canada. *Adoption Quarterly, 12*, 272–293. doi:10.1080/10926750903313302

Ross, L. E., Epstein, R., Goldfinger, C., Steele, L., Anderson, S., & Strike, C. (2008). Lesbian and queer mothers navigating the adoption system: The impacts on mental health. *Health Sociology Review, 17*, 254–266. doi:10.5172/hesr.451.17.3.254

Rueter, M., Keyes, M., Iacono, W. G., & McGue, M. (2009). Family interactions in adoptive compared to nonadoptive families. *Journal of Family Psychology, 23*, 58–66. doi:10.1037/a0014091

Ryan, S. (2000). Examining social workers' placement recommendations of children with gay and lesbian adoptive parents. *Families in Society, 81*, 517–528. doi:10.1606/10443894.1053.

Ryan, S. (2007). Parent–child interaction styles between gay and lesbian parents and their adopted children. *Journal of GLBT Family Studies, 3*, 105–132. doi:10.1300./J461v03n02_05

Ryan, S. D., Pearlmutter, S., & Groza, V. (2004). Coming out of the closet: Opening agencies to gay and lesbian adoptive parents. *Social Work, 49*, 85–95.

Ryan, S. D., & Whitlock, C. (2007). Becoming parents: Lesbian mothers' adoption experience. *Journal of Gay and Lesbian Social Services, 19*, 1–33. doi:10.1080/10538720802131642.

Schacher, J. S., Auerbach, C. F., & Silverstein, L. B. (2005). Gay fathers expanding the possibilities for us all. *Journal of GLBT Family Studies, 1,* 31–52. doi:10.1300/J461v01n03_02

Simmel, C., Barth, R. P., & Brooks, D. (2007). Adopted foster youths' psychosocial functioning: A longitudinal perspective. *Child & Family Social Work, 12,* 336–348. doi:10.1111/j.1365-2206.2006.00481.x

Stacey, J. (2006). Gay parenthood and the decline of paternity as we knew it. *Sexualities, 9,* 27–55. doi:10.1177/1363460706060687

Storsbergen, H. E., Juffer, F., van Son, M. J. M., & van Hart, H. (2010). Internationally adopted adults who did not suffer severe early deprivation: The role of appraisal of adoption. *Children and Youth Services Review, 32,* 191–197. doi:10.1016/j.childyouth.2009.08.015

Tan, T. X., & Baggerly, J. (2009). Behavioral adjustment of adopted Chinese girls in single-mother, lesbian-couple, and heterosexual-couple households. *Adoption Quarterly, 12,* 171–186. doi:10.1080/10926750903313336

Tasker, F., & Patterson, C. J. (2007). Research on lesbian and gay parenting: Retrospect and prospect. *Journal of GLBT Family Studies, 3,* 9–34. doi:10.1300/J461v03n02_02

Tornello, S. L., Farr, R. H., & Patterson, C. J. (2011). Predictors of parenting stress among gay adoptive fathers in the United States. *Journal of Family Psychology, 25,* 591–600. doi:10.1037/a0024480

Turner, C. S. (1999). *Adoption journeys: Parents tell their stories.* Ithaca, NY: McBooks Press.

Tyebjee, T. (2003). Attitude, interest, and motivation for adoption and foster care. *Child Welfare, 82,* 685–706.

U.S. Department of Health & Human Services. (2010). *The AFCARS report, preliminary FY 2009 estimates as of July 2010.* Retrieved from http://www.acf.hhs.gov/programs/cb/stats_research/afcars/tar/report17.html

van IJzendoorn, M. H., Juffer, F., & Poelhuis, C. W. K. (2005). Adoption and cognitive development: A meta-analytic comparison of adopted and nonadopted children's IQ and school performance. *Psychological Bulletin, 131,* 301–316. doi:10.1037/0033- 2909.131.2.301

Vandivere, S., & McKlindon, A. (2010). The well-being of U.S. children adopted from foster care, privately from the United States and internationally. *Adoption Quarterly, 13,* 157–184. 10.1080/10926755.2010.524871.

Von Korff, L., Grotevant, H., & McRoy, R. (2006). Openness arrangements and psychological adjustment in adolescent adoptees. *Journal of Family Psychology, 20,* 531–534. doi:10.1037/0893-3200.20.3.531

Whitten, K., & Weaver, S. (2010). Adoptive family relationships and healthy adolescent development: A risk and resilience analysis. *Adoption Quarterly, 13,* 209–226. doi:10.1080/10926755.2010.524873

Wrobel, G. M., Hendrickson, Z., & Grotevant, H. D. (2006). Adoption. In G. G. Bear & K. M. Minke (Eds.), *Children's needs III: Development, prevention, and intervention* (pp. 561–572). Bethesda, MA: National Association of School Psychologists.

Wrobel, G. M., Kohler, J. K., Grotevant, H. D., & McRoy, R. G. (2003). The family adoption communication (FAC) model: Identifying pathways of adoption-related communication. *Adoption Quarterly, 7*(2), 53–84. doi:10.1300/J145v07n02_01

Wrobel, G., & Neil, E. (2009). *International advances in adoption research for practice.* Chichester: Wiley.

Part II

Research: Understudied Topics and Groups

How Lesbians and Gay Men Decide to Become Parents or Remain Childfree

4

Nancy J. Mezey

Introduction

This chapter examines the understudied question of how lesbians and gay men choose to become parents or remain childfree. Although lesbians and gay men have been openly forming families with and without children over the past several decades (Pollack, 1995), few studies have examined lesbians' and gay men's decision-making processes about whether or not to become parents. Instead, scholarly and public discourse to date has focused primarily on lesbian and gay families *after* children enter into those families.

The limited research suggests that several factors shape how lesbians and gay men decide to become parents or remain childfree.[1] These factors include personal issues, support networks, work-related issues, and intimate partner relationships. Existing research also suggests that these factors are greatly shaped by structures of race, class, gender, and sexuality. In general, those with

greater race and class privilege are more likely to access material resources, receive greater support from family members, and intentionally decide to become parents. This chapter will review past literature on lesbian and gay parenting decisions, suggest new questions for further research, and discuss how studying lesbian and gay men's parenting decisions informs our understanding of families in general.

Understanding how lesbians and gay men engage in parent decision-making processes is important if we want to understand why, at this historical moment, lesbians and gay men are creating new families that may or may not include children. As the current American family landscape is in great flux (Baca Zinn, Eitzen, & Wells, 2011; Dunne, 2000), thinking about how lesbian and gay families shape and fit into that new landscape is crucial to understanding families today. Furthermore, understanding how lesbians and gay men decide to become parents or remain childfree allows us to understand the process of family formation from its genesis.

The chapter examines literature across a number of disciplines, particularly within the social and behavioral sciences. Each discipline—including gender and women studies, psychology, public health, queer studies, social work, and sociology—draws on different theoretical foundations. Such foundations include ecological theories (e.g., Chabot & Ames, 2004; Goldberg, 2010), identity theories (e.g., Berkowitz & Marsiglio, 2007), life course perspectives (e.g., Goldberg, 2010), feminist and multiracial feminist

---

[1] As discussed in earlier works (Mezey, 2008a, 2008b), I prefer the term "childfree" over the term "childless" because "childfree" suggests a positive state where women and men have chosen to be free from the responsibilities of child raising, rather than a negative state of something missing or lacking from a person's life.

N.J. Mezey, Ph.D. (✉)
Department of Political Science and Sociology,
Monmouth University, 400 Cedar Avenue,
West Long Branch, NJ 07764, USA
e-mail: nmezey@monmouth.edu

A.E. Goldberg and K.R. Allen (eds.), *LGBT-Parent Families: Innovations in Research and Implications for Practice*, DOI 10.1007/978-1-4614-4556-2_4, © Springer Science+Business Media New York 2013

perspectives (e.g., Berkowitz & Marsiglio, 2007; Mezey, 2008a), phenomenology (e.g., Gianino, 2008), social constructionism (e.g., Goldberg, 2010; Mezey, 2008a), and symbolic interactionism (e.g., Berkowitz & Marsiglio, 2007). All of these perspectives emphasize how parenting is socially, not biologically, constructed; however, each perspective also focuses on a slightly different aspect of the parenting decision-making process. Perspectives such as phenomenology, identity theory, and symbolic interactionism focus on micro-level interactions and the meaning of parenthood. The other perspectives focus on more macro-social processes. For example, a life course perspective takes a longitudinal focus, and ecological and multiracial feminist perspectives examine the connections between micro-level interpersonal interactions and meaning, and macro-level social institutions and inequalities. Multiracial feminism is distinct from the other perspectives in that it specifically examines the interconnections of race, class, and gender (Baca Zinn & Dill, 1996). Across the disciplinary spectrum, the most promising research incorporates an intersectional approach that encourages researchers to examine how structures of race, class, gender, and sexuality—as well as other factors discussed below—overlap to shape parenting decision-making processes (Boggis, 2001; Mezey, 2008a).

What We Know About Lesbian and Gay Parenting Decision-Making Processes

For the past two to three decades lesbians and gay men have been creating families while simultaneously experiencing positive support for, and negative barriers to prevent, the creation of their families (Berkowitz & Marsiglio, 2007; Hequembourg, 2007; Mallon, 2004; Stacey, 2006). Positive support comes largely from progressive individuals, organizations, and politicians who support lesbian, gay, bisexual, and transgender (LGBT) rights. Positive support also comes from medical professionals and adoption agencies that make reproductive technologies and adoption available to available to LGBT people.

Negative barriers come largely from conservatives who view LGBT people and their families as a threat to the moral fabric of society (Bernstein & Reimann, 2001). Negative barriers manifest themselves through legislation such as the Defense of Marriage Act (DOMA) both on federal and state levels, as well as amendments to state constitutions which prevent same-sex couples from marrying, that together have been instituted in 42 states in the USA (Alliance Defense Fund, 2008). Negative barriers also come in the form of heterosexism and homophobia within adoption and foster care systems (Mallon, 2004; Stacey, 2006). Furthermore, barriers exist on a psychological level, whereby some individuals believe that both "lesbian mother" and "gay father" are oxymorons, largely based on the assumptions that only "real" women (i.e., heterosexual women) can be nurturing parents (Berkowitz & Marsiglio, 2007; Lewin, 1993; Mallon, 2004; Stacey, 2006).

In the context of this mixed climate, several key factors—personal issues, access to support networks, work-related issues, and relationships with intimate partners—shape parenting decisions among lesbians and gay men. These factors, which are also shaped by structures of race, class, and gender, are discussed in the following sections.

Personal Issues

Three personal issues—that is, issues that occur within the individual experiences and thinking of lesbians or gay men—shape parenting decisions. These issues include (a) the desire to become a parent or remain childfree, (b) internalized homophobia, and (c) the ability and need to come out (i.e., reveal one's sexual identity to oneself and others) to negotiate multiple identities. Although personal in nature, these factors are shaped by outside forces, including one's position within hierarchies of race, class, gender, and sexuality. Thus, when examining the reasons why lesbians and gay men make particular parenting decisions, it is important to understand how macro-level social structural and institutional factors shape micro-level personal issues.

The Desire to Become a Parent or Remain Childfree

When lesbians or gay men want to become parents, or to remain childfree, they often work to turn those desires into a reality. In her study of 50 racially diverse gay men in Los Angeles, whom she interviewed between 1999 and 2003, Stacey (2006) identified a "passion-for-parenthood continuum" (p. 33) among the men. On one extreme of the continuum are what Stacey called "predestined parents"; these men were "compelled by a potent, irrepressible longing" (p. 33) to become parents. On the other extreme were "'parental refuseniks' for whom parenthood holds less than no appeal" (Stacey, 2006, p. 33). In general, the desire that these men had led them to pursue or not pursue fatherhood.

Similar findings were obtained by Gianino (2008) and Mallon (2004). Gianino (2008) conducted in-depth qualitative interviews with eight gay male parents to study how gay male couples transition from being childfree to becoming parents through adoption. He found that participants who became fathers recalled a strong desire to have children. Likewise, Mallon (2004) interviewed 20 gay men who had become fathers as "out" gay men during the 1980s. He concluded that the men whom he interviewed "felt such a compelling urge to become dads that they were willing to pursue their dream despite the lack of precedent, the lack of support, and the lack of opportunity" (p. 28). However, it is important to note that these studies only included gay men who had already become parents, and the gay men interviewed were mostly White and middle-class. Thus, this research does not provide insight into how some gay men who really want to become fathers are unable to because of economic and social barriers.

Other research does provide insight into how such barriers can alter people's parenting decisions despite what they may have originally desired (Berkowitz & Marsiglio, 2007; Mezey, 2008a). For example, Mezey (2008a) conducted a series of eight qualitative focus groups with a total of 17 lesbian mothers and 18 childfree lesbians of diverse race and class backgrounds in the Midwest. Five of the 35 women interviewed

who desired motherhood ultimately remained childfree. Similarly, four of the women interviewed who wanted to remain childfree ultimately became mothers. These outcomes were shaped largely by lesbians' different positions within race and class structures. In particular, lesbians privileged by race and class (i.e., White middle-class lesbians) were more likely to turn their parenting desires into realities because they had greater access than those less privileged to all of the factors discussed below: personal pride in their sexual identities, supportive family members, lesbian mother support networks, supportive partners, flexible jobs, financial stability, and access to physicians and adoption agencies.

Research by Stacey (2006), however, suggests that geographic location may intersect with race and class such that gay men of color and gay men from working-class backgrounds who live in areas with large and active lesbian and gay communities may be able to overcome economic and social barriers to become fathers. Despite coming from economically disadvantaged backgrounds and/or being racial-ethnic minorities, some of the gay men in Los Angeles whom she interviewed and who really wanted to become parents ultimately were able to fulfill that desire. As Stacey (2006) writes, affluent White couples

> Can literally purchase the means to eugenically reproduce White infants in their own idealized image .... In contrast, for gay men who are less privileged and/or uncoupled, public agencies provide a grab-bag of displaced children who are generally older, darker, and less healthy. (p. 39)

Thus, while Stacey (2006) found that race and class matter, *how* they matter may be different for different groups of lesbians and gay men depending on where in the USA they live.

It is also true that not all lesbians and gay men have a strong desire to parent or to remain childfree; some lesbians and gay men are quite ambivalent (Mezey, 2008a; Stacey, 2006). Stacey (2006) found that approximately half of the men she interviewed fell into the "ambivalent" category and therefore could be swayed toward, or away from, fatherhood depending on a variety of factors, most notably having a persistent partner. Mezey (2008a) also found that more ambivalent lesbians could be swayed by a number of factors either to become parents or to remain childfree. These factors included many of the issues that are addressed next.

Internalized Homophobia

A second personal issue that shapes lesbians' and gay men's parenting decisions is internalized homophobia. Because we live in a heterosexist and homophobic society (Stacey, 1996), many lesbians and gay men internalize societal messages that communicate that homosexuality is wrong or immoral; that lesbians and gay men make unfit parents; and that children will be harmed if they are raised by lesbians and gay men, particularly because children need both a mother and a father (Brown, Smalling, Groza, & Ryan, 2009; Gianino, 2008; Goldberg, 2010; Mallon, 2004). Because of internalized homophobia, lesbians and gay men may question their own right and ability to become parents. Such questioning often leads to personal doubt that presents a real barrier to becoming a parent (Brown et al., 2009; Gianino, 2008; Mallon, 2004).

In Berkowitz and Marsiglio's (2007) qualitative study of 19 childfree gay men and 20 gay fathers from Florida and New York, many of the childfree men displayed their internalized homophobia by voicing concerns about how people might treat or tease their potential children, particularly because of heterosexist norms, homophobic attitudes, and sexist understandings of men not being able to nurture children. Potential fathers also worried about how their family structure might negatively influence their children's experiences and life chances. Thus, internalized homophobia may have kept some of these ambivalent men from pursuing parenthood.

The Ability and Need to Come Out

Connected to internalized homophobia is the ability of lesbians and gay men to safely and comfortably come out. The coming out process is greatly shaped by one's social location determined by race and class (Espín, 1997; Goldberg, 2010;

Mezey, 2008b; Smith, 1998). Partially due to the long history of oppression in which White people have sexualized African-Americans in a variety of ways, many Black communities have developed a homophobic response to their gay and lesbian members (Greene, 1998). In addition, Latino culture places a high value on family honor, which is closely connected to the sexual purity of women (Espín, 1997). Furthermore, both Black and Latino communities are often closely tied with larger church communities. Thus, when lesbians and gay men of color come out, they may risk losing both their family and their community ties (Espín, 1997; Roberts, 2004).

Working-class, White lesbians also face difficulties coming out. Because working-class, White families might not want to overtly acknowledge their child's sexual identity, they may, similar to families of color, be willing to adopt a "don't ask, don't tell" practice whereby their lesbian or gay family member can remain part of the family unit as long as there is no open display or mention of one's sexual identity in front of the family (Mezey, 2008b).

While not always an easy process, coming out for middle-class, White lesbians and gay men holds fewer risks than for lesbians and gay men of color and/or working-class lesbians and gay men, because White, middle-class people in general hold greater economic and social power.[2] Furthermore, because White, middle-class lesbians and gay men come from families that are not necessarily strongly intertwined with larger communities, middle-class, White lesbians and gay men tend not to risk losing connection to communities outside their families if they come out (Brinamen & Mitchell, 2008).

Whether or not lesbians or gay men can come out to their family is important to their self-esteem and ability to feel comfortable within multiple identities. The necessity of negotiating multiple

---

[2] Middle-class includes those with at least a college degree, hold management-level positions, and earn a comfortable wage in which they can save some of their earnings. Working-class includes those with an associate's degree or less, who work at "blue collar" jobs and whose wages do not allow them to save much or any of their earnings (Mezey, 2008a).

identities becomes even stronger for lesbians and gay men who want to become parents. Regarding parenting decisions, the fear that lesbians and gay men have of coming out to their own parents can deter their decisions to become parents themselves (Brown et al., 2009; Mezey, 2008a, 2008b). The more accepting people's families are of their sexual identity, the easier it is for them to turn their parenting desires into a parenting reality. Drawing on qualitative responses that were part of a larger survey study of 182 mostly White, well-educated lesbian and gay adoptive parents across the country, Brown et al. (2009) found that a major barrier to becoming a parent was the negative response of their family. Ultimately, however, these respondents became parents, despite their parents' resistance. Similarly, Mezey (2008b) found that middle-class, White lesbians had the least struggle in terms of coming out and divulging their plans to become parents. While coming out for this group was stressful, on the whole middle-class, White lesbians found their families to be supportive of both their sexual identities and their desires to become mothers, leaving intact a supportive family network.

For lesbians and gay men of color, and for working-class lesbians and gay men, divulging a desire to parent is more difficult (Brinamen & Mitchell, 2008; Mezey, 2008b). In Mezey's (2008a, 2008b) study, lesbians of color, regardless of class, found coming out to their families stressful, particularly if they added the news that they wanted to become mothers. Lesbians of color who found that coming out and sharing their desire to parent might mean losing extended family support often delayed or abandoned their desires to become mothers. Working-class, White lesbians found that their families were often neutral, not fully embracing their lesbian parenting identities, but not rejecting them either (Mezey, 2008b). Given the race and class differences in how parents respond to lesbians and gay men coming out, and particularly coming out through the announcement of their desire to parent, it is not surprising that in Berkowitz and Marsiglio's (2007) study most of the fathers they studied were White and middle class. The childfree fathers, on the other hand, came from more diverse racial and class backgrounds than the fathers.

Despite similarities between the struggles or ease of coming out among lesbians and gay men, one difference by gender may be that while many lesbians appear to be coming out as a necessary step to becoming mothers, gay men seem to regard coming out as closing the door on becoming a parent (Brinamen & Mitchell, 2008; Mallon, 2004). Although there has been a large increase in the number of out gay men who have become parents, many gay men still perceive "gay father" to be an oxymoron. Therefore, for some gay men, coming out means deciding between being gay and being a father (Bergman, Rubio, Green, & Padron, 2010).

Historically, lesbian motherhood has also tended to be regarded as an oxymoron (Lewin, 1993). Yet the visibility of lesbian motherhood over the past several decades, along with the cultural expectation that women in general will become mothers (Hicks, 2006), may make coming out for lesbians seem more like a necessary step, rather than a closed door, to becoming a parent (Brinamen & Mitchell, 2008).

Clearly the above personal issues are experienced as just that—very personal. However, it is important to understand how the larger social context external to lesbians and gay men shape those personal issues. Berkowitz and Marsiglio (2007) found that the personal way in which gay men experienced the process of becoming fathers or remaining childfree was mediated by larger social factors including interactions with other people's children, as well as with lesbian mothers and gay fathers. For example, the death of a partner or family member and exposure to adoption or surrogacy organizations often sparked a "procreative consciousness" in gay men, leading them to want to become parents. In addition, gay potential parents needed to have substantial financial resources, resources that in general are reserved for those privileged by class.

Access to Support Networks, Information, and Resources

The second main factor that shapes lesbian and gay men's parenting decisions is access to support networks, information, and resources. Such support comes from accessing two major resources (a) lesbian and gay parent networks and (b) legal and medical information and services (Brown et al., 2009; Henehan, Rothblum, Solomon, & Balsam, 2007; Mezey, 2008a).

Lesbian and Gay Parent Networks

Support from other lesbians and gay men shapes lesbian and gay men's parenting decision-making processes. For lesbians and gay men—regardless of race or class—proximity to, and knowledge about and from other gay and lesbian parents, is very important to those who decide to become parents (Berkowitz & Marsiglio, 2007; Brown et al., 2009; Mallon, 2004; Mezey, 2008a). According to Brown et al. (2009), 21 (11.5%) of the 182 adoptive lesbian and gay parents in their study stated that the lack of knowledge that lesbians and gay men can adopt children was one of the biggest challenges to overcome in making the decision to become a parent. Other participants noted that had they known about gay friendly adoption agencies sooner, they would have had become parents earlier. Lesbians and gay men in places with larger lesbian and gay parent communities such as Los Angeles (Stacey, 2006) and New York City (Mallon, 2004) appear to have greater access to knowledge, role models, and support groups than those living in less urban areas (Goldberg, 2010).

In addition to geographic location, Mezey (2008a) also found that when making mothering decisions, race and class positions shape lesbians' access to lesbian support networks. She found that White, middle-class lesbians have greater access to lesbian-parent role models and support networks than do working-class lesbians and lesbians of color, particularly because lesbian "communities" are divided by race and class (Kennedy & Davis, 1993), as well as by mothering decisions (i.e., those who chose to become mothers and those who chose to remain childfree). For example, working-class, White lesbians in Mezey's (2008a) study reported that their communities were divided along lines of mothering decisions. In making parenting decisions,

therefore, they needed to decide if alienating lesbians with (or without) children was worth the risk of either becoming a parent or remaining childfree. Once they decided to become mothers, however, working-class, White lesbians were able—often with considerable effort on their part—to find and gain access into middle-class, White lesbian mother communities.

Working-class lesbians of color in this study, on the other hand, found their communities to be less divided by mothering decisions. However, those who wanted to become mothers could not always find or access other lesbians who had become mothers. Because they were not well integrated into lesbian parent networks, and therefore had limited knowledge about where to find or how to access necessary resources such as gay-friendly physicians, working-class lesbians of color often deferred or delayed their decisions to become mothers (Mezey, 2008a).

Middle-class lesbians, regardless of race, also had an easier time than their working-class counterparts in accessing other lesbians who were either childfree or mothers. Meeting other lesbians who were mothers gave them the confidence that they could make whatever choice they wanted, but also that they could access the resources they needed to become mothers (Mezey, 2008a). Some of the gay men in Berkowitz and Marsiglio's (2007) study also benefited from lesbian mother networks in that such networks helped them decide to become fathers.

Access to Legal and Medical Information and Services

An important question for lesbians and gay men who want to become parents is how to logistically achieve that goal (Agigian, 2004; Goldberg, 2010; Hequembourg, 2007; Mallon, 2004). Although there is evidence that some lesbians use heterosexual intercourse (Hequembourg, 2007; Mezey, 2008a), most lesbians become mothers through adoption, foster care, or donor (i.e., alternative) insemination (Agigian, 2004; Goldberg, 2010). If choosing the latter, lesbians generally purchase sperm through a sperm bank, many of which require the authorization and assistance of a physician (Agigian, 2004). Because men cannot get pregnant, heterosexual intercourse and donor insemination do not benefit gay men unless the woman with whom they are sharing their sperm agrees to carry and share the child born from that arrangement. Therefore, gay men often rely on adoption or surrogacy services to become fathers (Mallon, 2004). The result is that most lesbians and gay men need to access medical and/ or legal services to become parents.

Finding a physician who is willing to provide services to lesbians and gay men, however, is not always easy (Goldberg, Downing, & Richardson, 2009; Lasker, 1998). Because lesbians and gay men challenge people's definition of family as consisting of a connection between marriage and reproduction, they may receive discriminatory treatment by hospitals and fertility clinics (Goldberg et al., 2009). Lesbians have reported that some physicians will only inseminate heterosexual women in stable marriages (Lasker, 1998). Furthermore, once at a physician's office, lesbians sometimes find that some physicians discriminate in how they treat lesbians by asking the potential patients to undergo lengthy psychological exams to determine if they are fit parents (Lasker, 1998).

Some physicians also tend to ignore or mistreat accompanying partners. In their qualitative study of 30 heterosexual couples and 30 lesbian couples who had previously pursued fertility services to conceive, Goldberg et al. (2009) reported that health care professionals tended to only focus on the partner trying to get pregnant, thus ignoring and rendering invisible the non-trying partner, and leading some lesbians to question whether or not they wanted to use medical services (Goldberg et al., 2009). The poor social and emotional treatment (as opposed to the medical treatment) of lesbians by physicians may lead some lesbians to delay or dismiss their desires to become parents. Thus, having knowledge of which physician or adoption agency to go to in order to become a parent is key to helping lesbians and gay men realize their parenting desires.

Support networks also help lesbians and gay men access and negotiate legal services and systems.

Without such knowledge, lesbians and gay men—particularly those who live in states where adoption is difficult for lesbians and gay men, such as Arkansas, Florida, Utah, and Wisconsin (see http://www.hrc.org for a complete listing of laws related to adoption)—find the path toward adoption confusing or overwhelming. In one study of lesbians and gay adoptive parents, 25% of participants cited "restrictive state laws/practices" as a barrier to adopting children (Brown et al., 2009, p. 237). In addition to not being able to access such services, lesbians and gay men were afraid that the lack of legal support for their families would lead to a lack of legal protection for their children (Brown et al., 2009).

One way that lesbians try to protect their families legally is by using a donor through a sperm bank (Agigian, 2004). Not only does donor insemination allow lesbians to avoid heterosexual intercourse, but by using an anonymous donor lesbians eliminate the problem of the donor claiming custody of the child at a later date. A potential problem with using donor insemination, however, is that in order to access sperm and the means of being inseminated, lesbians often need to access physician-controlled medical services (Agigian, 2004), which, as previously discussed, can be challenging.

Even when lesbians and gay men can access gay-friendly medical and legal service providers, they often find that the financial cost associated with becoming a parent is prohibitively high. Because purchasing sperm and using physician's services, particularly more complex reproductive technologies, can be very costly and not usually covered by insurance, lesbians often begin to consider other routes to motherhood (Boggis, 2001) or decide to remain childfree (Mezey, 2008a). According to Agigian (2004), those with higher incomes are most likely to use donor insemination.

Similarly, private domestic adoption and international adoption can be very expensive, ranging between $5,000 and $40,000. Likewise, the use of surrogacy can range from $115,000 to $150,000 (Goldberg, 2010). Thus, for many lesbians and gay men, becoming a parent in a safe and legally protective way can be cost prohibitive. It is no accident, therefore, that most of the lesbians and gay men who participate in studies who have become parents through the use of adoption or reproductive technologies tend to be middle-class, well educated, and White (see e.g., Gianino, 2008; Mallon, 2004; Stacey, 2006).

Work-Related Issues

A third major factor that shapes parenting decision-making processes is represented by issues related to work. Although several studies have examined lesbians and gay men's experiences in paid employment (Reimann, 2001; Sullivan, 2004), only a handful of studies examine how work-related issues shape lesbians' and gay men's parenting decisions (Mezey, 2008a; Rabun & Oswald, 2009).

Work is important to the decision-making process because at minimum lesbians and gay men need to be able to pay for services that allow them to become parents through adoption or pregnancy. Middle-class lesbians and gay men have clear advantages over their working-class counterparts in that those who hold middle-class jobs not only earn a comfortable salary with some career satisfaction, but also their jobs often come with flexibility and solid benefits, including sick leave, vacation time, and health insurance (Kerbo, 2009). According to Mezey (2008a), these advantages give middle-class lesbians the ability to choose motherhood or remain childfree with the knowledge that they can have a secure income and be able to balance work and family, or work and other activities they enjoy (e.g., camping, traveling). Although middle-class lesbians of color voiced some concern about health insurance, they too enjoyed the comfort of a secure job similar to that of their White counterparts (Mezey, 2008a).

Working-class lesbians in Mezey's (2008a) study expressed much concern about how their work hindered their ability to become mothers. Because working-class jobs, and particularly those held by working-class lesbians of color, did not offer the same benefits as those occupied by lesbians in the middle class, working-class lesbians found that their jobs offered little flexibility,

limited career satisfaction, and inadequate health insurance, thus creating structural barriers that often forced them to choose between a job, education, and motherhood.

Therefore, lesbians in this study carefully considered work-related issues when trying to decide if they wanted to become mothers or remain childfree. For example, lesbians from working-class and middle-class backgrounds who wanted economic and personal freedom, and who had jobs that afforded them this freedom, often decided to remain childfree. They feared that if they become mothers, they would lose that freedom. On the other hand, lesbians who had jobs that they knew would allow them to balance work and family responsibilities—or who had committed partners with jobs that offered such opportunities—often decided to become mothers. By creating a system of opportunity and constraints based on structures of race and class, paid labor shapes mothering decisions by providing or denying lesbians the material means to help lesbians turn, or prevent them from turning, their parenting desires into reality (Mezey, 2008a).

It is important to consider how gay men's experiences might be similar to and/or different from lesbians' experiences. Studies like those conducted by Rabun and Oswald (2009), as well as Berkowitz and Marsiglio (2007), suggest that race and class matter in similar ways to gay men as they do for lesbians. For example, in their study of 14 childfree gay men who were mostly White, middle- or professional-class, and fell between the ages of 18 and 25 years, Rabun and Oswald (2009) found that while all of the men intended to become fathers, they asserted that they would only do so after they or their partners were financially secure. The men stated that they would achieve financial security by pursuing careers such as lawyers, physicians, professors, and engineers. The participants believed that these jobs would not only provide the economic security they needed to become fathers but also provide them with flexible schedules to accommodate their parental responsibilities.

Likewise, although they did not specifically study how paid labor shapes men's parenting decisions, Berkowitz and Marsiglio (2007) found that men with greater economic resources were in fact able to negotiate medical and legal institutions in ways that allowed them to become fathers. Because White men in general have the greatest access to high status, well-paying jobs in the USA (Andersen & Witham, 2011), it stands to reason that White, middle-class gay men will have greater access than working-class gay men and gay men of color to the social and material resources needed to fulfill desires to become fathers outside of heterosexual relationships. In fact, a study by Henehan et al. (2007) compared the social and demographic characteristics of gay men, lesbian, and heterosexual women and men who were childfree, as well those who were parents. Using data from 1,538 lesbians, gay men, and heterosexual women and men from across the USA, they found that their sample resembled the demographic profile of other studies of lesbians and gay men in that participants tended to be White, well-educated, and affluent.

Relationships with Intimate Partners

A fourth major factor that shapes whether or not lesbians and gay men will become parents or remain childfree involves the presence of and relationship with an intimate partner (Goldberg, 2010; Mallon, 2004; Mezey, 2008a; Stacey, 2006), and this factor is very much shaped by race, class, and gender. For those lesbians and gay men who want to become parents, having a willing and supportive partner makes the process easier. Similarly, a partner with a differing parenting desire, or no partner at all, can make the process more difficult, or derail the process all together.

Mezey (2008a) found that intimate partners were important in shaping the decision-making process, but that how they shaped the process depended largely on race and class positions. Her findings suggest that if lesbians who either wanted to have children, or who were ambivalent about becoming mothers, did not find the "right" partner at the "right" time, then they were likely to remain childfree. However, sometimes finding the "right" partner at the "right" time meant that

lesbians who thought they would remain childfree, or were unsure about becoming mothers, actually did become mothers. Furthermore, if a woman's desire to remain childfree or to become a mother was strong, then the mothering desire of her partner did not change her own path (Mezey, 2008a).

What is important to note, however, is that how lesbians determined who the "right" partner was, or what the "right" time was, was shaped largely by class structures. For working-class lesbians, the partner had to be financially stable and emotionally ready to have children. For middle-class lesbians, the partner only had to be emotionally ready. In addition, because of the large networks of "out" middle-class lesbians, middle-class lesbians did not fear leaving a partner who had a different mothering desire as much as working-class lesbians did, because middle-class lesbians assumed they could find another partner (Mezey, 2008a). Childfree Black lesbians, on the other hand, were more likely to stay with their partners even if their partners had differing parenting desires. The greater likelihood of Black lesbians staying with partners than White lesbians might have been true because of the limited options for finding a new partner within racially divided lesbian communities (Mezey, 2008a). Therefore, middle-class, White lesbians had greater economic and emotional flexibility that allowed them to rely less heavily on their partners than did lesbians of color and working-class lesbians in deciding to become mothers or remain childfree.

Regarding gay men, Stacey's (2006) study in Los Angeles found that finding the right partner at the right time may not hinder gay men's desires to have children if that desire is strong enough. This appeared to be true even for gay men who were disadvantaged by race and class. For example, one of the men Stacey interviewed was a Mexican immigrant who ran away from home when he was 15 years old. Once in the USA, this man worked at Taco Bell, put himself through high school, and ultimately ended up securing his US citizenship and a stable career as the manager of a furniture store. The man's passion for parenthood ultimately led him to leave a partner after several years in favor of adopting a child.

Future Directions: What We Need to Know About Lesbian and Gay Parenting Decision-Making Processes

As indicated above, there are gaps in the literature on lesbian and gay parental decision making. With a few important exceptions (see e.g., Berkowitz & Marsiglio, 2007; Mezey, 2008a; Stacey, 2006), the majority of research draws almost exclusively from middle- or upper-class samples of White lesbians and gay men. And with the exception of Mezey's (2008a) and Stacey's (2006) work, and to some extent the work of Berkowitz and Marsiglio (2007), studies that draw on samples with any kind of race or class diversity fail to explicitly examine that diversity as an integral part of their methodologies or analyses to understand how race and class shape decision-making processes. Therefore, the sampling and analyses included in most previous studies have a built-in bias that leaves major gaps in our understanding about how lesbians and gay men who face serious economic and social constraints decide to become parents or remain childfree. Furthermore, most research has focused on lesbians and gay men who ultimately decided to become parents, thus rendering those who decide to remain childfree an invisible or ignored population. Existing research is limited, therefore, in that it cannot explain what factors encourage people to remain childfree or prevent those who want to become parents from realizing that desire.

Perhaps because most research focuses on samples of people who are privileged by race and class, the underlying assumption of most research is that most lesbians and gay men who want to become parents can and do become parents. Without looking at lesbians and gay men who are childfree, racial-ethnic minorities, or working- or lower-class, current research tells only a partial story. Therefore, one of the most pressing questions for future research is, "What factors shape the parenting decision-making process of lesbians and gay men who are marginalized by race and class, as well as by other factors such as disability, nationality, and geographic location?"

In addition, studies that specifically compare the decision-making processes of lesbians and gay men would add to our understanding of how gender and sexual identities affect the decision-making process. Furthermore, a focus specifically on gay men, as well as on other understudied groups such as bisexual and transgender people, would add a wealth of knowledge to our understanding of parenting decision-making processes. Also needed are longitudinal studies to examine how well families fare once they make their parenting decisions. Are there any long-term differences, for example, in the quality of life that parents and children of diverse racial-ethnic and class backgrounds experience? If so, are those differences the result of the intersections not only of race and class but also because of sexuality and gender structures? What are the consequences of remaining childfree for those lesbians and gay men who contemplated parenthood but decided not to pursue that route for a variety of reasons?

How Does Studying Lesbian and Gay Men's Parenting Decisions Inform Our Understanding of Families in General?

Research on lesbian and gay parenting decision-making processes make four important contributions to our general understanding of families. First, such research focuses on the importance and socioeconomic implications of intentional parenting decision making. Data from 2001 indicate that approximately 49% of pregnancies among heterosexuals are unplanned. Approximately 50% of those pregnancies end in abortion, suggesting that half of unplanned pregnancies are unwanted (Finer & Henshaw, 2006). While there are no data to my knowledge concerning the number of unplanned pregnancies among lesbians and gay men in the *general population*, the studies on lesbians and gay men reviewed throughout this chapter suggest that nearly 100% of adult lesbians and gay men plan their parenthood.

What can we learn from intentional parenting decisions? According to Mezey (2008b), the fact that lesbians can choose motherhood is attractive to lesbians because having a choice means that motherhood is not an oppressive obligation to women. Some lesbians in her study argued that planned motherhood is good for women in general. Furthermore, if social problems such as increased abortion, increased financial struggles, and increased children in foster care systems stem from unplanned, and possibly unwanted pregnancies (Furstenberg, 2007), then studying the effects of intentional parenting decision making both on parents and children might offer some insight into how to create stable families for a variety of populations regardless of sexual identity.

Second, research on lesbians and gay men's parenting decision-making processes show that what we often consider to be innate or biological processes are in fact socially constructed. Studies on gay men and lesbians indicate that even the development of parenting desires grow out of the social context and experiences of those interviewed (see e.g., Brinamen & Mitchell, 2008; Mallon, 2004; Mezey, 2008a). In other words, while public opinion might label parenting desires as "biological urges," social constructionists understand those desires to develop out of particular social contexts (Brinamen & Mitchell, 2008; Mallon, 2004; Mezey, 2008a). Therefore, studies that use a social constructionist perspective to study parenting decision-making processes add to our body of knowledge of how parenting decisions are part of complex social processes, not simply a biological mandate.

Third, research on lesbian and gay men's parenting decision-making processes clearly indicates that economic, legal, and social support are critical to helping people making parenting decisions that fit with—or sometimes conflict with—their desires to become parents or remain childfree. Social support in the way of supportive families, communities, jobs, partners, and society in general helps lesbians and gay men create healthy families. If policy makers are interested in helping people create stable families, then they need to understand what kinds of social support are needed for all types of families to be healthy (Mezey & Sanford, 2009). Research on lesbian and gay men's parenting decisions not only provides insight into what kinds of support are needed but also provides a model for conducting research on other types of families, regardless of sexual identity.

Finally, research on lesbian and gay men's parenting decision-making processes sheds light on why and how diverse family forms develop at particular historical moments in time. Scholars have documented that we are living in a time in which there is great change in American families (Baca Zinn et al., 2011; Dunne, 2000). New family forms, or what Stacey (1996) calls "postmodern families"—including single-parent families, dual-income earning families, divorced and blended families, grandparent-headed families, and lesbian and gay families—now make up the fabric of the standard family landscape (Baca Zinn et al., 2011; Dunne, 2000). Disputes among conservative and progressive scholars in the form of the "family values debate" indicate that there are major differences in opinion as to why families are changing and the consequences of those changes (Dill, Baca Zinn, & Patton, 1998). While research on lesbian and gay families in general informs our understanding of *how* families are changing, research specifically on how lesbians and gay men decide to become parents or remain childfree informs our understanding of *why* families are changing. Answering this very basic question adds to our understanding of the multiple social processes that are coalescing to create such a diverse family landscape in the USA today.

References

Agigian, A. (2004). *Baby steps: How lesbian alternative insemination is changing the world.* Middletown, CT: Wesleyan University Press.

Alliance Defense Fund. (2008). *DOMAwatch.org* [Legal source for Defense of Marriage Acts information]. Retrieved from http://www.domawatch.org/stateissues/index.html

Andersen, M. L., & Witham, D. H. (2011). *Thinking about women: Sociological perspectives on sex and gender* (9th ed.). Boston, MA: Allyn & Bacon.

Baca Zinn, M., & Dill, B. T. (1996). Theorizing difference from multiracial feminism. *Feminist Studies, 22,* 321–331.

Baca Zinn, M., Eitzen, D. S., & Wells, B. (2011). *Diversity in families* (9th ed.). Boston, MA: Allyn & Bacon.

Bergman, K., Rubio, R. J., Green, R.-J., & Padron, E. (2010). Gay men who become fathers via surrogacy: The transition to parenthood. *Journal of GLBT Family Studies, 6*, 111–141.

Berkowitz, D., & Marsiglio, W. (2007). Gay men: Negotiating procreative, father, and family identities. *Journal of Marriage and Family, 69*, 366–381.

Bernstein, M., & Reimann, R. (2001). Queer families and the politics of visibility. In M. Bernstein & R. Reimann (Eds.), *Queer families, queer politics: Challenging culture and the state* (pp. 1–17). New York, NY: Columbia University Press.

Boggis, T. (2001). Affording our families: Class issues in family formation. In M. Bernstein & R. Reimann (Eds.), *Queer families, queer politics: Challenging culture and the state* (pp. 175–181). New York, NY: Columbia University Press.

Brinamen, C. F., & Mitchell, V. (2008). Gay men becoming fathers: A model of identity expansion. *Journal of GLBT Family Studies, 4*, 521–541. doi:10.1080/15504280802191772

Brown, S., Smalling, S., Groza, V., & Ryan, S. (2009). The experiences of gay men and lesbians in becoming and being adoptive parents. *Adoption Quarterly, 12*, 229–246.

Chabot, J. M., & Ames, B. D. (2004). "It wasn't 'let's get pregnant and go do it':" Decision making in lesbian couples planning motherhood via donor insemination. *Family Relations, 53*, 348–356.

Dill, B. T., Baca Zinn, M., & Patton, S. (1998). Valuing families differently: Race, poverty and welfare reform. *Sage Race Relations Abstracts, 23*(3), 4–30.

Dunne, G. A. (2000). Opting into motherhood: Lesbians blurring the boundaries and transforming the meaning of parenthood and kinship. *Gender and Society, 14*, 11–35.

Espín, O. M. (1997). *Latina realities: Essays on healing, migration, and sexuality.* Boulder, CO: Westview Press.

Finer, L. B., & Henshaw, S. K. (2006). Disparities in rates of unintended pregnancy in the United States, 1994 and 2001. *Perspectives on Sexual and Reproductive Health, 38*, 90–96.

Furstenberg, F. F., Jr. (2007). *Destinies of the disadvantaged: The politics of teenage childbearing.* New York, NY: Russell Sage Foundation.

Gianino, M. (2008). Adaptation and transformation: The transition to adoptive parenthood for gay male couples. *Journal of GLBT Family Studies, 4*, 205–243.

Goldberg, A. E. (2010). *Lesbian and gay parents and their children: Research on the family life cycle.* Washington, DC: American Psychological Association.

Goldberg, A. E., Downing, J. B., & Richardson, H. B. (2009). The transition from infertility to adoption: Perceptions of lesbian and heterosexual preadoptive couples. *Journal of Social and Personal Relationships, 26*, 938–963.

Greene, B. (1998). Family, ethnic identity, and sexual orientation: African-American lesbians and gay men. In C. J. Patterson & A. R. D'Augelli (Eds.), *Lesbian, gay,*

and bisexual identities in families: Psychological perspectives (pp. 40–52). New York, NY: Oxford University Press.

Henehan, D., Rothblum, E. D., Solomon, S. E., & Balsam, K. F. (2007). Social and demographic characteristics of gay, lesbian, and heterosexual adults with and without children. *Journal of GLBT Family Studies, 3*, 35–79.

Hequembourg, A. (2007). *Lesbian motherhood: Stories of becoming.* New York, NY: Harrington Park Press.

Hicks, S. (2006). Maternal men: Perverts and deviants? Making sense of gay men as foster careers and adopters. *Journal of GLBT Family Studies, 2*, 93–114.

Kennedy, E. L., & Davis, M. D. (1993). *Boots of leather, slippers of gold: The history of a lesbian community.* New York, NY: Routledge.

Kerbo, H. K. (2009). *Social stratification and inequality* (7th ed.). New York, NY: McGraw Hill.

Lasker, J. N. (1998). The users of donor insemination. In K. Daniels & E. Haimes (Eds.), *Donor insemination: International social science perspectives* (pp. 7–32). New York, NY: Cambridge University Press.

Lewin, E. (1993). *Lesbian mothers: Accounts of gender in American culture.* Ithaca, NY: Cornell University Press.

Mallon, G. P. (2004). *Gay men choosing parenthood.* New York, NY: Columbia University Press.

Mezey, N. J. (2008a). *New choices, new families: How lesbians decide about motherhood.* Baltimore, MD: The Johns Hopkins University Press.

Mezey, N. J. (2008b). The privilege of coming out: Race, class, and lesbians' mothering decisions. *International Journal of Sociology of the Family, 34*, 257–276.

Mezey, N. J., & Sanford, R. (2009). Family: Youth and adults. In T. Maschi, C. Bradley, & K. Ward (Eds.), *Forensic social work: Psychosocial and legal issues in diverse practice settings* (pp. 63–80). New York, NY: Springer.

Pollack, J. S. (1995). *Lesbian and gay families: Redefining parenting in America.* New York, NY: Franklin Watts.

Rabun, C., & Oswald, R. F. (2009). Upholding and expanding the normal family: Future fatherhood through the eyes of gay male emerging adults. *Fathering, 7*, 269–285. doi:10.3149/fth.0703.269

Reimann, R. (2001). Lesbian mothers at work. In M. Bernstein & R. Reimann (Eds.), *Queer families, queer politics: Challenging culture and the state* (pp. 254–271). New York, NY: Columbia University Press.

Roberts, K. A. (2004). *Religion in sociological perspective.* Belmont, CA: Thompson-Wadsworth.

Smith, B. (1998). *The truth that never hurts: Writings on race, gender, and freedom.* New Brunswick, NJ: Rutgers University Press.

Stacey, J. (1996). *In the name of the family: Rethinking family values in the postmodern age.* Boston, MA: Beacon.

Stacey, J. (2006). Gay parenthood and the decline of paternity as we knew it. *Sexualities, 9*, 27–55.

Sullivan, M. (2004). *The family of woman: Lesbian mothers, their children, and the undoing of gender.* Berkeley, CA: University of California Press.

Gay Men and Surrogacy

Dana Berkowitz

The visibility of gay fathers is on the rise, with growing numbers adopting children, sharing parenting with lesbian women, and having children through surrogacy arrangements (Gates, 2007; Goldberg, 2010a). The increase in the number of gay fathers who choose to construct their families outside of heterosexual unions is a result of a combination of factors that include but are not necessarily limited to: recent developments in reproductive technology, changing legalities in the adoption system, greater acceptance of lesbians and gay men, and broader changes in the diversity of American families (Goldberg, 2010a; Stacey, 1996). Changes in the sociohistorical context for gay men have increased the visibility of gay fathering, and gay fathers are much less likely to be viewed as the anomaly they once were (Berkowitz, 2007).

Despite their increasing visibility, there are a dearth of studies on gay fathers, particularly on the cohort of gay men who became parents after coming out rather than in the context of a previous heterosexual relationship (for exceptions see Berkowitz, 2007; Berkowitz & Marsiglio, 2007; Greenfeld & Seli, 2011; Lewin, 2009; Mallon, 2004; Stacey, 2006). Moreover, scholars understand very little about the diversity among gay fathers. Developing a more nuanced understanding

of gay fathers requires scholars to explore the diversity of structures, arrangements, and practices within these family constellations. For example, since there are several paths to parenthood for this emerging cohort of gay fathers—including domestic and international adoption, fostering, surrogacy arrangements, and creative kinship ties that often entail sharing parenting with a lesbian woman or women—studies of gay fathers need to better understand the unique family experiences embedded within each of these family forms.

This chapter provides an overview of the scholarship on one particularly understudied group of this new cohort of gay fathers—gay men who have become parents through the assistance of a surrogate mother (Bergman, Rubio, Green, & Padron, 2010; Goldberg, 2010a). Some of the questions that I address in this chapter are: For those gay men using surrogacy, how is the transition to parenthood unique when compared with adoption, fostering, and shared parenting with lesbian women? To what extent do gender, sexuality, social class, race, and ethnicity intersect in surrogacy arrangements? How does the importance of biological relatedness to the child shape the decision-making processes of those gay men pursuing surrogacy? How are the identities of the egg donor and/or surrogate mother implicated in the process of building a family and later, for doing family? Answering these fundamental questions about gay fathers and surrogacy provides a starting point for understanding the diversity in routes to gay parenthood and the variety of family structures formed. I expect that this chapter will

D. Berkowitz (✉)
Department of Sociology and Program in Women's and Gender Studies, Louisiana State University, 126 Stubbs Hall, Baton Rouge, LA 70803, USA
e-mail: dberk@lsu.edu

A.E. Goldberg and K.R. Allen (eds.), *LGBT-Parent Families: Innovations in Research and Implications for Practice*, DOI 10.1007/978-1-4614-4556-2_5, © Springer Science+Business Media New York 2013

be of value to researchers and students interested in the intersections of sexuality, gender, and reproduction. Lawyers, policy makers, educators, clinicians, and practitioners who work with sexual minority parents and assisted reproductive technologies may also see this chapter as a valuable source of information. Finally, this chapter should be of interest to current gay fathers who have used surrogacy and gay prospective fathers who are interested in pursuing surrogacy arrangements.

I begin by outlining some of the guiding theoretical perspectives that have been used to frame the scholarship on sexual minority parenting and assisted reproductive technologies. Next, I detail the different types of surrogacy arrangements and the demographic profiles of those gay men who use surrogacy. I review the few yet promising studies on gay fathers and surrogacy, exploring the rationales behind the men's choice to construct their family using this pathway; the relationships that develop between expectant fathers, surrogate mothers, and their children; and finally, the consequences for family formation. Then, I briefly discuss the emerging trend of reproductive outsourcing, detailing how gay men now have the option to travel abroad to less developed nations and purchase the services of a surrogate mother at a relatively low price. I consider the current legal issues facing gay fathers who use surrogacy and conclude by offering suggestions for research, theory, policy makers, and practitioners.

Theoretical Frameworks

Several intersecting and complementary theoretical perspectives have guided the scholarship on sexual minority parenting and surrogacy. Oftentimes these perspectives integrate one or more of the following: symbolic interactionism (Berkowitz, 2007; Berkowitz & Marsiglio, 2007), social constructionism (Stacey, 2006), feminism (Ehrensaft, 2005; Ryan & Berkowitz, 2009; Stacey, 2006) and intersectionality (Stacey, 2006). Symbolic interactionism assumes that human beings possess the ability to think and imbue their world with meaning. Such a perspective

has been used to emphasize how gay men develop their self-as-father identities and how meanings of self, parent, child, and family emerge from gay men's interactions with surrogates, egg donors, agencies, extended families, and interlopers (Blumer, 1969; Mead, 1934). Similarly, a social constructionist perspective turns the spotlight on the extent to which families, gender, and sexualities are socially and materially constructed (Oswald, Blume, & Marks, 2005). When gay fathers conceive children with egg donors and surrogates, they expose the socially constructed reality behind taken for granted assumptions about parenting, fathering, and family. Moreover, gay fathers actively disentangle heterosexuality from parenthood and in doing so disrupt fundamental notions about family. Gay men who choose to parent can challenge normative definitions of family, fatherhood, and even established gender and sexual norms of the mainstream gay subculture. Thus, viewing gay fathers' involvement with their children through these lenses illuminates the fluidity of family, gender, and sexuality.

Much of the work on sexual minority parenting has been spearheaded by feminist scholars who have long challenged "the ideology of the monolithic family and the notion that any one family arrangement is natural, biological, or functional in a timeless way" (Goldberg & Allen, 2007, p. 354). Feminist scholarship has been instrumental in highlighting how gay fathers who become parents through surrogacy do not represent the disintegration of family, but rather constitute new, creative, and valid family constellations. Nevertheless, I argue that further intersectional feminist analysis (Collins, 1990) is needed to better unpack how gay fathers who are able to use surrogacy are embedded within wider systems of economic, historical, and political structures. Throughout this chapter I will demonstrate how privilege and subordination intersect in gay families constructed through surrogacy in complex ways (Baca-Zinn, 1994). Taking seriously the interlocking systems of privilege and oppression in the lived experiences of gay fathers who use surrogacy illuminates how these men's class privilege and often White privilege, allows them to buy their way out of discriminatory adoptive policies and stake out a 9-month lease on a surrogate mother's womb to construct a genetically related, and sometimes a genetically engineered, child (Dillaway, 2008).

Gay Fathers Using Surrogacy

Surrogacy is an assisted reproductive technology (ART) in which the prospective parent(s) forge a contract with a woman to carry their child (Bergman et al., 2010). There are two different types of surrogacy arrangements: traditional genetic surrogacy and gestational surrogacy. Traditional genetic surrogacy is when the surrogate mother is implanted with the sperm of a man, carries the fetus to term, and births a child, of whom she is genetically related (Bergman et al., 2010). Gestational surrogacy, which is also called in vitro fertilization (IVF) surrogacy, occurs when another woman's ovum is fertilized by one of the man's sperm using IVF and the resulting embryo is transplanted into another woman's womb (Bergman et al., 2010). In the latter case, the surrogate who carries the fetus to term and births the child is not genetically related to the child. Gestational surrogacy has become increasingly more common and accounts for approximately 95% of all surrogate pregnancies in the USA (Smerdon, 2008).

In 2006, the Ethics Committee of the American Society for Reproductive Medicine concluded that requests for assisted reproduction should be treated without regard for sexual orientation. Some argue that this will prompt a rise in the number of gay men who become fathers through surrogacy arrangements (Golombok & Tasker, 2010). However, simply because the Ethics Committee issued a statement of sexual inclusivity does not necessarily require individual surrogacy agencies to comply with such an endorsement. For example, despite the fact that multiple organizational bodies have endorsed adoption by gays and lesbians *and* advocate for second parent adoption (e.g., the American Psychological Association and the American Academy of Pediatrics), the legal and interpersonal barriers that gay men and lesbians face in adopting have been well documented by scholars (Brodzinsky, Patterson, & Vaziri, 2002). Thus, the extent to which the committee's statement is effective in pressuring surrogacy agencies to work with gay men is unknown. Future research is needed that explores the practices and policies of individual surrogacy agencies and personnel.

Although it is impossible to provide a definitive number of gay men who have become fathers through surrogacy, *Growing Generations*, the oldest and largest agency specializing in surrogacy arrangements for gay men reports on its Web site that since its inception in 1996, it has since worked with approximately 1,000 clients (http://www.growinggenerations.com/). At the time of writing there have been only two empirical studies to date on gay men and surrogacy (Bergman et al., 2010; Greenfeld & Seli, 2011). In the first study, the authors recruited 40 different couples who became parents using gestational surrogacy through *Growing Generations* and explored how these men experienced the transition to parenthood (Bergman et al., 2010).[1] In the second study, the researchers recruited 15 gay men from *The Yale Fertility Center* who were in the process of using their sperm to facilitate gestational surrogacy. The program's mental health counselor interviewed each of these men and their partners ($N=30$ men) to assess the psychosocial impacts of their experience.

Aside from these two very recent studies, there is a noteworthy absence of empirical literature on gay men's use of surrogacy. Diane Ehrensaft (2000, 2005), a clinical and developmental psychologist who specializes in psychotherapy and consultation with families formed through assisted reproductive technologies, has written extensively about surrogacy in the context of both heterosexual and gay- and lesbian-parent families. There have also been a handful of empirical qualitative studies on gay fathers that have included men who became fathers through surrogacy in their samples (Berkowitz, 2007; Berkowitz & Marsiglio, 2007; Mitchell & Green, 2007;

---

[1] Bergman et al. (2010) never divulge how many of these 40 men were biological fathers.

Ryan & Berkowitz, 2009; Stacey, 2006). For example, Berkowitz (2007) and Berkowitz and Marsiglio (2007) conducted interviews with gay prospective parents and with gay men who became parents through multiple pathways, including adoption, fostering, kinship ties, and surrogacy. Ryan and Berkowitz (2009) used in-depth interviews with gay fathers and lesbian mothers to document the heteronormative dynamics that govern adoption, donor insemination, and surrogacy. In a paper drawing primarily on clinical case material, Mitchell and Green (2007) detailed the various decisions that lesbians and gay men make when using donor insemination (DI) and surrogacy to conceive children. In one of the few ethnographic studies of gay men's kinship practices, Stacey (2006) described a diverse sample of gay parents, many of whom became fathers through surrogacy. Finally, although not an empirical study per se, Arlene Istar Lev (2006), a social worker, chronicled her experiences meeting and interacting with gay fathers who have used surrogacy. The findings from these limited studies and clinical and experiential reports form the foundation of much of this chapter.

The High Cost of Surrogacy

Surrogacy arrangements can be made independently between a gay male couple (or individual) and a female surrogate without the assistance of an agency. Legally, however, this is quite risky and can create a host of potential legal problems regarding custody of the child (Lev, 2006). Prior to the recent rise of agencies like *Growing Generations*, which are willing to work with single gay men and gay couples, gay men were forced to find surrogate mothers through placing ads in newspapers or through other informal channels like inviting friends or family members to serve as surrogates (Lev, 2006). However, now, to minimize a host of possible legal complications, many gay men choose to work through an agency, despite the fact that this increases the cost of surrogacy exponentially (Lev, 2006). Working with an agency is beneficial in that agency personnel assist fathers with introductions to possible surrogate mothers, screen the

surrogate mother medically and psychologically, provide counseling for all involved parties, and help to navigate convoluted bureaucratic red tape (Lev, 2006). As stated above, commercial surrogacy, as mediated through an agency, is typically the most expensive route to parenthood for gay men and can range anywhere from $115,000 to $150,000 (http://www.growinggenerations. com). Commercial traditional surrogacy involves financing the participation of the surrogate, the services of an agency, physician services, legal fees, and health insurance to cover all procedures. In addition to the above expenses, commercial gestational surrogacy requires financing the participation of the egg donor, the services of both an egg donor agency and a surrogate agency, IVF physician services, and health insurance to cover all procedures. For gay men using this route there is an added layer of complexity in that they must also finance the necessary legal costs to ensure assignment of custody following the birth of their child (Golombok & Tasker, 2010).

The high costs of surrogacy mean that it is only an option for a small number of relatively affluent gay men—a fact that is illustrated by the demographic composition of the participants in the Bergman et al. (2010) study on gay men and surrogacy in which the authors interviewed one of the partners in 40 couples who had conceived children through surrogacy.[2] The mean household income out of the 40 men in their sample was $270,000, a number vastly above the national average[3] and far above the mean household income of gay men adopting children—$102,331, according to the 2000 U.S. Census (Gates, Badgett, Macomber, & Chambers, 2007). Moreover, 14 out of these 40 fathers already had children currently enrolled in a private preschool at an average cost of $8,764 annually, and 67% planned on sending their children to private schools in the near future. Furthermore, 68% of the men in the sample reported using some type of child-care assistance, ranging from au pairs, to nannies, to housekeepers.

---

[2] The Greenfeld and Seli (2011) study did not include any information about household income.

[3] This number in only reflective of the 37 out of 40 men who answered the question on income.

With regards to the racial and ethnic composition of the Bergman et al. (2010) sample, 80% were White, 7.5% were Asian, 7.5% were Latino, and 5% Middle-Eastern. In the Greenfeld and Seli (2011) sample, 90% (or 27 of the men) identified as White; only 10%, or three men, identified as Latino. Notably, there were no African-American men in either sample. The gay fathers in these samples are also different from gay men who become parents through adoption in terms of their racial and ethnic diversity. Using U.S. Census data, Gates et al. (2007) estimated that among gay male adoptive parents, 61% were White, 15% were African-American, 15% were Latino, 4% were Asian/Pacific Islander, 1% American Indian, and 4% reported some other race/ethnicity. Thus, although both studies are limited by a small sample and by the fact that recruitment occurred through *Growing Generations* (Bergman et al., 2010) and *The Yale Fertility Center* (Greenfeld & Seli, 2011), the demographic characteristics of these men highlight the extent to which surrogacy is a procreative pathway only available to a racially and economically privileged minority.

Thinking About Parenting: Surrogacy as an Option

Research has documented that gay men become parents for many of the same reasons as heterosexual men: Both cite the desire for nurturing children, the constancy of children in their lives, the achievement of some sense of immortality through children, and the sense of family that children help to provide (Bigner & Jacobsen, 1989; Mallon, 2004). However, the social and psychological dimensions of gay men's reproductive decision making are additionally complicated by internalized homophobia, anxieties about raising properly gendered (and heterosexual) children, and structural obstacles such as lack of information and navigating legal barriers (Berkowitz & Marsiglio, 2007; Brinamen & Mitchell, 2008; Goldberg, 2010a). Moreover, unlike the majority of their heterosexual counterparts who couple, become pregnant, and give birth, gay men who wish to parent must carefully

consider a variety of other variables when contemplating parenthood. Such considerations include deciding on how they should go about creating a family, i.e., whether it should be through adoption, foster parenting, kinship ties, or through surrogacy arrangements. Embedded in these decisions are issues of cost, access, and the extent to which a genetic relationship is perceived as important by men in their conceptualizations of family.

Oftentimes, those gay men who choose surrogacy are motivated by the higher degree of control they have in the process when compared with adoption, feel that the presence of a genetic link to their child is an important factor for the creation of family ties, and worry about the psychological stress a child may experience as a result of being adopted (Goldberg, 2010a; Lev, 2006). For example, one man told Lev (2006) that he chose surrogacy because "it was the only way our child would be born without sadness as a part of his life story, i.e., there was someone who had to give you up, didn't want you, couldn't care for you" (p. 76). In viewing an adopted child as always already wounded, or psychologically damaged, this man sets up a hierarchical pattern of families wherein those not formed through such privileged means like surrogacy are deemed less valuable. Scholars studying sexual minority parenting should be careful not to reproduce existing hierarchies in how they interpret research findings. Gay men's families constructed through surrogacy can be respected without treating them as any more privileged than families constructed through adoption, fostering, or kinship ties.

Even for those gay men who are open to adopting a child, depending on the laws of the state where they reside, adoption may either be prohibitive or laws governing adoption might be vague and unclear (Lev, 2006). For example, one gay father who lived in Florida reported that surrogacy was his best possible option for creating a family, given that Florida explicitly barred nonheterosexual adoption (Ryan & Berkowitz, 2009). Although most states do not have explicit statutes barring adoption by gay men (and at the time of writing the legalities in Florida are currently under appeal), the legal and interpersonal barriers that gay men and lesbians face in adopting have been well documented (Brodzinsky et al., 2002). One gay man in Lev's (2006) report explained that he and his partner "decided on surrogacy versus adoption because the laws are so vague that they could deny us a child strictly based on our orientation" (p. 76). Similarly, consider the following quote from another gay father who chose to use surrogacy:

> The thing about adoption is…that even though that child or those children are legally yours, they are never your children. And that is very frightening to me. That [we] would have this wonderful child or children through adoption and then at some point, something could happen, either through the courts or a change of the birth mother's mind…it is very unsettling to me and scared me. It scared me that the family we would create would be shaken by the birth mother or the genetic father coming back into our lives or the baby's life (Drew, gay father through surrogacy, as cited in Ryan & Berkowitz, 2009).

Reigning social norms establish biological relatedness as critical for defining family. Moreover, because gay men are often denied ceremonial and legal recognition of their families, the presence of a genetic link can be a meaningful symbol that validates their relationship to their child. Given these considerations, it should not be surprising that the presence of a genetic relationship is the most oft cited reason that gay men choose surrogacy (Lev, 2006).

The Family Tree: Gay Fathers, Surrogate Mothers, Egg Donors, and Their Children

Surrogacy is similar to DI in that it allows for one parent to be genetically related to the child and it involves a biological "other" to provide the other half of the genetic material. However, in the case of surrogacy, there is an added dimension not present in DI wherein another person—a female body—also carries the fetus to term and births the child. Thus, a critical difference between DI and surrogacy is that surrogacy always includes a physically present (female) body. However, despite this crucial departure, many of the complexities that accompany DI are also relevant in the context of surrogacy. For example, while surrogacy provides one parent a genetic link it also introduces a genetic asymmetry such that only one partner has a biological bond to the child

(Goldberg, 2010a). This of course may prompt couples to wonder how this biological connection will shape parent–child bonding and can even provoke jealous feelings in the partner who is not genetically related to the child (Ehrensaft, 2005). Moreover, questions about the source of the sperm can privilege one partner in a gay male couple. Although many gay fathers choose to find out whose sperm actually impregnated the surrogate (or, in many cases, the egg donor), some gay fathers report creatively bypassing this issue by mixing their sperm before insemination and choose not to find out whose sperm was ultimately responsible for conception following the birth of their child (Ryan & Berkowitz, 2009).

Given these complex negotiations, the decision of whose sperm should be used to impregnate the egg donor or surrogate is a significant one. Scholars know very little about gay couples' decision-making processes regarding whom of the two men should supply the sperm. Findings from studies with lesbian couples who use DI reveal that oftentimes this decision is predicated upon who has a greater desire to experience pregnancy and childbirth (Chabot & Ames, 2004; Goldberg, 2006)—a moot point of contention for gay couples. However, other issues surfaced with lesbian couples that may be similar for gay couples, such as fertility, health, and age considerations (Chabot & Ames, 2004; Goldberg, 2006). The Greenfeld and Seli (2011) study provides some initial evidence for how gay men using surrogacy make decisions about which partner should supply the sperm. In this sample, 12 couples, or 80%, deliberately chose who would inseminate the egg donor. Decisions were made with the following considerations in mind: six couples agreed that the older partner should provide the sperm, two couples had a partner who had already fathered children in a previous heterosexual relationship and thus thought that the other partner should have this opportunity as well, two couples chose the partner who had a stronger desire to be a biological parent, and two couples reported that they decided to go with the partner who had "better genes" (p. 227). In the remaining three couples, both partners had equivalent desires for biological parenthood and thus inseminated equal numbers of eggs. Two of these three couples produced twins who were half-siblings. With regards to the one couple who had a single child, the authors did not report whether the couple ultimately discovered who was the genetic parent.

Some research has suggested that choices about who should supply the sperm and have a genetic relationship to the child might be contingent upon one partner's belief that their family of origin is more likely to accept a child who is genetically related to them. In fact, there is some evidence that when only one parent has a genetic link to the child, some families of origin may be slow to accord full parental status to the other partner (Mitchell & Green, 2007). Sometimes families of the biological parent might see the child as belonging only to their own family, and families of the nongenetically related parent may neglect to see the child as a part of their family. Indeed, studies on lesbian women who became mothers through DI reveal that genetics matter for how families of origin relate to their grandchildren. For example, Gartrell et al. (2000) interviewed 84 lesbian parent-headed families and found that women reported a greater perceived investment from the families of origin of the mothers who had a biological tie to the child as compared to the families of origin of the mothers who were not biologically related to the child. Similarly, the nonbiological mothers in Hequembourg and Farrell's (1999) qualitative study on lesbian women who became parents though DI reported that their extended families were resistant to viewing them as legitimate mothers because they lacked both a biological and legal tie to their children. Future research is needed to see how gay men's families of origin relate to and bond with children conceived and birthed through surrogacy, particularly in those cases where a father is unable to secure a biological or legal relationship to the child.

Who Is the Surrogate Mother and/or Egg Donor?

Research with heterosexual and gay and lesbian couples has documented that parents who use assisted reproductive technologies like surrogacy are often motivated by the high level of control they have in choosing what their child will look like through carefully evaluating the characteristics of the surrogate mother and/or egg donor (Ehrensaft, 2005; Ryan & Berkowitz, 2009). For example, prospective parents often look for surrogates who resemble themselves or their partners in terms of race, ethnicity, religious affiliation, vocational interests, personal characteristics, and appearance (Mitchell & Green, 2007; Ryan & Berkowitz, 2009). The most common request from the men in Greenfeld and Seli's sample (2011) was for an egg donor who was tall, attractive, educated, and closely resembled the non-inseminating partner. Some gay prospective fathers have reported that as they evaluate their surrogates-to-be, they carefully cogitate on the importance of racial and ethnic matching, speculating how adding another dimension like racial differences to their already publicly perplexing family might confuse their child or encumber interactions with curious interlopers (deBoer, 2009; Ryan & Berkowitz, 2009). Prospective fathers often consider the extent to which they are willing to make what is already a conspicuous gay family even more conspicuous by becoming an interracial family (deBoer, 2009). Consider the following quote from a father in Ryan and Berkowitz's (2009) study:

> Well, on the website a lot of the women were 4 foot 2, Guatemalan women; it just wasn't going to work for us....We wanted to find a surrogate who was White and get rid of one other problem that these children, or child would have to deal with, you know, to be mixed race.

Making separate choices about an egg donor and a gestational surrogate allows intended parents to choose among a wider pool of egg donors, and the ability to select a donor whose physical, cultural, and biographical characteristics are more similar to themselves or their partners. Since there is a significantly smaller pool of gestational surrogates than egg donors, once the genetic concerns associated with the selection of the egg donor have been addressed, the choice of the surrogate is less constrained (Mitchell & Green, 2007). Thus, commercial surrogacy and egg donation makes it such that those men who can afford to do so "can literally purchase the means to eugenically reproduce White infants in their own idealized image, selecting desired traits in egg donors...with whom to mate their own DNA"

(Stacey, 2006, p. 39). In fact, in her advice to parents seeking assisted reproductive technologies, Ehrensaft (2005) writes that "you can feel that you have the whole world in your hands" as you "discover the power to craft the child that will be yours" (p. 42). This gives affluent gay men, who wish to become parents, the ability to regain control of their reproductive options. Those with the financial wherewithal literally have the purchasing power to procure a womb *and* produce a genetically engineered child (Dillaway, 2008).

Before actually meeting face-to-face, gay prospective parents thoughtfully peruse pamphlets and Web sites with pictures and descriptions of potential surrogates and/or egg donors (Ryan & Berkowitz, 2009). This initial screening of what Hertz (2002) has termed the "paper parent" happens within a context in which babies are increasingly viewed as precious commodities. Ehrensaft (2005) argues that this commodification is further magnified for those using assisted reproductive technologies since these intended parents have spent months, even years, searching for a donor or surrogate and draining financial resources paying for expensive procedures. For gay men, this process is further intensified since they are not only limited by the reproductive limits of their bodies, but have been told by religious, political, and cultural institutions that fatherhood was never an option for them. When viewed through a heteronormative lens, the idea of shopping for a child's features among potential egg donors or searching for a surrogate with the healthiest possible womb may be viewed as an unnecessary luxury akin to crafting a perfect child. However, for gay men using surrogacy, this process takes on a whole new meaning, as it is one of the few ways that they are able to manage the discord between dominant heterosexual reproductive scripts and their own reproductive experiences.

How Can We Trust Her? What Are Her Motives?

Surrogacy makes it such that the gay male couple, or the gay man, wait for a child to be birthed by a woman they may barely know. Moreover, because a surrogate mother cannot maintain the same anonymity that a sperm donor can, surrogacy involves an enormous amount of trust, even with accompanying legal protections. Some gay fathers may express anxiety about the child potentially developing a bond to the surrogate, while others may wonder about the woman's attachment to the child she is carrying (Ehrensaft, 2000; Lev, 2006). Some gay fathers have reported that an important criterion for a desirable surrogate was her ability to not bond with the child she is carrying (Lev, 2006).

Alongside an evaluation of the surrogate mother's biographical characteristics of age, race, physical attractiveness, medical history, intelligence, athleticism, and artistic ability, gay men also inquire about her motives. Although surrogates are reimbursed approximately $20,000, the majority report that they are not motivated solely by money, but rather by altruism, selflessness, and a desire to help a family have a child (Lev, 2006). Nonetheless, in a two-decade-old study done at the Infertility Center of New York, 89% of surrogate mothers admitted that they would not agree to serve as a surrogate mother unless they were paid a substantial fee (Dillaway, 2008). Thus, some researchers and social commentators assert that money is a substantial factor in motivating surrogate mothers, even if an altruistic motive is also present (Dillaway, 2008). People desiring children through surrogacy often grapple with whether the birth mother is motivated purely by financial means or by an inclination to help people in need of children (Ehrensaft, 2005). Gay men, having few other options for birthing children, may be especially worried about this motivation. However, in Stacey's (2006) ethnographic research on gay men and kinship, she found that some surrogates actually preferred to work with gay men because there was no mother in the picture who might potentially be dealing with feelings of jealousy, infertility, and exclusion. Moreover, unlike heterosexual couples, for which assisted reproductive technologies are usually a last resort, gay fathers turn to surrogacy joyfully as a pathway to parenthood. Because such assisted technologies are universally necessary for gay men who wish to create their own biological offspring, they carry none of the stigma or sense of failure of many infertile heterosexual couples (Mitchell & Green, 2007). Thus, theoretically it is possible that gay men might very well enjoy more harmonious relationships with surrogates, in the sense that "they did not arrive at surrogacy because of infertility and there is no symbolic or actual female for the surrogate to compete with or feel challenged by" (Goldberg, 2010a, p. 72).

The Surrogate Mother: A Present and Absent Figure

While the basis of commercial surrogacy is a financial arrangement, the realities are such that this is often a relationship pervaded by appreciation, mutual respect, and gratitude, with many gay fathers often forging deep bonds with their surrogates (Mitchell & Green, 2007). The notion of the birth mother who helps make the possibility of a baby come true weaves in and out of the entire life span of any family using surrogacy (Berkowitz, 2006; Mitchell & Green, 2007). The uniqueness of gay family formations can be seen at the time of pregnancy through the ways in which they attempt to manage the schism between dominant understandings of pregnancy and their experiences of it. Gay men have to place themselves in an experience that would not traditionally include either partner, particularly the nonbiologically related father. The limited empirical research on gay fathers who have used surrogacy suggests that they cultivate ways to share in the pregnancy experience of their surrogate. Some document their experience with scrapbooks or by giving their surrogate mother a video camera, while others use e-mail, skype, and webcams to keep up-to-date with belly growth, fetal development, ultrasound pictures, and doctors appointments (Berkowitz & Marsiglio, 2007). Even well after the pregnancy and birth, many gay fathers choose to have ongoing relationships with their surrogates, and in some cases, with their egg donors (Mitchell & Green, 2007). These relationships are sometimes maintained through letters, pictures, or in some cases the families stay distant friends. A few of

the fathers that Lev (2006) interviewed were so close with their surrogate that they named her godmother to their child. Although this pattern of designating the surrogate as a godmother was rather rare, the majority of gay fathers told Lev (2006) that they shared a distant, albeit caring relationship with their surrogates. Future research is needed to address how gay fathers and their surrogate mothers negotiate the childrearing boundaries that may result from this complex kinship arrangement.

The experiences of gay fathers show the contradictory status of the surrogate mother's (and egg donor's) relationship to the family as a simultaneously present and absent figure (Ehrensaft, 2005; Hertz, 2002). For some families, she is *present* through the recognition of the important contribution of her genetic material, her physical body, and her contribution to their family. But she can be *absent* in terms of a conventional social relationship to their kin (Ehrensaft, 2005). Although the paradoxical notion of presence and absence can be expected in any family arrangement that relies on assisted reproduction or adoption, it is especially evident in gay father-headed families because of the constant societal reminder that this third party was a necessity in creating their families.

Constructing Family Stories with and for Children

Like those families constructed through DI, surrogacy raises questions about a "symbolic other" necessary for the creation of a family that parents, children, extended family members, and other social actors must constantly negotiate. One commonality shared by families constructed through surrogacy and DI is that parents may struggle with how to tell their children the story of their inception. One way to do this is to celebrate a child's conception day, in addition to the child's actual birthday, as this becomes an important date that gay fathers who created their families though surrogacy are unique in knowing (Mitchell & Green, 2007). How gay fathers answer personal queries about their child's conception ultimately serves as a model for how their children will deal with similar situations and construct their own family stories. As these children grow older they cannot rely on a legacy of cultural givens, but rather must establish on their own the meanings and significance of their extended family (Mitchell & Green, 2007). Like their parents, children raised with an understanding of assisted reproductive technologies like that of surrogacy may be less inclined to conflate sex and reproduction, and thus may have a unique ability to challenge these taken for granted connections among their peers. Future research is needed on how children born to gay fathers and surrogate mothers negotiate dominant family ideology as they understand their family stories and communicate these stories to others.

How Does Life Change with the Transition to Parenthood?

Like all sexual minority parents, gay men who have become fathers through surrogacy face an adjustment to parenting "under the hegemonic shadow of the heterosexual paradigm" (deBoer, 2009, p. 333). Data from Bergman et al.'s study (2010) reveal that gay men who become parents using surrogacy experience similar life changes as heterosexual fathers. Many fathers in their study described shifting their schedules and their priorities to accommodate their child care responsibilities and their new role as parents. Fathers reported lessening work hours, switching jobs, and some even became stay-at-home dads. Sometimes these changes resulted in a decrease in household income. By decreasing their ties to paid labor and increasing their presence in the home, these men challenge socially constructed cultural narratives that assume men are incompetent nurturers and that gay men are antifamily and irresponsible.

Such findings are not unique to those gay men who become fathers through surrogacy. Studies conducted with gay fathers who became parents through adoption and fostering have documented similar findings (Lassiter et al. 2006; Mallon, 2004; Schacher, Auerbach, & Silverstein,

2005). However, other scholars have argued that the assumption that gay men's marginalized location from traditional family life means that gay fathers always resist and transform traditional notions of gayness, fathering, and family is overly reductionistic (Goldberg, 2010b). Such reasoning fails to account for the diversity within these families and the role of contextual variables like institutional support and the broader sociopolitical and legal milieu (Goldberg, 2010b). Take for example the fact that 68% of the men in Bergman et al.'s (2010) sample relied on hired help to assist with child care and domestic duties. Clearly, although many gay fathers challenge stereotypes of men as primary caregivers, many are also able to buy their way out of domesticity, a finding intimately tied to both their class position in society and their ability as male bodied parents to continue to rely on the privilege granted to the traditional father-as-breadwinner status. Moreover, because surrogacy is only available to an economically privileged minority of gay men, it seems reasonable to believe that a larger proportion of gay men who have become fathers through surrogacy are more likely to outsource domestic help than those who became fathers through adoption, fostering, or through kinship ties. Future research is needed to see if this is indeed the case.

Bergman et al. (2010) reported that one of the most striking findings from their study on gay men who became fathers through surrogacy was men's descriptions of heightened self-esteem from having and raising children. In addition, these men reported an increase in support and acceptance from both their families of origin and their partners' families of origin since they had become parents, even in cases where families of origin were not biologically related to new children—a finding similarly documented among new lesbian mothers (Goldberg, 2006). With the initiation of the parenting role comes a shift in adult gay children's relationships with their aging parents who often take pride in their new identities as grandparents (deBoer, 2009). Where this is certainly an experience shared by most parents, there is an added dimension for gay fathers since there is a lack of ceremonial and legal validation of their relationships. However, these findings contradict earlier work by Oswald (2002) who found that LGB parents perceived lesser support from their families of origin than heterosexual parents. That Oswald's study was conducted with nonmetropolitan parents of more marginalized social class backgrounds underscores the importance of untangling the class and regional dynamics that surface within different sexual minority headed households. Further research is needed to examine how interlocking systems of oppression and privilege differentially shape the transition to parenthood and the parenting experiences of gay fathers who use surrogacy.

Gay Fathers, Surrogacy, and Reproductive Outsourcing

Reproductive outsourcing is a relatively new but rapidly expanding enterprise. Couples and singles from the West can now travel to countries like India, Ukraine, Russia, and Guatemala and employ a foreign surrogate mother to gestate their baby. Where surrogacy has always been a practice marred with class distinctions, the emerging phenomenon of what some are calling fertility tourism (Smerdon, 2008) magnifies the inequality between commissioning parent and surrogate (and/or egg donor). It is not surprising then that many are skeptical of fertility tourism and see it as a system that allows "wealthy infertile couples to treat third parties from disenfranchised groups as 'passports' to reproduction" (Smerdon, 2008, p. 24).

India is quickly becoming the top destination spot for fertility tourists due to a number of interrelated factors like skilled medical professionals, liberal laws and regulations, and most importantly, low prices (Gentleman, 2008). Although there are no firm statistics on how many arrangements between Western commissioners and Indian surrogates exist, anecdotal evidence indicates a sharp increase in recent years. There are no federal or state regulations on which clients clinics can treat, and even though some clinics refuse to accept gay men and lesbians, others declare themselves to be LGBT friendly (Smerdon, 2008). Thus, gay men seeking surrogacy in India are at the mercy of individual clinicians and may even face the possibility of temporarily being pushed back into the closet. Those seeking such an arrangement may have to carefully decide if the low cost of a foreign womb is worth the high price of closeting themselves.

The emerging trend of reproductive outsourcing and fertility tourism poses many research questions for family scholars. For example, future research on gay fathers should explore how these men navigate the global bureaucracy of reproductive outsourcing. Furthermore, since the primary seduction of fertility tourism is its significantly lower cost, it is reasonable to presume that more and more gay men who value the presence of a genetic link to their children will consider this a viable procreative pathway. As the possibility of a biological child becomes more widely available to a new cohort of gay fathers, one cannot help but wonder what the consequences will be for local adoptable children, particularly those who are already deemed undesirable because of their race, ethnicity, age, or disability. Moreover, future research should ask how our shifting global reproductive economy will affect how less economically privileged gay men view the importance of a biological relationship for constructing family ties. Finally, as detailed below, this emerging global reproductive economy poses a host of legal issues that are yet to be resolved.

Legal Issues Facing Gay Surrogate Families

The legal context in the USA has changed dramatically in the past decade with regard to gay and lesbian couples and parents. Despite a number of advances, the legal landscape is still challenging terrain for many gay and lesbian parents. Although commercial surrogacy is highly regulated in the USA by private industry with "rigorous procedures such as psychological testing and interviews, genetic histories, and careful matching of donors and surrogates" (Bergman et al., 2010, p. 117), the federal government does not regulate surrogacy at all, and control and oversight of surrogacy arrangements is relinquished to individual state jurisdiction. Thus, those pursuing this procreative pathway are often left to navigate inconsistencies among states laws, legislative action, and court decisions (Smerdon, 2008). According to the Human Rights Campaign (2010a), six states currently allow individuals and couples to enter into surrogacy contracts: Arkansas, California, Illinois (gestational surrogacy only), Massachusetts, New Jersey (uncompensated surrogacy agreements only), and Washington (uncompensated surrogacy agreements only). The District of Columbia and 11 states prohibit surrogacy agreements in all or some instances. The District of Columbia, Nevada, New York, North Dakota, Texas, Utah, Virginia, and Florida prohibit surrogacy for all unmarried couples—thus prohibiting it for gay men; Indiana and Louisiana prohibit traditional surrogacy; and Michigan and Nebraska prohibit compensated surrogacy agreements. The remaining 34 states have vague or unclear laws and/or court case rulings on whether surrogacy agreements are allowed (Human Rights Campaign, 2010a).

Gay men who are considering surrogacy should be aware of these state-by-state regulations. Moreover, they should find an agency that is not only open to working with sexual minorities but also understands how to traverse the state-by-state surrogacy and Defense of Marriage Act (DOMA) laws. For example, the way that legal parentage under surrogacy works is such that the initial determination of parentage for a baby occurs within the state that a baby is born. So, if a heterosexual couple from New York, a state where surrogacy is illegal contracts with a surrogacy in California, that matches them with a surrogate in Louisiana, the initial determination of parentage would occur in Louisiana. However, the stakes would play out very differently for a gay couple in this scenario. Because Louisiana is referred to as a "super-DOMA" state (this means Louisiana does not allow same-sex couples those privileges granted to married couples), a same-sex couple would not be able to establish parentage in this state and would instead need to establish parentage for at least one of the partners in a different state (Goldberg, 2010a).

Adoption laws also vary by state and jurisdiction and very few states guarantee same-sex couples access to joint or *second-parent adoptions*. Second-parent adoptions allow the partner of a legal/biological parent to also adopt the child—thus becoming the second legally recognized parent (Pawelski et al., 2006). Second-parent adoptions are important for the safety and welfare of families in that they ensure that both parents have the ability to make emergency medical decisions for their children and are responsible for the financial support of their children even if the parents should separate (Pawelski et al., 2006). Currently, nine states (and DC) have statutes or appellate court rulings that guarantee gay and lesbian couples access to second-parent adoptions statewide, while perhaps as many as 18 other states have allowed second-parent adoptions by gay or lesbian parents in some jurisdictions (Human Rights Campaign, 2010b). In some cases second-parent adoption is not required, as two men can both be listed on the original birth certificate of a child born to a surrogate if a prebirth paternity judgment is obtained declaring both of them to be the sole parents (Pinkerton, 1998). This legal precedent was established when in 1998, Will Halm, a family law attorney specializing in surrogacy and egg donations, and the chair of *Growing Generations*, challenged the law in California. The California Supreme Court granted him and his partner the first ever pre-birth paternity judgment, naming the gay couple the legal parents of their son prior to his birth, thus eliminating the need for a second-parent adoption (Lev, 2006). Overall, the legal aspects surrounding surrogacy and sexual minority parents are for the most part rather unsettled. The courts fall terribly behind the realities of these families, regularly failing to protect them.

Suggestions for Research, Policy, and Practice

Commercial surrogacy is certainly one of the most high-tech and expensive paths to gay parenthood. The relatively high cost of surrogacy means that those men who create their families through this route typically have significantly higher incomes than men who may opt to become parents through adoption, fostering, or kinship ties. Gay men who become fathers using surrogacy are unique in that they are primarily White affluent men who have a biological tie to their child. These interlocking privileged positions can shield them from some of the vulnerabilities that gay men of Color, gay men with lesser incomes, and gay men who adopt all too often encounter. Nonetheless these men are similar to gay fathers in other contexts like adoption or fostering in that their path to parenting entails a great deal of thought, planning, and decision making.

Despite the growing body of scholarly work on gay fathers, we still know very little about the transition to parenthood and the parenting experiences of gay men who choose surrogacy. Future research should be conducted using comparative studies with samples of gay fathers in other contexts and with heterosexual fathers and mothers who became parents through surrogacy. Moreover, further research on gay families constructed through surrogacy is needed to better understand the extent to which the genetic connection between one of the fathers and the child affects the family dynamics, the division of domestic and paid labor, and relationships with family of origin. Scholars should also examine the degree and types of contact that exist between the surrogate and/or egg donor and the gay parents and their children after the birth of the child. Finally, additional work is needed to explore how gay fathers using surrogacy deal with their growing visibility in their diverse communities.

Further theorizing is required to better understand how constructions of race, family, and sociopolitical power are embedded in the relationships among gay fathers, surrogates, egg donors, and their children. As Rothman (1989) observed over two decades ago, surrogate motherhood was not brought to us by scientific progress; rather it was brought to us by brokers who saw the potential of a new market. Moreover, insomuch as our reproductive economy is becoming increasingly globalized, I urge scholars to better develop theories that situate sexual minority parenting within a feminist transnational framework that highlights the role of social structures and the state and can better account for the asymmetries and inequalities that are produced and sustained by flows of global capital (Kim, Puri, & Kim-Puri, 2005).

Policy makers need to be aware that gay men are having children through assisted reproductive technologies like that of surrogacy. As such, the rights afforded to heterosexual parents using surrogacy need to be extended to gay men, their partners, and their children. At a basic level, surrogacy agencies, lawyers, fertility specialists, and other health care professionals must work to communicate a philosophy of inclusion and acceptance for gay prospective fathers. Also, clinicians need to acknowledge that surrogate parenthood is increasingly common for gay men, both in the USA and abroad. Clinicians should assist gay men using surrogacy in their family planning, with special attention to the areas that uniquely define their transition to parenthood, like negotiating asymmetrical biological relatedness, obtaining co-parent or second parent adoptions, and exposure to heterosexist institutions and practices. Furthermore, for those couples who choose to have half of the eggs fertilized by one partner and half by the other, counseling should include considerations about the possible consequences that might result from this option. For example, the couple should be made aware of the genetic asymmetry that will result if they birth a single child, and of the possibility of having twins who share the same maternal genetics but different paternal genetics.

The parenting and family landscape is changing rapidly before our eyes and we now have extraordinary technological advances that combine eggs and sperm in what were until very recently unimaginable ways. Gay fathers choosing surrogacy are at the cutting edge of pushing society to reassess its assumptions and constructions about sex, reproduction, and parenthood. We can be certain that as more and more people are thinking about creative ways to have babies, the lessons learned from this emerging cohort of gay men who have become fathers through surrogacy will impact how we engage the new family forms of the twenty-first century.

References

Baca-Zinn, M. (1994). Feminist thinking from racial-ethnic families. In S. Fergusen (Ed.), *Shifting the center: Understanding contemporary families* (pp. 18–27). Boston: McGraw Hill.

Bergman, K., Rubio, R. J., Green, R. J., & Padron, E. (2010). Gay men who become fathers via surrogacy: The transition to parenthood. *Journal of GLBT Family Studies, 6*, 111–141. doi:10.1080/15504281003704942

Berkowitz, D. (2006). *Gay men: Negotiating procreative, father, and family identities*. (Unpublished doctoral dissertation). University of Florida, Gainesville, FL.

Berkowitz, D. (2007). A sociohistorical analysis of gay men's procreative consciousness. *Journal of GLBT Family Studies, 3*, 157–190. doi:10.1300/J461v03n02_07

Berkowitz, D., & Marsiglio, W. (2007). Gay men: Negotiating procreative, father, and family identities. *Journal of Marriage and Family, 69*, 366–381. doi:10.1111/j.1741-3737.2007.00371.x

Bigner, J. J., & Jacobsen, B. R. (1989). Parenting behaviors of homosexual and heterosexual fathers. *Journal of Homosexuality, 18*, 173–186. doi:10.1300/J082v18n01_09

Blumer, H. (1969). *Symbolic interactionism: Perspective and method*. Englewood Cliffs, NJ: Prentice-Hall.

Brinamen, C. F., & Mitchell, V. (2008). Gay men becoming fathers: A model of identity expansion. *Journal of GLBT Family Studies, 4*, 521–541. doi:10.1080/15504280802191772

Brodzinsky, D., Patterson, C., & Vaziri, M. (2002). Adoption agency perspectives on lesbian and gay prospective parents: A national study. *Adoption Quarterly, 5*, 5–23. doi:10.1300/J145v05n03_02

Chabot, J. M., & Ames, B. D. (2004). "It wasn't let's get pregnant and do it": Decision-making in lesbian couples planning motherhood via donor insemination. *Family Relations, 53*, 348–356. doi:10.1111/j.0197-6664.2004.00041.x

Collins, P. H. (1990). *Black feminist thought: Knowledge, consciousness, and the politics of empowerment*. New York: Routledge.

deBoer, D. (2009). Focus on the family: The psychosocial context of gay men choosing fatherhood. In P. L. Hammack & B. J. Cohler (Eds.), *The story of sexual identity: Narrative perspectives on the gay and lesbian life course* (pp. 327–346). New York: Oxford University Press.

Dillaway, H. E. (2008). Mothers for others: A race, class, and gender analysis of surrogacy. *International Journal of Sociology of the Family, 34*, 301–326.

Ehrensaft, D. (2000). Alternatives to the stork: Fatherhood fantasies in donor insemination families. *Studies in Gender and Sexuality, 1*, 371–397. doi:10.1080/15240650109349165

Ehrensaft, D. (2005). *Mommies, daddies, donors, surrogates: Answering tough questions and building strong families*. New York: Guilford Press.

Gartrell, N., Banks, A., Reed, N., Hamilton, J., Rhodas, C., & Deck, A. (2000). The National Lesbian Family Study: 3. Interviews with mothers of five-year-olds. *American Journal of Orthopsychiatry, 70*, 542–548. doi:10.1037/h0087823

Gates, G. (2007). *Geographic trends among same-sex couples in the U.S. Census and the American Community Survey*. Los Angeles: The Williams Institute.

Gates, G., Badgett, M. V. L., Macomber, J. E., & Chambers, K. (2007). *Adoption and foster care by gay and lesbian parents in the United States*. Washington, DC: The Urban Institute.

Gentleman, A. (2008). Foreign couples turn to India for surrogate mothers. *New York Times*. Retrieved from http://www.nytimes.com/2008/03/04/world/asia/04iht-mother.1.10690283.html

Goldberg, A. E. (2006). The transition to parenthood for lesbian couples. *Journal of GLBT Family Studies, 2*, 13–42. doi:10.1300/J461v02n01_02

Goldberg, A. E. (2010a). *Lesbian and gay parents and their children: Research on the family life cycle*. Washington, DC: American Psychological Association. doi:10.1037/12055-000

Goldberg, A. E. (2010b). Studying complex families in context. *Journal of Marriage and Family, 72*, 29–34. doi:10.1111/j.1741-3737.2009.00680.x

Goldberg, A. E., & Allen, K. R. (2007). Imagining men: Lesbian mothers' perceptions of male involvement during the transition to parenthood. *Journal of Marriage and Family, 69*, 352–365. doi:10.1111/j.1741-3737.2007.00370.x

Golombok, S., & Tasker, F. (2010). Gay fathers. In M. E. Lamb (Ed.), *The role of the father in child development* (pp. 319–340). Hoboken, NJ: Wiley.

Greenfeld, D. A., & Seli, E. (2011). Gay men choosing parenthood through assisted reproduction: Medical and psychosocial considerations. *Fertility and Sterility, 95*, 225–229. doi:10.1016/j.fertnstert.2010.05.053

Hequembourg, A., & Farrell, M. (1999). Lesbian motherhood: Negotiating marginal-mainstream identities. *Gender and Society, 13*, 540–555. doi:10.1177/089124399013004007

Hertz, R. (2002). The father as an idea: A challenge to kinship boundaries by single mothers. *Symbolic Interaction, 25*, 1–32. doi:10.1525/si.2002.25.1.1

Human Rights Campaign (2010a). *Surrogacy laws: State by state*. Retrieved from http://www.hrc.org/issues/2486.htm

Human Rights Campaign (2010b). *Second-parent adoption*. Retrieved from http://www.hrc.org/issues/2385.htm

Kim, S. H., Puri, J., & Kim-Puri, H. J. (2005). Conceptualizing gender-sexuality-state-nation: An introduction. *Gender and Society, 19*, 137–159. doi:10.1177/0891243204273021

Lassiter, P. S., Dew, B. J., Newton, K., Hays, D. G., & Yarbrough, B. (2006). Self-defined empowerment for gay and lesbian parents: A qualitative explanation. *The Family Journal, 14*, 245–252. doi:10.1177/1066480706287274

Lev, A. I. (2006). Gay dads: Choosing surrogacy. *Lesbian & Gay Psychology Review, 7*, 73–77.

Lewin, E. (2009). *Gay fatherhood: Narratives of family and citizenship in America.* Chicago: University of Chicago Press.

Mallon, G. P. (2004). *Gay men choosing parenthood.* New York: Columbia University Press.

Mead, G. H. (1934). *Mind, self, and society.* Chicago: University of Chicago Press.

Mitchell, V., & Green, R. J. (2007). Different storks for different folks: Gay and lesbian parents' experiences with alternative insemination and surrogacy. *Journal of GLBT Family Studies, 3*, 81–104. doi:10.1300/J461v03n02_04

Oswald, R. (2002). Resilience within the families of lesbians and gay men: Intentionality and redefinition. *Journal of Marriage and Family, 64*, 374–383. doi:10.1111/j.1741-3737.2002.00374.x

Oswald, R. F., Blume, L. B., & Marks, S. R. (2005). Decentering heteronormativity: A proposal for family studies. In V. Bengston, A. Acock, K. Allen, P. Dilworth-Anderson, & D. Klein (Eds.), *Sourcebook of family theories and methods: An interactive approach* (pp. 143–165). Newbury Park, CA: Sage.

Pawelski, J. G., Perrin, E. C., Foy, J. M., Allen, C. F., Crawford, M. D. M., & Kaufman, M. (2006). The effects of marriage, civil union, and domestic partnership laws on the health and well-being of children. *Pediatrics, 118*, 349–364. doi:10.1542/peds.2006-1279

Pinkerton, T. M. (1998). *Surrogacy and egg donation law in California.* Retrieved from http://www.surrogacy.com/legals/article/calaw.html

Rothman, B. K. (1989). *Recreating motherhood: Ideology and technology in a patriarchal society.* New York: W. W. Norton.

Ryan, M., & Berkowitz, D. (2009). Constructing gay and lesbian families 'beyond the closet'. *Qualitative Sociology, 32*, 153–172. doi:10.1007/s11133-009-9124-6

Schacher, S., Auerbach, C. F., & Silverstein, L. B. (2005). Gay fathers. Expanding the possibilities for all of us. *Journal of GLBT Family Studies, 1*, 31–52. doi:10.1300/J461v01n03_02

Smerdon, U. R. (2008). Crossing bodies, crossing borders: International surrogacy between the U.S. and India. *Cumberland Law Review, 39*, 15–85.

Stacey, J. (1996). *In the name of the family: Rethinking family values in the postmodern age.* Boston, MA: Beacon Press.

Stacey, J. (2006). Gay parenthood and the decline of paternity as we knew it. *Sexualities, 9*, 27–55. doi:10.1177/1363460706060687

Where Is the "B" in LGBT Parenting? A Call for Research on Bisexual Parenting

Lori E. Ross and Cheryl Dobinson

Introduction

In the context of a growing body of scholarship examining LGBT parenting and families, astonishingly little research has focused on the specific experiences of bisexual-identified parents. In her landmark book on lesbian and gay parenting, Goldberg (2010) notes that bisexual parenting experiences and perspectives are rarely acknowledged and explored, and that in most cases, inclusion of "bisexual" within the acronym "LGBT" is misleading, since when bisexual parents are included, they are simply collapsed together with the lesbian and/or gay parents in research samples, and may only include bisexual people with same-sex partners.

In this chapter, we attempt to address this gap in LGBT parenting research by (a) describing our recent literature search of multiple health and social sciences databases to establish the current state of the research on bisexual parenting; (b) reviewing related research and scholarship that has touched on the experiences of bisexual parents, including two studies conducted by our own team; (c) speculating about some of the key issues and concerns faced by bisexual parents, based on the available data; and (d) identifying key future directions for research in this field. We hope that this chapter will serve to encourage meaningful inclusion of bisexual parents in future research in the field of LGBT family science.

What Research Exists on Bisexual Parenting?

To establish the state of research in this area, we conducted a systematic literature review. Specifically, we searched the databases Medline, In Process Medline, Embase, CINAHL, PsycINFO, Gender Studies Database, Social Work Abstracts, Social Services Abstracts, Sociological Abstracts, Social Science Abstracts, and LGBT Life from start dates to August 2011. Keywords used for each database are available from the authors upon request. Of the 422 total abstracts identified in this search, only 7 reported any findings or considerations specific to bisexual parents (see Table 6.1 for a listing of these studies). Below, we will describe the key themes identified in this literature. First, however, we wish to consider the reasons that may underlie the lack of research on bisexual parenting, relative to research on lesbian and gay parenting.

L.E. Ross, Ph.D. (✉)
Department of Psychiatry, University of Toronto, 455 Spadina Ave., Suite 300, Toronto, ON M5S 2G8, Canada

Health Systems & Health Equity Research Group, Centre for Addiction & Mental Health, 455 Spadina Ave., Suite 300, Toronto, ON M5S 2G8, Canada
e-mail: l.ross@utoronto.ca

C. Dobinson, M.A.
Health Systems & Health Equity Research Group, Centre for Addiction & Mental Health, 455 Spadina Ave., Suite 300, Toronto, ON M5S 2G8, Canada
e-mail: cheryl_dobinson@sympatico.ca

A.E. Goldberg and K.R. Allen (eds.), *LGBT-Parent Families: Innovations in Research and Implications for Practice*, DOI 10.1007/978-1-4614-4556-2_6, © Springer Science+Business Media New York 2013

Table 6.1 Resources identified in a literature search of bisexual parenting and family issues, 2011

Article	Focus	# of bisexual participants	Bi-specific findings
Articles from database searches			
Anders (2005)	Married father of teenage boy discusses the process of coming out to his son, and the boy's acceptance.	First-person account	• Coming out to a teenage child can be a complex and intimidating process, but the son was already aware of his father's sexuality and was very accepting.
Brand (2001)	A Dutch married man and father of two recounts coming out with his wife's encouragement and support, and his exploration of sexuality with another openly bisexual married man.	First-person account	• Doesn't discuss interactions with children or their reaction to his coming out, other than it was extremely stressful to come out to his sons and their girlfriends.
Costello (1997)	Exploring bisexual, gay, and lesbian parents' expectations about their children's sexual identity development and the role they intended to play in that process.	5 self-identified bisexual people (out of 18 participants)	• Suggests that family has less difficulty accepting bisexuality than they would other minority identities when participants come out but are still in a heterosexual marriage or relationship and have children. • One bisexual parent believed his child would grow up to be bisexual because he believes that everyone is bisexual.
Goldberg (2007)	Qualitative study exploring how the adult children of LGB parents negotiate disclosure of their parents' sexual orientation.	2 self-identified bisexual women with bisexual mothers (out of 42 participants)	• No differences noted between bisexual participants and others, but bisexual identity of participants is noted in supporting quotations for the theme "I won't hide (anymore)." • Having had parents who were not out to them made queer children want to come out themselves.
Mallon (2011)	Review of literature and policy related to LGBT adoption.	N/A	• Notes the lack of research on how child welfare agencies manage applications from bisexual people, or bisexual peoples' experiences during the application process.
Murray and McClintock (2005)	Examined whether a parent's nondisclosure of his or her homosexuality or bisexuality negatively affects self-esteem and anxiety in children, as measured in adulthood.	5 raised by bisexual fathers, 2 by bisexual mothers (as per the participant's report of the parent's sexual orientation) (out of 99 participants)	• Mostly collapses bisexual sample with lesbian/gay, including all analyses related to the primary outcomes. • Reports proportion of participants who are themselves sexual minority identified: 43% of the participants raised by bisexual parents and 38% of the participants raised by gay/lesbian parents. Reports proportion of parents who divorced: 67% of the bisexual and 76% of the gay/lesbian parents.
Steele et al. (2008)	Purpose: to describe the mental health services used by women in the perinatal period and to identify potential correlates of mental health service.	14 self-identified bisexual women (out of 64 participants)	• Participants who conceived through sex with a man reported the highest rates of past year mental health service use and highest rates of unmet need for mental health services.

Materials identified from other sources, including reference lists of included articles, Internet searches and consultation with experts

Reference	Description	Sample	Key findings
Blanco (2009)	Part of the "Children in our lives" theme issue of the Bi Women newsletter.	First-person account	• Motherhood as a site for activism, including activism related to bisexual issues. • Examines how the daily realities of parenting can get in the way of active involvement in bisexual community.
Cahill et al. (2003)	Analysis of major U.S. policy issues affected LGBT people, their partners, and children.	N/A	• Bisexual parents face discrimination in child custody and visitation cases, where negative stereotypes about bisexual people are sometimes used to justify denying custody or limiting visitation. Two specific US cases are described in which bisexual parents were denied custody of their children.
Eady et al. (2009)	Draws from a qualitative study of lesbian, gay, bisexual, and trans adoption in Ontario to examine the experience of bisexual parents and prospective parents.	5 families including at least one parent who self-identified as bisexual (out of a total sample of 43 families)	• Bisexual participants anticipated and experienced that workers held stereotypic ideas about bisexuality that called into question their "fitness" as parents. • These experiences complicated decisions about whether or not to disclose their bisexual identities to workers (regardless of their partner status as different sex, same sex, or not partnered).
Firestein (2007)	Identifies key issues relevant to providing counseling to bisexual people.	Data drawn from a survey of over 2,000 self-identified bisexual and polyamorous people	• 38% of respondents reported that they were actively playing a part in raising children or stepchildren.
Gates et al. (2007)	Provides new information on gay, lesbian and bisexual adoption, and foster care from several U.S. government data sources.	Data from the National Survey of Family Growth (identity-based definition of sexual orientation)	• More bisexual than lesbian/gay individuals report a desire to have children. This is true for both men and women. • The authors also provided unpublished data from the same data set, indicating data showing that bisexual women were more likely to have given birth, and bisexual men more likely to have gotten someone pregnant, than their lesbian or gay counterparts, respectively (United States Department of Health and Human Services National Center for Health Statistics, 2002).
Johnson et al. (1987)	Describes parenting desires among a large nonclinical sample of lesbian and bisexual women.	424 self-identified bisexual women (together with 1,921 lesbians)	• 60.6% of bisexual women had considered having a child (58.8% of lesbians). • Bisexual women were more likely than lesbians to consider sex with a man as a potential method of conceiving, and less likely to consider donor insemination. • Only 2% of the total sample reported a successful pregnancy; all successful pregnancies among bisexual women resulted from sexual intercourse.
Lahey (1999)	Human rights, law, and sexuality issues in Canada.	N/A	• Suggests that bisexual identity is less "threatening" to the courts than lesbian and bisexual identity when it comes to custody and access; cites 3 cases in which bisexual parents were awarded custody.

(continued)

Table 6.1 (continued)

Article	Focus	# of bisexual participants	Bi-specific findings
Paiva et al. (2003)	Describes a study of sexuality and reproduction in 250 Brazilian men living with HIV.	38% reported sex with men at some time in their lives (number self-identifying as bisexual not reported)	• Desire for parenthood did not differ significantly between bisexual and heterosexual men.
Richman (2002)	"A study of meaning making and identity construction in child custody cases involving gay or lesbian parents."	N/A	• Describes 3 cases in which a parent petitioning for and trying to retain child custody was or was presumed to be bisexual. • Also notes the extent of erasure of bisexual identities in the family law system.
Ross et al. (2012)	Draws upon data from a mixed-methods study to examine the question of whether the experiences of bisexual mothers are comparable to those of lesbian mothers, with a particular focus on self-reported mental health, stress, and social support.	14 women who self-identified as bisexual; 14 women who reported a sexual minority identity and sex with a man in the past 5 years (incomplete overlap between these groups) out of a total sample of 64 sexual minority women	• Bisexual women reported poorer scores on assessments of mental health, substance use, social support, and experiences of perceived discrimination, relative to other women in the sample. • Differences were particularly pronounced for women who reported sexual activity with men in the past 5 years compared to women who did not. • Qualitative analyses highlighted experiences of invisibility and exclusion.
Wells (2011)	A mother discusses how her concerns as a parent were central in her shift toward a bisexual identity.	First-person account	• Highlights how parenting desires and/or experiences may be important in bisexual identity development.

Why Are Bisexual People Invisible in LGBT Parenting Research?

Before examining the invisibility of bisexual people in LGBT parenting research, it is first necessary to define the term "bisexual" for the purposes of our work. Sexual orientation is typically defined along one or more of the following axes: sexual attraction, sexual behavior, and self-identification (Parks, Hughes, & Werkmeister-Rozas, 2009). As noted by Laumann, Gagnon, Michael, and Michaels (1994), there is often discordance between these three domains: for example, a significant proportion of individuals reporting sexual activity with both men and women do not endorse a sexual minority identity (e.g., Meyer, Rossano, Ellis, & Bradford, 2002).

Bisexuality has been defined and measured in various ways, beginning with Kinsey's famous 7-point scale (within which bisexual individuals would fall between points 1 and 5, depending on the relative frequency of their heterosexual versus homosexual contacts; Kinsey, Pomeroy, & Martin, 1948; Kinsey, Pomeroy, Martin, & Gebhard, 1953). Subsequently, the Klein Sexual Orientation Grid (Klein, 1993) was developed to enable a more comprehensive assessment of multiple domains of an individual's sexual orientation (including, but not limited to, attraction, behavior, and self-identification) for one's past, present, and ideal selves. This enabled identification of bisexual individuals on the basis of any one of his seven dimensions (e.g., not only those who self-identify as bisexual but also those who report sexual behavior with or attraction toward both men and women).

In light of the scarcity of research on this topic, we have chosen to utilize a broad definition of bisexuality which includes all those who identify as bisexual and/or who report lifetime attraction toward or sexual experiences with men and women (and for some bisexual people, transgender individuals as well). While we acknowledge that the breadth of this definition limits our capacity to draw specific conclusions, at this stage, we are limited by the extant research. However, wherever possible, we note the definition of bisexuality employed by authors of the original studies included in our review.

The absence of specific investigation into the experiences of bisexual parents is consistent with the relative lack of bisexual-specific research in the areas of LGBT psychology, health, social work, and other social sciences. For example, within the extensive body of research examining mental health disparities associated with minority sexual identities (see King et al., 2008 for a meta-analysis), only recently have studies begun to separate out bisexual individuals from their lesbian and gay counterparts. Importantly, when this is done, most studies show that across specific health outcomes, disparities are most pronounced for the bisexual group, relative to both gay/lesbian and heterosexual comparators (e.g., Goldsen, Kim, Barkan, Balsam, & Mincer, 2010). Indeed, a growing body of evidence suggests that bisexual identity and/or reports of sexual activity with both men and women are associated with poor outcomes across a variety of health indicators (Brennan, Ross, Dobinson, Veldhuizen, & Steele, 2010; Steele, Ross, Dobinson, Veldhuizen, & Tinmouth, 2009). Experience of exclusion from both heterosexual and gay/lesbian communities is one factor that has been postulated to account for these differences (Ross, Dobinson, & Eady, 2010).

This invisibility in research cannot be attributed to small numbers of bisexual people available to participate in research. As Yoshino (2000) has reviewed, all of the major studies of adult sexuality published between 1948 and 1994 found that bisexuality (variously defined on the basis of identity or behavior) is at least as common, or more common, than exclusive homosexuality. Although more recent North American epidemiological research suggests that the relative prevalence of bisexuality versus homosexuality may depend on gender (with bisexuality being more common than exclusive homosexuality among women but not men; see Mosher, Chandra, & Jones, 2005; Statistics Canada, 2004), it is clear that there is not a substantial difference in the prevalence of bisexuality versus exclusive homosexuality in the population as a whole.

Considering the prevalence of bisexuality, and that the little available literature in other disciplines suggests important distinctions between bisexual and gay/lesbian people, why is there such a striking lack of research in the area of bisexual parenting? We argue that social constructionist theoretical perspectives, both as they apply to the social construction of sexual identities, and to the social construction of family, may be relevant. Social constructionist theory examines how power and other social processes influence the creation of meaning, theories, and common knowledge (Kitzinger, D'Augelli, & Patterson, 1995; Ross et al., 2010). This is in contrast to essentialist paradigms which assume that phenomena such as sexual identities are biologically determined and immutable (Fassinger & Arseneau, 2007). In contemporary White European cultures, sexual orientation is typically constructed to be dichotomous in nature, with the only legitimate options being heterosexuality or homosexuality (Barker & Langdridge, 2008). This is a form of structural monosexism (i.e., beliefs, actions, and structures that promote or presume heterosexuality or homosexuality to the exclusion of bisexuality; Yoshino, 2000). This monosexist construction renders bisexuality (a) invisible, (b) irrelevant, and (c) illegitimate. We consider each of these constructions in turn.

The social invisibility of bisexual people and communities has been documented in analysis of media portrayals (Meyer, 2009). With respect to media in the UK, Barker and her colleagues note "that there is very little overt media representation of bisexuality" (Barker, Bowes-Catton, Iantaffi, Cassidy, & Brewer, 2008, p. 145). Indeed, when a character shifts from having different-sex to same-sex relationships (or vice versa), that person's sexual orientation is portrayed as having changed—bisexuality is rarely mentioned, nor does it appear to be considered as an option for characters in film or television. Consider, for example, the award-winning film *Brokeback Mountain* (Lee, 2006) in which the two lead characters are consistently described as gay in media reviews and analysis, despite the fact that both also have female partners.

Qualitative research has captured the implications of this bisexual invisibility as it relates to the experiences of bisexual people. For example,

in our study of 55 bisexual people from Ontario, Canada, participants described the extent to which bisexual invisibility contributed to challenges in everyday interactions with important people in their lives, as well as struggles in coming to terms with their bisexual identities (Ross et al., 2010). These experiences are consistent with first person accounts included in some of the earliest anthologies related to bisexuality (e.g., Hutchins & Kaahumanu, 1991; Weise, 1992), suggesting surprisingly little shift in the intervening decades with respect to social (in)visibility of bisexuality.

Invisibility of bisexual identity can take different forms depending upon the partnership status of an individual bisexual person. For example, bisexual people with same-sex partners are often invisible as bisexuals, but visible as nonheterosexual and therefore are recognized within the broader lesbian/gay/bisexual community. Bisexual people with different-sex partners, on the other hand, are often invisible both as bisexual and as nonheterosexual. This is particularly the case if they are partnered with someone who identifies as heterosexual or if they participate in normative institutions such as marriage or family building (Ross, Siegel, Dobinson, Epstein, & Steele, 2012). Further, bisexual parents with different-sex partners may experience or perceive exclusion from the lesbian or gay community due to the assumption of "heterosexual privilege"; that is, the assumption that by virtue of their ability to "pass" as heterosexual, bisexual people do not experience discrimination on the basis of sexual orientation. Implications of this assumption for different-sex partnered bisexual parents are further discussed below.

Bisexual identities are often also constructed to be irrelevant. That is, there is an implicit assumption that the experiences of bisexual people will be the same as those of either heterosexual or gay/lesbian individuals, depending on the sex of their current partner (if they are partnered) (Yoshino, 2000). As described above, this assumption has been noted in LGBT research, wherein bisexual individuals are routinely collapsed into categories with lesbian/gay individuals, as though there is no important conceptual or theoretical distinction between them (Rodriguez Rust, 2009). Our systematic literature review found that this assumption pervades the majority of research on LGBT parenting, in which bisexual people (particularly those who are parenting with a same-sex partner) are most often collapsed together with gay or lesbian participants, without any analysis of the ways in which their experiences or outcomes may be different. Experiences of same-sex partnered bisexual people are assumed to be the same as those of lesbian/gay individuals, and therefore lumped under the "lesbian/gay" umbrella (Ulrich, 2011). Different-sex partnered bisexual people, on the other hand, are often considered by many in the lesbian and gay community to experience "heterosexual privilege" associated with their different-sex partnerships, which complicates access to support within these communities (Ault, 1994).

With respect to the social construction of bisexuality as illegitimate, those who do not fit into heterosexual or lesbian/gay categories are constructed to be in some way abnormal, unhealthy, or unstable. For example, there is a pervasive belief that bisexuality exists only as a transition stage to a "true" lesbian/gay identity (Firestein, 1996), and research in psychology and other fields has long perpetuated the lack of legitimacy of bisexual identities (see Brewster & Moradi, 2010 for critiques of some of this work). In a telephone survey examining attitudes toward various marginalized or politicized communities, Herek (2002) found that probes regarding attitudes toward bisexual people yielded more negative affect than those regarding almost any group, including people with AIDS, lesbian and gay people, and people of various racial and ethnic minority groups.

Monosexist constructions of bisexuality as an illegitimate sexual identity, taken together with social constructions of family that prioritize the heterosexual, nuclear family model, may contribute to stigmatizing assumptions about the "fitness" of bisexual people as parents. Two common assumptions about bisexuality in particular may conflict with social constructions of family in this manner. First, the assumption that bisexual people are unable to maintain long-term monogamous relationships, together with the assumption that polyamory is in some way damaging to children, may produce the conclusion that bisexual people will be unable to model healthy relationships for their children (see Chap. 8, for a discussion of experiences of polyamorous parents). Others have examined the ways in which the constructs of "family" and "parent" are desexualized (Oliver, 2010), to the extent that sexual minority parents might bear "an additional layer of scrutiny of their parenting, that of being (presumably) a sexually active adult while parenting" (Weber, 2010, p. 381). Common constructions about bisexuality position this orientation as overly sexualized, to the degree that healthy, committed relationships are considered impossible or undesirable for bisexual people (Ulrich, 2011). As a result, the identity of "bisexual parent" appears to sexualize the notion of family, offending those who purport to operate in defense of "family values." For example, in our qualitative study of the experiences of bisexual people applying for adoption, one couple described the concerns of adoption workers about who would be caring for the children while a polyamorous bisexual woman married to a man spent time with her female partner (Eady, Ross, Epstein, & Anderson, 2009).

Second, the prevailing belief that bisexuality is a transitional identity and therefore that bisexual people are psychologically unstable or immature, together with assumptions that individuals with mental health challenges are unable to parent appropriately (Nicholson, Sweeney, & Geller, 1998), may call into question the mental "fitness" of bisexuals to parent. We observed this assumption in action at a recent workshop on LGBT adoption, when workers stated that based on their training, they understood bisexuality to be a transition stage and so would have concerns about whether a bisexual-identified person would be "mature" enough to be a suitable candidate for adoption.

These assumptions must be considered in the context of a hostile social environment, which historically (and in some regions, currently) has dictated a need for research aiming to "prove" the adequacy of LGBT people as parents to assist in custody cases, access to adoption and fertility services, and other political battles. As Epstein (2009) has discussed, 30 years ago, the vast majority of lesbians who sought custody of their children in the courts lost; many more likely relinquished custody to avoid having to go through the courts. Recently, proponents of Proposition 8 in the state of California drew heavily upon (unsubstantiated) fears about the impact of same-sex marriage on the well-being of children (Bajko, 2010; Langbein & Yost, 2009). In such an environment, researchers might have concern (whether conscious or not) that investigations about bisexual parents, constructed as psychologically unstable and sexually deviant, might uncover data suggesting "inadequate" parenting by members of LGBT communities— results that could have dangerous political consequences. However, both scholars and community activists have called for a shift in research paradigms away from those which construct differences as deficits, and toward models that explore and celebrate the ways in which LGBT people may parent differently from our heterosexual counterparts (e.g., Epstein, 2009; Goldberg, 2010; Stacey & Biblarz, 2001). As we challenge monosexist social constructions about bisexual identity, research exploring the unique issues and experiences of bisexual parents is warranted, and truly overdue.

What Do We Know About the Experiences of Bisexual Parents?

In this section, we draw from the six studies identified in our literature review, two recent relevant studies conducted by our team, six additional sources identified through consultations with bisexual community leaders and academics, and the results of a broader Internet search of non-peer reviewed material, including books, first person accounts, and community newsletters. Based upon these diverse data sources, we speculate about some of the key issues and experiences of bisexual parents that may be worthy of additional research. We have organized these ideas into the following themes (a) statistics regarding the number of bisexual parents; (b) outcomes

in children of bisexual parents; (c) disclosure of bisexual identity; (d) experiences of bisexual people with systems and supports; (e) health and well-being of bisexual parents; and (f) relationships between parenting/parenting desires and bisexual identity development. Below, we discuss each of these themes in turn.

Statistics Regarding the Number of Bisexual Parents

One of the earliest studies to report specific findings about bisexual parents examined parenting desires among bisexual women and lesbians recruited in a nonclinical setting (Johnson, Smith, & Guenther, 1987). The authors found that more than 50% of each sexual orientation group had considered having a child since identifying as lesbian or bisexual. The preferred means for having a child differed between the two groups, with lesbians more likely to favor adoption or donor insemination and bisexual women more likely to consider intercourse with a man. However, in this early study, only 2% of the participants reported success in having a child at the time that they were surveyed.

More recent data suggest that many bisexual people have, or want to have, children, and indeed that bisexual men and women may be more likely than gay men or lesbians to have children. For example, in a survey of over 2,000 bisexual people (all of whom also identified as polyamorous), 38% reported actively playing a part in raising children or stepchildren (Firestein, 2007). These numbers are consistent with data from the National Survey of Family Growth, in which both bisexual men and women were more likely than their gay and lesbian counterparts to report that they desired children (Gates, Badgett, Macomber, & Chambers, 2007) and that they had given birth (44.8% of bisexual women vs. 34.9% of lesbians) or gotten someone pregnant (26.6% of bisexual men vs. 15.8% of gay men) (United States Department of Health and Human Services National Center for Health Statistics, 2002). Finally, a study of 250 Brazilian men with HIV found that there was no difference between the bisexual and heterosexual men in their sample with respect to their desire to father children: Just under half of the total sample reported that they wished to have children in the future (Paiva, Filipe, Santos, Lima, & Segurado, 2003). Thus, available data indicate that at least as many bisexual people as gay/lesbian people have children or desire to parent.

Outcomes in Children of Bisexual Parents

There is a vast body of literature examining a variety of outcomes in the children of lesbian and gay parents (Tasker, 2005). This research has primarily been used to demonstrate that children raised in families headed by same-sex couples are "just like" those raised by heterosexual families, to protect the custody rights of lesbian and gay parents in the courts and support adoption rights and access to assisted reproduction services. Children of bisexual parents appear to have been largely left out of this dialogue: They may be invisible among both those families presumed to be lesbian- or gay-parent led, and those families presumed to be heterosexual led. In an article reviewing considerations for those who might encounter LGBT parents in the family court system, Tye (2003) notes the lack of specific research on the children of bisexual (as well as transgender) people, concluding that studies identified in his review "that have specifically included bisexual or transgender categories have shown no significant differences that would negatively affect parenting capacity" (p. 94).

Children of bisexual parents are likely to be affected by heteronormative systems, such as schools (Sears, 2005), as well as homophobic reactions to disclosure of a parent's sexual orientation (Snow, 2004), just as children of gay and lesbian parents are. Although we were not able to identify any research exploring the school experiences of children of bisexual parents specifically, research on the experiences of children of LGBT parents more broadly suggests that school-aged children who bully others on the basis of parental sexual orientation do not have a sophisticated

understanding of these concepts: Children may experience violence and harassment on the basis of any perception that they or their families deviate from sexual or gender norms, regardless of whether or how they actually do (Epstein, Idems, & Schwartz, 2009). While more research is needed, it is likely that children of bisexual parents share many of the same anxieties as children of lesbian/gay parents. In particular, the children may have concerns regarding the potential discovery of their parents' sexual orientation, resulting assumptions about their own sexual orientation, and bullying or harassment that they may then experience.

Our search identified only two studies reporting data related to outcomes in children raised by bisexual people; both specifically examining the actual or anticipated sexual identity of children raised by bisexual parents. In the first, Costello (1997) conducted a qualitative study to examine how LGB parents conceptualize their children's sexual orientations. Of her total sample of 18 participants, 5 identified as bisexual. The overall conclusion of this study was that LGB parents are "willing [to] actively … foster a sexual identity different from their own" (Costello, 1997, p. 63) in their children, and there is no indication in the author's argument that this conclusion is likely to differ depending on the specific sexual orientation of the sexual minority parent. However, only 1 of the 18 participants reported anticipating that their child was likely to not be heterosexual; this bisexual father expressed that he expected that his daughter would be bisexual, as he considered this to be the universal, essential sexual orientation.

The second study to report on the sexual orientation of children raised by bisexual parents was conducted by Murray and McClintock (2005). These authors studied the outcomes in adult children of LGB people who had concealed their sexual orientation during the participants' childhoods. Of the 36 participants who reported an LGB parent, 7 reported having at least one bisexual parent (7 bisexual fathers and 2 bisexual mothers). Only a few of the outcomes presented in this study are reported separately for participants with bisexual versus lesbian or gay parents. However, the authors do report the proportion of participants who are themselves sexual minority identified (43% of the participants raised by bisexual parents and 38% of the participants raised by gay/lesbian parents). No statistical significance testing was conducted, as this was not a primary outcome of interest in this study.

Although the body of research examining outcomes in children of lesbian and gay parents has been rightly critiqued for its focus on establishing similarities with children raised by heterosexual parents (Stacey & Biblarz, 2001), it is curious that the children of bisexual parents are largely invisible in this debate. This omission could be because the presumed "danger" to children is implicitly understood to be associated with same-sex sexual behavior, rather than sexual minority identity, thus rendering the parent's specific identity irrelevant. Perhaps as a result of this assumption, much of the research on LGBT parenting has focused on the structure of the couple relationship (i.e., same sex), rather than the specific sexual orientation of the partners. As discussed below, it may also be that bisexuality less frequently arises as an issue in the courts, perhaps due to parents' strategic choices about how to present their identities (e.g., opting for a better-understood lesbian or gay identity, rather than a socially contested bisexual one). However, as indicated by the emerging literature on strengths of children raised by lesbian and gay parents (Goldberg, 2007; Stacey & Biblarz, 2001), there may be advantages to being raised by bisexual parents that are worthy of study. For example, in one first-person account, the daughter of a bisexual father describes herself as knowing more about the world and being more open-minded than her friends, as a result of her father's sexual identity (Jones & Jones, 1991). Additional research with the children of bisexual parents, drawing upon a lens that explores and celebrates potential differences associated with being raised by a bisexual parent, would be of interest.

Disclosure of Bisexual Identity

Disclosure of bisexual identity may be a primary issue that distinguishes experiences of bisexual parents from those of their lesbian and gay counterparts. Unlike heterosexual and gay/lesbian identity, bisexual identity cannot be presumed based on the gender of one's current sexual or romantic partner. As such, invisibility of bisexual identity is a challenge faced by many bisexual people, regardless of whether they are currently in a same-sex or different-sex relationship (if they are partnered). A consequence of this invisibility is the need to explicitly disclose one's bisexual identity to anyone in one's personal or social circle one wishes to make aware. In the family and parenting context, this might include one's partner, children, and members of the child's social circle (e.g., the parents of friends, teachers, or daycare personnel), among others.

One of the primary relationship concerns of bisexual people relates to issues around disclosure of bisexual identity to partners and potential dating partners (e.g., McClellan, 2006; Ross et al., 2010). As a result of the commonly held belief that bisexual people are incapable of committed, monogamous relationships, such disclosure may spur insecurities about fidelity and may discourage potential dating partners from pursuing the relationship (McClellan, 2006). In the context of same-sex partner relationships, disclosure is further complicated by the biphobia that exists within some pockets of the broader lesbian and gay community (Yoshino, 2000): Some bisexual people have reported being turned down even for a first date solely on the basis of their bisexuality (Ross et al., 2010). Similarly, disclosure in the context of different-sex partnered relationships can be challenging as a result of homophobic or biphobic attitudes and beliefs on the part of heterosexual-identified partners or potential dating partners (Li, Dobinson, & Ross, 2012). As a result of these challenges, some bisexual people may choose not to disclose; however, partner support of bisexual identity has been cited by bisexual people as an important factor in maintaining a state of emotional well-being (Ross et al., 2010). For example, in his first-person account of coming out as bisexual in the Netherlands, Brand (2001) describes the key role of the support of his wife in his coming out process. Strategies for and implications of disclosure and nondisclosure of bisexual identity to partners merit additional research; of particular interest will be whether and how parenting or desire to parent may affect these experiences.

Some first-person accounts (e.g., Anders, 2005) describe positive experiences of disclosure of bisexual identity to older (i.e., preteen and teenaged) children. We could identify no research exploring experiences of bisexual parents disclosing or wishing to disclose their identity to younger children. For monogamous bisexual people, disclosure of identity to young children may be challenging depending on the child's developmental stage: While many young children can quite easily understand differences in family constellations (i.e., families with two mommies, two daddies, or other combinations relevant to LGBT-led families), the concepts of romantic partnerships or sexual identity may be more difficult to grasp, particularly if one's story of bisexual identity also requires the child to understand a temporal sequence (i.e., having had partners of another gender sometime in the past). Further, while excellent age-appropriate resources are available to assist in discussions about lesbian- and gay-led families [e.g., children's stories such as *And Tango Makes Three* (Richardson, 2005)], we are aware of no such resources discussing bisexual parent-led families. Research is needed to understand experiences of disclosure of bisexual identity of a parent from the perspective of both parents and children.

Like many lesbian, gay, and trans parents, bisexual parents may also wish to disclose their identity to other important figures in their children's lives, including teachers or childcare providers. We could identify no research that has specifically examined experiences of bisexual people in this regard. Although research and resources are available that purport to speak to issues for "LGBT" parents (e.g., Ryan & Martin, 2000; Youth Leadership and Action Program of COLAGE, 2003), these presume that the experiences of bisexual parents (and in many cases, trans parents as well) will simply echo what is known about the experiences of lesbian and gay parents. While bisexual parents likely share with lesbian and gay parents the impact of societal homophobia

and heterosexism on these disclosures, they may additionally be affected by common monosexist attitudes and beliefs, as described above. Research is needed to understand these experiences, and particularly to examine whether experiences might differ depending on whether parents are same-sex partnered, different-sex partnered, multiple partnered, or not partnered. For example, do same-sex partnered bisexual parents feel it is necessary or desirable to disclose their bisexual identity, when by virtue of its composition their family is already read as queer? How do different-sex partnered bisexual parents experience having their children's teachers, their children's friends' parents, and so on, assume them to be heterosexual? How do race, class, and other marginalized identities additionally interact with these issues to influence decisions about disclosure?

Our literature review identified two empirical studies examining experiences of disclosure for bisexual parents. Neither of these studies examined experiences of bisexual parents disclosing their identities to their children or others in the parenting sphere; rather, they both considered the extent to which parenting or family experiences might have an impact on experiences of disclosure in other settings. In the study by Costello (1997) described above, the analysis of participants' narratives related to coming out to their families of origin includes a quote from a bisexual-identified participant who came out to her parents to prepare them for a forthcoming episode of the *Geraldo* show on bisexuality, on which she was to appear. Costello speculated as follows:

> Unlike all the other subjects, she came out in the context of a marriage to a person of the opposite sex. She was already 35 and the mother of a 2-year-old child. Much of the threat to parental values which undergirds the coming out trauma was thus attenuated in her case, which would explain why her parents may not have reacted with much distress to her announcement of bisexuality. (p. 72)

As such, Costello (1997) speculates that the experiences of bisexual people coming out to their families of origin may be influenced by the extent to which they conform to socially constructed notions of family (being married to a different-sex partner, with children).

Goldberg (2007) conducted a qualitative study with 42 adults raised by LGB parents, to investigate their experiences of disclosure of their parent's sexual orientation. Of the sample of 42 women, 2 were raised by a bisexual mother. One of the themes of the study was "I won't hide (anymore)," wherein participants reported that having had their parents not disclose their orientation, or ask the children not to disclose about their parents' identities, during childhood, motivated them to disclose about their families and avoid secrecy as adults. A quote from a bisexual participant raised by a bisexual mother is provided in support of this, although the theme is also supported with data from participants with parents of other orientations. Taken together, these data suggest that research is warranted to examine whether and how the parenting and family relationships of bisexual people may affect their decisions to disclose and experiences of identity disclosure for both parents and children.

Experiences of Bisexual People with Systems and Supports

We could find little literature examining the implications of disclosure of bisexual identity within social structures and systems related to child care and child rearing. With respect to legal and child custody matters, Cahill and the National Gay and Lesbian Task Force Policy Institute (2003) note that "bisexual parents face discrimination in child custody and visitation cases, where negative stereotypes about bisexual people are sometimes used to justify denying custody or limiting visitation" (p. 74). The authors went on to describe a 2001 custody case from Mississippi, in which custody was awarded to the heterosexual father instead of the bisexual mother, and "the morality of the mother's lifestyle" (p. 75) was noted as one important factor in the judge's decision. In the Canadian context, Lahey (1999) suggests that bisexual parents do not face the same barriers in custody and access that lesbian and gay parents often do. She described three cases in which a parent's bisexuality was a consideration in a custody decision, and in all three cases

custody was awarded to the bisexual parent (two mothers and one father). She concluded that bisexual identity may be perceived as "less threatening" (p. 134) by the courts, relative to a lesbian or gay identity. As Richman (2002) notes, however, bisexuality is considered much less frequently than homosexuality in the family courts. Based on her review of the legal literature Richman reports: "Even when a litigant self-identified as bisexual, she or he was thought of and treated as homosexual" (p. 301).

Mallon (2011) has recently noted the lack of research examining experiences of bisexual people in the adoption system. However, experiences in our Canadian study of adoption by bisexual-identified people suggest that stereotypes and beliefs about bisexual parents may create significant, though not insurmountable, barriers for them in their attempts to prove their worth as parents or potential parents (Eady et al., 2009). For this secondary analysis of our study of 43 LGBT individuals or families who had adopted or applied to adopt a child in Ontario, we examined in depth the interviews of the 5 participants who identified as bisexual, to identify key themes and experiences. Taken together, these narratives suggest that many adoption workers have little understanding about bisexuality and bring common negative or stereotypical beliefs and assumptions to their encounters with bisexual potential parents. In particular, the dual assumption that bisexual people are not capable of committed, monogamous relationships and therefore cannot create a stable home for a child was both experienced and anticipated by these participants as they negotiated the child welfare system. For example, one participant, a single bisexual woman, opted not to disclose her past male partners and to identify herself as lesbian throughout the adoption process, anticipating that her adoption worker would believe these stereotypes about bisexuality, and as such would be more supportive of her if she believed her to be a lesbian.

There is also a lack of research examining the extent to which bisexual people experience a community of parenting support. Some bisexual people may feel discomfort in predominantly heterosexual parenting spaces, due to concerns about homophobia or heterosexism. However, they may also find LGBT-specific parenting spaces, if they are available in their communities, to be unwelcoming. For different-sex partnered bisexual people, receiving peer support from same-sex parents may be challenging due to a lack of shared experiences, for example, with respect to methods of conceiving a child or experiences negotiating the school system as an in/visibly queer family. Further, bisexual parents with different-sex partners may experience or perceive a lack of community among lesbian or gay parents due to the assumption of "heterosexual privilege," as described above. In particular, lesbian and gay people, as well as some service providers, may think that different-sex partnered bisexual parents do not require or merit accommodations that attempt to address concerns related to sexual orientation (e.g., LGBT-specific parenting programs and resources). The extent to which bisexual parents access parenting supports within both LGBT and heterosexual parenting communities requires further research, including research to determine whether parents' current partner status (same sex, different sex, none, or multiple) is a determinant of perceived or received support.

Health and Well-Being Among Bisexual Parents

We could identify no literature other than that published by our own team (Ross et al., 2010; Steele, Ross, Epstein, Strike, & Goldfinger, 2008) that has examined the health or mental health of bisexual parents. Steele et al. (2008) examined patterns of mental health service utilization among a sample of 64 sexual minority women who were currently attempting to conceive a child, pregnant, or parenting a child less than 1 year of age. Approximately 22% of the sample identified as bisexual. Although most analyses in this study involved pooling all of the sexual minority women, the authors examined mode of conception as a potential predictor of mental health service utilization. These analyses revealed that participants who conceived through sex with a man (regardless of their sexual identity) had the highest rates of past year mental health service use (57.1% vs. 37.1% for those who conceived with the aid of a sperm bank and 15.0% for those who conceived via a known donor). Women who conceived through sex with a man also reported the highest rates of unmet need for mental health services (35.5% vs. 17.6% and 25% for women who conceived via a sperm bank and known donor, respectively).

In a subsequent analysis of the same data set, we examined the mental health and social support of the 14 bisexual-identified participants and the 14 participants who reported sex with men in the past 5 years [there was some, but incomplete, overlap between these two groups (Ross et al., 2012)]. Bisexual-identified women reported significantly poorer scores on instruments assessing overall mental health, anxiety, and relationship satisfaction, relative to other sexual minority women. Women who reported sex with men in the past 5 years similarly reported poorer scores on assessments of overall physical health, overall mental health, depression, anxiety, drug use, social support, and perceived discrimination. Qualitative interviews were also conducted with five bisexual-identified women and eight women who reported sex with men in the past 5 years (these women endorsed a variety of sexual identities; most commonly bisexual, Two-Spirit, and queer). Examination of the interview data highlighted experiences of invisibility and exclusion, which may contribute to the observed poor health outcomes. In particular, women who were partnered with men described the complex emotions they experienced in response to their experiences as passing for a "normal" heterosexual, nuclear family in the context of pregnancy or parenting. It may be that different-sex partnered bisexual women are particularly likely to experience invisibility and exclusion from the broader LGBT community, which in turn may have important implications for their mental health.

The findings of these two studies are consistent with research indicating that bisexual people in the general population typically have poorer health and mental health outcomes than those of people of other sexual orientations (e.g., Goldsen et al., 2010; Hughes, Szalacha, & Mcnair, 2010; Tjepkema, 2008), as well as research identifying the early parenting years as a time of risk for mental health problems in predominantly heterosexual samples (Yonkers, Vigod, & Ross, 2011). Qualitative research suggests that experiences of invisibility and exclusion may contribute to the mental health disparities experienced by bisexual people (Ross et al., 2010). However, research is required to examine how this is experienced specifically in a parenting context, as well as how experiences of poor health and mental health may be related to parenting decisions and experiences for bisexual people (e.g., choosing whether or not to have children in the context of poor physical or mental health; implications for health-related quality of life among bisexual parents).

Parenting and Bisexual Identity Development

Finally, there is some evidence, albeit very limited, that parenting and parenting desires may play a role in bisexual identity development or sexual activity for some sexual minority women. For example, one bisexual participant in a mixed-methods study of sexual minority mothers by Ross et al. (2012) described her present choice to be in a primary relationship with a man as being predominantly about her desire to have children. In a first-person account in a community newsletter, Wells (2011) described how her desire to connect with someone committed to nurturing her child led her to shift away from her previous lesbian identity to consider potential male partners. In another issue of this same newsletter, a bisexual mother described how motherhood acts as an important site for her political activism: Concern about the world her daughter would grow up to inhabit, as well as a desire to educate her about social justice issues, led her to become more involved than she might otherwise have in various activist and advocacy activities, including activities related to queer and bisexual issues (Blanco, 2009). At the same time, she considered the extent to which the daily realities of parenting can reduce one's involvement in and

connection to bisexual communities. The extent to which other bisexual women, as well as bisexual men, experience these same advantages and challenges of parenting in relation to bisexual community involvement requires study.

Where Do We Go from Here? Future Directions

In summary, our systematic literature review has identified a striking lack of research on the experiences of bisexual parents. Further, our review of the broader literature suggests a number of potential issues and concerns that may be unique to or differentially experienced by bisexual parents. Research specifically attending to the experiences of bisexual parents is therefore warranted. While this will ideally take the form of studies specifically focused on research questions relevant to bisexual parents and family issues, we also encourage researchers working in the area of LGBT parenting more broadly to identify opportunities to contribute to this body of knowledge. In particular, we encourage researchers to include sufficient numbers of bisexual parents in their studies to permit for stratified analyses, to identify issues that are unique to bisexual parents. Also, greater representation of bisexual parents in future research may reveal potentially interesting and important differences between bisexual parents and other sexual minority (e.g., lesbian/gay identified) parents.

We have identified here several important areas for future research on bisexual parenting and family issues. However, it will be necessary for such research to carefully consider the diversity of experiences encapsulated within the umbrella of bisexual identity or experience. For example, some bisexual people (like some heterosexual, lesbian, and gay people) may conceptualize family in ways that run counter to the socially constructed nuclear family model. In other words, some bisexual people may choose not to marry or have children; may raise children to whom they are not biologically related; or may raise children in the context of alternative family forms, such as polyamorous families. The extent to which choices in this regard are related to personal constructions of bisexual identity is worthy of study. This means that examination of the ways in which bisexual identity informs beliefs and decisions about family and parenting is an important area of study, including among those bisexual people who are not parenting in the traditional contexts typically captured in parenting and family studies research.

Critical in future research will be consideration of the further diversity within the broad category of bisexual parents, and careful definition/description of who is included within the category of bisexual. For example, we have defined bisexuality very broadly to include those who identify as bisexual, and those who report attraction to and/or sexual activity with both men and women; the experiences of individuals who do endorse a bisexual identity versus those who do not may differ. Experiences of male, female, and trans bisexual people are similarly likely to differ significantly based on socially constructed ideas about gender and parenting, as well as gendered notions of sexuality. As noted above, partner status of bisexual parents may also determine their experiences in important ways. Intersections with other important identities, including race, class, and ability, among others, will shape the ways in which bisexuality affects parenting and family experiences. It is notable that very few of the first-person accounts about experiences of bisexual parenting have taken up these important intersections (see Jones & Jones, 1991 for an exception). Consideration of these complex and rich intersections will help to illuminate the breadth of parenting and family experiences within the bisexual community.

Acknowledgment We wish to acknowledge the contributions of the following individuals: Sheila LaCroix for her assistance with the literature search, Allison Eady and Sarah James-Abra for assistance with screening abstracts and manuscript preparation, Margaret Robinson for helping to identify additional sources and providing helpful feedback on an earlier draft, and participants in the academic_bi yahoo group, whose discussions informed our thinking about potentially unique issues and experiences for bisexual parents. This work was supported by the Canadian Institutes of Health Research (CIHR), Award HPI-66922, and grants from the Institute of Gender and Health (IGH), Canadian Institutes of Health Research (CIHR 2005-11-HOA-1988721), the Fonds Quebecois de Recherche sur la Societe et la Culture (FQRSC 111796) awarded to the research team SVR (http://www.svr.uqam.ca). L. Ross is supported by a New Investigator Award from CIHR and the Ontario Women's Health Council, Award NOW-84656. In addition, support to CAMH for salary of scientists and infrastructure has been provided by the Ontario Ministry of Health and Long Term Care. The views expressed here do not necessarily reflect those of the Ministry of Health and Long Term Care.

References

Anders, M. (2005). Miniature golf. *Journal of Bisexuality,* 5, 111–117. doi:10.1300/J159v05n02_13

Ault, A. (1994). Hegemonic discourse in an oppositional community: Lesbian feminists and bisexuality. *Critical Sociology, 20,* 107–122. doi:10.1177/089692059402000306

Bajko, M. S. (2010, January 14). Children key in Prop 8 trial. *Bay Area Reporter.* Retrieved from http://www.ebar.com/news/article.php?sec=news&article=4473

Barker, M., Bowes-Catton, H., Iantaffi, A., Cassidy, A., & Brewer, L. (2008). British bisexuality: A snapshot of bisexual representations and identities in the United Kingdom. *Journal of Bisexuality, 8,* 141–162. doi:10.1080/15299710802143026

Barker, M., & Langdridge, D. (2008). II. Bisexuality: Working with a silenced sexuality. *Feminism & Psychology, 18,* 389–394. doi:10.1177/0959353508092093

Blanco, M. C. (2009). What I did on my ten-year vacation. *Bi Women, 27*(1), 1–6. Retrieved from http://www.robynochs.com/Bi_Women/Bi_Women_V27-1_DJF_09_web.pdf

Brand, K. (2001). Coming out successfully in the Netherlands. *Journal of Bisexuality, 1,* 59–67. doi:10.1300/J159v01n04_05

Brennan, D. J., Ross, L. E., Dobinson, C., Veldhuizen, S., & Steele, L. S. (2010). Men's sexual orientation and health in Canada. *Canadian Journal of Public Health, 101,* 255–258.

Brewster, M. E., & Moradi, B. (2010). Perceived experiences of anti-bisexual prejudice: Instrument development and evaluation. *Journal of Counseling Psychology, 57,* 451–468. doi:10.1037/a0021116

Cahill, S., Gay, N., & Institute, Lesbian Task Force Policy. (2003). *Family policy: Issues affecting gay, lesbian, bisexual, and transgender families.* New York, NY: National Gay & Lesbian Task Force.

Costello, C. Y. (1997). Conceiving identity: Bisexual, lesbian and gay parents consider their children's sexual orientations. *Journal of Sociology and Social Welfare, 24,* 63–89.

Eady, A., Ross, L. E., Epstein, R., & Anderson, S. (2009). To bi or not to bi: Bisexuality and disclosure in the adoption system. In R. Epstein (Ed.), *Who's your daddy? And other writings on queer parenting* (pp. 124–132). Toronto, ON: Sumach Press.

Epstein, R. (2009). *Who's your daddy and other writings on queer parenting*. Toronto, ON: Sumach Press.

Epstein, R., Idems, B., & Schwartz, A. (2009). Reading, writing and resilience: Queer spawn speak out about school. In R. Epstein (Ed.), *Who's your daddy? And other writings on queer parenting* (pp. 215–232). Toronto, ON: Sumach Press.

Fassinger, R. E., & Arseneau, J. R. (2007). "I'd rather get wet than be under that umbrella": Differentiating the experiences and identities of lesbian, gay, bisexual, and transgender people. In K. J. Bieschke, R. M. Perez, & K. A. DeBord (Eds.), *Handbook of counseling and psychotherapy with lesbian, gay, bisexual, and transgender clients* (2nd ed., pp. 19–49). Washington, DC: American Psychological Association.

Firestein, B. A. (1996). Bisexuality as paradigm shift: Transforming our disciplines. In B. A. Firestein (Ed.), *Bisexuality: The psychology and politics of an invisible minority* (pp. 263–291). Thousand Oaks, CA: Sage Publications.

Firestein, B. A. (2007). *Becoming visible: Counseling bisexuals across the lifespan*. New York, NY: Columbia University Press.

Gates, G. J., Badgett, M. V. L., Macomber, J. E., & Chambers, K. (2007). *Adoption and foster care by gay and lesbian parents in the United States*. Los Angeles, CA: The Williams Institute.

Goldberg, A. E. (2007). Talking about family: Disclosure practices of adults raised by lesbian, gay, and bisexual parents. *Journal of Family Issues, 28*, 100–131. doi:10.1177/0192513X06293606

Goldberg, A. E. (2010). *Lesbian and gay parents and their children: Research on the family life cycle*. Washington, DC: American Psychological Association.

Goldsen, K. I., Kim, H. J., Barkan, S. E., Balsam, K. F., & Mincer, S. L. (2010). Disparities in health-related quality of life: A comparison of lesbians and bisexual women. *American Journal of Public Health, 100*, 2255–2261. doi:10.2105/AJPH.2009.177329

Herek, G. M. (2002). Heterosexuals' attitudes toward bisexual men and women in the United States. *Journal of Sex Research, 39*, 264–274. doi:10.1080/00224490209552150

Hughes, T., Szalacha, L. A., & Mcnair, R. (2010). Substance abuse and mental health disparities: Comparisons across sexual identity groups in a national sample of young Australian women. *Social Science & Medicine, 71*, 824–831. doi:10.1016/j.socscimed.2010.05.009

Hutchins, L., & Kaahumanu, L. (Eds.). (1991). *Bi any other name: Bisexual people speak out*. Boston, MA: Alyson.

Johnson, S. R., Smith, E. M., & Guenther, S. M. (1987). Parenting desires among bisexual women and lesbians. *The Journal of Reproductive Medicine, 32*, 198–200.

Jones, B., & Jones, P. (1991). Growing up with a bisexual dad. In L. Hutchins & L. Kaahumanu (Eds.), *Bi Any Other Name: Bisexual people speak out* (pp. 159–166). Boston, MA: Alyson.

King, M., Semlyen, J., Tai, S. S., Killaspy, H., Osborn, D., Popelyuk, D., et al. (2008). A systematic review of mental disorder, suicide, and deliberate self harm in lesbian, gay and bisexual people. *BMC Psychiatry, 8*, 70. doi:10.1186/1471-244X-8-70

Kinsey, A. C., Pomeroy, W. B., & Martin, C. E. (1948). *Sexual behavior in the human male*. Oxford, England: Saunders.

Kinsey, A. C., Pomeroy, W. B., Martin, C. E., & Gebhard, P. M. (1953). *Sexual behavior in the human female*. Philadelphia, PA: W. B. Saunders.

Kitzinger, C., D'Augelli, A. R., & Patterson, C. J. (1995). Social constructionism: Implications for lesbian and gay psychology. In A. R. D'Augelli & C. J. Patterson (Eds.), *Lesbian, gay and bisexual identities over the lifespan* (pp. 136–161). New York, NY: Oxford University Press.

Klein, F. (1993). *The bisexual option* (2nd ed.). New York, NY: Harrington Park Press.

Lahey, K. A. (1999). *Are we 'persons' yet?: Law and sexuality in Canada*. Toronto, ON: University of Toronto Press.

Langbein, L., & Yost, M. A. (2009). Same-sex marriage and negative externalities. *Social Science Quarterly, 90*, 292–308. doi:10.1111/j.1540-6237.2009.00618.x

Laumann, E. O., Gagnon, J. H., Michael, R. T., & Michaels, S. (1994). *The social organization of sexuality: Sexual practices in the United States*. Chicago, IL: University of Chicago Press.

Lee, A. (Director) (2006). *Brokeback Mountain [Motion Picture]*. Alliance Atlantis: Universal City, CA.

Li, W., Dobinson, C., & Ross, L. E. (2012). *Unique issues bisexual people face in intimate relationships: A descriptive exploration of lived experience*. Unpublished manuscript.

Mallon, G. P. (2011). The home study assessment process for gay, lesbian, bisexual and transgender prospective adoptive and foster families. *Journal of GLBT Family Studies, 7*, 9–29. doi:10.1080/1550428X.2011.537229

McClellan, D. L. (2006). Bisexual relationships and families. In D. F. Morrow & L. Messinger (Eds.), *Sexual orientation & gender expression in social work practice: Working with gay, lesbian, bisexual, & transgender people* (pp. 243–262). New York, NY: Columbia University Press.

Meyer, M. D. E. (2009). 'I'm just trying to find my way like most kids': Bisexuality, adolescence and the drama of One Tree Hill. *Sexuality & Culture, 13*, 237–251. doi:10.1007/s12119-009-9056-z

Meyer, I. H., Rossano, L., Ellis, J. M., & Bradford, J. (2002). A brief telephone interview to identify lesbian and bisexual women in random digit dialing sampling. *Journal of Sex Research, 39*, 139–144. doi:10.1080/00224490209552133

Mosher, W. D., Chandra, A., & Jones, J. (2005). Sexual behavior and selected health measures: Men and women 15–44 years of age, United States, 2002. *Advance Data from Vital and Health Statistics; no 362.* Hyattsville, MD: National Center for Health Statistics.

Murray, P. D., & McClintock, K. (2005). Children of the closet: A measurement of the anxiety and self-esteem of children raised by a non-disclosed homosexual or bisexual parent. *Journal of Homosexuality, 49,* 77–95. doi:10.1300/J082v49n01_04

Nicholson, J., Sweeney, E. M., & Geller, J. L. (1998). Mothers with mental illness: I. The competing demands of parenting and living with mental illness. *Psychiatric Services, 49,* 635–642.

Oliver, K. (2010). Motherhood, sexuality, and pregnant embodiment: Twenty-five years of gestation. *Hypatia, 25,* 760–777. doi:10.1111/j.1527-2001.2010.01134.x

Paiva, V., Filipe, E. V., Santos, N., Lima, T. N., & Segurado, A. (2003). The right to love: The desire for parenthood among men living with HIV. *Reproductive Health Matters, 11,* 91–100.

Parks, C. A., Hughes, T. L., & Werkmeister-Rozas, L. (2009). Defining sexual identity and sexual orientation in research with lesbians, gay men, and bisexuals. In W. Meezan & J. L. Martin (Eds.), *Handbook of research with lesbian, gay, bisexual and transgender populations* (pp. 71–99). New York, NY: Routledge.

Richardson, J. (2005). *And Tango makes three.* New York, NY: Simon & Schuster Books for Young Readers.

Richman, K. (2002). Lovers, legal strangers, and parents: Negotiating parental and sexual identity in family law. *Law and Society Review, 36,* 285–324.

Rodriguez Rust, P. C. (2009). No more lip service: How to really include bisexuals in research on sexuality. In W. Meezan & J. I. Martin (Eds.), *Handbook of research with lesbian, gay, bisexual, and transgender populations* (pp. 100–130). New York, NY: Taylor & Francis.

Ross, L. E., Dobinson, C., & Eady, A. (2010). Perceived determinants of mental health for bisexual people: A qualitative examination. *American Journal of Public Health, 100,* 496–502. doi:10.2105/AJPH. 2008.156307

Ross, L. E., Siegel, A., Dobinson, C., Epstein, R., & Steele, L. S. (2012). 'I don't want to turn totally invisible': Mental health, stressors and supports among bisexual women during the perinatal period. *Journal of GLBT Family Studies, 8*(2), 137–154.

Ryan, D., & Martin, A. (2000). Lesbian, gay, bisexual, and transgender parents in the school systems. *School Psychology Review, 29,* 207–216.

Sears, J. T. (2005). *Youth, education, and sexualities: An international encyclopedia* (Vol. 1: A-J). Westport, CT: Greenwood Press.

Snow, J. E. (2004). *How it feels to have a gay or lesbian parent: A book by kids for kids of all ages.* Binghamton, NY: Harrington Park Press.

Stacey, J., & Biblarz, T. J. (2001). (How) does the sexual orientation of parents matter? *American Sociological Review, 66,* 159–183.

Statistics Canada (2004, June 15). First information on sexual orientation. *The Daily.* Retrieved from http://www.statcan.gc.ca/daily-quotidien/040615/dq040615b-eng.htm

Steele, L. S., Ross, L. E., Dobinson, C., Veldhuizen, S., & Tinmouth, J. M. (2009). Women's sexual orientation and health: Results from a Canadian population-based survey. *Women & Health, 49,* 353–367. doi:10.1080/03630240903238685

Steele, L., Ross, L. E., Epstein, R., Strike, C., & Goldfinger, C. (2008). Correlates of mental health service use among lesbian and bisexual mothers and prospective mothers. *Women & Health, 47,* 95–112. doi:10.1080/03630240802134225

Tasker, F. (2005). Lesbian mothers, gay fathers, and their children: A review. *Journal of Developmental and Behavioral Pediatrics, 26,* 224–240.

Tjepkema, M. (2008). Health care use among gay, lesbian and bisexual Canadians. *Health Reports, 19,* 53–64. Retrieved from http://www.statcan.gc.ca/pub/82-003-x/82-003-x2008001-eng.html

Tye, M. C. (2003). Lesbian, gay, bisexual, and transgender parents: Special considerations for the custody and adoption evaluator. *Family Court Review, 41,* 92–103. doi:10.1111/j.174-1617.2003.tb00871.x

Ulrich, L. (2011). *Bisexual invisibility: Impacts and recommendations.* San Francisco, CA: San Francisco Human Rights Commission.

United States Department of Health and Human Services, National Center for Health Statistics. (2002). *National Survey of Family Growth, Cycle VI.* Analyses conducted by Naomi Goldberg, The Williams Institute.

Weber, S. (2010). A stigma identification framework for family nurses working with parents who are lesbian, gay, bisexual, or transgendered and their families. *Journal of Family Nursing, 16,* 378–393. doi:10.1177/1074840710384999

Weise, E. R. (Ed.). (1992). *Closer to home: Bisexuality & feminism.* Seattle, WA: Seal Press.

Wells, J. (2011). Tuxedo shirts. *Bi Women, 29,* 8. Retrieved from http://biwomenboston.org/2010/12/01/tuxedo-shirts/.

Yonkers, K. A., Vigod, S., & Ross, L. E. (2011). Diagnosis, pathophysiology and management of mood disorders in pregnant and postpartum women. *Obstetrics and Gynecology, 117,* 961–977. doi:10.1097/AOG.0b013e31821187a7

Yoshino, K. (2000). The epistemic contract of bisexual erasure. *Stanford Law Review, 52,* 353–461.

Youth Leadership and Action Program of COLAGE. (2003). *Tips for making classrooms safer for students with lesbian, gay, bisexual, transgender and/or queer parents.* COLAGE. Retrieved from http://pride.lusu.ca/pdf/Educators/safe_classrooms.pdf.

7

Jordan B. Downing

Transgender-Parent Families

As part of the LGBT (lesbian, gay, bisexual, transgender) community, transgender individuals encounter many of the same challenges in developing families as lesbian and gay individuals do, such as societal discrimination and legal recognition. However, transgender parents face unique concerns and issues that differ significantly from lesbian and gay parents. For instance, transgender parents often encounter various forms of transphobia, medical pathologization, and lack of adequate health-care services. Furthermore, within this broad context of systemic discrimination, the timing of transitioning from one's gender assigned at birth to one's self-identified gender influences family development and process. For example, depending on whether an individual transitions before having children or when they are already parents will impact how children relate to their parents' transgender identification. For individuals who transition in the midst of parenting, their developmental process of "coming out" occurs alongside their partners' and children's own developmental progressions. Thus, in such contexts, all family members interactively adapt to interpersonal and intrapersonal changes in the midst of one parent transitioning.

Although a growing body of empirical research has begun to explore issues and concerns relating specifically to transgender individuals (e.g., Hines, 2007; Newfield, Hart, Dibble, & Kohler, 2006; Pinto, Melendez, & Spector, 2008; Sanchez & Vilain, 2009), very little empirical work has examined transgender-parent families. Personal autobiographical accounts (e.g., Boylan, 2003) and theoretically and clinically informed literature (e.g., Lev, 2004) have shed light on the complexities of family development and process within transgender-parent families. For instance, as transgender individuals transition from their gender assigned at birth to their self-identified gender, they often experience major shifts in their intimate relations and family life (Hines, 2006a; Lev, 2004). Furthermore, developing one's transgender identity, and coming out as transgender, is a unique process often entailing name changes, medical changes, bodily changes, and gender expression changes (Hill, 2007). Studying transgender-parent families is therefore particularly complex given the diversity of gender identities that may be included under the rubric of "trans." For the purposes of this chapter, the term "trans" will be used as an umbrella term to encompass a broad range of gender-variant identities and expressions [e.g., male to female (MTF), female to male (FTM), transsexual, transgender (Lev, 2010)].

J.B. Downing, M.A. (✉)
Department of Psychology, Clark University,
950 Main St, Worcester, MA 01610, USA
e-mail: jdowning@clarku.edu

A.E. Goldberg and K.R. Allen (eds.), *LGBT-Parent Families: Innovations in Research and Implications for Practice*, DOI 10.1007/978-1-4614-4556-2_7, © Springer Science+Business Media New York 2013

In the current chapter, I review the limited literature on trans-parent families, exploring individual and family processes that may occur in the context of trans-parent families. Drawing on research and theory from across a variety of disciplines, areas for future research are highlighted throughout. Focus is given to examining the following four areas (a) how trans-parent families may destabilize traditional notions of normative gendering within family relationships, (b) how discrimination may impact trans individuals and their families, (c) how "transitioning" within the context of a previously heterosexual or same-sex relationship may shape identity and family formation for trans parents, their partners, and their children, and (d) how issues of social location with regard to race, class, and geography may shape the experience of trans-parent families.

Redefining the Heteronormative Family

In considering how trans-parent families transgress the heteronormative nuclear family ideal, queer theory and theories on intersectionality are particularly useful theoretical frameworks for addressing the particularities of trans-parent families (e.g., Diamond & Butterworth, 2008; Warner, 2004). Through deliberate resistance to stable identity categories, queer theory provokes a rethinking of the very social categories of how people define themselves (Warner, 1993). Queer theory also emphasizes the transgressive power of resisting normative gender and sexuality (Butler, 1990; Halberstam, 2005). An intersectionality framework emphasizes how intersecting social constructs such as socioeconomic status, race, and geographical location shape individual subjectivities (Cole, 2009). Thus, within the context of trans-parent families, an intersectionality framework can help to move beyond a focus on defining the trans experience or trans-parent experience to a more dynamic focus on the diverse developmental processes and contextual factors shaping trans-parent families. Thus, attending to processes of transitioning (Hines,

2006b) and processes of identity and family development within specific contexts provides for a nuanced understanding of diverse trans subjectivities and their family members.

In considering trans-parent family development, it is important to consider how different gender identifications of trans individuals (e.g., MTF, FTM, gender queer) may uniquely shape family formation and processes (Tye, 2003). For example, an FTM parent's transitioning to a male identity may provoke a rethinking of what it means to engage in "mothering" and "fathering" within the family, which in turn may shape how children construct their own masculinity and femininity. How parenting practices and family formations are created, socially accepted, and marginalized may differ depending on whether one identifies as MTF, FTM, or gender queer. Further, contextual factors, such as race, class, and geographic location, shape how trans people develop and experience their gender identities either prior to becoming parents or within the context of parenting.

Trans people transgress gender normative notions that one's masculine or feminine gendering is a "natural" expression of one's biological sex. In doing so, they destabilize dominant constructions of "maleness" and "femaleness" as inherent characteristics of men and women. Trans parents, in particular, are uniquely positioned to challenge hegemonic gender practices deeming certain partnering and parenting behaviors as inherently "masculine" and "feminine" (Ryan, 2009). Trans individuals most directly transgress normative gender identity development, and as a result, they may be particularly invested in developing parenting relationships in ways that do not rely on gendered norms for constructing divisions of labor.

For instance, in a qualitative study of 10 FTM trans people, Ryan (2009) explored how previously identified lesbian women may uniquely define and practice "fathering." Ryan emphasized how some of the FTM individuals in her study did not rely on traditional notions of masculinity and fathering which are often enacted by men in heterosexual relationships (Ryan, 2009). However, Ryan asserts, despite potentially feeling liberated from normative gendering in shaping parenting practices, some trans men may fear being perceived as less authentically male as a result of not being able to procreate through heterosexual sex with their female partners (Ryan, 2009). Such instances demonstrate the complex ways in which gender may be uniquely constructed, and deconstructed, within the context of trans-parent families.

Furthermore, as a result of experiencing discrimination by families of origin, trans individuals may construct families in ways that do not rely on biological kinship relations (Maguen, Shipherd, Harris, & Welch, 2007). For instance, Maguen et al.'s (2007) study of disclosure practices of 156 trans individuals begins to address some of the ways in which trans people may structure family relations that extend beyond biologically related kin. Their findings indicated that trans participants (86% of which were MTF) were more likely to disclose their gender identity to friends and intimate partners before disclosing to family of origin (particularly siblings and mothers). Participants actively developed support networks and chosen families that consisted of personal friends and loved ones who were identity affirming. Thus, similar to gay- and lesbian-parent families, trans-parent families may expand traditional notions of the family by developing new support networks that function as "families of choice" (Oswald, 2002; Weston, 1991). However, unlike gay and lesbian individuals, finding a social support network that can become a chosen family may be particularly difficult for trans people given the prevailing stigma, marginalization, and discrimination that trans people face—even from within the LGBT community (Ryan, 2009). Moreover, FTM individuals tend to "pass" as men more easily than MTF individuals "pass" as women (Lev, 2004). Thus, FTM people who easily fit within the male/female binary may experience less societal stigma, more support from families of origin, and less of a desire or need to create chosen families.

Further, understanding how trans parents' gender identities shape children's experiences can help shed light on how children navigate their own developmental processes in relation to their parents. Given trans parents' potentially greater openness to a diversity of gender presentations and behaviors, they may be particularly open with regard to gender role expectations for their children (Ryan, 2009). For instance, Ryan's study of 10 FTM trans parents highlighted how trans men actively resisted prescribing gender normative rules for their children (Ryan, 2009). Thus, trans parents may be particularly attuned to allowing their children to explore a variety of masculine and feminine behaviors and expressions as their children develop their own gender identities. Conversely, however, children within trans-parent families may feel particularly pressured to conform to traditional notions regarding male and female gendering to legitimate the healthy and "normal" functioning of their family (Lev, 2010). Thus, rather than subverting gender norms, children may experience pressure from their social environment, parents, and peers to conform to gender normative behavior (Lev, 2010).

Lastly, just as trans parents must negotiate decisions regarding coming out to people who may not be aware of their trans status, decisions regarding when and to whom to come out may be particularly salient to children of trans parents. Depending on the extent to which the trans parent is openly and visibly trans will impact how children negotiate such disclosure practices. For instance, in contexts where the trans parent is visibly gender variant or gender nonconforming, children may have less agency as to the timing and contexts in which coming out about their trans-parent family status is initiated. Future research is needed that explores how trans parents and partners openly or more subtly provide messages to their children as to how to negotiate such processes of disclosure regarding the trans-parent status. Overall, a greater understanding of various family dynamics and processes within trans-parent families can help speak to the unique ways in which trans parents, and their partners and children, construct potentially novel notions of what it means to be a family outside of the heteronormative, gender normative nuclear family ideal.

Impact of Discrimination on Partnering and Parenting

Trans individuals develop their identities and families within the context of micro- as well as macro-level societal discrimination and stigmatization (Devor, 2002; Lev, 2004; Maguen et al., 2007). Trans individuals face unique forms of discrimination and transphobia due to transgressing normative gender identities and expressions (Spade, 2007). Specifically, trans people face legal discrimination, lack of health-care services, employment discrimination, and lack of general societal acceptance (Hill, 2007; Shelley, 2008; Tye, 2003). For instance, with regard to employment discrimination, it is estimated that 13–56% of trans people have been fired, 13–47% have been denied employment, and 22–31% have been harassed, verbally or physically (Badgett, Lau, Sears, & Ho, 2007). Not only do they face greater stigmatization than gay and lesbian individuals, but they may also be at a greater risk for hate crimes, particularly ones that are seriously assaultive (Kuehnle & Sullivan, 2001). For example, Kuehnle and Sullivan's (2001) study of 241 gay, lesbian, and transgender individuals' experiences of victimization indicated that MTF transgender individuals sustained more serious personal injuries as compared to lesbian and gay individuals.

Societal Discrimination

Trans parents, in particular, may experience unique forms of societal discrimination depending on their sexual orientation and gender identity. Similar to previous generations of gay men who viewed coming out as antithetical to parenthood (Berkowitz & Marsiglio, 2007), marginalizing discourses and practices may prevent some trans individuals from seeing parenthood as a realistic option despite their desires to become parents. Those individuals who do pursue parenthood may encounter various forms of discrimination. For example, Ryan's (2009) qualitative study of 10 FTM parents illuminated how some FTM parents, who identified as queer or as gay men, had to navigate homophobia as well as transphobia. In this way, they experienced marginalization based on both their sexual orientation and gender identification.

Understanding the impact of societal marginalization on family formation and development is particularly important given that experiencing discrimination may impact psychological well-being and mental health (Bockting, 2009), which in turn, may impact relationship satisfaction, parenting, and children's well-being (Short, 2007). Of particular interest is how children being raised within the context of trans-parent families may be impacted by discrimination related to their parents' gender identity. Research that sheds light on the impact of discrimination and bullying on children of gay and lesbian parents (see Goldberg, 2010) provides a helpful context for understanding the potential consequences of stigmatization of children within trans-parent families. For instance, Bos and Gartrell's (2010) study on the impact of homophobic stigmatization on 78 adolescents of lesbian parents suggests that although stigmatization was associated with more behavior problems, these problems were negated when adolescents had positive and close relationships with their mothers. Such findings are important to consider when studying trans-parent families. For instance, children growing up within the context of trans-parent families may experience stigmatization based on their parents' nonnormative gender identity. How much children confront such stigma will depend on both their unique social context and how visible and out their parent is as trans. However, experiencing stigmatization alone may not lead to any negative impact on children's well-being if the parent–child relationship remains strong and supportive. Further, depending on whether or not children are in relatively LGBT affirmative environments (schools, neighborhoods, communities, states) will impact the extent to which children confront discrimination based on their parents' gender status. Future research is needed to explore how children may be impacted by possible stigmatization and marginalization, examining the ways in which trans-parent families may work to buffer the effects of personal and societal discrimination.

Institutionalized Discrimination

Institutionalized forms of discrimination may impact trans-parent families as well. For instance, individuals who have transitioned prior to becoming parents and are currently partnered in same-sex relationships may have to contend with discriminatory legal laws within states which prevent same-sex couples from coadopting (Gates, Badgett, Macomber, & Chambers, 2007). Such stressors regarding legal parental status may have implications for the mental health of both trans parents and their partners. Research on same-sex parent families suggests that there are negative mental health effects of needing to be concerned with one's parental legal rights (Shapiro, Peterson, & Stewart, 2009). Within the context of trans-parent families, an MTF prospective adoptive parent who has chosen to pursue adoption with her female partner may not be able to coadopt their child at the time of placement as a result of heterosexist laws in states which prohibit coadoption by same-sex couples. Thus, some trans parents may be concerned about their legal parental rights, particularly in contexts where they are not biologically related to their child, and such concerns may in turn lead to worse mental health outcomes. Future research is needed that explores how supportive legal environments for trans-parent families may impact the overall mental health and well being of parents.

Legal regulations may further impact trans-parent families in the context of separation and child custody disputes (Lev, 2004; Ryan, 2009). Similar to gay and lesbian individuals who may lose custody of their children due to heterosexist discriminatory laws that do not recognize same-sex unions, trans people may find themselves in similarly unsupportive legal terrain. The legal landscape for child custody cases with trans parents is still relatively unchartered territory in terms of established precedent (Ryan, 2009). However, trans individuals are at risk in custody cases given the lack of explicit laws in the USA declaring that a parent's transgender status should not be considered a factor in determining child custody. Ironically, one partner's transitioning may actually help previously identified same-sex couples to access heterosexual privilege in divorce cases. For instance, in the context of a previously identified lesbian relationship, legally changing one's sex to male may actually lead to a swifter and easier divorce in states that do not recognize same-sex marriage (Conant, 2010). Future research is clearly needed that examines how discriminatory legal and social environments impact the viability of relationship dissolution in the context of trans-parent families.

Transitioning During Parenthood

Families in which one parent transitions in the midst of parenting encounter unique challenges and dynamics as partners and children navigate the shifting gender identification of one parent. Much of the extant research on transitioning within the contexts of relationships has focused primarily on partnered relationships, rather than parenting relationships (e.g., Samons, 2009). Trans individuals who transition within the context of parenthood face unique concerns and developmental processes with regard to coming out to their partners and children (Lev, 2004). Further, although some individuals transition to a uniquely gender-variant or outwardly visible trans presentation, other trans people are more concerned with "passing", with the ultimate goal of fitting within the male/female binary (Lev, 2004). For those individuals who wish to identify as men and women, their nonnormative gender identity development may not be visibly obvious to others post-transitioning. Trans men, in particular, may have an easier time being visibly "read" as male by others and may even choose not to disclose their trans identity to their children (Ryan, 2009). Thus, children may not necessarily be aware of their parents' transitioning if their parents transitioned prior to becoming parents and chose not to come out to their children. It is yet unclear how disclosing one's transgender identification, as well as the timing and pace of a parent's transitioning, might impact children's adjustment.

As trans individuals develop their gender identities and expressions, interpersonal tensions may emerge in the context of intimate relationships (Hines, 2006a; Lev, 2004). Trans people may experience initial rejection, anger, hurt, or confusion by partners and family members who are non-accepting of or uncomfortable with their developing gender identity (Lev, 2004). Such challenges in relationships and support have implications for overall well-being. For instance, research suggests that the greater number of individuals that trans people come out to regarding their trans identity, the greater level of social support they may experience, which in turn can have implications for increased perceptions of well-being (Maguen et al., 2007). Significantly, in Maguen et al.'s (2007) study, the majority of participants disclosed their transgender identity to spouses and friends first before turning to other more distant personal relationships. Such findings highlight how intimate and close relationships may play a particularly important role in providing social support for transgender individuals throughout their transitioning. Within the trans-parent context, such social support may be all the more necessary in buffering the negative effects of marginalizing discourses and practices that stigmatize trans-parent families.

Within the discipline of sociology, Hines' (2006a) study of transgender practices of partnering and parenting relationships begins to shed light on how transitioning may be interpersonally negotiated within intimate and familial relationships. Through in-depth case studies of three transgender individuals, Hines qualitatively explored how transitioning impacts partnering and parenting relationships. Although Hines' focus was only on three individuals (drawn from a larger study consisting of 30 trans adults, most of whom were not parents), her study begins to address the complexities of how trans identity construction may be enacted within the contexts of intimate relationships. In particular, her analysis suggests changes in gender presentation and identification may provoke changes in sexual desire and intimacy. For instance, one trans participant in Hines' study felt increasingly comfortable with his body post-transitioning and thereby felt more interested in developing a satisfying sexual relationship. Further, Hines' analysis indicated that developing nonnormative gender (and sexual) identities allowed some participants to move beyond stereotyped gender roles as they began to develop more equal relationships. Within the family context, specifically, Hines' analysis highlights how transitioning within the context of parenting may not only help affirm the transitioning partner's identity, but also facilitate an increase in authentic and open communication between the trans parent and child. Thus, as intimate relationships are renegotiated, couple dynamics may shift, which in turn may impact parent–child interactions. Hines' study illustrates how participants perceived transitioning less as an individualized process, and more as a family process. That is, decisions concerning disclosure, name changes, and gender presentation were considered in relation to concerns and care for the children's needs and adjustment (Hines, 2006a).

Such qualitative empirical findings support Lev's (2004) clinically informed model of transgender "family emergence" (p. 271) whereby families go through four primary stages of family development (a) discovery and disclosure, (b) turmoil, (c) negotiation, and (d) finding balance. Lev's model highlights that transitioning within a family context may indeed entail periods of distress or family turmoil; however, families can actually grow deeper and stronger as the trans parent is fully integrated into the family. Indeed, having partner involvement throughout the transitioning stage may have positive outcomes for transitioning (Blanchard & Steiner, 1983), and therapists and medical practitioners can help facilitate support between partners throughout transitioning within a family context. Such support would help alleviate the personal distress that trans people may face who delay transitioning due to fears of rejection by their partners or losing their children (Lev, 2004; Lewins, 1995).

Previous research that has examined transitioning within the context of intimate relationships often has focused on MTF individuals within the context of previously heterosexual relationships (e.g., Samons, 2009). Thus, in terms of understanding partner experiences of transitioning, the perspectives and concerns of heterosexual-identified wives have often been emphasized rather than a more comprehensive exploration of a variety of relationships, partnering experiences, and gender identifications. Clinically focused literature and medical/therapeutic practices have tended to assume that in the case of MTF individuals who are married to women, with or without children, divorce is an inevitable outcome of transitioning (Lev, 2004; Samons, 2009). Such assumptions can lead clinicians to prematurely encourage couples to separate rather than fully exploring possible areas of relationship growth and change.

Any expectation of divorce or separation as an inevitable or necessary result of transitioning prematurely assumes that trans people cannot sustain (the same) intimate relationships throughout and after transitioning (Lev, 2004). Indeed, maintaining relationships through transitioning is not only a possibility but also a reality which many researchers and clinicians have failed to recognize and support within medical and therapeutic contexts (Lev, 2004). Clinically informed literature has begun to shed light on the potential positive aspects of transitioning within the context of intimate relationships (e.g., Samons, 2009). Although transitioning within the context of a relationship, and particularly a parenting relationship, may be stressful on the relationship, partners have shown resiliency and support throughout transitioning processes (Samons, 2009). Indeed, clinicians who are knowledgeable about and sensitive to transitioning experiences and trans issues may play a crucial role in helping partners and children adjust to the trans parent's gender identification (Lev, 2004). However, isolation and lack of services may be significant stressors impacting transitioning experiences (Joslin-Roher & Wheeler, 2009). Thus, empirical research as well as clinically informed research has consistently emphasized the importance of social support and contextual factors that shape how transitioning impacts partnering and parenting relationships.

In the context of relationships where one partner transitions during the course of the relationship, non-trans partners may go through unique identity shifts as they negotiate their partner's transitioning. For example, a qualitative study of nine lesbian-, bisexual-, and queer-identified partners of transgender men indicated that non-trans partners often engaged in a process of self-exploration following their partner's transitioning (Joslin-Roher & Wheeler, 2009). Some lesbian women felt the need to reevaluate their own identification as lesbians after their partners came out as trans men (Joslin-Roher & Wheeler, 2009). Given that many trans men may transition within the context of lesbian relationships, female partners may have to reconcile their sexual orientation identification as lesbian or queer as a result of their partner's shift to a male identity. Lesbian-identified women may thereby find themselves publicly situated within a heterosexual binary within which they do not personally identify (Lev, 2003). Thus, it is conceivable that such shifts in identity may be further complicated within the context of parenting. For example, in situations in which one parent transitions in the midst of parenthood, both parents and children may need to adjust to the shifting social positioning of the family at large (e.g., the shift from a same-sex parent family to a heterosexual-parent family).

Thus, just as non-trans partners adjust to their partners' transitioning, children ultimately go through interpersonal and intrapersonal changes as well as they understand and renegotiate their parents' gender identity. Significantly, how children negotiate their parents' transitioning may differ dramatically depending on the child's developmental age. For instance, a 5-year-old child will clearly have a different experience of a parent's transitioning compared to a teenager. Preliminary research suggests that younger children may have the easiest time adapting to their parents' shift in gender identity (White & Ettner, 2004). White and Ettner's (2004) study of therapists' ratings of children whose parents were in the midst of transitioning indicated that, compared to preschoolers, adolescents had the most difficult time adapting to their parents' transitioning. Adolescents may be particularly attuned to societal norms that stigmatize transgender parents. Furthermore, their parents' transitioning may more acutely evoke feelings of loss as they renegotiate their trans parents' shifting gender identity. Importantly, trans people who are adapting well to transitioning, and whose partners and children are also adapting well, may not be in therapy; thus, their experiences may not be captured by such research that is derived from within a clinical context.

Importantly, how one identifies in terms of gender and sexual orientation may have quite different psychological, relational, and family consequences. For instance, within the context of a heterosexual marriage, a previously identified heterosexual man may, post-transition, identify as a lesbian woman. In doing so, she has repositioned her gender identification while remaining partnered with a woman (Lev, 2004). Further, within the heterosexual/homosexual binary, she has also shifted her sexual orientation identification. Such a change may have significant personal and family consequences as she proceeds to identify as a lesbian within a sociocultural context that continues to marginalize, stereotype, and discriminate against lesbians. Raising children within the context of a lesbian-parent relationship context may entail unique challenges (e.g., discrimination) and benefits (e.g., more flexible work/family divisions). On the other hand, within the context of a previously lesbian relationship, one partner may transition from a female to a male gender identity and in doing so shift the relationship to a more socially accepted status as heterosexual (Ryan, 2009). Thus, the overall family dynamics, as well as social acceptance of the family, may change depending on the parents' particular type of trans identification. Children may, therefore, find that they are negotiating a shift from a more stigmatized family status (same-sex parent family) or, on the other hand, to a more visibly heteronormative family formation (with a mother and father). However, if the trans parent transitioned in a context in which community members are aware of the transitioning, trans-parent families that have been repositioned within the heterosexual binary may not garner the heterosexual privilege typically afforded heterosexual couples. Thus, future research is needed to explore how a shift in gender and sexual orientation identification of a trans parent impacts overall family dynamics and societal acceptance.

Race, Class, and Social Context

The processes of transitioning and identifying as transgender within a family context may differ significantly depending on one's social positioning with regard to such variables as race, socioeconomic status, and geographical location. The process by which transitioning and living transgender become recognized, accepted, and refuted is contextually situated at an individual and relational level as well as at a larger socio-institutional level (e.g., employment possibilities, health-care needs, and community acceptance). For instance, trans individuals who lack adequate social support, legal recognition, and general societal acceptance may be at risk for greater mental health issues. Newfield et al.'s (2006) study of 446 FTM participants indicated that trans participants who had received hormone therapy had significantly higher quality of life scores compared to those who had not received testosterone. However, mental health providers and medical practitioners can act as gatekeepers, preventing individuals from receiving the hormone treatment that they request (Tye, 2003). Indeed, overt discrimination by health-care providers may prevent trans people from receiving appropriate care (Tye, 2003). Sex-reassignment surgery, in particular, can be very costly and without insurance companies covering such procedures, trans individuals may not be able to seek the services they request. In contrast, within the Netherlands sex-reassignment surgery is covered by state health insurance (Tye, 2003), thereby helping to facilitate transitioning for individuals regardless of socioeconomic status. Thus, if insurance companies do not reimburse for treatments within the USA, only those individuals who have the financial means to pay for such treatments will receive adequate care. Individuals from a lower socioeconomic status may therefore have a more difficult time developing a self-affirming gender identity, which has consequences for overall psychological well-being and family well-being (Newfield et al., 2006).

Such issues accessing adequate health care as a result of medical gate-keeping or low financial means have significant implications for trans-parent families. For instance, trans parents who lack economic resources, but desire a full transition to a male or female identity, may ultimately present as more gender ambiguous than they would otherwise desire. Such barriers to health care, which may put them at greater risk for psychological distress, may, in turn, impact their partnering and parenting practices as well as their children's overall well-being. Thus, a huge area for empirical research entails examining how socioeconomic status may impact trans-parent families. Clinically informed literature suggests that class barriers that make transitioning too cost-prohibitive may have negative consequences for both the trans parent and overall healthy family development (Lev, 2004). Empirical research is needed that explicitly examines working-class trans-parent families. Such research could help elucidate the intersections of class and nonnormative gendering within trans-parent families.

Racial identity and marginalization might uniquely intersect with nonnormative gendering within the context of trans-parent families. Theorizing about "the" transgender experience may risk marginalizing people of color whose experiences may not be captured by such presumably all-inclusive categories (Roen, 2001). Indeed, for certain racial or ethnic groups, one's racial identity, rather than gender identity, may be more salient within certain contexts (Roen, 2001). Roen's (2001) case study of three gender liminal[1] Maaori individuals in New Zealand suggested that some trans people may resist identifying with medical discourses on transsexuality to maintain traditional cultural values. Thus, racial and cultural minorities may uniquely reconcile tensions between their racial, cultural, and gender identities as they develop gender nonconforming identities. Further, transitioning may have quite different ramifications and meanings (both at the individual subjective level and societal level), depending on how that individual is

positioned racially and socioeconomically. For instance, Mezey's (2008) ethnographic study of lesbian women's coming out experiences and perceptions of parenthood indicated that coming out to families of origin was easier for those lesbians with race and class privilege, which, in turn, made it easier for them to decide to become parents. Prospective trans parents may feel similarly restrained or emboldened to become parents given race and class positioning. For instance, racially marginalized and lower socioeconomic status trans people may be less likely to disclose their trans identity to family members and thereby gain their support which would make deciding to parent easier. Future empirical research is needed, however, to explore how racial minority status and socioeconomic status interactively influence levels and types of social support for trans individuals. Thus, research that utilizes an intersectionality perspective is particularly needed to fully address such issues of race and class in shaping trans-parent family development.

Attending to issues of race, class, and sociocultural positioning will help elucidate the unique experiences of trans-parent families within specific social contexts. Further, across research on trans people and their families, issues of geography typically remain unspoken beyond acknowledgment of country or regional context. Internet-based research, which has the potential to derive samples from quite diverse geographical regions, suggests that trans people are very much developing their lives, support networks, and families within rural as well as urban contexts (Newfield et al., 2006). As Halberstam (2005) emphasized in her theorizing of queer and trans identities, the notion that rural environments are inevitably hostile environments for nonconforming individuals eclipses a broader range of desires and choices regarding how trans people choose to live within different contexts. Thus, beyond merely developing a research sample that is geographically diverse, research is needed that centrally considers the impact of geographical location on trans-family development. For instance, recent research on gay and lesbian individuals and families suggests the importance of understanding how geographical location, and

---

[1] Roen intentionally uses the term "gender liminal" rather than "transgender" given that transgender theorizing has often eclipsed the experiences of racial minorities who are gender nonconforming.

rural contexts in particular, shape sexual minority experiences of belonging and family (Oswald & Culton, 2003). Creating affirming social environments for trans-parent families, however, may be particularly difficult given the greater stigmatization of trans individuals who must contend with prevailing normative discourse regarding parenting and family.

Conclusion

Trans-parent families are currently transgressing normative notions of family formation. Similar to research on same-sex parent families, research that explores how gendered divisions of labor are enacted within trans-parenting contexts has the potential to illuminate family processes that radically expand dominant perceptions of traditional mothering and fathering. For example, this work could explore how trans parents and their partners construct their children's gender in ways that may draw on and subvert normative gendering. Although little empirical work has examined trans-parent families, relevant empirical research as well as clinically and theoretically informed literature on trans individuals and parents has begun to shed light on the unique factors shaping trans-parent family development. Trans people and their families are creating and sustaining families within the context of systemic discrimination. Such discrimination may impact trans-parent families differently depending on the availability of social support as well as the specific social context within which they live. For instance, having a close network of family and friends may help to buffer the potential negative psychological impact of marginalizing discourses and practices regarding trans-parent families. Importantly, there are also an increasing number of support resources for trans-parent families and their children [e.g., the KOT (Kids of Trans) resource guide, which was developed by COLAGE, an organization developed by and for people with one or more lesbian, gay, bisexual, transgender, or queer parents; Canfield-Lenfest, 2008]. Future research that elucidates family processes and development can help provide greater visibility and validation to

trans parents as well as their partners and children. Further research is needed that moves beyond the clinical context and utilizes theoretical approaches and research methods that examine a diversity of gender identifications, as well as race, class, and sociocultural factors that shape trans-parent families.

References

Badgett, L., Lau, H., Sears, B., & Ho, C. (2007). *Bias in the workplace: Consistent evidence of sexual orientation and gender identity discrimination.* Los Angeles, CA: The Williams Institute.

Berkowitz, D., & Marsiglio, W. (2007). Gay men: Negotiating procreative, father, and family identities. *Journal of Marriage and Family, 69,* 366–381. doi:10.1111/j.1741-3737.3007.00371.x

Blanchard, R., & Steiner, B. W. (1983). Gender reorientation, psychological adjustment, and involvement with female partners in female-to-male transsexuals. *Archives of Sexual Behavior, 12,* 149–157. doi:10.1007/BF01541558

Bockting, W. O. (2009). Transforming the paradigm of transgender health: A field in transition. *Sexual and Relationship Therapy, 24,* 103–107. doi:10.1080/14681990903037660

Bos, H., & Gartrell, N. (2010). Adolescents of the USA National Longitudinal Lesbian Family Study: Can family characteristics counteract the negative effects of stigmatization? *Family Process, 49,* 559–572. doi:10.1111/j.1545-5300.2010.01340.x

Boylan, J. F. (2003). *She's not there: A life in two genders.* New York, NY: Broadway Books.

Butler, J. (1990). *Gender trouble: Feminism and the subversion of identity.* New York, NY: Routledge.

Canfield-Lenfest, M. (2008). *Kids of trans resource guide.* (*COLAGE* publication). Retrieved from http://www.colage.org/resources/kot/

Cole, E. R. (2009). Intersectionality and research in psychology. *American Psychologist, 64,* 170–180. doi:10.1037/a0014564.

Conant, E. (2010, April 13). The right to love—and loss. *Newsweek.* Retrieved from http://www.thedailybeast.com/newsweek/2010/04/13/the-right-to-love-and-loss.html

Devor, H. (2002). Who are "we"? Where sexual orientation meets gender identity. *Journal of Gay and Lesbian Psychotherapy, 6,* 5–21. doi:10.1300/J236v06n02_02

Diamond, L. M., & Butterworth, M. (2008). Questioning gender and sexual identity: Dynamic links over time. *Sex Roles, 59,* 365–376. doi:10.1007/s11199z-008-9425-3

Gates, G., Badgett, M. V., Macomber, J. E., & Chambers, K. (2007). *Adoption and foster care by gay and lesbian parents in the United States.* Washington, DC: The Urban Institute.

Goldberg, A. E. (2010). *Lesbian and gay parents and their children: Research on the family life cycle*. Washington, DC: American Psychological Association.

Halberstam, J. (2005). *In a queer time & place: Transgender bodies, subcultural lives*. New York, NY: New York University Press.

Hill, D. B. (2007). Trans/gender/sexuality: A research agenda. *Journal of Gay & Lesbian Social Services: Issues in Practice, Policy & Research, 18*, 101–109. doi:10.1300/J041v18n02_06

Hines, S. (2006a). Intimate transitions: Transgender practices of partnering and parenting. *Sociology, 40*, 353–371. doi:10.1177/0038038506062037

Hines, S. (2006b). What's the difference? Bringing particularity to queer studies of transgender. *Journal of Gender Studies, 15*, 49–66. doi:10.1080/09589230500486918

Hines, S. (2007). Transgendering care: Practices of care within transgender communities. *Critical Social Policy Special Issue, 27*, 462–486. doi:10.1177/0261018307081808

Joslin-Roher, E., & Wheeler, D. P. (2009). Partners in transition: The transition experience of lesbian, bisexual, and queer identified partners of transgender men. *Journal of Gay & Lesbian Social Services, 21*, 30–48. doi:10.1080/10538720802494743

Kuehnle, K., & Sullivan, A. (2001). Patterns of anti-gay violence. An analysis of incident characteristics and victim reporting. *Journal of Interpersonal Violence, 16*, 928–943. doi:10.1177/088626001016009005

Lev, A. I. (2003). Couples in transition: When one is trans and other is not. *In the Family, 8*, 18–23.

Lev, A. I. (2004). *Transgender emergence: Therapeutic guidelines for working with gender-variant people and their families*. New York: Haworth Press.

Lev, A. I. (2010). How queer!—The development of gender identity and sexual orientation in LGBTQ-headed families. *Family Process, 49*, 268–290. doi:10.1111/j.1545-5300.2010.01323.x

Lewins, F. (1995). *Transsexualism in society: A sociology of male-to-female transsexuals*. South Melbourne, Australia: Macmillan.

Maguen, S., Shipherd, J. C., Harris, H. N., & Welch, L. P. (2007). Prevalence and predictors of disclosure of transgender identity. *International Journal of Sexual Health, 19*, 3–13. doi:10.1300/J514v19n01_02

Mezey, N. J. (2008). The privilege of coming out: Race, class, and lesbians' mothering decisions. *International Journal of Sociology of the Family, 34*, 257–276.

Newfield, E., Hart, S., Dibble, S., & Kohler, L. (2006). Female-to-male transgender quality of life. *Quality of Life Research, 15*, 1447–1457. doi:10.1007/s11136-006-0002-3

Oswald, R. (2002). Resilience within the family networks of lesbians and gay men: Intentionality and redefinition. *Journal of Marriage and Family, 64*, 374–383. doi:10.1111/j.1741-3737.2002.00374.x

Oswald, R., & Culton, L. (2003). Under the rainbow: Rural gay life and its relevance for family providers. *Family Relations, 52*, 72–79. doi:10.1111/j.1741-3729.2003.00072.x

Pinto, R. M., Melendez, R., & Spector, A. (2008). Male-to-female transgender individuals building social support and capital from within a gender-focused network. *Journal of Gay & Lesbian Social Services: Issues in Practices, Policy & Research, 20*, 203–220. doi:10.1080/10538720802235179

Roen, K. (2001). Transgender theory and embodiment: The risk of racial marginalization. *Journal of Gender Studies, 10*, 253–263. doi:10.1080/09589230120086467

Ryan, M. (2009). Beyond Thomas Beatie: Trans men and the new parenthood. In R. Epstein (Ed.), *Who's your daddy? And other writings on queer parenting* (pp. 139–150). Toronto, Canada: Sumach Press.

Samons, S. L. (2009). Can this marriage be saved? Addressing male-to-female transgender issues in couples therapy. *Sexual and Relationship Therapy, 24*, 152–162. doi:10.1080/14681990903002748

Sanchez, F. J., & Vilain, E. (2009). Collective self-esteem as a coping resource for male-to-female transsexuals. *Journal of Counseling Psychology, 56*, 202–209. doi:10.1037/a0014573

Shapiro, D. N., Peterson, C., & Stewart, A. J. (2009). Legal and social contexts and mental health among lesbian and heterosexual mothers. *Journal of Family Psychology, 23*, 255–262. doi:10.1037/a0014973

Shelley, C. A. (2008). *Transpeople: Repudiation, trauma, healing*. Toronto, ON: University of Toronto Press.

Short, L. (2007). Lesbian mothers living well in the context of heterosexism and discrimination: Resources, strategies and legislative change. *Feminism & Psychology, 17*, 57–74. doi:10.1177/0959353507072912

Spade, D. (2007). Methodologies of trans resistance. In G. Haggerty & M. McGarry (Eds.), *A companion to lesbian, gay, bisexual, transgender, and queer studies* (pp. 237–261). New York, NY: Blackwell.

Tye, M. C. (2003). Lesbian, gay, bisexual, and transgender parents: Special considerations for the custody and adoption evaluator. *Family Court Review, 41*, 92–103. doi:10.1177/1531244502239355

Warner, M. (1993). *Fear of a queer planet: Queer politics and social theory*. Minneapolis, MN: University of Minnesota Press.

Warner, D. N. (2004). Towards a queer research methodology. *Qualitative Research in Psychology, 14*, 321–337. doi:10.1191/1478088704qp021oa

Weston, K. (1991). *Families we choose: Lesbians, gays, kinship*. New York, NY: Columbia University Press.

White, T., & Ettner, R. (2004). Disclosure, risks and protective factors for children whose parents are undergoing a gender transition. *Journal of Gay and Lesbian Psychotherapy, 8*, 129–145.

"These Are *Our* Children": Polyamorous Parenting

8

Maria Pallotta-Chiarolli, Peter Haydon, and Anne Hunter

Introducing Polyfamilies

Anne: What do you think requires further research [about polyfamilies?]

Pete: Apart from everything? (PolyVic poly-parenting group)

Children raised in polyamorous families (or polyfamilies) have parents who may be bisexual, gay, lesbian, heterosexual, or transgendered; are of diverse cultures and social classes; are in openly negotiated intimate sexual relationships with more than one partner; and may all live together or in various abodes (Anapol, 2010; Pallotta-Chiarolli, 2010a, 2010b). Thus, the definitional parameters of polyfamilies are broad and inclusive of LGBT group marriages/relationships, wherein multiple LGBT adult sexual partners live together communally with children, and open marriages/relationships where one or more of the LGBT adults may have more than one partner. Polyfamilies are also inclusive of both polyamorous families wherein various LGBT adults may seek external partners and polyfidelitous families wherein the LGBT adults agree to only be in sexual relationships with each other and not be open to relationships outside the group. Researchers and family service providers need to be mindful of these multiple and sometimes shifting configurations of nonnormative intimacies and queer multi-parent families (Anapol, 1992, 2010; Barker & Langdridge, 2010; Pallotta-Chiarolli, 2010a). Indeed, a strong link between bisexuality and polyamory has been identified in the existing research such that bisexual individuals often have partners of diverse genders (Anderlini-D'Onofrio, 2009; Pallotta-Chiarolli, 2010a).

Polyamorous parenting is an underresearched area and very few health and education resources are available to support polyfamilies. This chapter will make visible the "non-normative intimacies" (Roseneil & Budgeon, 2004, p. 138) of polyamory within which children are being raised, and thus supports the need for research from the standpoint of "actual" families rather than through the traditional family lens (Erera, 2002). It is also a continuation of the research being undertaken with underrepresented "queer multiparent families": LGBT parents who challenge "oppressive master narratives that legitimize and normalize heteronormative, nuclear families" (Vaccaro, 2010, p. 443) and two-parent households (see also Goldberg, 2010).

The thematic framework of this chapter is the double-edged sword familiar to all queer family configurations. On the one hand, polyfamilies suffer from a lack of presence which disadvantages

M. Pallotta-Chiarolli, Ph.D. (✉)
Social Diversity in Health and Education, School of Health and Social Development, Deakin University, 221 Burwood Highway, Burwood, VIC 3125, Australia
e-mail: mariapc@deakin.edu.au

P. Haydon, B.A. • A. Hunter, B.A.
PolyVic, Melbourne, VIC, Australia
e-mail: peteyak1960@gmail.com; hippolytahunter@gmail.com

A.E. Goldberg and K.R. Allen (eds.), *LGBT-Parent Families: Innovations in Research and Implications for Practice*, DOI 10.1007/978-1-4614-4556-2_8, © Springer Science+Business Media New York 2013

them in terms of legal, economic, societal, and institutional rights and acceptance. On the other hand, fears of misunderstanding, demonization, and othering by health, education, and legal service providers make polyfamilies reluctant to disclose their families or even their very existence to the wider societal matrix in which they exist and operate. In this chapter, this duality of lack of visibility and fear of disclosure and its interconnections will be examined in the context of formal societal structures such as education, health, and the law; less formal networks such as family, friends, neighbors, and social groups; and the nebulous but powerful sea of mass media in which we all swim.

Two main channels of research will be reviewed: the relatively sparse academic research available on the subject, and the findings garnered from a discussion group conducted with polyamorous parenting members of a polyamory social and support group, PolyVic, in Victoria, Australia, which holds regular meetings and social events such as picnics. Upon invitation to participate in an audio-taped discussion to collect data for this chapter, 13 polyparents (9 women and 4 men aged between 35 and 50) attended and selected pseudonyms for themselves.

The lack of existing research will be highlighted throughout to identify what is unknown or understudied and propose some directions for further research. The perspectives and experiences of the PolyVic parenting group will provide further insights into what polyparents would like health and education providers and the wider community to know about their families; what further research they feel needs to be undertaken; and what kinds of resources they would like to have available. Indeed, the PolyVic parenting group voices many ongoing experiences and perspectives consistent with the findings of previous research, from the early 1970s to as recently as 2010.

In writing this chapter, we were also mindful of the concerns of health researchers and health-service providers working with nonnormative families that "there is far too much emphasis on the supposed deficits and problems with diverse families, and insufficient attention to their strengths and abilities" (Erera, 2002, p. 213).

Indeed, Erera (2002) argues that many of the problems and pressures experienced by "diverse families" are due to factors outside the family itself, imposed by a social environment that stigmatizes, discriminates, and particularly in the case of polyfamilies, makes invisible. Hence, this chapter will present the strengths and abilities of polyfamilies and consider the impact of an external social environment that is nonsupportive or ignorant of their actual families (see also Anapol, 2010; Sheff, 2010). In response to these external ascriptions, Kentlyn (2008) explains how the home of queer or nonnormative families becomes both a "safe" and a "scrutinized" space: "[The] private space of the queer home can be seen to embody the tension between a safe space to be queer in, but also a place where the subversive performance of gender, sexuality and family comes under scrutiny" (pp. 327–328). Our review of existing research and our empirical research with the PolyVic polyparenting group will incorporate an ongoing analysis of the tensions and interweavings between external surveillance and regulation, and the safety and privacy of the polyhome (Foucault, 1978).

Research Meta-Issues

Before addressing specific issues of concern for polyfamilies, we outline three meta-issues of research absence that are identifiable throughout the available research such as in Maria's qualitative research with 94 polyamorous parents, their adult children, and polyamorous and/or bisexual young adults in the USA and Australia (Pallotta-Chiarolli, 2010a, 2010b). First, it becomes immediately obvious that there is a lack of presence of polyfamilies in academic discourse which also reflects the lack of awareness of polyfamilies in social, legal, health, and educational realities. Due to the absence of theorizing and data about polyfamilies and their children, we must use the analytical literature on children from same-sex parent families to help articulate and explain what children from polyfamilies go through—although children in polyfamilies may face even more heightened levels of invisibility and stigmatization. But as similarities and differences between same-sex parent families and polyfamilies are complex, we refer to this research only where clearly applicable.

Second, the research that has been conducted has been limited by its reliance on White middle-class samples. Maria recognizes that this is a major limitation in her own previous research (Pallotta-Chiarolli, 2002, 2006, 2010a, 2010b) which reflects the wider concern that most research methods fail to access larger representations of people of diverse socioeconomic, cultural, and religious locations, and transgendered identities (Noel, 2006; see also Haritaworn, Chin-ju, & Klesse, 2006; Sheff, 2006; Sheff & Hammers, 2011). Most polyamorous research participants, including those in the PolyVic polyparenting group, were White, middle-class, college-educated individuals who identified as male or female and had high levels of cyberliteracy which allowed them to participate in social and support groups, particularly online, and thereby find themselves participating in our research (Noel, 2006). This concern is indicative of Sheff and Hammers' (2011) contention that race, education, and class privileges provide valuable buffers from the myriad potential negative outcomes associated with sexual and relational nonconformity.

Third, in the available research projects and writings, the perspectives, experiences, and insights of children and adults who have grown up in polyfamilies are largely absent; how these experiences affected their well-being, later relationships, and education is also absent. Researchers such as Strassberg (2003) consider this lack a major hindrance to the development of legal, health, and educational policies and practices that support these children and their families.

Substantive Themes in the Research

Having outlined the three major limitations within the available research, this section will now present the four major themes that have been addressed in the literature. These four themes are (a) issues of disclosure and exposure to one's children and external systems such as schools; (b) internal

polyfamily environments and their impact on children; (c) the need for polyfamily-friendly health, welfare, and legal services; and (d) polyfamilies in the media and popular culture. Quotes from the PolyVic polyparenting discussion group are presented to illustrate these themes.

Issues of Disclosure and Exposure

A major overriding theme arising in research and writings about polyfamilies is how "out" parents should be to their children and to external systems, communities, and individuals. In turn, this will affect how "out" their children should or will be in systems, communities, and to peers at school and elsewhere.

Disclosure to Children

Consider this quote by Robyn, a mother of two teenaged boys, who was a member of the PolyVic parenting discussion group:

> When we did disclose, talk to them and share with them, it was at a point where they would be going "Are mum and dad having an affair?" … .So it was at a point where we had to say, "Mum and Dad love each other, this is safe, we love you, and any time we have a relationship with someone let's remember the values of how to have a healthy relationship. … People do things different, well this is just another one of those things that we do differently." And they were like … "Let's have some pizza." (laughter)

In the above, Robyn discusses her experience of when and how she disclosed her polyamory to her children. How and when to disclose to children and its possible ramifications were a major concern of all polyparents in the discussion group, and this theme is also reflected in the available research such as the Polyamory Survey conducted by Loving More, an American-based organization with its own magazine, which elicited over 5,000 responses in 2001/2002. In her analysis of sections of this survey (Pallotta-Chiarolli, 2002, 2006), Maria found that about 29% of respondents were biological parents of children under 18, 16% were legal guardians of children under 18, 18% were biological parents of children over the age of 18, and 4% were legal guardians of children over the age of 18. Despite these percentages, only about 30% of parent/guardian respondents had told their children about their poly relationships or their desire to be in one, and all parents feared that disclosure to children would place children in difficult situations of whether or not to disclose to outside peers and adults. Of those who did disclose or whose children were growing up in openly polyamorous families, about 45% of the parents reported having received affirming and unproblematic responses from their children. Another 15% of the parents reported having received negative responses wherein children were distressed about or rejecting their family structure and its potentially negative reception in the wider society, and 40% had received neutral responses, as in children did not seem interested in engaging with discussions about the family structure (Pallotta-Chiarolli, 2002, 2006).

A related issue that has been discussed to some degree in research and certainly requires further study is the association between children's age and developmental context and the results of disclosure to children. It consistently appears that the age/maturity level of the child is a significant factor that parents endeavor to take into account when making decisions about disclosure/exposure to parental partnerships (see Constantine & Constantine, 1976; Davidson, 2002; Pallotta-Chiarolli, 2010a; Strassberg, 2003). Generally, it appears that preschool youngsters can handle disclosure in a more matter-of-fact way, while school-age children, who have had exposure to normative constructions of families within schools and among a wider range of peers and mainstream media discourses, tend to experience varying degrees of embarrassment and discomfort and may feel conflicted when hearing outsiders' discriminatory remarks about their parents. Adolescents are likely to experience the strongest anxieties and confusions as they are facing puberty issues in regards to their own sexualities, relationships, and identities, and may feel increased sensitivity to peer attitudes against nonnormative sexualities and families. They are also the most

likely age group to keep their polyfamilies secret, given that they are also more aware of wider dominant moral, political, or social discourses that construct cultural understandings of what constitutes a healthy family (Watson & Watson, 1982; Weitzman, 2006, 2007).

Overall, a major anxiety that most polyparents talked about in all the available research is the fear that being out about their families would lead to harassment and stress for their children. Many tried to prepare their children for the consequences of their public disclosure and provided them with verbal, mental, and emotional strategies to counteract or deflect negativity so that they would be active agents rather than passive victims in educational and health institutions (Boden, 1990). Both the pros and cons of disclosure to children were prominent discussion points in the PolyVic polyparenting group:

Robyn: Sometimes I think "Oh have I made life harder for them?" And yet I can't go against what I feel has sat well with myself and therefore I have confidence that they'll get through.

Juliet: Yeah, but look at it like the immune system you know, to challenge and strengthen the immune system. … you don't cotton-wool your children in any way, just give them what comes up in life, and protect them.

Daryl: [But] they're kind of expected to be an activist for something they didn't start.

Many polyfamilies and their children feel like border dwellers, constantly navigating their positions between home and the external world. Drawing from Wright's (2001) work with lesbian-parent families, we can begin to articulate the ongoing tension children may experience between their selves within their families, "which feels 'normal' and safe and nurturing," and their experience outside their families, "in which they often feel invisible or vilified… [in] a society that enforces conformity" (p. 288). Having access to other knowledge and ways of being, and joining in the questioning of "normal" constructions of family, may place children of polyfamilies permanently on the borders of society because of their "edge identities" (Bersten, 2008, p. 9).

It requires decisions from children on how to define and construct their sexual and intimate relationships with peers within the normative social space of schools, clubs, friendship groups, as well as recognize that they will most likely experience some degree of marginalization and harassment. It may also lead to self-questioning dilemmas for parents border dwelling between a philosophy of raising their children with a broader understanding of sexuality, family, and relationships, and a protective concern that their children may be ostracized because of this philosophy.

This discussion of bordering arose in the PolyVic polyparenting group, especially concerning the emergence of the child beyond the world of the family and into a potential stress of ambiguity and duality:

Daryl: We've been open with our kids and they know what's going on and they're all happy and fine about that but when other kids ask them, "What's going on there?" they're gonna see that the situation is not exactly the same as their family situation. My kids are gonna have to explain something. … I imagine they probably already have to some of their friends and that's probably going to get back to their families and then there'll be some misunderstanding and some explanation will be needed to be done there.

Passing as Normal and Keeping Secrets

Many polyparents in the available literature (see Pallotta-Chiarolli, 2010a, 2010b; Sheff, 2010) and in our PolyVic research worried about the effects of disclosing their poly relationships to their children because of the overwhelming invisibility of their families. This concern is a prime example of the deleterious effects of the interconnection between lack of visibility and fear of disclosure. Wright (2001) explains how feeling that the outside world has no way to understand or talk about their kind of family can create a sense of unreality for children, "as if one is seeing something that others cannot see"; this realization of invisibility and lack of acceptance

can "plant the seed of fear in the child's heart" (p. 288). To protect children from this cognitive and emotional dissonance, and to protect themselves as parent members of local communities and recipients of legal, health, and educational services, many polyfamilies will pass as monogamous to their own children. The alternative imposes a difficult either/or decision for parents: either allow children to "go public," with attendant risks to the children, or risk damaging the children by expecting them to keep a secret.

Thorson's (2009) work on communication privacy management (CPM) offers some insight into and strategies in the negotiation of these dilemmas. CPM addresses how parents and children negotiate "information ownership" and privacy rules and enact "protection and access rules" (Thorson, 2009, p. 34) for any processes of disclosure. Jeremy, a father of two school-aged children discussed his and his children's strategies of CPM in the polyparenting discussion group:

> I work in a Catholic school. They don't know anything about me. I don't want them to know anything, you know?. … And so it's the same with our children. They'll get to the point of going, "With this person I can share this, and with this person I don't" ….We trust in their commonsense.

Thus, polyfamilies need to consider and negotiate which forms of passing and CPM may work best in their specific contexts. Using terms constructed by Richardson (1985) in her work with women who were in secret relationships with married men, the following strategies were adopted by polyfamilies: withdrawing from potentially harmful external settings as much as possible; compartmentalizing, segregating, or bordering the worlds of home and external settings; cloaking certain realities so that they are invisible or pass as normative; or fictionalizing certain aspects of one's life and family. Indeed, polyparenting may involve working with one's children to redefine, reconstruct, and/or fictionalize the family for the outside world (Arden, 1996; Sheff, 2010; Trask, 2007).

Maria's previous research has explored how polyfamilies will pass, border, or pollute (see Douglas, 1966) in external settings and spaces such as in schools (Pallotta-Chiarolli, 2010a, 2010b).

For example, some families will choose to pass as heterosexual or possibly as same-sex couple parent families. For instance, they will give existing known normative labels such as "auntie," "godparent," and "friend" to polyfamily members to avoid external scrutiny of and discrimination against their polyhome. For some polyfamilies, these strategies of editing, scripting, and concealment provide protection and the ability to live out family realities with little external surveillance or interference (Kentlyn, 2008; Kroeger, 2003). Although these findings fit in with the broader literature on LGBT life in general, and parenting/families in particular (see Barker & Langdridge, 2010; Garner, 2004; Goldberg, 2010; Wright, 2001), we assert that what polyfamilies are going through may be more difficult than what happens for monogamous or coupled LGBT persons in general due to the even greater levels of invisibility and/or stigmatization.

Polluting Public Spaces

Some polyparents and their children see themselves as polluting outside worlds by coming out and presenting their relationships as legitimate and worthy of official affirmation. Thus, they not only claim public space but also compel institutions to adapt to new and expanding definitions of family. Proactive polyparents speak of a plurality of resistances (Foucault, 1978) including subversive strategies such as gaining positions of parent power and decision making in schools and other communities, or establishing solid working relationships and friendships within neighborhood, church, and school communities. These strategies consolidate their security, and give access to policy making, community thinking, and action, as well as making it possible to forge strong trusting bonds with other "deviant" minority persons in the community (Pallotta-Chiarolli, 2006, 2010a, 2010b).

Nevertheless, as Sheff (2010) found in her qualitative research with 71 polyamorous adults in the USA, the reality or potential of external stigmatization in any interaction outside the polyhome may require children to manage the stigma of their parents' relationships, and for which parents

"express remorse about the pain their relationships have caused the children" (p. 178). A strategy used to alleviate this was "stigma management" (Sheff, 2010, p.178) whereby parents strived to make the family and polycommunity a space/place of intimacy, positive role models, and support to diminish the impact and significance of external stigmatization. The members of the PolyVic polyparenting group discussed at length the issue of managing external stigmatization and discrimination:

Anne: Having to deal with the judgement of people outside about the impact that your polyamory is having on your family.

Robyn: It's also good to teach your child that she should do what she wants and … not be worried about what other people think of her as well.

Daryl: We had a bunch of kids over from the scout group last night and I don't know if all of the families'd be cool about it. … I know at least three of the families are okay but at least one of them I'm thinking, they're going to find out, they might be a bit weirded out about it.

The "Poster-Child Mentality"

Children with polyparents who are out may feel the pressure to "closet" any facets of themselves in public spaces and institutions that may be constructed as flaws emanating directly from polyparenting. They may feel compelled to display how "normal" and unpolluted they themselves are, or they develop what Garner (2004) calls the "poster-child mentality" (p. 29) in her discussion of children with LGB parents:

> We fear normal won't be good enough. So instead, we strive for perfect. Anything less leaves weak spots for critics to poke holes though our argument that our families are worthy of social acceptance. … [Children] grow tired of having to constantly watch what they do or say. They experience anxiety about getting caught with their guard down and fear it could result in someone exploiting their families' vulnerabilities. All these consequences take their toll on children's self-esteem and self-worth. (pp. 2–3)

Children of polyfamilies may feel the need to pollute/pass as perfect to signify the success of the family (Pallotta-Chiarolli, 2010a; Sheff, 2010). Again, this is also found in families headed by same-sex couples (see Goldberg, 2007), a process that Garner (2004) describes as "straightening up for the public" (p. 179) and that could be termed "monogamizing for the public" in relation to polyfamilies. As Garner notes, "Our families currently lack the 'luxury' to be as openly complicated, confusing, or dysfunctional as straight families" (p. 6).

Much more research is required into the existence and extent of the poster-child mentality in children of polyfamilies. Most offspring from out polyfamilies and most out polyparents concluded, in Maria's research and in other studies such as Sheff's (2010), that despite problems and potential dilemmas, the positives of living in a polyfamily generally outweighed the negatives. This dilemma of weighing up the dangers and the positives of having children polluting their schools with knowledge and "sassiness" about their polyfamilies was part of the PolyVic polyparenting group discussion. In the following, Eve, a mother of a preschooler, shared her concerns with parents of school-aged children:

Eve: And what happens when someone at school says "Oh your mum's a slut!"?
Robyn: Yeah! (laughter) Just say, "Yeah that's right! Yeah."
Juliet: That's probably empowering for the teenager to be able to do.
Eve: It depends on the teenager.

Self-monitoring of one's behavior according to real or imagined external scrutiny (Foucault, 1978) may also mean that some children will pass as perfect to their own families to avoid distressing their loved ones. Thus, they may conceal from their parents any anxiety, harassment, or negativity from school and peers (Garner, 2004).

"If I'm Out to My Kids, Do I Risk Losing Them?"

A theme that has consistently arisen in research since the 1970s is the question of whether parents should disclose their polyamorous lifestyles to children knowing that children may then disclose to external health, education, and social services, and thereby risk being taken away from their families (see Watson & Watson, 1982). A study by Walston (2001), which elicited 430 polyamorous respondents to an online survey, found that 32% of the polyparents expressed concern that polyamory would affect future child custody while 4% of the polyparents said polyamory had affected their child custody to some degree.

The concern that living in a polyfamily might be considered justification for legally removing children from a parent's custody also arose in Pallotta-Chiarolli's (2010a, 2010b) research wherein 13% of the polyparent respondents had experienced (or knew someone who had experienced) discrimination in contact with Child Protective Services (Pallotta-Chiarolli, 2002, 2006). Many parents stressed the need for families to collect documentation and legal papers to protect themselves and their children should any situation arise at school or with child and social welfare services (Anapol, 2010). Thus, these consistent findings across research reports again raise the question: To what extent is the low rate of visibility of polyfamilies due to their concealment from outside structures such as health, education, and family services for fear of the ramifications of disclosure? (see Easton & Liszt, 1997; Sheff, 2010).

The fear of losing custody or access to one's children was voiced strongly in the PolyVic parenting group:

Eve: How do I give [my daughter] that gift of self-confidence without society telling her that her family's sick and wrong, and without someone calling in social services at some point?
Nigel: I went through a process with DHS [Department of Health Services] last year. And my fear is that it was only because of the person who got involved in the case – the case manager - that everything was fine. My partners and I decided to be completely open because we felt that if while the staff were talking to our kids this all came out, then

it'd be "Oh there's something that they think is wrong, so what's going on there?" … .And we just reassured this person that we don't have sex in front of the children. … I felt very threatened. … running the risk of losing the family. … yeah it was just this constant fear of "How do we approach this?" And just having to second-guess: "Ok if we do A will B happen?"

"Will My Kid's School Understand?"

What negotiations and silences surround polyamorous families within school communities? How do children from polyamorous families experience school? Apart from Pallotta-Chiarolli (2010a, 2010b), these questions remain unasked in most recent research with polyamorous families (see e.g., Hill, 1997; Walston, 2001). The little research there shows that sensationalized stereotypes about nonmonogamous relationships conspire with silence about diverse family realities to perpetuate ignorance, misrepresentation, and stigmatization in school settings (Pallotta-Chiarolli, 2006). Parents in polyfamilies have to make a decision about how much information to give to their children's schools. Many simply decide to give a minimum of functional information, as evidenced by this discussion in the PolyVic parenting group:

Robyn: We just haven't talked about it to the school.

Juliet: It's nothing that the school has to know about, I'd say.

Bronwyn: It hasn't come up. … we had a funny circumstance recently when [a partner] came with me to pick up the kids, and the girls just ran over to her and said "Are you coming for a sleepover?" and there's been other people which they've said that to at after-school care. I haven't had any comments. If I had a comment I would address it. The children haven't been asked any questions.

Some schools may try to suppress polyamory issues that they feel are inappropriate or will be badly received by other children and their families:

Nigel: One of my children was told at [secondary] school not to discuss poly or my bisexuality with any school friends or on the school grounds at all. … they would be ostracised or they'd be picked on, that it was not relevant for school. … it came from the year level co-ordinator. … The advice was ignored [by my daughter] (laughter) which I'm quite proud of. … [We were] quite offended. We actually contacted the teacher and said "No, that's wrong. We will be encouraging our daughter to be herself and to do what she wants."

Researching Internal Polyfamily Environments

A second theme that has received scant attention is children's experiences of living in polyfamilies, the internal machinations of polyfamilies, and their influence on children's development and future as adults (see Iantaffi, 2009). What becomes evident in the following sections are the numerous benefits of polyparenting for both children and adults; yet these remain largely unknown in public settings and in service provision to families.

The Benefits for Children of a Polyfamily Structure

Some early research on polyfamilies found how children may actually benefit from their experiences in this family structure. For example, the 1970s saw some attempts at researching and documenting the experiences and well-being of children from group marriages (one form of polyfamily where three or more adults live together and are sexually intimate with at least two other members of that group) (Constantine & Constantine, 1972, 1973, 1976; Francoeur, 1972). A pioneering study of 40 children from 12 group marriage families by Constantine and Constantine (1976) found that children enjoyed a permissive environment, extending to their schooling, which was community run or cooperative with other communes. They concluded that any difficulty children faced in adapting to polyparenting was exacerbated by the lack of positive and supportive services and the prevalence of prejudice.

A consistent finding in research with polyparents since the 1970s is their strong emphasis on nonsexist practices, particularly encouraging girls to be assertive in resolving interpersonal relationships (see e.g., Eiduson, Cohen & Alexander, 1973). Similarly, members of the PolyVic polyparenting group also talked of raising their children in non-misogynist and non-heteronormative ways.

Polyparent participants in the most recent published research (Sheff, 2010) highlight five benefits of their family structures: (a) emotional intimacy with children due to fostering honesty and a sex-positive environment; (b) the greater amount of shared resources (such as financial) and resource persons; (c) more personal time due to "the ability to distribute parenting" (p. 174); (d) greater attention for children due to the availability of adults; (e) more positive role-model adults who communicate, negotiate, and have varying skills and interests. Participants in the PolyVic polyparenting group discussed similar positives, such as opportunities for those interested in parenting to become carers for children:

Lisa: [Being a] tribal aunt's been a really cool thing and very empowering.
Eve: [My child] has an oddfather, not a godfather … and he's a fairy oddfather. And he's part of our extended poly family.
Pete: Or [you can have a] fairy oddmother.

New Kinship Terms

The above section of transcript from the discussion group also points to how polyfamilies are constructing new kinship terms (such as "fairy oddmother"), or reintroducing pre-Industrial or non-Western kinship terms (such as "tribal aunt") perhaps sparked by the growing Western appreciation (and perhaps romanticization) of traditional indigenous communities and lifestyles (Anderlini-D'Onofrio, 2009). It is unclear from the available research whether these kinship terms are being invented or introduced by children or parents but they do represent an emerging shared discourse among polyfamilies and in poly-communities in providing appropriate and affirming family and kinship terms as points of identification and belonging.

"It Takes a Village": Shared Child Rearing

The above discussion on the invention or re-introduction of kinship terms indicates a significant facet of polyparenting which requires much more research: the concept and practice of shared parenting or "tribal" parenting (Anapol, 1992, 2010; Anderlini-D'Onofrio, 2009; Iantaffi, 2006, 2009). Some polyparents see poly as the new extended family, with greater ease of parenting than found in the nuclear, two-parent family, and they celebrate the benefits of diverse communal parenting and shared responsibility:

Bronwyn: Huge advantage to the children to have adults that are willing to share of themselves … it takes a village to raise a child. They have input from a variety of adults with a variety of beliefs, a variety of religious backgrounds, of political views, just all sorts of things that they bring as an adult to children's life.
Eve: The [mainstream] attitude's kind of, "Oh why aren't YOU looking after YOUR child?" whereas in this kind of poly community I think you often find that it's "these are our children" … collaborative parenting.

Anapol (2003) believes that children could be much better educated in polyamorous families, because with a larger number of adults "pooling their resources and their expertise, children would have direct access to a diverse group of tutors as well as educational software, videos, and databases" (p. 4, see also Anapol, 1992, 2010). One disadvantage of this collaborative polyparenting identified in prior research is that children become attached to partners of their parents, and, should they later leave, the children experience the "resultant separation anxiety and grief" (Sheff, 2010, p. 177). Based on her interviews and a review of the existing research, Sheff (2010) concluded that polyamorous parents used a strategy of "emotional protection" such as striving to ensure the partners make long-term or lifelong commitments to the children, as well as helping children learn the skills required to "manage loss or transition" (p. 177).

The Need for Polyfamily - Friendly Health, Welfare, and Legal Services

The third theme that emerges across the available research is the pathologization and problematization of polyfamilies, multisexual parents, and their children by legal, welfare, and health-service providers, and the lack of substantial research into what polyfamilies require from these services and systems (Davidson, 2002; Strassberg, 2003; Weitzman, 2006, 2007). Below, Pete, a parent of two children who were now in their 20s, discusses his experiences with a counselor when his children were much younger:

> In the 90s I attended a counselor who obviously thought that polyamory was a problem. I was pretty committed to working with her at the time. I was living a polyamorous life, although I hadn't heard the word. She suggested I try monogamy cos she didn't think that I was polyamorous – that lasted about eight months …. Ultimately that process with her confirmed that I really was polyamorous, and that some therapists really don't get polyamory (laughter).

Weber (2002) found that 38% of a sample of polyamorous people who had participated in counseling or therapy had not revealed their polyamory to their health-service providers, and 10% of those who did reveal it experienced a negative response. Even if the providers were open-minded and willing to learn about polyamory, clients had to use some of their paid session time to educate the professional. As

Firestein (2007) writes in relation to bisexuality and polyamory in the health sector, and as is evident in the growing membership and variety of discussions on listservs such as Polyfamilies and Polyparenting: "Our clients are no longer coming to us because they want to be 'normal.' They are coming to us because they want to be whole" (Firestein, 2007, p. xiii; see also Weitzman, 2006, 2007).

Polyfamilies in the Media and Popular Culture

The fourth major theme that has been consistent throughout the available research is the need to incorporate positive representations of polyamorous families in texts, media, and popular culture for both polyparents and their children. These representations will then provide public points of reference and examples that would facilitate both wider societal visibility and polyfamilies' confidence to disclose to their own children and the external society.

Eve: We have mass-media representation of lying and cheating and how to do it properly.

Pete: It's not easy, but a documentary to foster public discussion and public awareness of polyamory would be great.

Maia: Media representation with characters that I can identify with?

Eve: Yeah. Positive representation, not "laugh at" and "bitch about."

In the Polyamory Survey, around 98% of respondents supported "the creation of positive images on TV, in books and movies of people living in poly relationships." In relation to educational issues, when asked, "How strongly do you support the creation of positive images in high school curriculum of people living in poly relationships?", about 94% of respondents indicated support (Pallotta-Chiarolli, 2002, 2006). These findings again raise the question: to what extent is the ongoing low degree of disclosure to one's children and outside social institutions due to the lack of positive images in popular culture that provide a discourse that affirms polyfamilies and thereby the emotional and social health and well-being of their children (Pallotta-Chiarolli, 2010a)?

A detailed discussion and critical analysis of the few available films that deliberately or inadvertently address polyfamilies and their children can be found in Pallotta-Chiarolli (2010a). In the available research and our own polyparenting group discussion, polyparents expressed their desire for films and television programs with poly representations not linked to crime or pathology, as well as personal accounts, biographical writings, and opinion pieces describing polyparenting. For example, Easton and Liszt (1997) devote a chapter to child rearing for bisexual, nonmonogamous, and polyamorous mothers, showing the creative options for raising children in polyamorous households (see also Bear, 1998; Iantaffi, 2006, 2009; Taormino, 2008; Trask, 2007). In most personal writings on children in polyamorous families, and as has been discussed earlier in this chapter, the focus is on the positives these children experience growing up in such homes: "Children are equipped with lots of support and self-esteem, and (probably) more information than their peers, [who] might even benefit from a more unconventional home environment" (Arden, 1996, p. 251; see also Halpern, 1990; Nearing, 1996; Newitz, 2006; West, 1996). Thus, there is a need for more personal writings and other texts on how polyfamilies address internal and external challenges in relation to children, and how adults who have been raised in polyfamilies reflect back on their experiences.

Books for Children, Adolescents and Young Adults

Many polyparents and their offspring called for novels as well as picture books for children. Maria's own novel for adolescents, young adults, and adults, *Love You Two* (Pallotta-Chiarolli, 2008) with its multicultural, multisexual, and multipartnered characters, is based on her research over 15 years. The central character is Pina who discovers her mother is polyamorous.

This sets off a chain of events and encounters with people who disrupt, subvert, and agentically construct their own sexual identities and families according to their own needs (see Lambert, 2009 for a review).

Two other recent teen/young adult novels have also touched upon polyamory in young people: Prodan's (2008) *The Suicide Year* and *A Queer Circle of Friends* by Lees (2006). Indeed, Lees' three main characters, who are already between, beyond, and on the borders of gender and sexual binaries, construct a polyamorous relationship based on honesty and negotiation. Throughout the book, their poly relationship is a secure and sexually and emotionally satisfying given.

Two children's picture books that can be used to introduce and discuss polyfamilies are *Six-Dinner Sid* (Moore, 1991) and Else-Marie and her *Seven Little Daddies* (Lindenbaum, 1991). "Six-dinner Sid" could easily be defined as a polyamorous cat that lives with six different families. Lindenbaum's (1991) book is about Else-Marie's family, which comprises one normal-size mother and seven tiny, identical daddies whom she loves. However, when her mother announces that she has to work overtime and that Else-Marie's daddies will pick her up at playgroup, thereby outing her family's structure and her fathers' stature, the child spends an anxious day imagining all the dreadful things that could happen when her school friends discover how unusual her family is. However, her fears prove ungrounded.

Films for Young Adults

It is important that popular films be made available for young people to see representations of polyamorous possibilities. A recent film marketed for teenagers and young adults via its New York urban school setting and soundtrack, *Take the Lead* (2006), is based on the real-life story of dance teacher Pierre Dulaine, who gives a group of "problem kids" a second chance by exploring their dance skills and entering them into a city competition. One of the subplots in this film is how the rivalry between two boys, Ramos and

Danjou, over the affections of Sasha, develops into a joyful threesome both emotionally and in the dance competition.

YouTube has made possible the wide dissemination of a short film for young adults called *Boyfriends*, produced by Robert Anthony Hubbell (http://www.robertanthonyhubbell.com). It is the story of a 16-year-old boy, Will, whose girlfriend tells him she loves him but is in love with someone else as well, their friend Brian. She introduces the idea of polyamory to him and the audience through Deborah Anapol's (1992) book, *Love without Limits*. The ending shows a happy resolution, accompanied by the *Polyamory Song* sung by David Roves which explains how the world will see them as "mad" and "bad." However, the music is whimsical and flippant, perhaps indicating that the young people will ably deal with such marginalization.

General Film and Television Representations of Polyamory

Because of their social currency, films for general audiences containing positive depictions of polyamory can have a great influence in creating visibility, awareness, understanding, and legitimation of polyamory, thereby also assisting polyfamilies to feel more confident in disclosing their family forms. Positive presence in the media and popular culture can thus allow for the normalization of polyfamilies and their children, and thereby reduce the current need for passing, secret keeping, and bordering strategies. To date, most representations of polyamory in film have not even acknowledged the term itself, let alone provided positive representation. For example, many films resolve the dilemma of multiple loves through death, thereby using what Maria calls the "poly potential" as a romantic narrative device with which to "up" the drama/trauma quotient and elicit more heart-rending and gut-wrenching responses from the audience. This occurs toward the end of the following films: *Pearl Harbor* (2001), *Marie-Jo and Her Two Loves* (2002), and 2012 (2010).

Some films venture beyond this death device, or at least depict polyparents as "good" regardless

of whatever other situations they may be in. For example, in *Ordinary Decent Criminal* (2003), the polyamorous thief Michael is depicted as a devoted father in various situations with his children. *Films like Splendor* (1999), *French Twist* (2003), and *December Bride* (1997) incorporate pregnancy and having babies in a polyfamily structure, where fathers have to grow to adjust to responsible poly relations and polyparenting while the women are already comfortably and confidently in that space.

A final film of note is the *Brazilian Me You Them* (2001). Based on the true story of a woman with three male partners and four children, it explores the economic hardships in a drought-ridden rural area that require the whole family to work together to survive. This film gains its power by eschewing Hollywood glamorization or demonization of these relationships, presenting raw, real, and multidimensional love, sensuality, and negotiation.

In television, HBO's popular *Big Love*, set within a Mormon religious context, explores both positives and challenges of polygamy, including external stigmatization, children's mixed responses to polyparents, how children handle peer-group curiosity at school, and the internal differences within Mormon polygamy, ranging from cult-like rural fundamentalism to urban, modern socioeconomic settings.

In summary, we are beginning to see film and television representations of polyamorous parenting, albeit most of them using death, devastation, and dark humor. What we require are positive media representations of polyamory for polyparents and their children. Finally, we need film and television scripts that actually use terms like "polyamory" or "polyfidelity."

Future Directions: What Polyparents Want

Based on the available research and our discussion group, we next present what polyamorous parents report as needing and wanting to support their families' and children's health and well being. The identification of these needs is important in providing a framework within which we can ensure that future research, policy, and practice directly address polyfamilies' requirements.

More Research and More Polydiversity in the Research

A major need identified by polyfamilies is for further research to be undertaken in all areas of polyfamilies. For example, we need statistical data and demographics on how many polyfamilies there are and how they are constituted. We also require qualitative research on how polyfamilies raise children and the impact on children's lives now and in their adulthood. Also, how do polyfamilies navigate external settings such as schools, health services, and local communities. Our discussion group identified some other specific issues such as the rates of domestic violence in polyfamilies; the mental health of polyfamily members; how polyfamilies organize legal and property issues and arrangements; the impact of polyparenting on children's adult lives in general; and their relationship configurations and negotiations in particular.

Legitimization and Resource Development in Educational, Health, and Legal Systems

As has already been discussed in this chapter, polyparents call for more resources, professional development for service providers, and polyfriendly policies and legislation in all educational, health, welfare, and legal services that will support and legitimate their relationships and families. Blue, a polyparent in the PolyVic discussion group, echoed the thoughts of many polyfamilies in believing these legal shifts will eventually occur, albeit too slowly:

> It will take groups like this [PolyVic], and more discussions, and activism, and us going "Um … hello? We're voters and we pay our taxes and you're ignoring us. And you're outlawing us, in fact" … but it'll take longer than my lifetime to get to that acceptance point.

In particular, polyfamilies call for the awareness of their existence in schools via policies, pedagogies, and pastoral care to cater for the specific needs and recognize the specific skills and insights of their children:

Robyn: For our children to be able to share their journey with other people in a school environment or a church environment or any environment would be more ideal than having to be … careful.

In Conclusion: From "Normality" to "Diversity"

Throughout this chapter, we have provided an overview of the limited available research and our recent empirical findings from the PolyVic polyparenting discussion group which explored the overarching interconnected themes of the lack of polyfamily visibility and the fear of disclosure by polyfamilies. We also discussed how these themes were manifested within the polyhome and in raising children; in interactions with education, health, and legal services; and the place of media, popular culture, and texts. In concluding this chapter, we wish to espouse the need to adopt a mental and societal orientation to "diversity" rather than "normality" as a framework within which these themes and sites are situated. A framework of diversity prepares people for a wide variety of circumstances, structures, genders, sexualities, and ethnicities, and all the combinations thereof, and helps do away with the piecemeal approach wherein polyfamilies are currently ignored, erased, or rendered invisible.

A model of diversity can focus on healthy behaviors rather than healthy "situations," and on principles of providing good care rather than principles of providing the "right" family structure. This model helps refocus social perception away from a constant duologue of normality and deviance and toward a complex multiple dialog where the ultimate goal is the interaction of healthy individuals within healthy communities. Coalitions and bridges, inclusive of social and educational movements, are required at the crossroads of various social justice issues that affect families across the range of nationality, race, class, (dis)ability, age, gender, and sexual identities. These collaborations must include the "questioning and reconceptualizing [of] relationship and families" and "engage all of us in creating sustainable relationships, families and communities" (Noel, 2006, pp. 616–617).

We conclude this chapter with the words and work of Valerie White (2007), a lawyer and member of the Boston poly support and discussion group Family Tree, who often supports polyfamilies in legal situations. She asks why children raised in a stable polyclan are considered to be in a worse situation than children from modern "blended" families—with stepparents, absent parents, stepsiblings, and half-siblings—who may have to deal with much chaos and change:

> As more and more polyamorous people find each other and establish intentional families they will produce a cohort of young people who are confident, ethical, self-actualizing, open-minded and secure. Two of them live at my house. (p. 13)

Acknowledgment To the wonderful group of parents from PolyVic who participated in the discussion for this chapter and to Jess Heerde who assisted in the preparation of this chapter.

References

Anapol, D. (1992). *Love without limits: The quest for sustainable intimate relationships*. San Rafael, CA: Intinet Resource Center.

Anapol, D. (2003). *The future of the family and the fate of our children*. Retrieved from http://www.lovewithoutlimits.com/future_family.html

Anapol, D. (2010). *Polyamory in the 21st century: Love and intimacy with multiple partners*. New York, NY: Rowman and Littlefield.

Anderlini-D'Onofrio, S. (2009). *Gaia and the new politics of love: Notes from a poly planet*. Berkeley, CA: North Atlantic Books.

Arden, K. (1996). Dwelling in the house of tomorrow: Children, young people and their bisexual parents. In S. Rose & C. Stevens (Eds.), *Bisexual horizons: Politic, histories, lives* (pp. 244–257). London, UK: Lawrence & Wishart.

Barker, M., & Langdridge, D. (2010). *Understanding non-monogamies*. London, UK: Routledge.

Bear, P. D. (1998). Our children. *Loving More Magazine, 14*, 28–29.

Bersten, R. (2008). Marginalia: Living on the edge. *Gay and Lesbian Issues and Psychology Review, 4*(1), 9–18.

Boden, D. (1990). The world as it happens: Ethnomethodology and conversation analysis. In G. Ritzer (Ed.), *Frontiers of social theory: The new synthesis* (pp. 185–213). New York, NY: Columbia University Press.

Constantine, L., & Constantine, J. (1972). Where is marriage going? In J. S. DeLora & J. R. DeLora (Eds.), *Intimate lifestyles: Marriage and its alternatives* (pp. 44–46). Pacific Palisades, CA: Goodyear.

Constantine, L., & Constantine, J. (1973). *Group marriage: A study of contemporary multilateral marriage*. New York, NY: Macmillan.

Constantine, L., & Constantine, J. (1976). *Treasures of the island: Children in alternative families*. Beverly Hills, CA: Sage.

Davidson, M. (2002). Working with polyamorous clients in the clinical setting. *Journal of Human Sexuality, 5*. Retrieved from http://www.ejhs.org/volume5/polyoutline.html

Douglas, M. (1966). *Purity and danger: An analysis of concepts of pollution and taboo*. New York, NY: Ark.

Easton, D., & Liszt, C. A. (1997). *The ethical slut*. San Francisco, CA: Greenery Press.

Eiduson, B. T., Cohen, J., & Alexander, J. (1973). Alternative in childrearing in the 1970s. *American Journal of Orthopsychiatry, 43*, 720–731.

Erera, P. I. (2002). *Family diversity: Continuity and change in the contemporary family*. Thousand Oaks, CA: Sage.

Firestein, B. A. (Ed.). (2007). *Becoming visible: Counseling bisexuals across the lifespan*. New York, NY: Columbia University Press.

Foucault, M. (1978). *The history of sexuality: An introduction* (Vol. 1). New York, NY: Pantheon.

Francoeur, R. T. (1972). *Eve's new rib: Twenty faces of sex, marriage and family*. New York, NY: Harcourt, Brace, Jovanovich.

Garner, A. (2004). *Families like mine: Children of gay parents tell it like it is*. New York, NY: Harper Collins.

Goldberg, A. (2007). (How) does it make a difference? Perspectives of adults with lesbian, gay and bisexual parents. *American Journal of Orthopsychiatry, 77*, 550–562. doi:10.1037/0002-9432.77.4.550

Goldberg, A. (2010). *Lesbian and gay parents and their children: Research on the family life cycle*. Washington, DC: American Psychological Association.

Halpern, E. L. (1990). If love is so wonderful, what's so scary about MORE? In M. Munson & J. P. Stelboum (Eds.), *The lesbian polyamory reader: Open relationships, non-monogamy and casual sex* (pp. 157–164). New York, NY: Harrington Park Press.

Haritaworn, J., Chin-ju, L., & Klesse, C. (2006). Poly/logue: A critical introduction to polyamory. *Sexualities, 9*, 515–529. doi:10.1177/1363460706069963

Hill, B. (1997). An unscientific yet highly significant survey of polydom via the net. *Loving More Magazine, 11*, 22–25.

Iantaffi, A. (2006). Polyamory and parenting: Some personal reflections. *Lesbian and Gay Psychology Review, 7*(1), 70–72.

Iantaffi, A. (2009). Houses full of love: Bringing up children in polyamorous relationships. In R. Epstein (Ed.),. *Who's your daddy? and other writing on queer parening* (pp. 346–359). Toronto: Sumach Press

Kentlyn, S. (2008). The radically subversive space of the queer home: 'Safety house' and 'neighbourhood watch'. *Australian Geographer, 39*, 327–337. doi:10.1080/00049180802270523

Kroeger, B. (2003). *Passing: When people can't be who they are*. New York, NY: Public Affairs.

Lambert, S. (2009). Bisexuality emerges in teen/young adult fiction. *Examiner*. Retrieved from http://www.examiner.com/examiner/x-17829-Bisexual-Examiner~y2009m9d12-Bisexuality-emerges-in-teenyoung-adult-fiction-Love-You-Two

Lees, L. (2006). *A queer circle of friends*. East Lansing, MI: LisaLees.

Lindenbaum, P. (1991). *Else-Marie and her seven little daddies*. New York, NY: Henry Holt.

Moore, I. (1991). *Six-dinner Sid*. New York, NY: Simon and Schuster.

Nearing, R. (1996). Poly political animals speak. *Loving More Magazine, 8*, 22–23.

Newitz, A. (2006). Love unlimited. *New Scientist (1971), 2559*(7), 44–47.

Noel, M. J. (2006). Progressive polyamory: Considering issues of diversity. *Sexualities, 9*, 602–620.

Pallotta-Chiarolli, M. (2002). Polyparents having children, raising children, schooling children. *Loving More Magazine, 31*, 8–12.

Pallotta-Chiarolli, M. (2006). Polyparents having children, raising children, schooling children. *Lesbian and Gay Psychology Review, 7*(1), 48–53.

Pallotta-Chiarolli, M. (2008). *Love you two*. Sydney, Australia: Random House.

Pallotta-Chiarolli, M. (2010a). *Border families, border sexualities in schools*. New York, NY: Rowman & Littlefield.

Pallotta-Chiarolli, M. (2010b). To pass, border or pollute: Polyfamilies go to school. In M. Barker & D. Langdridge (Eds.), *Understanding non-monogamies* (pp. 182–187). London, UK: Routledge.

Prodan, L. (2008). *The suicide year*. Round Rock, TX: Prizm Books.

Richardson, L. (1985). *The new other woman*. New York, NY: The Free Press.

Roseneil, S., & Budgeon, S. (2004). Cultures of intimacy and care beyond 'the family': Personal life and social change in the early 21st century. *Current Sociology, 52*, 135–159. doi:10.1177/0011392104041798

Sheff, E. (2006). Poly-hegemonic masculinities. *Sexualities, 9*, 621–642. doi:10.1177.1363460706070003

Sheff, E., & Hammer, C. (2011). The privilege of perversities: Race, class and education among polyamorists and kinksters. *Psychology and Sexuality, 2*, 198–223

Sheff, E. (2010). Strategies in polyamorous parenting. In M. Barker & D. Langdridge (Eds.), *Understanding non-monogamies* (pp. 169–181). London, UK: Routledge.

Strassberg, M. I. (2003). *The challenge of postmodern polygamy: Considering polyamory*. Retrieved from https://culsnet.law.capital.edu/LawReview/backIssues/31-3/Strassberg14.pdf

Taormino, T. (2008). *Opening up: A guide to creating and sustaining open relationships*. San Francisco, CA: Cleis Press.

Thorson, A. R. (2009). Adult children's experiences with their parent's infidelity: Communicative protection and access rules in the absence of divorce. *Communication Studies, 60*, 32–48. doi:10.1080/10510970802623591

Trask, R. (2007). PolyParents, polyKids. *Loving More Magazine, 37*, 16–17.

Vaccaro, A. (2010). Toward inclusivity in family narratives: Counter-stories from queer multi-parent families. *Journal of GLBT Family Studies, 6*, 425–446. doi:10.1080/1550428X.2010.511086

Walston, J. (2001, August). *Polyamory: An exploratory study of responsible multi-partnering*. Paper presented at the Institute of 21st-Century Relationships Conference, Washington, DC.

Watson, J., & Watson, M. A. (1982). Children of open marriages: Parental disclosure and perspectives. *Alternative Lifestyles, 5*(1), 54–62.

Weber, A. (2002). Survey results: Who are we? And other interesting impressions. *Loving More Magazine, 30*, 4–6.

Weitzman, G. D. (2006). Therapy with clients who are bisexual and polyamorous. *Journal of Bisexuality, 6*(1/2), 138–164. doi:10.1300/J159v06n01_08

Weitzman, G. D. (2007). Counseling bisexuals in polyamorous relationships. In B. A. Firestein (Ed.), *Counseling bisexuals across the lifespan* (pp. 312–335). New York, NY: Columbia University Press.

West, C. (1996). *Lesbian polyfidelity*. San Francisco, CA: Booklegger Publishing.

White, V. (2007). Thinking about children. *Loving More Magazine, 37*, 12–13.

Wright, J. M. (2001). Aside from one little, tiny detail, we are so incredibly normal: Perspectives of children in lesbian step families. In M. Bernstein & R. Reimann (Eds.), *Queer families, queer politics: Challenging culture and the state* (pp. 272–292). New York, NY: Columbia University Press.

Race and Ethnicity in the Lives of Sexual Minority Parents and Their Children

Mignon R. Moore and Amy Brainer

The great diversity of sexual minority communities[1] in the USA and other parts of the world has received limited attention in the academic literature on same-sex parenting. Such research has been dominated by studies that emphasize the experiences of higher-income, well-educated, White lesbians living in Western nations (Biblarz & Savci, 2010). In this chapter, we analyze characteristics of racial and sexual minority families in the USA and internationally, revealing the substantial geographic, socioeconomic, and other types of variations in these households. We use an intersectional framework within the field of sociology (Choo & Ferree, 2010; Collins, 2000; Moore, 2012) to highlight race, class, gender, and sexuality as mutually constitutive in the lives of sexual minority parents and their children. While race and sexuality also intersect for families in the dominant or "unmarked" categories (heterosexual and White), our focus in this chapter is on those groups for whom race and sexual minority status are overtly salient in the ways they structure inequalities in society and influence pathways to and experiences of family formation (Greene, 1997). As much as this review provides important variation in the experiences of sexual minority families, it also challenges the academic community to substantially broaden its scope when studying same-sex parenting.

In the second edition of *Black Feminist Thought: Knowledge, Consciousness and the Politics of Empowerment*, Patricia Hill Collins (2000) conceptualizes sexuality in three ways: as a free-standing system of oppression similar to oppressions of race, class, nation, and gender; as an entity that is manipulated within each of these distinctive systems of oppression; and as a social location or conceptual glue that binds intersecting oppressions together and helps demonstrate how oppressions converge. In her later work,

---

[1] We use "sexual minority" to refer to individuals whose sexual relationships and identities are minoritized politically within their societies, families headed by such individuals, and communities formed around this shared minority status. We use more specific terms such as "lesbian," "gay," and "Two-Spirit" when citing research about people who use these terms to describe themselves. It should be noted that these are not mutually exclusive categories; for example, in research studies that refer to "LGBT parents," "T" (transgender and transsexual) parents may also identify themselves as lesbian, gay, or bisexual (or as some other sexual identity). For demographic information, we rely heavily on U.S. Census data, which classifies partnered households as "same sex" or "heterosexual" based on the gender of the adults living in the home (some caveats about this classification system are offered in our section on International Contexts). While "same-sex households" are often read as lesbian and gay households, it is important to recognize that household members may identify themselves as lesbian, gay, bisexual, or none of these, and that sexual minorities and gender variant people are found in both same- and different-sex households.

M.R. Moore, Ph.D. (✉)
Department of Sociology, University of California Los Angeles, Box 951551, 264 Haines Hall, Los Angeles, CA 90095-1551, USA
e-mail: moore@soc.ucla.edu

A. Brainer, M.A.
Department of Sociology, University of Illinois-Chicago, Harrison Street, Chicago, IL 60607-7140, USA
e-mail: amybrainer@gmail.com

Black Sexual Politics: African Americans, Gender, and the New Racism (Collins, 2004), sexuality is further theorized through the lens of heterosexism, which she identifies as a freestanding system of power similar to racism, sexism, and class oppression that suppresses heterosexual and homosexual African-American women and men in ways that foster Black subordination.

Each of these conceptualizations reveals the ways intersecting oppressions rely on sexuality to mutually construct one another. As we will demonstrate in this chapter, Collins' (2004) application of the intersectionality paradigm to the study of Black women's sexuality is also a useful way to conceptualize sexuality as one of several social locations racial and sexual minority parents inhabit. In today's social and political climate, sexual minority group interests are often analyzed and advocated for in ways that privilege the particular interests of higher-income Whites within those groups. When these interests are constructed as separate from and even oppositional to the interests of (presumably heterosexual) racial minority groups, it is sexual minority people of color and their families who are especially harmed (Cahill, 2010; Romero, 2005).

The study of race is also important within the larger discourses of diversity politics. For example, Hicks (2011) argues that ignoring race and racism in relation to lesbian, gay, and queer parenting is an example of White racial privilege. In his analysis of in-depth interviews with lesbian, gay, and queer parents (also see Chap. 10), the author describes one White gay father who claimed that race was a "nonissue" for him and his two adopted Vietnamese sons. However, Hicks notes that this White gay father could not possibly know all the ways his sons will be positioned racially by others. The literature we review rejects a color-blind view of race as a "nonissue" for parents and families and instead acknowledges the significance of race/ethnicity as well as nationhood in sexual minority family formation.

There are three key components of this chapter. We begin with descriptive information about the size, location, and other demographic characteristics of racial minority same-sex couple-headed families in the USA. The next section examines pathways to and experiences of parenting for racial and sexual minority families living in the USA, as well as White same-sex parents of racial minority children. In the final section, we shift our attention to sexual minority parenting in international contexts and explore some of the theoretical challenges presented by this expanding field of vision. The chapter concludes with a number of practical implications that emerge from this literature and points to directions for future research.

Demographic Characteristics of U.S. Racial Minority Same-Sex Partner Families

The demographic information we present is drawn from a variety of sources, including 2000 U.S. Census data; the 2000 Black Pride Survey, administered by the National Gay and Lesbian Task Force and distributed to 2,700 Black lesbian, gay, bisexual, and transgender (LGBT) people in nine cities; and a survey conducted by the Human Rights Campaign in 2007–2008 that purposively sampled African-American, Latina/o, and Asian and Pacific Islander American LGBT communities (Cahill, 2010; Cahill, Battle, & Meyer, 2003; Cianciotto, 2005; Dang & Frazer, 2004; Dang & Vianney, 2007; Gates, Lau, & Sears, 2006; Romero, 2005). Our focus on these specific racial/ethnic and sexual minority groups reflects the limits of available data, as other racial and sexual minority populations (such as indigenous sexual minority families) are not represented in the data in sufficient numbers to sketch their demographic characteristics.

African-Americans

According to Dang and Frazer's (2004) report on data from the 2000 U.S. Census, Black same-sex partner households (defined as same-sex partner households in which at least one person identifies as Black or African-American) are 14% of all same-sex partner households, a proportion that closely mirrors the population of Black households in the USA. Seventy-nine percent of these families (all of which were headed by two women or two men) were headed by two Black women or two Black men and 21% were interracial households. Characteristics of these families were more similar to characteristics of the broader population of Black families in the USA than to those of White same-sex couple-headed families. Specifically, Black same-sex couples reported parenting at rates similar to Black different-sex couples and significantly higher than White same-sex couples. Fifty-two percent of Black female same-sex couples and 36% of Black male same-sex couples were raising at least one child under the age of 18, compared to 32% of White female same-sex couples and 18% of White male same-sex couples. Black same-sex couples were also more than twice as likely as White same-sex couples to be parenting at least one nonbiological child, including adopted and fostered children and children of relatives.

Many Black same-sex partnered families were residing in smaller, more rural cities and towns. Of the top 10 metropolitan areas with the highest proportions of Black same-sex households, all 10 were in the South. This pattern is consistent with residential patterns among the total population of Black families in the USA, 54% of whom were residing in the South at the time of the 2000 Census (Dang & Frazer, 2004). Same-sex couples in which both partners are Black reported lower median annual household income ($41 K) than same-sex couples in which one partner was Black ($58 K) and same-sex couples in which both partners were White ($64 K). Same-sex couples in which one or both partners are Black were also less likely to own their homes (52%) than were same-sex couples in which both partners are White (71%). These findings mirror larger patterns of racial disparities in wealth and income in the USA (Campbell & Kaufmann, 2006; Oliver & Shapiro, 1997).

Dang and Frazer (2004) highlight numerous public policy implications that emerge from these data. Because Black same-sex couples are more economically disadvantaged on average than are White same-sex couples, at the same time that they are more likely to be raising children, they are disproportionately harmed by certain laws that limit access of sexual minorities to certain rights and benefits. Such policies make it more difficult for adults to include children they co-parent with a same-sex partner on their health insurance plans and protect them in other ways. Cahill et al. (2003) make a similar argument based on their analysis of the 2000 Black Pride Survey. Given high rates of parenting among survey respondents, and evidence that racial and economic disparities among LGBT people mirror those of the larger society, Cahill et al. (2003) frame same-sex marriage, fostering, and adoption as matters of racial and economic justice. They observe that laws prohibiting same-sex fostering and adoption are most prevalent in southern states with the largest Black populations and the highest rates of parenting among Black same-sex couples.

Dang and Frazer (2004) and Cahill et al. (2003) further argue that antigay parenting policies threaten the Black community as a whole by reducing the pool of potential foster and adoptive parents for Black children who are overrepresented in the foster care system. Black children who enter the foster care system remain there longer, are moved more often, and receive the least desirable placements of any group of children. When prospective parents are not permitted to foster or adopt because of their sexual minority status, the outcome for many Black children is continued upheaval and non-placement (Washington, 2008). By situating the concerns of same-sex parents and their children not only in relation to issues of gender and sexuality but also in relation to larger structures of racial and economic inequality, these scholars are expanding the discourse around sexual minority parenting in needed directions.

Hispanic and Latina/o Americans

According to a 2005 report, 12% of all same-sex partner households in the 2000 U.S. Census include at least one Hispanic partner. This percentage is likely to have increased in the last decade, given the accelerated growth of Hispanic and Latina/o populations in the USA (Passel & Cohn, 2008). Cianciotto's (2005) analyses of U.S. Census data revealed that Hispanic same-sex partners were twice as likely as non-Hispanic, White same-sex partners to be raising children. Among interethnic same-sex couples in which one partner was Hispanic, 54% of female couples and 41% of male couples were raising one or more children under 18. For same-sex couples in which both partners were Hispanic, parenting rates increased to 66% of female couples and 58% of male couples. Hispanic same-sex partners were raising children at nearly the same rates as Hispanic different-sex partners and shared many other characteristics in common with the overall population of Hispanic Americans. Same- and different-sex Hispanic American couples resided in the same areas of the country, with large concentrations in Arizona, California, Florida, and Texas, all states that have, at one point in time, passed constitutional amendments banning same-sex marriage.

Hispanic same-sex partner households in the U.S. Census reported a lower median annual household income ($37 K) and lower rates of home ownership (48%) than did non-Hispanic White same-sex partner households ($64 K and 71%, respectively). Same-sex couples in which both partners were Hispanic received public assistance at higher rates (10% of women, 6% of men) than interethnic same-sex couples in which only one partner was Hispanic (6% of women, 3% of men) and same-sex couples in which both partners were non-Hispanic White (3% of women, 2% of men). Of all these groups, families headed by two Hispanic women were most likely to qualify for Temporary Assistance for Needy Families (TANF). However, heterosexual marriage promotion, fatherhood promotion, faith-based initiatives, and paternity requirements for TANF promoted under the Bush administration made it more difficult or impossible for many of these mothers and their children to access needed benefits (Cahill, 2010; Cianciotto, 2005).

A key component of Cianciotto's (2005) report is its discussion of immigration and citizenship. Among interethnic same-sex couples in which one partner is Hispanic, 6% of women and 8% of men were noncitizens; among same-sex couples in which both partners were Hispanic, those percentages rose to 38% of women and 51% of men (compared to just 2% of women and 3% of men in non-Hispanic White same-sex households). Cianciotto notes that U.S. immigration policy is largely based on the principle of "family unification," which allows US citizens and permanent residents to sponsor their spouses and other close family members for immigration purposes. Family unification policies are heterosexually defined and do not include provisions for same-sex partners and families headed by same-sex couples. The Defense of Marriage Act (DOMA) prevents US citizens and permanent residents from sponsoring their noncitizen same-sex partners, putting many binational same-sex couples in the difficult position of living apart, moving outside the USA, or finding ways to stay together illegally under a constant threat of deportation. Binational same-sex couples who are parents must additionally protect the welfare of their children without adequate support from the State. Research on immigration, citizenship, and mixed-status families needs to be better integrated with research on sexuality minority parents and their children, for whom these issues are a central concern.

Asian and Pacific Islander Americans

The 2000 U.S. Census showed 38,203 Asian and Pacific Islander (hereafter API) Americans in households headed by a same-sex couple. Between 3% and 4% of all same-sex partner households included at least one API partner (Gates et al., 2006). In 2005, the largest ever nationwide survey of LGBT API Americans was administered by the National Gay and Lesbian Task Force Policy Institute (Dang & Vianney, 2007). Of the 860 API survey respondents, 4% reported living with one or more children under 18 and 3% were biological parents of those children.

In 2000 U.S. Census data reported on by Gates et al. (2006), API same-sex partner households were shown to have more in common with API different-sex partners than with White same-sex partners. Like API different-sex couples, API same-sex couples are ethnically diverse and reside in areas of the country that have large populations of API Americans, with the top three states being California, New York, and Hawaii. API same-sex couples reported higher levels of education than their non-API counterparts, yet earned less on average ($55 K median household income) and were less likely to own their homes (52%) than same-sex couples in which both partners are non-Hispanic White. This pattern is consistent with research by Campbell and Kaufmann (2006) showing a penalty for API Americans in translating educational attainment into income and wealth. Disparities between API same-sex couples and non-Hispanic White same-sex couples are reflective of racial disparities in the broader US population.

Similar to findings for Hispanic and Latina/o Americans, immigration and citizenship emerged as key issues for LGBT APIs. API LGBT survey respondents ranked immigration as the number one issue facing all APIs in the USA, and one of the top four issues facing API LGBT Americans (other top issues were hate violence/harassment, media representations, and marriage equality) (Dang & Vianney, 2007). Census data show that there are 35,820 binational same-sex couples living in the USA, and in 45% of these cases, the foreign partner is Asian. Thus, it is estimated that approximately 16,000 Asian nationals are currently affected by immigration policies that prevent their US-citizen partners from petitioning for them to remain in the country (Romero, 2005). According to a 2004 report by the Asian American Federation of New York, also based on 2000 U.S. Census data, approximately one-third of all API lesbians and gays living in New York, San Francisco, and Los Angeles are noncitizens. Victor Romero (2005) argues that "family unification" is a long-held value among Asian Americans and one that directly challenges the anti-Asian legacy of U.S. immigration law. But not all API families are protected under the principle of family unification. API lesbian and gay couples and their children are still feeling the legacy of immigration law that constructs certain groups (formerly Asians, now lesbians and gays)

as unassimilable. Romero challenges the larger API community to think carefully about its values and history and to throw its weight behind measures that would extend unification to *all* Asian and Pacific Island families, including those API families that include same-sex couples.

Implications for Studying Sexual Minority Parenting

In surveying the demographic characteristics of racial and sexual minority populations, we have determined that a number of new analytic approaches to the study of same-sex parenting are warranted. Several scholars have argued that same-sex parenting and related laws and policies should be framed as matters of racial and economic justice, with close attention to intersections of race, gender, sexuality, and social class (Cahill et al., 2003; Cahill & Jones, 2001; Cianciotto, 2005; Dang & Frazer 2004). Immigration and citizenship need to be more central to the study of sexual minority family formation (Cianciotto, 2005; Dang & Vianney, 2007; Romero, 2005). These analytic shifts require scholars to rethink the issues that are relevant to sexual minority parents and their children and to include such issues as racial disparities in homeownership and income, access to welfare benefits, and family unification in our academic conferences and papers, clinical practice, advocacy, and other work on behalf of sexual minority parents, families, and communities. Intersections of race, gender, sexuality, and social class highlighted in this section inform multiple dimensions of family life and are evident in the research studies discussed throughout this chapter, including pathways to and experiences of parenting, as we explore next.

Racial Variance in Pathways to and Experiences of Parenting

In the literature on same-sex parents and their children, many researchers have focused narrowly on those pathways to and experiences of parenting that are most prevalent among White, middle- and upper-income lesbians and gay men, such as alternative insemination through in vitro fertilization and co-adoption in the context of a same-sex relationship. Pathways to parenting that are more common among working-class and racial minority families receive less attention, often because of how researchers define their samples (Moore, 2011b). This omission has persisted despite evidence that a majority of parents in same-sex relationships are working class, and upper-income White gay couples are the least likely group among all same-sex couples to be parenting (Rosenfeld, 2010).

Here we consider two pathways to parenting that remain under-examined in the literature on same-sex parent families: parenting children from a prior heterosexual union and taking on the role of a mother or father to children in the extended family or racial community. We discuss how multiple minority statuses shape these pathways as well as the parenting experiences that follow, drawing examples from research on African-American and Jamaican lesbian mothers, American Indian Two-Spirit parents, and Black and Latino gay fathers. We then consider a third pathway to same-sex parenting, interracial adoption, and discuss how race matters in the lives of White parents who adopt racial and ethnic minority children.

Parenting Children from a Prior Heterosexual Relationship: The Case of Lesbian Mothers

Many researchers have framed their studies of lesbian motherhood in certain ways as to make the results comparable to those of other empirical studies of family structure and family process in heterosexual two-parent families. Such an analogous research design makes it easier to address central assumptions in the literature regarding the division of household labor and the distribution of childcare and childrearing tasks (Gartrell et al., 1999, 2000; Patterson, 1995). Research on lesbian-headed families also tends to be framed around long-held assumptions about lesbian identity, particularly the idea that lesbians as a

group are egalitarian in their distribution of paid work, housework, and childcare, and that they organize their households and interact with each other in ways that support this principle (Dunne, 2000; Sullivan, 2004). Unfortunately, restricting samples so that they only include women who take on a lesbian identity before becoming parents biases research studies, and the literature more generally, toward the experiences of White, middle- and upper-income lesbians, who are better able to afford costly insemination procedures and who are more likely to support the ideological principles of egalitarian feminism (Moore, 2011a). Maintaining such a narrow definition of who is a lesbian parent does a disservice to our understanding of the complexities of lesbian motherhood because it overrepresents the less common route to a lesbian identity status and lesbian family formation. That is, the majority of today's mothers who identify as lesbian became parents by bearing a child in the context of a prior heterosexual relationship (Morris, Balsam, & Rothblum, 2002).

In her research on African-American lesbian families, Moore (2008, 2011a) found that many women who had become mothers in the context of prior heterosexual unions continued to make a concentrated effort to satisfy the societal definition of a "good mother" that is implicitly linked to heterosexuality. This expectation produced a conflict for these mothers, who had to contend not only with the construction of lesbian identity as deviant but also with negative stereotypes around race and Black women's sexuality. Their sexual orientation forced a sexual self into visibility in the context of motherhood, which frightened some and went against a politics of silence in this arena (for more information on the politics of silence, see Hammonds, 1997; Hine, 1989).

Makeda Silvera (1995), writing about lesbian motherhood for Jamaican women in the USA, says that it is the "sexual mother" that frightens the community and forces family members to close their eyes. She recalls one of the biggest criticisms she experienced from family and friends was that in openly raising her daughters as a Black lesbian in her racial community, she was flaunting her sexuality "like a red rag, a flag on a pole" (Silvera, 1995, p. 315). She says they could tolerate her as a lesbian and as a mother, but not as a lesbian mother living with a woman lover. This was "counter-culture, counter-Black, counter-mother" (p. 316). Silvera's (1995) experience and Moore's (2008, 2011a) research both illuminate the centrality of race to discourses about motherhood. While lesbian mothers across marginalized racial groups may struggle to be viewed as "good mothers," the standards to which they are held are shaped not only by gender and sexuality but also by constructions of race, racism, and intraracial group dynamics.

Accounting for racial variance in pathways to and experiences of parenting reveals the substantial diversity of mothering experiences among lesbian-identified women. Just as importantly, it introduces new frameworks for research and analysis of lesbian parenting and parenting more broadly, which explore how parenting discourses are gendered as well as racialized.

Parenting in Extended Families and Communities

In many racial and ethnic communities, family responsibilities, including the provision of financial and emotional support, elder and child caretaking, and other household duties, are shared throughout social networks that may involve extended family and friends' participation in a variety of familial roles (Meyers, Han, Waldfogel, & Garfinkel, 2001; Wilhelmus, 1998). Research on Black families has shown that kinship arrangements commonly include multigenerational family structures as well as other types of extended family households (Mays, Chatters, Cochran, & Mackness, 1998). Several researchers have found that Latina/o and Asian immigrant families sustain complex networks that join households and communities—even across geographic borders—to provide assistance and support after immigration (Itzigsohn, Cabral, Medina, & Vazquez, 1999; Vidal de Haymes, Kilty, & Segal, 2000). Sexual minority family members are also a part of these multigenerational and extended family networks. In addition to their own biological,

foster, or adopted children, many lesbian and gay people are "parenting" other children in their family networks by providing financial and emotional support to siblings, nieces and nephews, and grandchildren (Mays et al., 1998; Moore, 2011a). These parenting and family arrangements are not showing up in research studies that define same-sex parenting more narrowly.

Some scholars have begun to integrate sexual minority parent and family research with the broader literature on racial and ethnic minority families. Mays et al. (1998) build on literature on multigenerational African-American households and extended kin networks to analyze questionnaires returned by a national sample of more than 1,000 African-American lesbian women and gay men. Among the quarter of respondents who reported living with one or more children under 18, many lived with and assumed parenting responsibilities for grandchildren, nieces and nephews, younger siblings, and other children in their extended family networks. The researchers argue that exclusion of lesbian and gay people from family networks is disadvantageous for all members of the family, as it cuts off the flow of financial and emotional contributions that lesbian and gay people give and receive.

Other research reveals that many people are assuming parenting roles to contribute not only to their extended family networks but also to their broader racial and ethnic communities. Gilley (2006) spent 6 years living and working with members of two southwestern organizations for Native people who identify themselves as Two-Spirit. His work explores many dimensions of what it means for contemporary Indian people to "become" Two-Spirit through a synthesis of male and female qualities, and gay and Native identities. Historically, one of the most important roles Two-Spirit people assume is that of teacher and caregiver for children. Two-Spirit people teach children (especially girls) about Indian ceremonies and other cultural practices, and care for children when their parents are not able to do so. In Gilley's research, Two-Spirit men cared for nieces, nephews, and other family members, supervised organizations for local teens, and reached out in formal and informal ways to support gay Indian youth. In keeping with their Two-Spirit identity, the men were called upon to stand in as both male and female role models for young people. The men did not describe their parenting activities in terms of a personal desire to have children or form a nuclear family together with a same-sex partner. Instead, their parenting roles were virtually indistinguishable from their obligations to the larger family, community, and tribe. By teaching children and youth about Indian culture, Two-Spirit people positioned themselves as integral to Indian life.

A second example of parenting to sustain the larger community emerges from Lewin's (2009) research on gay fathers. Drawing from interviews with 95 gay fathers in Chicago, Los Angeles, Iowa City, and the San Francisco Bay area, Lewin analyzed the meanings gay men attach to their parenting roles and aspirations as they move across spaces defined as "gay" and those defined as related to "family" (and thus "not gay" by conventional standards). Among other meaning-making strategies, gay men in this research constructed fatherhood as "the right thing to do" in moral terms, often in response to stereotypes of gay men as morally deficient. While gay fathers across racial and ethnic categories shared how their particular heritage and family traditions shaped both their desire to be parents and their approach to childrearing, for Black gay fathers, the moral impetus for fatherhood took on a special urgency, framed as a responsibility that extended beyond their immediate circle of kin. While non-Hispanic White gay men as well as racial and ethnic minority gay men described fatherhood as "doing the right thing," for Black gay fathers, this included doing the right thing for the broader racial community by caring for Black children who might otherwise languish in the foster care system. Lewin's research shows the salience of race even in patterns that occur across racial groups. While non-Hispanic White gay men and racial and ethnic minority gay men used similar narrative constructs to describe their parenting, these took on different contours for Black gay fathers, who were most likely to connect their parenting narratives to larger issues of systemic racism and the survival of Black children and youth.

Latino gay dads in Lewin's (2009) and Mallon's (2004) research also stressed the significance of sharing an ethnic heritage with their children, drawing on biologized notions of kinship to construct their families, and placing importance on the intergenerational transmission of Latino culture. Many of the parenting activities described by these Latino gay fathers—such as observation of special holidays and other ethnic group traditions—are similar to those performed by indigenous and immigrant women whom Billson (1995) and Espiritu (2001) have recognized as being "keepers of the culture." As keepers of the culture, women are held responsible not only for bringing up their own children but also for sustaining the larger racial, ethnic, and often transnational community. Theories of gendered parenting roles relative to the preservation of culture and community would be greatly enriched by the inclusion of sexual minority parent experiences and practices.

Transracial Adoption

Transracial adoption is the placement of a child who is of one race or ethnic group with adoptive parents of another race or ethnic group. In the USA, transracial adoption occurs primarily (though not exclusively) when White adults adopt racial minority children born in the USA or abroad. As the numbers of sexual minority parent-headed families increase, so do the numbers of White sexual minority parents raising racial minority children (Farr & Patterson, 2009). Racial minority lesbians and gay men have pointed out that race matters in lesbian and gay communities as much as it matters in the broader society (Greene, 1997). That race matters is something that parents of color know through life experience. White sexual minority parents who are raising racial minority children may or may not understand race in this way.

In Mallon's (2004) interview study of gay fathers living in Los Angeles and New York, White gay fathers varied in how much or how little they felt race mattered for their families. Some made special efforts to prepare their children and families to deal with racism and to connect their children with a larger racial or ethnic community, while others did not feel that this was necessary, or engaged with race only superficially, viewing it primarily as an issue of "culture." For example, one White gay father who had adopted two Latino children said that he did not do much about "instilling the native culture" in his children other than eating in Mexican restaurants (Mallon, 2004, p. 119). The literature on transracial adoption shows that the inability and/or unwillingness of parents to address questions about race, racial inequality, and ethnicity with their children may produce barriers for children's successful racial/ethnic identity integration (Samuels, 2009; Spencer & Markstrom-Adams, 1990; Viladrich & Loue, 2009). Children have a more difficult time when they lack access to role models who have been able to successfully integrate racial identities with other identities (Spencer, 1983; Spencer & Markstrom-Adams, 1990). A growing body of research shows that race and color consciousness, not "color blindness," is the best practice approach to transracial adoption (Quiroz, 2007; Samuels, 2009). Thus, White sexual minority parents who adopt racial minority children need to be prepared to engage with questions about race and racial inequality, or these issues may be neglected or subsumed into a discourse of cultural diversity as they were for some of the fathers in Mallon's study.

Intersections of race and sexuality are highlighted in Richardson and Goldberg's (2010) research on White lesbian adoptive mothers of racial and ethnic minority children. Richardson and Goldberg interviewed 20 White lesbian couples (40 women) pre- and post-adoption, asking about the challenges these women faced with regard to multiple minority statuses and their preparedness to deal with such challenges. Prior to adoption, many mothers expressed concern about the discrimination their child might face, including discrimination from members of their own families and communities who held racist and homophobic views. Many of these concerns were realized as early as 3 months post-adoption, when most couples had encountered negative feedback related to the child's race. Mothers in this research

also described positive experiences pre- and post-adoption and identified particular strengths they perceived themselves to have as lesbian parents forming multiracial families. While their perspectives on and experiences of race varied, overall these mothers espoused a color conscious rather than a color-blind ideology with regard to transracial adoption.

Stephen Hicks (2011) argues that transracial adoption by lesbian, gay, and queer parents forces us to consider how race might be relevant to the ways parenting is conceptualized and carried out. Questions of adoption, foster care, and race are related to those of resemblance and belonging—what it means to "look like" family. In interviews with lesbian adoptive couples creating multiracial families, Hicks shows the importance to many of these mothers of "looking like" a family with regard to skin color, often in anticipation of how their family might be perceived by others. While lesbian and gay parenting has a capacity to destabilize notions of racial inheritance and biological bonds, and while parents explicitly challenge these ideals, they should also be acutely aware of ways in which racism may be expressed through insistence upon "likeness/fit" as a criterion for family formation.

Implications for Studying Sexual Minority Parents

In this section, we have reviewed work on pathways to and experiences of parenting among racial and sexual minority families, as well as White lesbian and gay parents of racial minority children. Collectively, these cases reveal the limitations of current definitions of same-sex parenting, which tend to focus narrowly on families formed through pregnancy or adoption in the context of a same-sex relationship and preexistent lesbian or gay identity. This approach excludes the majority of working-class and racial minority same-sex parents, who enter into and experience parenting in other ways (such as parenting children from a prior heterosexual union or caring for children of relatives). In addition, many lesbian and gay family scholars have focused primarily or exclusively on how gender and sexuality shape same-sex parenting, but have not considered how race and culture also shape parenting discourses and practices. Researchers focusing on populations outside the USA have raised closely related critiques of current definitions and approaches to same-sex parenting, as we explore in the final section of this chapter.

Sexual Minority Parenting in International Contexts

Studies of sexual minority parents in international contexts are important to consider, as this research reveals the rich diversity of sexual minority families globally and provides new approaches to theory, clinical practice, and public policy that emerge from the unique experiences and perspectives of these households. Three themes surface in this international literature. First, we stress the importance of moving away from the typological approach common in family scholarship, which classifies parents and households as *either* "heterosexual" *or* "same sex." This distinction is artificial for many subjects in the studies we review and one that has seriously limited the scope of family research in Africa, Asia, and other parts of the world. Second, we problematize another feature of this typological approach: the *ranking* of "same-sex" parents against "heterosexual" parents, using sameness as a criterion for equality and a measure of parental success (e.g., the more similar to heterosexual parents they are shown to be, the more deserving same-sex parents are of equal treatment). We take inspiration from studies of sexual minority parents in rural Indian and indigenous New Zealand communities who are not seeking sameness with heterosexuals, but rather emphasizing those traits that make their families unique. Third, we stress the role of the State in shaping the life chances of sexual minority parents and their children. In earlier sections of this chapter, we highlighted the impact of State policies and practices in the USA, such as welfare reform, on racial and sexual minority families. Here, we expand this analysis to consider how heteronormative definitions of

family are constructed and enforced in different geopolitical contexts, citing examples from Japan and Chile. These examples offer a glimpse of the diverse forms heteronormative policies and practices can take. We conclude that further research is needed which considers socio-legal and citizenship issues for sexual minority parents living under different forms of governance.

Rethinking the Distinction Between "Heterosexual" and "Same-Sex" Parents

Wekker's (2006) ethnographic research on women engaged in "the *mati* work" in Paramaribo, Suriname, is especially instructive with regard to the limitations of a heterosexual/same-sex typology for analyzing parenting. Mati refers to love and sexual intimacy between women, conceived of as a pleasing behavior rather than as the basis of an individual or collective identity. Over a period of 10 years, Wekker immersed herself in the lives of 25 working-class Afro-Surinamese women, who ranged in age from 23 to 84 at the start of the research. Wekker found that women who mati usually have children by men and maintain sexual relationships with the fathers of their children, often in exchange for men's financial contributions to their households. Their primary emotional and romantic attachments, however, are to other women, and most rely on the help of other women to bring up their children. Women doing "the mati work" described their relationships with men as primarily transactional, and their relationships with women as more passionate, imbued with strong feelings of infatuation, desire, love, jealousy, and expectations of fidelity. These women did not, however, think of themselves as essentially different from women who form relationships exclusively with men.

Wekker (2006) uses the case of Afro-Surinamese women who mati to show the limitations of the Western concept of homosexual identity. We use it here to show the limitations of the concept of same-sex parenting. Women who mati are actively parenting with other women and are finding sexual and romantic fulfillment in these same-sex relationships; however, they do not adopt a lesbian identity or see themselves as belonging to a community based on their sexual object choice, nor do they necessarily discontinue all sexual relations with men. Wekker's findings are consistent with reports that in African and other non-Western societies, women who are engaged in same-sex relationships "have" men to fulfill certain functions, one of them being to reproduce (Aarmo, 1999; Potgieter, 2003). Conventional approaches to defining and studying same-sex parenting have not accounted for these kinds of arrangements.

In addition, many women outside of the USA who have same-sex desires enter into or remain in heterosexual marriages concurrently with their same-sex relationships. Drawing on her ethnographic research with *lala* (lesbian) identified women in Beijing, Engebretsen (2009) presents three case studies to highlight a range of lala family arrangements. One woman in the study remained heterosexually married and mothered a child in the context of this marriage, while also dating her lala partner. Two other lalas created a marriage-like relationship with one another and merged families, sharing care work for elderly parents. In the third case, a self-identified *chunde T* (pure T; similar, though not equivalent, to "stone butch") chose to marry a gay male friend to satisfy her parents. Those who married men were able to maintain what Engebretsen calls "hetero-marital face," but found it difficult to form and keep lasting same-sex relationships because of the demands their marital and family arrangements placed on them. The women who formed a marriage-like relationship with one another found more lasting satisfaction in that relationship, but expressed deep regret at their inability to have a child together. Engebretsen does not conclude that any one of these family arrangements is superior to or ultimately more satisfying than the others. Instead, she critiques Western discourses that prioritize certain marital ideologies and relationship strategies, without fully recognizing the diversity of nonnormative sexualities globally.

By classifying households as *either* heterosexual *or* same sex, family scholars exclude those

households where parenting arrangements are shared among multiple adults who may be romantically and/or sexually connected to one another. The international literature shows that these arrangements are much more common than family scholars account for given existing typologies, and the studies we reviewed require family scholars to think more broadly about what sexual minority parenting might look like. A broader approach is also needed in research on US populations, where the heterosexual/same-sex distinction is no less problematic [see, for example, scholarship by Pfeffer (2010) on transsexual and transgender families, and by Moss (2012) on bisexual and polyamorous families in the USA, which raise similar concerns about how these families are classified].

Moving Beyond "Sameness" as a Measure of Parental Success

The international literature on sexual minority parenthood reveals that many of these adults do not seek "sameness" with heterosexuals as a way to legitimate their parenting—a common trope in discourses about lesbian and gay parenting in the USA (Biblarz & Stacey, 2010). Instead, they make conscious choices to parent differently from those around them and pursue different goals for their children's futures. In Swarr and Nagar's (2003) case study of a sexual minority female couple raising two daughters in rural India, the couple chose not to arrange marriages for their daughters despite familial and community pressure to do so. They also made the decision not to adopt a son, which would have ensured their own later life social security. These mothers explained that they wanted their daughters to receive an inheritance so that they would have the option not to marry; if they had a son, he would receive the entire inheritance. They connected their vision for their daughters' future independence to their own struggles for independence from compulsory heterosexual marriage, and their desires to transform marriage and family to make these institutions fairer for women and sexual minorities.

Glover, McKree, and Dyall (2009) used focus group interviews to study fertility issues and access to reproductive technologies in Maori (New Zealand indigenous) communities. Among *takatapui* (nonheterosexual) women interviewed, the issue of sperm donation was discussed at length. Some takatapui women reported that they preferred gay male sperm donors because they wanted to limit the influence of heterosexuality on their children, and because they wanted to pass on the "gay gene" if such a thing should exist. The significance of these comments becomes more apparent when we consider the social and political climate in New Zealand, where the largest sperm bank banned gay donors until 2006. After the ban was lifted, a Professor of Genetics at New Zealand's Canterbury University said people who received sperm from gay men should be informed that a "gay gene" might be passed to their children (Glover et al., 2009, p. 305). In a context where discourse around the possible existence of a "gay gene" has been used to directly attack sexual minority communities, takatapui mothers and prospective mothers are offering a subversive counter-discourse by constructing the "gay gene" not as a social menace, but as a positive and desirable trait.

When taken together, the two themes we have presented—rethinking the distinction between same-sex and heterosexual parents, and moving beyond "sameness" as a measure of parental success—produce alternative ways of conceptualizing the particular needs, desires, and social roles of sexual minority parents. Many of these adults have not constructed an individual or collective identity based on sexual object choice, and they do not see themselves as belonging to a different social category than people who prefer different-sex partners. However, they see themselves as making efforts to instill particular values in their children that may differ from some of the more traditional values in their cultures of origin. Neither identity-based social movements nor comparative research that measures same-sex parenting, against heterosexual parenting, is likely to hold significant meaning for these parents. While exposing the limits of existing paradigms, studies of non-Western sexual minority

parenting focus on the aspects of individuals' lives that parents and families themselves find most salient.

The Role of the State in Regulating Same-Sex Parents and Their Children

Drawing on 6 years of ethnographic research in the Japanese lesbian community, including multiple life histories with 10 lesbian women ranging in age from mid-20s to early 50s, Chalmers (2002) argues that the processes of marriage, childbearing, and childrearing consolidate Japanese women's status as adults, "whole people", and full citizens in contemporary Japan. She traces the contemporary idealization of Japanese motherhood to the Meiji period, the institutionalization of the concept of *ryosai kenbo* (good wife, wise mother) and the accompanying ideology of the "mothering instinct," which the Japanese government promoted as a part of the process of modernization. She additionally notes the relationship between institutionalized heterosexuality and children's citizen status. A Japanese child is classified as "legitimate" only if the child is acknowledged by the household head, defined as the child's father. Although attempts to equalize birth status were made in 1995, legitimate children continue to accrue social advantages as they navigate the household registration system, the education system, and other social institutions. In 1993, the Prime Minister of Japan was quoted as saying, "discrimination against children out of wedlock, in order to promote respect for legal marriage, is a reasonable distinction to make" (Chalmers, 2002, p. 115). A mother's marital status therefore matters greatly not only for her own social standing but also for the social standing of her children. For the lesbian women in Chalmers' study, the social penalty attached to being an unwed mother caused equal or greater anxiety than the social penalty attached to being a lesbian. Some of these women chose to enter or remain in marriages to men because they wanted their children to have socio-legal legitimacy.

Herrera (2009) uses ethnographic fieldwork and in-depth interviews with 29 Chilean lesbian mothers ranging in age from 25 to 72 to explore how lesbians in Chile understand and carry out parenthood. Her respondents were acutely aware of their erasure through State policies and practices, such as the absence of any legal recognition or protection for same-sex relationships, and the denial of adoption and reproductive technologies to lesbians. Many of these women hid their sexual orientation from their families and communities (and especially from their ex-husbands) because they feared losing custody of their children. They saw their motherhood and their lesbian relationships and identities as compatible, yet recognized that they would be viewed and treated as "bad mothers" within the court system because of their lesbian sexuality. Herrera (2009) notes that a legitimate fear of having one's children taken away "profoundly marks the way [Chilean lesbians] experience motherhood" (p. 50).

Research studies like those by Chalmers (2002) and Herrera (2009) highlight the role of the State in regulating same-sex parents across societies and the diversity of forms this regulation can take. Through such constructs as illegitimate children and unfit mothers, courts of law and other State apparatuses are shaping the life chances of same-sex parents and their children, in many cases excluding them from full citizenship. Family scholars have begun to use the lens of citizenship to analyze lesbian and gay parenthood in the USA (see, for example, Lewin, 2009; Ryan-Flood, 2009). This conversation needs to be expanded to include sexual minority parents who are creating families under a variety of forms of governance and taking on unique socio-legal challenges in their respective national contexts.

Implications for Studying Sexual Minority Parents

Raewyn Connell (2007) argues for a transformation of social science disciplines through the inclusion of sources of knowledge production that originate from "the global south"—regions outside the dominant European and North American metropole. Theoretical approaches advanced from these areas have the potential to speak to and about European and North American life by challenging us theoretically and in ways that are relevant to the study of populations within as well as outside the USA. This work offers a contribution to the field of sexuality studies more broadly as well as to the study of specific sexual minority populations by destabilizing the same-sex/heterosexual typology and the problematic measurement of same-sex parents against their heterosexual counterparts, advancing new understandings of sexuality and the State. We have tried to show key ways that international research can inform our analytic approach to sexual minority parenting. Further research in international contexts is needed to develop our understanding of sexual minority family formation and to expand the theory, practice, and policy decisions concerning these families.

Directions for Future Research

An emerging body of work on racial and sexual minority parents demands more of scholars in several areas. To make the conversation about sexual minority parenting more inclusive and comprehensive, researchers need to be cognizant of how methods and sampling have shaped what we know, and do not know, about sexual minority parents and their children. Social scientists must rethink definitions of "same-sex parenting" and parenting in general, to account for the variety of ways in which people create families and bring children into those families. Current definitions exclude many common practices, such as parenting children from prior heterosexual unions, bearing and rearing children in the context of ongoing heterosexual marriages or transactional sexual arrangements maintained concurrently with same-sex relationships, and parenting children in extended family and community networks. By relying on narrow definitions of who "counts" as a sexual minority parent (often defined as subjects who entered into a lesbian or gay identity *prior* to becoming parents through artificial insemination or adoption), researchers implicitly bias the data toward White, middle-class families, who are more likely to conform to such definitions, but less likely to be parenting than racial and sexual minority families.

Social science researchers also need to recognize a wider range of issues that are of key concern to sexual minority parents. Issues of immigration and citizenship are not often included in public conversations about same-sex parenting, yet are profoundly important to many racial minority same-sex parents and their children. How the State constructs sexual citizen subjects has implications for parenting and family formation within and across societies in ways that scholars are just beginning to analyze. Sexual minority parenting might be framed as an issue of racial and economic justice, yet political and legal debates tend to focus exclusively on the gender and sexual orientation of parents, without regard for the racial implications of laws and policies about same-sex marriage, fostering, and adoption. In addition to rethinking who counts as a sexual minority parent, as we have argued above, researchers need to rethink the issues that are shaping the quality of life for sexual minority parents and their children, and pay more attention to such issues as immigration law and welfare reform, which are ranked as important by families themselves.

By accounting for the racial variance in pathways to and experiences of parenting, and by expanding our research beyond White, Western populations, this chapter also opens up new entry points into some of the central debates within family and sexuality studies. Issues of sameness and difference are raised by Biblarz and Stacey (2010) in their article on the ways gender and sexuality of parents relate to children's well-being. They argue that having outcomes equivalent to those of heterosexual parents is an inherently problematic way to legitimate same-sex parenting. Studies discussed in the present work extend this line of reasoning. Rather than seeing heterosexual parenting as the benchmark for success, some racial and sexual minority parents consciously alter their parenting styles in pursuit of *different* outcomes for their children. Parents and families in much of this work challenge heteronormativity in deeper ways than a discourse of "sameness" can accomplish.

The work we have reviewed lends empirical support to intersectionality theories that motivate us to move beyond additive models of structural location. Racial and sexual minority families interact with their social worlds in ways that are not reducible to theories of race and racism, or to theories of sexuality and heterosexism. Reintegrating racial and sexual minority parents and their children into research, practice, and policy promises to expand our knowledge about the population of same-sex parent-headed families, at the same time that it enriches existing theories and questions, and offers new possibilities for moving forward as a field.

Acknowledgment The first author received support for this work from the University of California, Los Angeles, Center for Health Improvement of Minority Elderly/ Resource Centers for Minority Aging Research, under NIH/NIA Grant P30-AG02-1684.

References

Aarmo, M. (1999). How homosexuality became 'un-African': The case of Zimbabwe. In E. Blackwood & S. Wieringa (Eds.), *Female desires: Same-sex relations and transgender practices across cultures* (pp. 255–280). New York, NY: Columbia University Press.

Asian American Federation of New York. (2004). *Asian Pacific American same-sex households: A census report on New York, San Francisco and Los Angeles*. Retrieved from http://www.aafny.org/cic/report/GLReport.pdf

Biblarz, T., & Savci, E. (2010). Lesbian, gay, bisexual, and transgender families. *Journal of Marriage and Family, 72*, 480–497. doi:10.1111/j.1741-3737.2010.00714.x

Biblarz, T., & Stacey, J. (2010). How does the gender of parents matter? *Journal of Marriage and Family, 72*, 3–22. doi:10.1111/j.1741-3737.2009.00678.x

Billson, J. M. (1995). *Keepers of the culture: The power of tradition in women's lives*. Lanham, MD: Lexington Books.

Cahill, S. (2010). Black and Latino same-sex couple households and the racial dynamics of antigay activism. In J. Battle & S. Barnes (Eds.), *Black sexualities: Probing powers, passions, practices and policies* (pp. 243–268). Piscataway, NJ: Rutgers University Press.

Cahill, S., Battle, J., & Meyer, D. (2003). Partnering, parenting, and policy: Family issues affecting Black lesbian, gay, bisexual, and transgender (LGBT) people. *Race and Society, 6*, 85–98. doi:10.1016/j.racsoc.2004.11.002

Cahill, S., & Jones, K. T. (2001). *Leaving our children behind: Welfare reform and the gay, lesbian, bisexual, and transgender community*. New York, NY: Policy

Institute of the National Gay and Lesbian Task Force. Retrieved from http://www.thetaskforce.org/downloads/reports/fact_sheets/WelfareFactSheet.pdf.

Campbell, L. A., & Kaufmann, R. L. (2006). Racial differences in household wealth: Beyond black and white. *Research in Social Stratification and Mobility, 24*, 131–152. doi:10.1016/j.rssm.2005.06.001

Chalmers, S. (2002). *Emerging lesbian voices from Japan*. New York, NY: Routledge.

Choo, H. R., & Ferree, M. M. (2010). Practicing intersectionality in sociological research: A critical analysis of inclusions, interactions, and institutions in the study of inequalities. *Sociological Theory, 28*, 129–149. doi:10.1111/j.1467-9558.2010.01370.x

Cianciotto, J. (2005). *Hispanic and Latino same-sex couple households in the United States: A report from the 2000 Census*. New York, NY: The National Gay and Lesbian Task Force Policy Institute. Retrieved from http://www.lgbtracialequity.org/publications/HispanicLatinoHouseholdsUS.pdf

Collins, P. H. (2000). *Black feminist thought: Knowledge, consciousness, and the politics of empowerment*. New York, NY: Routledge.

Collins, P. H. (2004). *Black sexual politics: African Americans, gender, and the new racism*. New York, NY: Routledge.

Connell, R. (2007). *Southern theory: Social science and the global dynamics of knowledge*. Boston, MA: Polity.

Dang, A., & Frazer, S. (2004). *Black same-sex households in the United States: A report from the 2000 census*. New York, NY: The National Gay and Lesbian Task Force Policy Institute and the National Black Justice Coalition. Retrieved from http://nbjc.org/assets/BCRNationalReport.pdf

Dang, A., & Vianney, C. (2007). *Living in the margins: A national survey of lesbian, gay, bisexual and transgender Asian and Pacific Islander Americans*. New York, NY: The National Gay and Lesbian Task Force Policy Institute. Retrieved from http://www.thetaskforce.org/downloads/reports/reports/API_ExecutiveSummaryEnglish.pdf

Dunne, G. A. (2000). Opting into motherhood: Lesbians blurring the boundaries and transforming the meaning of parenthood and kinship. *Gender and Society, 14*, 11–35. doi:10.1177/089124300014001003

Engebretsen, E. L. (2009). Intimate practices, conjugal ideals: Affective ties and relationship strategies among lala (lesbian) women in contemporary Beijing. *Sexuality Research & Social Policy, 6*, 3–14. doi:10.1525/srsp.2009.6.3.3

Espiritu, Y. L. (2001). We don't sleep around like white girls do: Family, culture, and gender in Filipina American lives. *Signs: Journal of Women in Culture and Society, 26*, 415–440. doi:10.1086/495599

Farr, R., & Patterson, C. (2009). Transracial adoption by lesbian, gay, and heterosexual couples: Who completes transracial adoptions and with what results? *Adoption Quarterly, 12*, 187–204. doi:10.1080/10926750903313328

Gartrell, N., Banks, A., Hamilton, J., Reed, N., Bishop, H., & Rodas, C. (1999). The National Lesbian Family Study: 2. Interviews with mothers of toddlers. *American Journal of Orthopsychiatry, 69*, 362–369. doi:10.1037/h0080410

Gartrell, N., Banks, A., Reed, N., Hamilton, J., Rodas, C., & Deck, A. (2000). The national lesbian family study: 3. Interviews with mothers of five-year-olds. *American Journal of Orthopsychiatry, 70*, 542–548. doi:10.1037/h0087823

Gates, G., Lau, H., & Sears, R. B. (2006). Asians and Pacific Islanders in same-sex couples in the United States: Data from census 2000. *Amerasia Journal, 32*, 15–32.

Gilley, B. J. (2006). *Becoming two-spirit: Gay identity and social acceptance in Indian country*. Lincoln, NE: University of Nebraska Press.

Glover, M., McKree, A., & Dyall, L. (2009). Assisted human reproduction: Issues for takatapui (New Zealand indigenous non-heterosexuals). *Journal of GLBT Family Studies, 5*, 295–311. doi:10.1080/15504280903263702

Greene, B. (1997). *Ethnic and cultural diversity among lesbians and gay men*. Thousand Oaks, CA: Sage.

Hammonds, E. M. (1997). Toward a genealogy of Black female sexuality: The problematic of silence. In M. J. Alexander & C. T. Mohanty (Eds.), *Feminist genealogies, colonial legacies, democratic futures* (pp. 170–182). New York, NY: Routledge.

Herrera, F. (2009). Tradition and transgression: Lesbian motherhood in Chile. *Sexuality Research & Social Policy, 6*, 35–51. doi:10.1525/srsp.2009.6.2.35

Hicks, S. (2011). *Lesbian, gay and queer parenting: Families, intimacies, genealogies*. Basingstoke, UK: Palgrave Macmillan.

Hine, D. C. (1989). Rape and the inner lives of Black women in the Middle West: Preliminary thoughts on the culture of dissemblance. *Signs: Journal of Women in Culture and Society, 14*, 912–920. doi:10.1086/494552

Itzigsohn, J., Cabral, C. D., Medina, E. H., & Vazquez, O. (1999). Mapping Dominican transnationalism: Narrow and broad transnational practices. *Ethnic and Racial Studies, 22*, 316–339. doi:10.1080/014198799329503

Lewin, E. (2009). *Gay fatherhood: Narratives of family and citizenship in America*. Chicago, IL: The University of Chicago Press.

Mallon, G. P. (2004). *Gay men choosing parenthood*. New York, NY: Columbia University Press.

Mays, V., Chatters, L., Cochran, S., & Mackness, J. (1998). African American families in diversity: Gay men and lesbians as participants in family networks. *Journal of Comparative Family Studies, 29*, 73–87. http://soci.ucalgary.ca/jcfs/issues.

Meyers, M. K., Han, W. J., Waldfogel, J., & Garfinkel, I. (2001). Child care in the wake of welfare reform: The impact of government subsidies on the economic well-being of single-mother families. *The Social Service Review, 75*, 29–59. doi:10.1086/591881

Moore, M. R. (2008). Gendered power relations among women: A study of household decision making in Black, lesbian stepfamilies. *American Sociological Review, 73*, 335–356. doi:10.1177/000312240807300208

Moore, M. R. (2011a). *Invisible families: Gay identities, relationships, and motherhood among Black women.* Berkeley, CA: University of California Press.

Moore, M. R. (2011b). Two sides of the same coin: Revising analyses of lesbian sexuality and family formation through the study of Black women. *Journal of Lesbian Studies, 15*, 58–68. doi:10.1080/10894160.2010.508412

Moore, M. R. (2012). Intersectionality and the study of Black, sexual minority women. *Gender and Society, 26*, 33–39. doi:10.1177/0891243211427031

Morris, J. F., Balsam, K. F., & Rothblum, E. D. (2002). Lesbian and bisexual mothers and nonmothers: Demographics and the coming-out process. *Journal of Family Psychology, 16*, 144–156. doi:10.1037/0893-3200.16.2.144

Moss, A. R. (2012). Alternative families, alternative lives: Married women doing bisexuality. *Journal of GLBT Family Studies, 8.*

Oliver, M., & Shapiro, T. (1997). *Black wealth/white wealth: A new perspective on racial inequality.* New York, NY: Routledge.

Passel, J. S., & Cohn, D. V. (2008). *US population projections, 2005–2050.* Washington, DC: Pew Research Center. Retrieved from http://pewhispanic.org/files/reports/85.pdf

Patterson, C. J. (1995). Lesbian mothers, gay fathers, and their children. In A. R. D'Augelli & C. J. Patterson (Eds.), *Lesbian, gay, and bisexual identities over the lifespan: Psychological perspectives* (pp. 262–290). New York, NY: Oxford University Press.

Pfeffer, C. (2010). 'Women's work'? Women partners of transgender men doing housework and emotion work. *Journal of Marriage and Family, 72*, 165–183. doi:10.1111/j.1741-3737.2009.00690.x

Potgieter, C. A. (2003). Black South African lesbians: Discourses on motherhood and women's roles. *Journal of Lesbian Studies, 7*, 135–151. doi:10.1300/J155v07n03_10

Quiroz, P. (2007). *Adoption in a color-blind society.* Lanhan, MD: Rowman & Littlefield.

Richardson, H. B., & Goldberg, A. E. (2010). The intersection of multiple minority statuses: Perspectives of White lesbian couples adopting racial minority children. *Australian and New Zealand Journal of Family Therapy, 31*, 340–353. doi:10.1375/anft.31.4.340

Romero, V. (2005). Asians, gay marriage, and immigration: Family unification at a crossroads. *Indiana International & Comparative Law Review, 15*, 337–347.

Rosenfeld, M. J. (2010). Nontraditional families and childhood progress through school. *Demography, 47*, 755–775. doi:10.1353/dem.0.0112

Ryan-Flood, R. (2009). *Lesbian motherhood: Gender, families and sexual citizenship.* Basingstoke, UK: Palgrave MacMillan.

Samuels, G. M. (2009). 'Being raised by white people': Navigating racial difference among adopted multiracial adults. *Journal of Marriage and Family, 71*, 80–94. doi:10.1111/j.1741-3737.2008.00581.x

Silvera, M. (1995). Confronting the 'I' in the eye: Black mother, Black daughters. In K. Arnup (Ed.), *Lesbian parenting: Living with pride and prejudice* (pp. 311–320). Charlottetown, NS: Gynergy Books.

Spencer, M. B. (1983). Children's cultural values and parental child rearing strategies. *Developmental Review, 3*, 351–370. doi:10.1016/0273-2297(83)90020-5

Spencer, M. B., & Markstrom-Adams, C. (1990). Identity processes among racial and ethnic minority children in America. *Child Development, 61*, 290–310. doi:10.2307/1131095

Sullivan, M. (2004). *The family of woman: Lesbian mothers, their children, and the undoing of gender.* Berkeley, CA: University of California Press.

Swarr, A. L., & Nagar, R. (2003). Dismantling assumptions: Interrogating 'lesbian' struggles for identity and survival in India and South Africa. *Signs: Journal of Women in Culture and Society, 29*, 491–516. doi:10.1086/378573

Vidal de Haymes, M., Kilty, K. M., & Segal, E. A. (2000). *Latino poverty in the new century: Inequalities, challenges, and barriers.* London, UK: Haworth Press.

Viladrich, A., & Loue, S. (2009). Minority identity development. In S. Loue (Ed.), *Sexualities and identities of minority women* (pp. 1–18). New York, NY: Springer.

Washington, T. (2008). Throwing Black babies out with the bathwater: A child-centered challenge to same-sex adoption bans. *Hastings Race and Poverty Law Journal, 6*, 1–54.

Wekker, G. (2006). *The politics of passion: Women's sexual culture in the Afro-Surinamese diaspora.* New York, NY: Columbia University Press.

Wilhelmus, M. (1998). Mediation in kinship care: Another step in the provision of culturally relevant child welfare services. *Social Work, 43*, 117–126.

Stephen Hicks

It might seem strange, at first, to include a chapter on gender in a section on neglected areas of research. After all, doesn't a lot of the research on LGBT parents and their children talk about questions of gender identity or role? While this is true in many cases (see, for example, Green, 1978; Hoeffer, 1981; Ricketts, 1991; Skeates & Jabri, 1988), the version of gender addressed is largely one to do with parental role and its supposed effects upon child development. That is, a rather static view of gender as having merely to do with a role or identity is employed. Nevertheless, it is important to remember that much of this early research into lesbian, gay, or transgender parenting was produced in response to concerns about supposed damaging effects upon children, including notions that gender development would be negatively impacted. This work was a necessary and important contribution in a climate in which lesbians, for example, had been losing custody or residence of their children solely upon the basis of their sexuality (Hunter & Polikoff, 1976). But it also means that some of the research questions addressed were about reassuring readers that LGBT parents provide "balanced" gender role models and that their children do not develop "abnormal" gender identities.

There is little work in the field of LGBT parenting research that asks critical questions about

what "gender" actually means and, relatedly, how it is put to use. Ferree (2010) reminds us that feminist scholarship has questioned reified and individualized versions of gender, since a more critical account:

> rejects gender as a static norm or ideal (the so-called *gender-role*), and instead defines gender as a social relation characterized by power inequalities that hierarchically produce, organize, and evaluate masculinities and femininities through the contested but controlling practices of individuals, organizations, and societies. (p. 424)

In this chapter, I propose an analysis of gender as an interactional *practice* that occurs within social relations that have to do with expectations and prescriptions, which are morally and hierarchically motivated. This means that I reject notions of gender as a mere role or identity and ask, instead, how it is put to use in the delimiting of acceptable ways to be "female/male" and in the promotion of heteronormative ideas. My chapter begins by asking how gender is conceptualized, and it goes on to review existing research in terms of what this has to say about the gender identity and role of, first, LGBT parents and, second, their children—or, more precisely, I investigate the *versions* of gender constructed in the research. The studies considered here are mainly focused on lesbian, gay, and trans parents, because although bisexual parents are considered in two of the pieces reviewed, there is little specific attention given to bisexuality in this field. I go on to analyze research that attempts to critique gender norms, before drawing from my

S. Hicks, Ph.D. (✉)
School of Nursing, Midwifery, and Social Work,
University of Salford, Salford, M6 6PU, UK
e-mail: s.hicks@salford.ac.uk

A.E. Goldberg and K.R. Allen (eds.), *LGBT-Parent Families: Innovations in Research and Implications for Practice*, DOI 10.1007/978-1-4614-4556-2_10, © Springer Science+Business Media New York 2013

own research into foster care and adoption by lesbians and gay men (Hicks, 2008, 2011), to ask how to reconceptualize gender as social and political interaction. That is, I ask how to avoid a fixed view of gender and the tendency to compare LGBT parents with, and expect them to live up to, gendered normativities. Here, I hope to shift reified views of gender, in favor of an approach that asks how gender is enacted and attributed in talk, text, and practice.

What Is "Gender?"

The word "gender" was initially used by sexologists working with transsexuals (e.g., Money, 1978; Stoller, 1968) and by feminists (e.g., Oakley, 1972; Rubin, 1975) to describe a role, identity, or social category based upon biological sex difference. Later definitions variously define gender as a form of institutional and social relations, in which knowledge about women and men is produced and used to sustain division and inequality, and as a social practice that must be enacted and negotiated within everyday life. This means that not only has the word "gender" been theorized in very different ways but it is a social concept related to questions of power and the institution of heterosexuality, rather than merely describing a characteristic acquired in childhood. As Woodward (2011) argues:

> Gender is embodied and lived through everyday interactions and, although it is characterised by the endurance of inequalities such as patriarchy, it is also subject to change and is a fluid concept, which can be negotiated and transformed as well as reinstated. (p. 4)

In relation to LGBT parents, however, "gender" has mainly been used in more usual ways; that is, to refer to a natural/biological state, an identity, or a role. Opponents of LGBT parenting, for example, refer to "natural" differences between women and men and the need for all children to have parents that reflect, and provide role models of, these differences. In the UK, Patricia Morgan (2002), a sociologist associated with the Institute for Economic Affairs, the Institute for the Study of Civil Society, and the

Christian Institute—all promoters of the married, heterosexual family—argues that "intact marriage might be regarded as 'the gold standard for child rearing'" (p. 44) and that the children of gay or lesbian parents are likely to suffer a confused gender and sexual identity. In the USA, Lynn Wardle, a professor of law who supported the 1996 Defense of Marriage Act and is opposed to gay adoption, argues that children have a "need for dual-gender parenting" (Wardle, 1997, p. 852) to avoid confusion, and that there are "gender-linked differences in child-rearing skills; men and women contribute different (gender-connected) strengths and attributes" (p. 857).

Some research has responded to such claims by evaluating the gender identity and role of the children of LGBT parents to show "normal" development and outcome. Green's (1978) analysis of 37 children raised by lesbian or transsexual parents, for example, suggests typical gender development and the absence of what is clinically defined as "gender identity disorder" (Green, 1998, p. 2). Tasker and Golombok (1997) argue, based upon their longitudinal, comparative study of 25 adults with lesbian parents and 21 adults with heterosexual mothers, that although those from lesbian households were more likely to consider a relationship with someone of the same gender, they were no more likely than individuals living with a heterosexual mother to develop a gay, bisexual, or lesbian identity in adulthood. While research of this type has been vital in helping to challenge the views of those who argue against LGBT parenting, it may also be criticized for measuring those parents against a heteronormative standard and failing to question the notion of expected gender or sexual identity development.

Supporters of LGBT parenting also employ views of gender as a fixed role, identity, or measurable variable in their work. For example, Biblarz and Stacey's (2010) meta-analysis of studies from 1993 to 2008 concludes that existing research has "not identified any gender-exclusive parenting abilities" (p. 16), but goes on to suggest that there may be some "findings of difference that might conceivably derive from parental gender" (p. 13). They propose the possibility that "two women parent better on average than a woman and a man, or at least than a woman and a man with a traditional division of family labor," and also that single parents are able to "foster more androgynous parenting practices" (p. 17). However, the authors advocate for the examination of gender "as distinct from the number, marital status, sexual orientation, or biogenetic relationship of parents" and suggest that it is possible to "isolate the variable of parental gender" (Biblarz & Stacey, 2010, p. 5) to test for its effects.

The problem with these perspectives on gender is that they reify a social practice or set of expectations, so that gender becomes measurable and "thing-like," with all other contextual and interactional matters disappearing from the picture. An alternative perspective, one concerned with gender *practices*, considers the ways in which it is enacted or performed in everyday life, how such performances are context dependent, and the hierarchical, heteronormative expectations of gender as a social system. For example, ethnomethodological theories of gender argue:

> a person engaged in virtually any activity may be held accountable for performance of that activity as a *woman* or a *man* … to "do" gender is not always to live up to normative conceptions of femininity or masculinity; it is to engage in behavior *at the risk of gender assessment*. (West & Zimmerman, 1987, p. 136)

This is a crucial point, since it recognizes not only that gender is about social prescription and proscription but also that many people—including heterosexuals—do not live up to normative ideas about what is expected of women and men. Feminist and queer theorists have also suggested that gender distinctions are part of the maintenance of heterosexual superiority. The production of gender is intimately connected to what Butler (1990) terms "compulsory heterosexuality" (p. 31), so that notions of the feminine/masculine are imagined to be opposite, discrete, yet complementary forms.

Sociological perspectives on gender remind us that *each of us* is required to perform gender everyday, and "role" actually refers to expectations or prescriptions for appropriately masculine or feminine forms. What most people do in everyday life is what Kessler and McKenna

(1985) term "gender attribution" (p. 2), a process by which we are compelled to assign each person into one of two expected categories, female or male. They argue that "the element of social construction is primary in all aspects of being female or male" (Kessler & McKenna, 1985, p. 7), including supposed sex differences. Notions about what is properly masculine or feminine are treated as behavioral or psychological characteristics, attributed differently to men and women. Thus, for example, women are assumed to be the "naturally" better carers/parents. Instead, Kessler and McKenna talk about gender assignment (attribution of a gender category at birth), identity ("an individual's own feeling of whether she or he is a woman or a man," p. 8), and role ("a set of expectations about what behaviors are appropriate for people of one gender," p. 11).

As is the case for everyone, LGBT parents must take up or enact gender in everyday life. They must be taken for a woman or a man and, while this expectation does not necessarily imply willing adherence to gender norms, it does mean that any perceived deviance from the norm will be problematized. The breaching of gender role expectations will usually result not in any questioning of the gender order, but in stigmatization of the individual, group, or category (LGBT parents) that they are taken to represent. Ethnomethodological theorists, such as Kessler and McKenna (1985), also argue that it is important to examine gendered subjectivity as practiced within an everyday context, rather than in the abstract, and so I return to this point in relation to LGBT parenting toward the end of the chapter. But first, it is necessary to consider in more depth how gender is analyzed in the existing research on LGBT parents and their children.

Gender in Existing Research on LGBT Parents and Their Children

Gender and LGBT Parents

Many LGBT parents talk about the constraining effects of gender. For example, in a focus group-based study of 25 gay fathers based in New York, Boston, and Connecticut, the majority reported "gender role strain" (Benson, Silverstein, & Auerbach, 2005, p. 3), based upon the perceived need to conform to expectations about masculinity. In other studies, gay dads talk about being made to feel that the care of children ought to be carried out by women (Doucet, 2006; Lewin, 2009; Mallon, 2004; Riggs, 2010). Lesbian mothers also state that, in some contexts, they are positioned as gender nonconformists; for example, in some people's reactions to a two-mother family (Dalton & Bielby, 2000), or in surprised responses to butch-identified lesbians who become mothers (Epstein, 2002; Pelka, 2009). Epstein's (2002) interviews with lesbian mothers who identify as butch reveal assumptions that mothers are assumed to be typically female/"feminine" or unremarkably gendered. As she argues, "Butch pregnancy and motherhood disrupt notions of coherent butch identity and butch mothers are subject to the cruelty that can result from a lack of willingness to see beyond these notions" (Epstein, 2002, p. 47).

Ryan's (2009) interviews with 10 female-to-male trans parents also suggest that "what trans men juggle is not the supposed baffling conundrum of how someone born female could be a father, but the rigid rules of gendered family life set up by other people" (p. 140). Trans parents in both Hines' (2007) and Ryan's (2009) research reported that they experienced prejudicial and negative reactions from some people who did not accept their gender determination or the notion that they may be suitable parents.

These gender configurations—gay dads, two mothers, butch moms, transgender parents—are all treated by some as unusual or even abnormal because they are perceived to challenge expectations about standard, heterosexual roles, including the notion that children ought to be parented by a caring/nurturing mother and a providing father. In this way, LGBT parents disrupt expected social categories in terms of gender and parenting. While this means that they may be subject to opprobrium, such disruptions also help to transform gender prescriptions. LGBT parents recognize, however, that the opportunities for gender transformation are limited. Gender presentation is context dependent, and so there will be situations in which gender nonconformity is embraced and others in which to do so might be unsafe, unwise, or difficult for parents and children. As the literature considered in this section reveals, LGBT parents both "do" and "undo" gender simultaneously.

Gay Fathers and Gender

Parenting and caring activities among gay men are sometimes taken as evidence of gender dissidence, since "nurturing, caretaking, and domestic activities [are] simultaneously more necessary for gay men and less likely to be threatening to their masculine identity" (Stacey, 2006, p. 47). Based upon interviews with 29 gay fathers in the greater Los Angeles area, Stacey (2011) argues that most expressed a mix or range of gendered positions not always tied to notions of masculinity. Other studies also suggest gay dads blend male/female roles or take up androgynous ones (Bigner & Bozett, 1990; Bozett, 1989). There are instances of "degendered parenting" in the literature (Benson et al., 2005, p. 19), where gay men reject standard notions about the proper roles of mothers/fathers. Schacher, Auerbach, and Silverstein (2005), too, suggest situations in which the "gender role distinctions between 'mommy' and 'daddy' [are] obsolete" (p. 44). Yet this largely has to do with gay fathers' desires to avoid typically gendered divisions of labor within the home. In other contexts, particularly more public ones—schools, workplaces, community groups, health settings, social spaces, childcare facilities, and so on—gay dads have to weigh how much they are prepared to challenge gender assumptions and are particularly conscious about the fact that their children have to negotiate conventionally gendered expectations.

In her ethnography based upon individual, couple, and group interviews with 118 "primary, caregiving fathers" (p. 12), of which 9 were gay men, Doucet (2006) argues that gay dads are able to recognize both masculine and feminine aspects within themselves. But, at the same time, such ideas are actually heavily gendered. For example, Bernard, a participant in Doucet's research, says:

> I do some things that are typical of fathering. I throw a ball and play catch, mini golf, take him on the roller coaster, watch movies, play sports. But I also do non-typical things. I let him cry; I am

physically demonstrative. I want to break that generational cycle. I let him play with dolls, watch
women superheroes ... (p. 123)

While Doucet's (2006) analysis recognizes
the "border crossings" (p. 123) engaged in by gay
fathers who wish to break down some of the sup-
posedly female/male aspects of identities and
activities, at the same time, a concern with the
"doing" of gender reveals the ways in which
Bernard's speech actually *genders* activities, so
much so that going on a roller coaster or watch-
ing a movie is associated with "fathering." His
talk demonstrates an acute awareness of gendered
expectations, which he wishes to challenge.
Bernard uses ideas about the "generational cycle"
in interesting ways here. He wants to "break that
... cycle" so that he does not model typical ways
of being a man to his son, but at the same time,
Bernard imagines that his nontypical behaviors
will be passed on. The notion of gender as somehow modeled by parents and taken up by children
remains intact.

Doucet (2006), however, also notes occasions
at which "gay fathers ... have to demonstrate that
they can blend into parenting settings so that gender and sexuality lose critical significance" (p.
205). Lewin's (2009) research with 95 gay fathers
in Chicago, San Francisco, Los Angeles, and
Iowa City also found that they had to contend
with notions that parenting was essentially maternal but, at the same time, most of her respondents
rejected the idea that they were "mothering" to
emphasize their masculinity. In Mallon's (2004)
study of 20 gay men who became fathers through
foster care or adoption, most reported that they
had to contend with others', and sometimes their
own, views that men ought not to care for children, and also that such caring work is generally
devalued because it is primarily undertaken by
women. One couple reported that their ability or
willingness to perform caring and household
tasks had been commented upon by heterosexual
neighbors, whereby women were generally
approving but men seemed to feel that the gay
couple had made things difficult for them; that is,
the performance of childcare and household
duties by gay men implied that all men ought to
be able to do these tasks.

Lesbian Mothers and Gender

Lesbian mothers, similarly, both "draw upon and
resist dominant cultural practices, scripts, and
assumptions" (Dalton & Bielby, 2000, p. 57)
concerning expected gender roles and identities.
Lewin (1993), who interviewed 135 women (73
lesbian and 62 heterosexual single mothers)
residing in the San Francisco Bay Area, argues
for more commonalities, rather than differences,
between the two groups, suggesting that:

a lesbian who becomes a mother has effectively
rejected the equation of homosexuality with unnat-
uralness and the exclusion of the lesbian from the
ranks of "women." In this sense, finding a way to
become a mother constitutes a form of resistance
to the gender limitations, and particularly to the
constructions of sexual orientation, that prevail in
the wider culture. Curiously, though, this act of
resistance is achieved through compliance with
conventional expectations for women, so it may
also be construed as a gesture of accommodation.
(p. 74)

Lewin (1993) thus argues, not that lesbian
mothers are simply "the same" as heterosexual
ones, but rather that both share in a "system of
meaning that envelops motherhood in our culture"
(p. 182). In some senses, she suggests, lesbian
mothers occupy an expected gender role in a way
that *any woman who is a not a mother* does not.

Sullivan's (1996) research with 34 lesbian
co-parent couples in the San Francisco Bay Area
found a mixture of responses to the notion of gender
roles. Most couples described their household labor,
including parenting, as equally shared rather than
divided by role, but five had a full-time breadwinner/
stay-at-home caregiver configuration in which
the stay-at-home parent was more dissatisfied and
anxious about domestic arrangements. In later
research, Sullivan (2004) theorizes lesbian families
as "free of historically produced, socially enforced
gender conventions" (p. 6), yet her respondents
actually create and hold on to gender difference
within their talk. For example, Danielle, a participant in Sullivan's research, says:

I think that [Nathan]'ll have a different view of
women, not even so much from me but from Lee
[her partner]. Because Lee can do anything.
I mean, she cooks, she cleans, she builds, she does
gardening...I think Nathan's going to, I don't think

that Nathan's not going to lose not having a man. I think that he's um, you know, he's going to have the loss on some level of not knowing who his father is and not having that person here in his life, but Lee puts my brother-in-law to shame! (p. 86)

As with the example of Bernard, Danielle's talk is acutely conscious of gender and its implications, and she too takes up the idea of passing on a positive gender role to her son. Danielle's talk both challenges expected gender roles ("Lee can do anything") and reflects worries about male role models in relation to Nathan. While Sullivan (2004) argues in her study that lesbian parenting "may disrupt the cycle of gender reproduction" (p. 79), Danielle's talk nevertheless relies on the notion of gender role models, even though she proposes nontraditional ones. Both Danielle and Bernard feel accountable for gender identity/ presentation.

Egalitarian Roles?

There is evidence in some research that lesbian or gay parents challenge gendered assumptions through attempts to develop more egalitarian ways of living and dividing up household roles and tasks (Ciano-Boyce & Shelley-Sireci, 2002; Goldberg, 2010a; Sullivan, 1996, 2004; Weeks, Heaphy, & Donovan, 2001). Dunne (2000) argues, based upon interviews with 29 UK lesbian couples with children conceived through donor insemination, that the absence of polarized gender roles leads to the "construction of more egalitarian approaches to financing and caring for children" (p. 13). However, this notion of the egalitarian family is questioned elsewhere. Carrington's (1999) ethnography based upon interviews and observations of 26 lesbian and 26 gay families in the San Francisco Bay Area, for example, concludes that "lesbigay families are neither as egalitarian as they would like to believe nor as we would prefer that others believe" (p. 11). In fact, much of the research that suggests egalitarian shared parenting amongst LGBT families is based upon the experiences of White, middle-class, urban respondents.

Moore's (2008, 2011) research with Black mothers in New York (32 from lesbian stepfamilies and 8 who had children via alternative insemination) argues that notions of gendered egalitarianism may be tempered by actual family practices in which Black women strongly value economic independence. In addition, biological mothers, particularly in stepfamilies, undertake significantly more household chores and budget management, but as a way to retain status and respectability. The control of certain household or caring tasks acts as a way to confirm an identity as a "good" mother and to control, or have a deciding voice, in how a household is run. Moore (2011) argues that Black women value autonomy and economic independence over notions of egalitarian division of labor, and that her respondents saw these as crucial to the success of their relationships. Given that Black lesbians are also more likely than Whites to experience poverty, lack of opportunity, and social stigmatization, then these questions about respectability and financial autonomy are highly relevant.

The notion of egalitarianism is also problematized in further studies where social class is taken into account. Gabb's (2008) research, based upon diaries, interviews, and observations of 14 lesbian parents and their 10 children in the North of England, and Taylor's (2009) interviews with 60 gay and lesbian parents in the UK suggest the notion is a largely middle-class one, derived from research that does not ask questions about class or that is based solely upon middle-class samples. Gabb and Taylor both suggest that questions to do with poverty or lack of opportunity may mean, for example, that a lesbian couple who appears to occupy traditionally gendered homemaker/breadwinner roles may derive some sense of ordinariness or respectability from this arrangement, an important dynamic in a social context that is otherwise stigmatizing. They may also lack the choice or opportunity to adopt what is considered to be a more egalitarian model of family life, since this model is sometimes derived from research with couples in which both partners work part time or can afford to pay for day care (Dunne, 2000; Sullivan, 2004; Weeks et al., 2001).

Gender and the Children of LGBT Parents

In relation to the children of LGBT parents, two linked themes concerned with gender are key: the question about whether those children develop "normal" gender identities and the question about whether LGBT parents provide adequate gender role models. Before asking some critical questions about both of these ideas, it is helpful to review relevant studies on these points.

Children's Gender Development

In response to suggestions that the children of LGBT parents will develop "abnormal" gender roles and identities, researchers have argued that they do not exhibit any gender confusion, and that their parents or families offer adequate role models (Freedman, Tasker, & di Ceglie, 2002; Golombok, Spencer, & Rutter, 1983; Green, 1978, 1982, 1998; Green, Mandel, Hotvedt, Gray, & Smith, 1986; Patterson, 1992; Tasker & Golombok, 1997). However, while these authors have concluded that the gender development of children of LGBT parents is very similar to that of children of heterosexual parents, there is also evidence that those parents are careful not to impose rigid gender roles or expectations upon their children (Biblarz & Stacey, 2010; Fulcher, Sutfin, & Patterson, 2008; Hill, 1987; Hoeffer, 1981; Kweskin & Cook, 1982; MacCallum & Golombok, 2004). Further, studies, such as those of Tasker and Golombok (1997), point out that children's gender behavior is not simply modeled on their parents, since they evaluate this in relation to what they understand to be culturally appropriate.

Kane's (2006) analysis of interviews with 42 heterosexual, lesbian, and gay parents of preschool-aged children, primarily based in southern and central Maine, is relevant here, as she considers parental perceptions of children's gendered attributes and behaviors. She argues that many of these parents showed negative responses to expressions of perceived femininity in their sons, most of which are to do with fears about sons becoming "a sissy" (p. 161) or "fear that a son either would be or would be perceived as gay"

(Kane, 2006, p. 162). Kane notes that heterosexual fathers were more likely to see any perceived femininity/homosexuality in sons as a reflection upon themselves (or upon their own masculinity). Lesbian, gay, and heterosexual female parents, however, said that they felt accountable to others for their sons' perceived masculinity. LGBT parents may be particularly conscious that they are held accountable to others for their child's perceived gender identity/role, and they may be acutely aware of not wishing to impose nonstandard ideas about gender onto their children, since they know that their children have to live in a gender-conforming world.

Gender Role Models

The question about whether LGBT parents are able to provide their children with adequate "gender role models" is a major theme of existing research. Gender role theory (see Mischel, 1966; Parsons, 1956) holds that children learn about being a woman/man from interactions with, and their modeling of, two parents—a father and a mother. These ideas are drawn upon by commentators opposed to all nonheterosexual or nonnuclear (heterosexual, two-parent) families. Morgan (2002), for example, suggests that gender confusion "seems to be rife, with daughters of lesbian mothers more likely to value and exhibit male sex-typed traits, and sons more female-valued traits" (p. 78). It is worth pausing to look at this claim for a moment, since Morgan's conclusions are based in part upon research by Hoeffer (1981), which also used social learning theory to suggest that children acquire a sex role. Hoeffer studied the chosen toy preferences of children (aged 6–9) of 20 lesbian and 20 single, heterosexual mothers in the San Francisco Bay Area. Putting aside for a moment very serious qualms about toy preference as an indicator of gender role, Hoeffer reported that there were no significant differences between the two groups of children, and that most chose traditionally gender-typed toys. She also argued that some lesbian mothers were less likely to insist that their children play with traditionally gender-typed toys, but this is turned—in Morgan's account—into "rife" gender confusion. Thus, it is important to remember that, for commentators like Morgan, *any* questioning of expected gender roles is a bad thing.

Clarke's research (Clarke, 2006, 2007; Clarke & Kitzinger, 2005) has suggested that gay and lesbian parents frequently are forced into defensive responses to gender role theory, whereby they emphasize that their children have contact with both women and men and that they will present balanced gender roles. In lesbian-parent families, for example, "male presence is routinely positioned as a producer of normative gender and sexual identities, and of normative subjects more generally" (Clarke, 2007, p. 342). Feminist critiques of gender/sex role socialization theory have also argued that it is very limited to assume that gender is taken on by children through learning from their parents; this theory sees gender as fixed, passively learned, and a static thing to be imitated (Berk, 1985; Davies, 1989; Stanley & Wise, 1993). For example, Thorne's (1993) ethnographic observation of gendered play, in public elementary schools in California and Michigan, suggests that children produce gender, "actively and collaboratively, in everyday life" (p. 4), and that gender is "not something one passively 'is' or 'has'" (p. 5), rather it is performed variously, depending upon activity and context. Thorne argues, for example, that assertions about gender differences between girls and boys actually refer to *averages*, but within-gender variation is actually greater than differences between boys and girls taken as groups. This crucial point may also be applied to LGBT parents: There are many differences, rather than commonalities, in gender presentation or ideas among members of those categories.

Gender role theory is also problematic because it promotes the idea that men and women naturally perform discrete but complementary tasks, and so reinforces the notion that caring for children is a woman's role or responsibility. This is part of the way in which gender role theory is heteronormative, since this supposed complementarity of roles is based upon a female and male parent, and upon the prohibition of non-heterosexual ways of life. That is, gender role difference is not natural; it must be upheld and reiterated.

How Does Gender Matter?

Biblarz and Stacey's (2010) meta-analysis makes an important contribution to the literature because it argues, "claims that children need both a mother and father are spurious because they attribute to the gender of parents benefits that correlate primarily with the number and marital status of a child's parents since infancy" (p. 17). But, at the same time, they note there may be some advantages to growing up in a nontraditionally gendered family, such as more egalitarian and shared parenting among lesbian couples, less emphasis on gender conformity among gay male parents, and less "gender chauvinism" (Biblarz & Stacey, 2010, p. 14) among sons of lesbian mothers.

I have chosen to focus on this piece briefly because, in assuming gender in order to look for its effects, Biblarz and Stacey (2010) actually make gendered assumptions, treating lesbian families as examples of "fatherlessness" (p. 6), treating gay and lesbian families as automatically gendered male/masculine and female/feminine, treating some parenting behaviors as "feminine" or "masculine" (p. 11), and talking about "feminine socialization" of women or the "masculine development" of boys (p. 12). These problems are highlighted in the section of Biblarz and Stacey's article that deals with gay fathers. They argue that gay male parents "appear to adopt parenting practices more 'feminine' than do typical heterosexual fathers" (Biblarz & Stacey, p. 12). I argue, however, that gay fathers are described or identify themselves in such terms because they talk and act using ideas, practices, or props usually associated with women/mothers, not because of any essential feminine aspects to a caring/parenting role or because of their sexuality. Biblarz and Stacey acknowledge this, since they talk about adoption of "feminine…parenting practices," but they also claim that "gay male parents challenge dominant practices of masculinity, fatherhood, and motherhood more than lesbian co-mothers depart from normative femininity or maternal practice" (pp. 12–13).

This latter argument may be limited, however, because gay fathers always appear more gender deviant than lesbian mothers within a category ("parent/carer") that is usually regarded as feminine. In addition, while there are some gay dads who challenge dominant gendered ideas, not all do, and, conversely, there are lesbian mothers who disrupt normative femininity or question standard notions of motherhood. More importantly, these notions depend upon context and upon the ways in which a gendered subjectivity is enacted and interpreted.

In her response to Biblarz and Stacey's (2010) piece, Goldberg (2010b) questions "whether gender can ever be truly studied and understood independent of both the immediate (familial) environment and the broader (e.g., societal and legal) context," and also asks, "whether the gender that we observe in one environment or context is truly equivalent to the gender that we observe in another" (p. 29). She reminds us that gender conformity may be taken up by gay/lesbian parents in some contexts because of their concerns about safety or social opprobrium, and she raises the limitations of seeing lesbian families as essentially all-female or gay families as all-male environments. The gendered worlds of children, and their parents, are likely to be much more complicated than this. In another response, Tasker (2010) similarly argues that much of what Biblarz and Stacey refer to has to do with attitudes toward and norms about, rather than core aspects of, gender.

It may appear strange to some readers that I have chosen to focus on the work of Biblarz and Stacey (2010) here, since their research has clearly challenged heteronormative and gendered presumptions about who is fit to parent (Biblarz & Stacey, 2010; Stacey & Biblarz, 2001). But my point is that, even in research that actively supports LGBT parenting, there are problematic notions of gender. To assume gender as a measurable variable is to reify it, that is, to turn a complex set of social expectations, behaviors, and reactions into an entity. This has the consequences of seeing gender as the determinable cause of other behaviors and of reading certain behaviors as somehow automatically gendered. What this means is that questions about how and why gender is enacted within particular scenes are removed from the picture, and it is to these questions that I now turn.

"Doing" Gender in LGBT Parents' Lives

Gay and lesbian applicants who wish to foster or adopt children frequently report that they are expected to reassure social work representatives about their balanced gender role models, even where they disagree with or dispute the notion (Cocker, 2011; Hicks & McDermott, 1999; Riggs, 2007, 2010, 2011; Ross, Epstein, Anderson, & Eady, 2009). In my own research, based upon interviews with 15 lesbian and gay parents, I spoke to a gay adoptive couple, Peter and Pete, who told me their social worker asked them about "stereotypical roles," and that, although they "tried to argue it for a while," they "just had to give up." They said, "we just went along with it … it was a defeat. …Those gender roles used to get on [our] nerves really" (Hicks, 2011, pp. 123–124). A lesbian adoptive couple, Nita and Clare, also spoke in similar terms, explaining that their preference to adopt girls was considered a problem:

> **Clare:** [Our social worker] asked us whether … well, there's something on the form where it asks about, "Are jobs allocated or do you have roles that are …?" So we said how we didn't have male and female roles and how we thought it really important for children not to, and all that sort of stuff … and the other thing that came up with gender was that we wanted girls.
> **Nita:** Yes we talked quite a lot about that really, because she wanted us not to say that …
> **Steve:** What did you have to say in the end?
> **Clare:** At the beginning of the assessment, [the social worker] said there was no problem, she said, "Oh yes, it's really common for people to say they only want boys or they only want girls. … No problem"-sort of thing, but it wasn't until. … Well, I got the impression that it was when she went back and she had team meetings and people played devil's advocate with the Panel … and she then became sort of more and more anxious about it and pushed it, and certainly the second social worker pushed it as well, so that was when we …
> **Nita:** … caved in! (Hicks, 2011, p. 188)

This sense of "defeat/giving up/caving in" is important as it highlights how gender performance is dependent upon context and upon questions of power. The institutional order of state foster care/adoption social work requires that the question of gender role models be addressed in relation to gay and lesbian applicants, and those applicants, as well as some social workers, who, in other contexts, are opposed to notions of gender role, must conform since they are held accountable. And while there is resistance to gender norms here, a standard and institutional discourse dominates, one in which adherence to a moral order that upholds expected gender roles is required.

Mark, a gay foster carer, presented himself as "a man who happens to be gay" (Hicks, 2011, p. 125), and said that his sexuality is often "not really relevant ... I'm the dad rather than the gay dad" (p. 132). Yet, at the same time, Mark was expected by others to address gender roles and to identify women in his everyday life, and he articulated a managed identity, in which his being gay was relevant but not always introduced by him into everyday scenes. This has to do with gauging of safety and comfort, whether there is a perceived need to protect fostered or adopted children from the views of others, and the desire to participate in normative practices and conversations at times. Mark's gender presentation is also about wanting to be seen as an "ordinary" man/father, and it has to do with challenging what he described as stereotypical views of *gay* dads as effeminate or suspicious.

Similar examples occur in Symons' (2002) film, *Daddy & Papa: A Story about Gay Fathers in America*. In one scene, Zac, the adopted son of Johnny and William, is seen playing in high heels. The couple comments:

> **Johnny:** People went out of their way to point out to us that Zac was one hundred percent boy, but once in a while he threw us a curveball ... When he developed an attachment to the neighbor's girl's high heels, it was a whole new ballgame ...
> **William:** If he did more traditionally feminine things, people would tie that to the fact that he has two dads. It's probably just internalized homophobia, but when stuff like that happens in public, I feel a little bit of—shame. (Symons, 2002)

William's confession of shame, here, is linked directly to the notion of a failed gender presentation, even though much narrative work has already been done to situate Zac as a proper boy (the couple even jokes about bringing up a "jock,"

and their language employs sports metaphors). But William's talk shows that he is painfully aware of those who would argue that gay parents produce gender-confused kids. William understands that a gender system that requires boys *not* to play with high heels is wrong, yet he blames his own "internalized homophobia" for his shameful reaction. Rather than question the gender order, he turns the concern in on himself—it is his psychological problem that dominates and results in feelings of shame. That is, he makes it into a psychological problem, one that identifies subjection to the gender order. He takes up a position, an affect, within gendered discourse, one in which femininity—especially in a boy—equals failure.

Lesbian and trans parents, similarly, refer to conventional gendered identities at times. Mamo's (2007) study of assisted conception among 36 lesbian, gay, bisexual, and queer women argues that "reproduction does not represent liberation from gender norms and the sexual and reproductive order, nor does it merely reinforce that order" (p. 57), since these parents both rejected but also relied upon notions of gender roles. Thomas Beatie's (2008) autobiographical account, detailing his pregnancy as a transgender man, works hard to establish that he was "never confused about ... gender identity—I always knew, long before I could articulate it, that I was really male" (p. 6). That is, at times a more conventional or "natural" approach to gender is taken up in LGBT parents' narratives. In relation to trans people, for example, Prosser (1998) argues that "transsexual and transgendered narratives alike produce not the revelation of the fictionality of gender categories but the sobering realization of their ongoing foundational power" (p. 11), since, to be taken for a "proper" person or parent, one has to be taken for a man or a woman.

The Everyday Presence of Gender

I have argued in this chapter that gender is a system that requires and reinforces the notion of different sexes (male/female) and roles, and that this has particular significance for LGBT parents, since the care of children is widely viewed as a feminine/heterosexual preserve and questions of sexuality/parenting are read through a gendered lens. Where LGBT parents or their children are perceived to question standard gender in some way, then it is the individual or group, rather than the gender order, that is subject to stigma. LGBT parents may be imagined, for example, to be insufficiently masculine/feminine, or, in the case of gay or lesbian couples, to represent "too much" of either, and to pass on such gender "abnormality" to their children. I have argued that this is, in part, why much of the existing research on LGBT parents aims to show "normal" gender development in children, to counter such gender stereotypes. This kind of argument, however, may actually reinforce standard notions of gender development, and, at the same time, reiterate the notion of gender as an entity, identity, or role (usually fixed in childhood), rather than a set of social practices and processes that have to do with power, knowledge, and expectation.

In his sociological study of transsexuality, Bogdan (1974) reminds us that it "is important for social scientists to understand their position, that they manufacture realities. The creation of perspectives with their reifying vocabularies is not a scientific issue. It is a moral and political issue" (p. 233). It is for this reason that I have argued that *all* research on LGBT parents presents a particular account or version of gender, rather than describing some kind of factual entity. Bogdan (1974) goes on to argue that we grow up:

> in a society that emphasizes a strictly dichotomous image of sex roles and, through the mass media, holds up clearly defined prototypes of these roles. The existence of these prototypes in the form of tightly constructed sex images insures that most people will feel inadequate in their attempts to measure themselves with in [sic] these terms. (p. 223)

LGBT parents identify those moments when they are made to feel most "inadequate" in gendered terms, yet, at the same time, they also identify the possibilities for challenging standard gender. As Khor (2007) argues, they "are 'doing gender' but less in the sense of conforming to gender expectations as in the sense of construct-

ing new norms for themselves, and being at the same time aware of gender norms" (p. 68). Nevertheless, we live in a social order that requires the taking up of gendered subjectivities–one in which living in a nontraditionally gendered, or even a non-gendered, way is made very difficult, and is something that LGBT parents are acutely conscious of, especially in relation to their children. LGBT parents talk about awareness of accountability for their, or their children's, perceived gender, and they raise issues that have to do with context and a concern for their children, to identify the ways in which gender enactment has to do with questions of personal safety or comfort. At some points they may speak of, or enact, the challenging of stereotypically gendered roles/identities at times, but at others they may try to "pass" in more conventionally gendered ways. This tells us that gender is not fixed, it is performed, and it has to do with power relations of hierarchy that may have damaging consequences for LGBT parents and their children if not carefully managed.

My perspective in this chapter has been based upon the argument that *each of us* is required to perform gender everyday, and that "role" in fact refers to expectations or prescriptions for appropriately masculine or feminine forms. A sociological and critical account of gender asks how and why gender is enacted differently dependent upon context, and how the production of ideas about a person's gender is always a dialogic process, one in which hierarchical and moral distinctions are produced. It also highlights the powerful effects of gendered ideas in the everyday lives of LGBT parents, but it ought, too, to provoke us to ask more difficult questions: that is, whether we really need gender and how we might challenge its damaging effects.

References

Beatie, T. (2008). *Labor of love: The story of one man's extraordinary pregnancy*. Berkeley, CA: Seal Press.

Benson, A. L., Silverstein, L. B., & Auerbach, C. F. (2005). From the margins to the center: Gay fathers reconstruct the fathering role. *Journal of GLBT Family Studies, 1*(3), 1–29. doi:10.1300/J461v01n03_01

Berk, S. F. (1985). *The gender factory: The apportionment of work in American households.* New York, NY: Plenum Press.

Biblarz, T. J., & Stacey, J. (2010). How does the gender of parents matter? *Journal of Marriage and Family, 72,* 3–22. doi:10.1111/j.1741-3737.2009.00678.x

Bigner, J. J., & Bozett, F. W. (1990). Parenting by gay fathers. In F. W. Bozett & M. B. Sussman (Eds.), *Homosexuality and family relations* (pp. 155–175). New York, NY: Harrington Park Press.

Bogdan, R. (Ed.). (1974). *Being different: The autobiography of Jane Fry.* New York, NY: Wiley.

Bozett, F. W. (1989). Gay fathers: A review of the literature. In F. W. Bozett (Ed.), *Homosexuality and the family* (pp. 137–162). New York, NY: Harrington Park Press.

Butler, J. (1990). *Gender trouble: Feminism and the subversion of identity.* New York, NY: Routledge.

Carrington, C. (1999). *No place like home: Relationships and family life among lesbians and gay men.* Chicago, IL: University of Chicago Press.

Ciano-Boyce, C., & Shelley-Sireci, L. (2002). Who is Mommy tonight? Lesbian parenting issues. *Journal of Homosexuality, 43*(2), 1–13. doi:10.1300/J082v43n02_01

Clarke, V. (2006). 'Gay men, gay men and more gay men': Traditional, liberal and critical perspectives on male role models in lesbian families. *Lesbian & Gay Psychology Review, 7,* 19–35.

Clarke, V. (2007). Men not included? A critical psychology analysis of lesbian families and male influence on child rearing. *Journal of GLBT Family Studies, 3,* 309–349. doi:10.1300/J461v03n04_01

Clarke, V., & Kitzinger, C. (2005). 'We're not living on planet lesbian': Constructions of male role models in debates about lesbian families. *Sexualities, 8,* 137–152. doi:10.1177/1363460705050851

Cocker, C. (2011). Sexuality before ability? The assessment of lesbians as adopters. In P. Dunk-West & T. Hafford-Letchfield (Eds.), *Sexual identities and sexuality in social work: Research and reflections from women in the field* (pp. 141–162). Farnham, UK: Ashgate.

Dalton, S. E., & Bielby, D. D. (2000). 'That's our kind of constellation': Lesbian mothers negotiate institutionalized understandings of gender within the family. *Gender and Society, 14,* 36–61. doi:10.1177/089124300014001004

Davies, B. (1989). *Frogs and snails and feminist tales: Preschool children and gender.* Sydney, Australia: Allen & Unwin.

Doucet, A. (2006). *Do men mother? Fathering, care, and domestic responsibility.* Toronto, ON: University of Toronto Press.

Dunne, G. A. (2000). Opting into motherhood: Lesbians blurring the boundaries and transforming the meaning of parenthood and kinship. *Gender and Society, 14,* 11–35. doi:10.1177/089124300014001003

Epstein, R. (2002). Butches with babies: Reconfiguring gender and motherhood. *Journal of Lesbian Studies, 6*(2), 41–57. doi:10.1300/J155v06n02_06

Ferree, M. M. (2010). Filling the glass: Gender perspectives on families. *Journal of Marriage and Family, 72,* 420–439. doi:10.1111/j.1741-3737.2010.00711.x

Freedman, D., Tasker, F., & di Ceglie, D. (2002). Children and adolescents with transsexual parents referred to a specialist gender identity development service: A brief report of key developmental features. *Clinical Child Psychology and Psychiatry, 7,* 423–432. doi:10.1177/1359104502007003009

Fulcher, M., Sutfin, E. L., & Patterson, C. J. (2008). Individual differences in gender development: Associations with parental sexual orientation, attitudes, and division of labor. *Sex Roles, 58,* 330–341. doi:10.1007/s11199-007-9348-4

Gabb, J. (2008). *Researching intimacy in families.* Basingstoke, UK: Palgrave Macmillan.

Goldberg, A. E. (2010a). *Lesbian and gay parents and their children: Research on the family life cycle.* Washington, DC: American Psychological Association.

Goldberg, A. E. (2010b). Studying complex families in context. *Journal of Marriage and Family, 72,* 29–34. doi:10.1111/j.1741-3737.2009.00680.x

Golombok, S., Spencer, A., & Rutter, M. (1983). Children in lesbian and single-parent households: Psychosexual and psychiatric appraisal. *Journal of Child Psychology and Psychiatry, 24,* 551–572.

Green, R. (1978). Sexual identity of 37 children raised by homosexual or transsexual parents. *The American Journal of Psychiatry, 135,* 692–697.

Green, R. (1982). The best interests of the child with a lesbian mother. *The Bulletin of the American Academy of Psychiatry and the Law, 10,* 7–15.

Green, R. (1998). Transsexuals' children. *International Journal of Transgenderism, 2*(4). Retrieved from http://www.wpath.org/journal/www.iiav.nl/ezines/web/IJT/97-03/numbers/symposion/ijtc0601.htm

Green, R., Mandel, J. B., Hotvedt, M. E., Gray, J., & Smith, L. (1986). Lesbian mothers and their children: A comparison with solo parent heterosexual mothers and their children. *Archives of Sexual Behavior, 15,* 167–184.

Hicks, S. (2008). Gender role models…who needs 'em?! *Qualitative Social Work, 7,* 43–59. doi:10.1177/1473325007086415

Hicks, S. (2011). *Lesbian, gay & queer parenting: Families, intimacies, genealogies.* Basingstoke, UK: Palgrave Macmillan.

Hicks, S., & McDermott, J. (Eds.). (1999). *Lesbian and gay fostering and adoption: Extraordinary yet ordinary.* London, UK: Jessica Kingsley Publishers.

Hill, M. (1987). Child-rearing attitudes of black lesbian mothers. In Boston Lesbian Psychologies Collective (Ed.), *Lesbian psychologies: Explorations and challenges* (pp. 215–226). Urbana, IL: University of Illinois Press.

Hines, S. (2007). *TransForming gender: Transgender practices of identity, intimacy and care.* Bristol, UK: Policy Press.

Hoeffer, B. (1981). Children's acquisition of sex-role behavior in lesbian-mother families. *American Journal of Orthopsychiatry, 51*, 536–544.

Hunter, N. D., & Polikoff, N. D. (1976). Custody rights of lesbian mothers: Legal theory and litigation strategy. *Buffalo Law Review, 25*, 691–733.

Kane, E. W. (2006). 'No way my boys are going to be like that!': Parents' responses to children's gender nonconformity. *Gender and Society, 20*, 149–176. doi: 10.1177/0891243205284276

Kessler, S. J., & McKenna, W. (1985). *Gender: An ethnomethodological approach*. Chicago, IL: University of Chicago Press.

Khor, D. (2007). 'Doing gender': A critical review and an exploration of lesbigay domestic arrangements. *Journal of GLBT Family Studies, 3*(1), 35–72. doi:10.1300/J461v03n01_03

Kweskin, S. L., & Cook, A. S. (1982). Heterosexual and homosexual mothers' self-described sex-role behavior and ideal sex-role behavior in children. *Sex Roles, 8*, 967–975.

Lewin, E. (1993). *Lesbian mothers: Accounts of gender in American culture*. Ithaca, NY: Cornell University Press.

Lewin, E. (2009). *Gay fatherhood: Narratives of family and citizenship in America*. Chicago, IL: University of Chicago Press.

MacCallum, F., & Golombok, S. (2004). Children raised in fatherless families from infancy: A follow-up of children of lesbian and single heterosexual mothers at early adolescence. *Journal of Child Psychology and Psychiatry, 45*, 1407–1419. doi:10.1111/j.1469-7610.2004.00324.x

Mallon, G. P. (2004). *Gay men choosing parenthood*. New York, NY: Columbia University Press.

Mamo, L. (2007). *Queering reproduction: Achieving pregnancy in the age of technoscience*. Durham, NC: Duke University Press.

Mischel, W. (1966). A social-learning view of sex differences in behavior. In E. Maccoby (Ed.), *The development of sex differences* (pp. 56–81). Stanford, CA: Stanford University Press.

Money, J. (1978). Determinants of human gender identity/role. In J. Money & H. Musaph (Eds.), *Handbook of sexology: History and ideology* (pp. 57–79). New York, NY: Elsevier.

Moore, M. R. (2008). Gendered power relations among women: A study of household decision making in black, lesbian stepfamilies. *American Sociological Review, 73*, 335–356. doi:10.1177/000312240807300208

Moore, M. R. (2011). *Invisible families: Gay identities, relationships, and motherhood among black women*. Berkeley, CA: University of California Press.

Morgan, P. (2002). *Children as trophies? Examining the evidence on same-sex parenting*. Newcastle upon Tyne, UK: The Christian Institute.

Oakley, A. (1972). *Sex, gender and society*. London, UK: Temple Smith.

Parsons, T. (1956). Family structure and the socialization of the child. In T. Parsons & R. F. Bales, in collaboration with J. Olds, M. Zelditch, Jr., & P. E. Slater (Eds.), *Family: Socialization and interaction process* (pp. 35–131). London, UK: Routledge & Kegan Paul.

Patterson, C. J. (1992). Children of lesbian and gay parents. *Child Development, 63*, 1025–1042.

Pelka, S. (2009). Sharing motherhood: Maternal jealousy among lesbian co-mothers. *Journal of Homosexuality, 56*, 195–217. doi:10.1080/00918360802623164

Prosser, J. (1998). *Second skins: The body narratives of transsexuality*. New York, NY: Columbia University Press.

Ricketts, W. (1991). *Lesbians and gay men as foster parents*. Portland, OR: National Child Welfare Resource Center for Management and Administration, University of Southern Maine.

Riggs, D. W. (2007). *Becoming parent: Lesbians, gay men, and family*. Teneriffe, Australia: Post Pressed.

Riggs, D. W. (2010). *What about the children! Masculinities, sexualities and hegemony*. Newcastle upon Tyne, UK: Cambridge Scholars Publishing.

Riggs, D. W. (2011). "I'm not gay, but my four mums are": Psychological knowledge and lesbian-headed families. *Radical Psychology*, *9*(2). Retrieved from http://www.radicalpsychology.org/vol9-2/riggs.html

Ross, L. E., Epstein, R., Anderson, S., & Eady, A. (2009). Policy, practice, and personal narratives: Experiences of LGBTQ people with adoption in Ontario, Canada. *Adoption Quarterly, 12*, 272–293. doi:10.1080/10926750903313302

Rubin, G. (1975). The traffic in women: Notes on the "political economy" of sex. In R. Reiter (Ed.), *Toward an anthropology of women* (pp. 157–210). New York, NY: Monthly Review Press.

Ryan, M. (2009). Beyond Thomas Beatie: Trans men and the new parenthood. In R. Epstein (Ed.), *Who's your daddy? and other writings on queer parenting* (pp. 139–150). Toronto, ON: Sumach Press.

Schacher, S. J., Auerbach, C. F., & Silverstein, L. B. (2005). Gay fathers expanding the possibilities for us all. *Journal of GLBT Family Studies, 1*(3), 31–52. doi:10.1300/J461v01n03_02

Skeates, J., & Jabri, D. (Eds.). (1988). *Fostering and adoption by lesbians and gay men*. London, UK: London Strategic Policy Unit.

Stacey, J. (2006). Gay parenthood and the decline of paternity as we knew it. *Sexualities, 9*, 27–55. doi:10.1177/1363460706060687

Stacey, J. (2011). *Unhitched: Love, marriage, and family values from West Hollywood to Western China*. New York, NY: New York University Press.

Stacey, J., & Biblarz, T. J. (2001). (How) does the sexual orientation of parents matter? *American Sociological Review, 66*, 159–183.

Stanley, L., & Wise, S. (1993). *Breaking out again: Feminist ontology and epistemology* (2nd ed.). London, UK: Routledge.

Stoller, R. (1968). *Sex and gender: On the development of masculinity and femininity*. London, UK: Karnac Books.

Sullivan, M. (1996). Rozzie and Harriet? Gender and family patterns of lesbian coparents. *Gender and Society, 10,* 747–767. doi:10.1177/089124396010006005

Sullivan, M. (2004). *The family of woman: Lesbian mothers, their children, and the undoing of gender.* Berkeley, CA: University of California Press.

Symons, J. (2002). (Producer & Director). *Daddy & papa: A story about gay fathers in America [Motion picture].* Harriman, NY: New Day Films. Producer & Director.

Tasker, F. (2010). Same-sex parenting and child development: Reviewing the contribution of parental gender. *Journal of Marriage and Family, 72,* 35–40. doi:10.1111/j.1741-3737.2009.00681.x

Tasker, F. L., & Golombok, S. (1997). *Growing up in a lesbian family: Effects on child development.* New York, NY: Guilford Press.

Taylor, Y. (2009). *Lesbian and gay parenting: Securing social and educational capital.* Basingstoke, UK: Palgrave Macmillan.

Thorne, B. (1993). *Gender play: Girls and boys in school.* Buckingham, UK: Open University Press.

Wardle, L. D. (1997). The potential impact of homosexual parenting on children. *University of Illinois Law Review, 1997,* 833–920.

Weeks, J., Heaphy, B., & Donovan, C. (2001). *Same sex intimacies: Families of choice and other life experiments.* London, UK: Routledge.

West, C., & Zimmerman, D. H. (1987). Doing gender. *Gender and Society, 1,* 125–151.

Woodward, K. (2011). *The short guide to gender.* Bristol, UK: Policy Press.

The "Second Generation": LGBTQ Youth with LGBTQ Parents

11

Katherine Kuvalanka

Do lesbian, gay, bisexual, transgender, and queer (LGBTQ)[1] parents have LGBTQ children? Yes, they do—sometimes—just as heterosexual and gender conforming parents do. Yet, research on the psychosocial development of LGBTQ youth has focused exclusively on adolescents from heterosexual- and gender-conforming-parent families. This line of inquiry has revealed that LGBTQ identity formation can be a lengthy and arduous process for some LGBTQ youth (Savin-Williams, 1996), as they may internalize negative, heterosexist messages from society and, often, family (Morrow, 2004). In turn, some LGBTQ youth experience feelings of isolation (Williams, Connolly, Pepler, & Craig, 2005), which may contribute to increased risk for mental health problems, such as depression and substance abuse (Morrow, 2004). It is unknown, however, whether these findings can be generalized to "second generation" youth—that is, LGBTQ youth with LGBTQ parents. Perhaps having an LGBTQ parent might ease one's own coming out process;

on the other hand, second generation youth may be "doubly marginalized" (Goldberg, 2007, p. 127), as a result of societal discrimination in relation to both their own and their parents' identities.

Youth and young adults who report nonheterosexual and gender nonconforming identities, and who also have LGBTQ parents, have been included in a few existing studies (e.g., Bailey, Bobrow, Wolfe, & Mikach, 1995; Kosciw & Diaz, 2008; Tasker & Golombok, 1997). The experiences of these individuals as second generation, however, have received very little attention in the family and social science literatures, despite calls for research on this population (Goldberg, 2007; Mooney-Somers, 2006). One reason for this lack of attention is, perhaps, that researchers have been wary of highlighting the existence of LGBTQ youth with LGBTQ parents for fear their studies will be utilized as evidence for arguments against LGBTQ parenting (Stacey & Biblarz, 2001). Given that LGBTQ parents face institutionalized discrimination (e.g., some states, such as Mississippi and Utah, continue to deny same-sex couples the opportunity to adopt children; National Gay and Lesbian Task Force, 2011), these concerns are valid. Furthermore, there are still relatively few studies of children with LGBTQ parents in general, due in part to the challenge of accessing LGBTQ-parent families (Stacey & Biblarz, 2001); thus, recruitment of second generation youth, a subgroup of an already difficult-to-access population, is likely an even greater challenge for researchers.

Although little empirical research exists on their experiences, nonacademic writers and queer

---

[1] The labels *LGBTQ* and *queer* are used throughout the chapter to refer to all nonheterosexual and gender nonconforming identities in general, even though social science research has not included all participants with these identity labels equally. More specific terms (e.g., *lesbian*) are used when referring to individual study samples or self-reported labels of study participants.

K. Kuvalanka, Ph.D. (✉)
Department of Family Studies and Social Work,
Miami University, 101F McGuffey Hall, Oxford,
OH 45056, USA
e-mail: kuvalanka@muohio.edu

A.E. Goldberg and K.R. Allen (eds.), *LGBT-Parent Families: Innovations in Research and Implications for Practice*, DOI 10.1007/978-1-4614-4556-2_11, © Springer Science+Business Media New York 2013

activists have been discussing the second generation—and providing many of them with community and support—for more than 15 years (COLAGE, 2010; Garner, 2004; Kirby, 1998). Systematic examination of the experiences of the second generation, however, may be beneficial in that challenges—as well as advantages—that are unique to this population could be revealed (Goldberg, 2007). For example, although second generation youth may face societal discrimination in relation to both their own and their parents' sexual orientation or gender identities, they may have more familial support and role modeling to help them cope than LGBTQ youth with heterosexual parents (Kosciw & Diaz, 2008). Thus, studies focusing on second generation youth could help family professionals understand the needs of these individuals and their families and how to better support them (Mooney-Somers, 2006). Moreover, exploring how the second generation might—or might not—benefit from having LGBTQ parents could provide important lessons for *all* parents of LGBTQ youth, in that there may be certain parental behaviors that prove to be more salient to these youth than their parents' identity as LGBTQ.

In this chapter, I will first present the primary theoretical framework, social constructionism, that has been used to frame this area of study (Kuvalanka & Goldberg, 2009) and that guides my present discussion of the second generation. I will then review what is currently known about the experiences of second generation individuals from both academic (e.g., Kuvalanka & Goldberg, 2009) and nonacademic (e.g., Garner, 2004) sources, including preliminary findings from my current research, based upon in-depth interviews with 30 LGBTQ young adults with LGBTQ parents. Lastly, I will address future research directions for expanding our knowledge and understanding of the second generation and their families.

Theoretical Perspective

A social constructionist approach views families, sexuality, and gender as socially and materially constructed (Oswald, Blume, & Marks, 2005) and contests the heteronormative practice of legitimating only those relationships that are based on biological and legal ties (Dunne, 2000). A social constructionist perspective does not reduce sexual feelings and gender identity to essential qualities with which a child is born; rather, a diverse range of factors are acknowledged as impacting behavior and identity, including biological (Hines, 2004) and social processes (Kitzinger, 1987). According to a social constructionist approach, individuals use their available social context to understand, create meaning out of, and assign labels to their experiences, behaviors, and identities. Sexual identity formation in particular is understood as an interactive and continual process that occurs between the individual and his or her social environment (Horowitz & Newcomb, 2001). From this perspective, some children of LGBTQ parents may ultimately identify as LGBTQ because of shared genetic or biological influences, and/or social processes in their environment that permit gender nonconformity and/or same-sex exploration without fear of punishment or censure (Kuvalanka & Goldberg, 2009). Likewise, the unique familial environment of second generation youth may ultimately influence their coming out processes, such that they may experience coming out as different (i.e., easier or harder) from some LGBTQ youth with heterosexual and gender conforming parents, because of their parents' sexual/gender identities (Kuvalanka & Goldberg, 2009).

According to a social constructionist framework, interpretations are necessarily shaped by individuals' everyday interactions with peers, family members, and others in our immediate social context. Further, the broader historical, cultural, and ideological contexts, and the meanings and ideologies that are dominant within these contexts, also have significant influence in this regard (Crotty, 1998; Schwandt, 2000). Therefore, in understanding how second generation youth develop and make sense of their sexual and/or gender identities, we must consider the dominant—and possibly conflicting—ideologies and institutions that shape their experiences. For example, the dominant cultural narrative is that heterosexuality and gender conformity is privileged in society, affording heterosexual and gender conforming individuals symbolic and practical benefits, such as greater relationship recognition and support at both interpersonal and institutional levels (Oswald et al., 2005). Second generation youth may internalize this narrative, as they may have perceived and experienced discrimination based on their parents' and their own sexual orientation and/or gender identities. At the same time, they may construct alternative, resistant narratives about sexual orientation and gender identity, insomuch as their parents may have served as positive nonheterosexual and/or gender nonconforming role models. Thus, a social constructionist perspective facilitates theorizing of the ways in which both society and family have an influence on how second generation youth subjectively construct and make meaning of their LGBTQ identities. For example, according to a social constructionist perspective, whether/how parents share expectations for their children's eventual sexual and gender identities, parents' own level of internalized homophobia, and the societal narrative that "gay parents raise gay kids" are all hypothesized to have an influence on the child's ease of identity formation.

What Do We Know About the Second Generation?

The experiences of second generation individuals have been highlighted in newspaper articles (e.g., Kirby, 1998) and queer anthologies (Epstein, 2009; Howey & Samuels, 2000; Sonnie, 2000). Some empirical research has also been conducted (Garner, 2004; Kuvalanka & Goldberg, 2009). Prior to describing some of these diverse sources, I will provide a brief overview of the literature on the gender development and sexual orientation of children with LGBTQ parents in general, as it provides a foundation for inquiry into the experiences of second generation youth. The literature suggests that in many ways, the gender and sexuality development of children from nonheterosexual-parent families appears to unfold similarly

to that of children of heterosexual parents, but that in some ways, their development may be uniquely shaped by having LGBTQ parents. The limitations of this literature, however, should be kept in mind, in that it has focused primarily on White, well-educated, lesbian-parent families.

Gender Development of Children with LGBTQ Parents

Parental sexual orientation has not proven to be an effective indicator of successful child development, as studies comparing children with LGBTQ parents and those raised by heterosexual parents have revealed few differences in cognitive functioning and school achievement, behavioral adjustment, and social and emotional development (see Biblarz & Savci, 2010). Researchers have generally explored two aspects of gender development among children with LGBTQ parents: gender identity and gendered role behavior. *Gender identity* concerns self-identification as female or male, and *gendered roles* refers to those behaviors and attitudes that are regarded by a particular culture as appropriately female or male (Bem, 1974). Assessment of gendered role behavior to determine whether or not children are developing satisfactorily assumes there are behaviors and roles that are appropriate and "normal" for females and males, and, therefore, affirms and reinforces gender-role stereotypes (Fitzgerald, 1999). Nevertheless, studies document no differences regarding gender identification between children of lesbian parents and children of heterosexual parents (Golombok, Spencer, & Rutter, 1983; Gottman, 1990; Green, Mandel, Hotvedt, Gray, & Smith, 1986) and have found "appropriate" displays of gendered behaviors/attitudes among children of lesbian parents (Brewaeys, Ponjaert, Hall, & Golombok, 1997; Golombok et al., 2003; Gottman, 1990; MacCallum & Golombok, 2004). A few studies, however, have found some group differences in gendered role behavior and attitudes; for example, Green et al. (1986) reported that girls of lesbian mothers were more likely to prefer some boy-typical activities (e.g., playing with trucks) and to aspire to male-typed careers (e.g., engineer, astronaut) compared to daughters of heterosexual mothers. Children of lesbian mothers have also been found to hold less traditional gendered role attitudes than children of heterosexual parents, while lesbian mothers have also reported more liberal attitudes about gender than heterosexual parents (Sutfin, Fulcher, Bowles, & Patterson, 2008).

Sexual Orientation of Children with LGBTQ Parents

Some studies that have explored sexual orientation identification of children with LGBTQ parents have done so seemingly in the interest of determining whether these children are more likely to identify as nonheterosexual than children of heterosexual parents. This line of inquiry seems to suggest that it is "bad" if children turn out to be nonheterosexual (Fitzgerald, 1999); indeed, according to the heteronormative cultural ideal, healthy (i.e., "normal") sexuality development is equated with heterosexuality (Oswald et al., 2005). Nevertheless, until studies utilizing large, representative samples are conducted, the question of whether children of LGBTQ parents are more likely to identify as LGBTQ than children of heterosexual and gender conforming parents will remain unanswered. The existing research, however, suggests that the vast majority of youth and adults with LGBTQ parents identify as heterosexual and/or demonstrate no differences from youth and adults with heterosexual parents in regard to experiences of same-sex attraction (Bailey et al., 1995; Gottman, 1990; Tasker & Golombok, 1997; Wainright, Russell, & Patterson, 2004).

One study, however, did reveal complex findings regarding the sexual orientation of children of lesbian parents. Tasker and Golombok (1997) compared 25 young adults with lesbian mothers with 21 young adults with heterosexual mothers. Findings revealed no significant differences between groups with respect to sexual identity or experiences of same-sex sexual attraction. However, young adults from lesbian families were more likely to have considered the possibility of having a same-sex relationship and to have actually been involved in a same-sex relationship. Tasker and Golombok suggested that having a lesbian mother appeared to broaden young adults' views about their potential sexual relationships (i.e., they were open to the possibility of entering into a same-sex relationship). Indeed, Goldberg (2007) reported in her study of 42 adults with lesbian, gay, and bisexual (LGB) parents that some participants felt that growing up with a nonheterosexual parent led them to develop "less rigid and more flexible notions and ideas about sexuality" (p. 557).

Three studies (Cohen & Kuvalanka, 2011; Gabb, 2004; Mitchell, 1998) examined what lesbian mothers aimed to teach their children about sexuality-related topics, and found that many of the lesbian mothers reported that they intentionally sought to teach diverse notions of sexuality, so that their children would know that there are options beyond heterosexuality. Notably, these findings seem to be distinct from much of the research on heterosexual parents (Heisler, 2005; Martin, 2009). For example, Martin (2009) explored how heterosexuality was reproduced and normalized by 600 mothers (all of whom identified as heterosexual, except for two who identified as bisexual) with very young children. Martin found that most of the mothers in her study assumed their children to be heterosexual, described adult and romantic relationships to children as exclusively heterosexual, and did not discuss with their children the existence of nonheterosexual sexual orientations. LGBTQ parents' experiences of having nonheterosexual and/or gender nonconforming identities may influence their intentions to teach their children more diverse notions of sexual orientation. Further, LGBTQ parents who have experienced stigmatization in relation to their LGBTQ identities may want their children to learn about sexual orientation in a different, more positive and accepting way, devoid of shame and stigma (Mitchell, 1998).

A handful of studies have investigated LGBTQ parents' preferences for their children's sexual orientations and have found that these parents have diverse perspectives in this regard (e.g., Costello, 1997; Gartrell et al., 2000; Javaid, 1993). Javaid (1993) asked lesbian and heterosexual mothers about their attitudes regarding their children's sexual behavior and life choices. Seven out of 13 lesbian mothers expressed "an acceptance of, but not preference for, homosexual behavior in their children" (Javaid, 1993, p. 241), while three reported homosexuality to be more acceptable for their daughters than their sons, and three preferred that their children be heterosexual. Notably, all of the heterosexual mothers in Javaid's study reported that they preferred their children to be heterosexual and that they would be "disappointed" (p. 241) if their children identified as nonheterosexual. All of the 18 LGB parents interviewed by Costello (1997) said they would accept their children's eventual sexual orientation identities regardless of what they might be, while 4 went on to state a preference for their children to be nonheterosexual, and 4 preferred that their children identify as heterosexual. Those who preferred heterosexuality for their children discussed the societal discrimination that nonheterosexual individuals face.

It seems that LGBTQ parents' experiences as sexual minorities in a society that privileges heterosexuality influence their hopes and fears for their children in regard to sexual orientation. In line with a social constructionist perspective, some LGBTQ parents may create familial environments that are in some ways different from, as well as similar to, the familial environments provided by some heterosexual parents. Sexual minority parents may be more cognizant of the potential for their children to eventually assume a sexual orientation identity other than heterosexual. As in heterosexual-parent families, LGBTQ parents' feelings about this possibility may have implications for their children's own sexual orientation development. Children with LGBTQ parents may internalize their parents' openness to—or possibly anxiety about—the children's anticipated sexual orientation identities (Kuvalanka & Goldberg, 2009).

But what happens when the child of a LGBTQ parent actually does come to identify as nonheterosexual or gender nonconforming? In her self-reflective commentary, Mooney-Somers (2006), a psychology researcher and second generation lesbian daughter of a gay father, asserts that there are ways in which the experiences of the second generation may be sufficiently different from those of the first generation, warranting empirical research on this population.

Defining the Second Generation

The term "second generation" was coined in the early 1990s by Dan Cherubin, a gay man with a lesbian mother (Kirby, 1998). In his coming out about his own and his mother's sexual orientation identities, he encountered negative reactions from others, including lesbian and gay parents themselves (Garner, 2004). For example, when Cherubin marched in a gay pride parade holding a sign that read "Gay Son of Gay Moms," he encountered negative, seemingly homophobic expressions on the faces of LGBTQ parents (Garner, 2004, p. 176). Apparently, Cherubin embodied the opposite of what LGBTQ parents were trying to portray at that time: that LGBTQ parents raised "normal" children—and "normal" meant "heterosexual" (Garner, 2004). Indeed, when Cherubin served on an educational panel about LGBTQ families, a lesbian mother and co-panelist, who had fought for custody of her two young children, said to him: "Nothing personal, Dan, but you're my worst nightmare" (Kirby, 1998, p. 2). As a result of his experiences, Cherubin created an organization for LGBTQ youth and adults with LGBTQ parents and named it "Second Generation." Soon afterwards, he partnered with COLAGE, a national organization run by and for individuals with one or more LGBTQ parents, to expand the network of support for "second gen-ners" (COLAGE, 2010).

Cherubin's and others' experiences as second generation LGBTQ youth are shared in the groundbreaking book by writer and queer family activist Abigail Garner (2004), *Families Like Mine: Children of Gay Parents Tell It Like It Is*. During the course of conducting research for her book, Garner interviewed more than 50 young adults with LGBTQ parents, some of whom also identified as LGBTQ. In her chapter titled

"Second Generation: Queer Kids of LGBT Parents," Garner highlights the diversity of experiences among this group:

> Although "second generation" is an umbrella term for all LGBT kids with LGBT parents, there is no definitive second generation family experience that represents them all …. A lesbian daughter of politically active lesbian mothers, for example, will have a different second generation experience than a daughter raised by a closeted gay dad. (p. 179)

Thus, the term "second generation" refers to all nonheterosexual and/or gender nonconforming individuals with one or more nonheterosexual and/or gender nonconforming parent—the experiences of whom are just beginning to be acknowledged and understood.

Identifying Advantages and Challenges for Second Generation Youth

As stated, empirical literature on this population is scarce but emerging. Kuvalanka and Goldberg (2009), in the first in-depth study of second generation individuals that has been reported in the social science literature, examined the experiences of 18 LGBTQ young adults with lesbian and bisexual mothers. Many of Kuvalanka and Goldberg's (2009) findings echoed and extended those of Garner (2004), lending credence to her pioneering discussion of the diverse experiences of the second generation. Kuvalanka and Goldberg's study was a secondary data analysis, based upon data drawn from two separate qualitative research projects that the authors had each previously conducted. A total of 78 young adults with LGB parents were recruited, 21 of whom happened to identify as LGBTQ by adulthood.[2]

Subsequently, 18 of the 21 second generation participants (ages 18–35 years; $M = 23.2$ years) were deemed eligible for inclusion in the secondary data analysis.[3] Regarding gender, 11 participants identified as female, three as male, three as genderqueer, and one as "gender ambiguous." Regarding sexual orientation, seven participants identified as bisexual, five as queer, three as gay, one as lesbian, one as "mildly bisexual," and one as a "tranny-dyke." Seventeen participants had lesbian mothers and two had bisexual mothers (1 participant had one lesbian and one bisexual mother).

Potential Advantages for Second Generation Youth

Both Garner's (2004) and Kuvalanka and Goldberg's (2009) research revealed that having nonheterosexual parents when one identifies as LGBTQ may be potentially beneficial, in that some participants felt they had a less arduous coming out process than they might have had if they had heterosexual parents. For example, some of Kuvalanka and Goldberg's participants said that they were able to discover their own nonheterosexual or gender nonconforming identities sooner, in that having a nonheterosexual parent allowed them to explore and question their sexual/gender identities at a younger age than other youth, which facilitated their own self-discovery. More generally, participants from both studies believed that having LGBTQ parents had given them broader conceptualizations of the potential sexual or gender identity options available to them, including those that go beyond the traditional binaries of gay/straight and female/male. Furthermore, many of them also did not worry about rejection upon disclosure of their identities to their LGBTQ parents. As Charlie, a gay man with a lesbian mother, explained: "I didn't have that added fear of rejection from my mother,

---

[2] These were convenience samples; thus, the relatively high proportion of LGBTQ-identified participants could be attributed to the method of recruitment and the focus of the studies. For example, second generation individuals may be especially inclined to be members of COLAGE, an advocacy organization for children of LGBTQ parents, and to participate in studies that investigate the experiences of LGBTQ-parent families, as they may be interested from multiple perspectives: children of LGBTQ parents and as possible future LGBTQ parents themselves.

[3] Three participants from Goldberg's original study were not included, because (a) after reading through transcripts, it was determined that one participant had participated in both researchers' studies and (b) two participants in Goldberg's subset were considerably older than the rest of the participants (48 and 50 years old; 13 years older than the next oldest participant).

because no matter what, it was always like, there's no way she can reject me" (Kuvalanka & Goldberg, 2009, p. 912).

Perhaps, then, for some second generation individuals, their parents' identification, support, and acceptance may neutralize society's powerful homonegative messages and serve to foster greater self-acceptance and self-esteem. Indeed, for some participants, their uniquely supportive and affirmative familial environments led them to construct their own emergent identities as normal and acceptable (Garner, 2004; Kuvalanka & Goldberg, 2009). Further, some of Garner's interviewees felt they benefited from having a strong connection to the LGBTQ community from a young age, and from having a deep understanding of LGBTQ history and culture. Garner posited that it is beneficial for second generation individuals to grow up with "out" and "proud" parents, who can serve as positive role models, thus lessening the development of internalized homophobia among these youth: "LGBT parents … have the opportunity to pass on a priceless gift to their second generation children: pride in discovering their authentic selves" (p. 192).

Potential Challenges for Second Generation Youth

Several participants in both Garner's (2004) and Kuvalanka and Goldberg's (2009) research discussed the unique challenges they faced as second generation youth. For example, some participants said they felt pressure from their LGBTQ parents and others to be heterosexual and gender conforming, and some delayed coming out as LGBTQ due to fears of fulfilling critics' assertions that "gay parents raise gay kids." David, who identified as bisexual, shared how this stereotype affected his sexual identity formation: "I do feel to some extent I didn't want to be gay because that just proves the stereotype true that gay parents will raise a gay child and shouldn't be allowed to have children" (Kuvalanka & Goldberg, 2009, p. 911). In relation to this, some participants also expressed annoyance and feelings of disempowerment as a result of the commonplace assumption that their sexual or gender identities were necessarily related to their

parents' sexual orientations. Amy, who identified as queer, revealed:

> That's something that's really been pushed on me—like, "You're like this because of your mom," which feels, like, really disempowering in a lot of ways. And I think that is probably the thing that has hurt the most … just this feeling of like, my claim to my identity is being taken away. (Kuvalanka & Goldberg, 2009, p. 911)

Other participants in the Kuvalanka and Goldberg (2009) study reported that they initially did not want to be LGBTQ, or that they had specific concerns related to their own sexual/gender identities, after witnessing the prejudice and discrimination that their parents had endured. For example, Tom, who identified as gay, had grown up hearing his heterosexual father and stepmother make homophobic comments about his lesbian mother, which in turn made Tom wary of coming out to them. Thus, second generation youth are inevitably confronted with the heterosexism their parents have faced (Mooney-Somers, 2006), and some, if not most, understand they may face similar struggles, which may cause ambivalence or fear about coming out to family, friends, and society. These experiences reveal that having a LGBTQ parent is not guaranteed protection against the influence of societal heteronormativity.

Interestingly, Kuvalanka and Goldberg (2009) reported that several of their participants said they did not turn to their lesbian/bisexual mothers for support during their sexual and gender identity formation. In particular, sons of lesbian/bisexual mothers tended to look elsewhere for support. In addition to the obvious gender difference between mothers and sons, sons may also be hesitant to discuss their emerging sexualities with their mothers because of their perception that aspects of gay male culture (e.g., pornography) may clash with their mothers' (lesbian feminist) political sensibilities (Jensen, 2004). Furthermore, it seemed that some mothers' internalized homophobia and shame may have inhibited open discussions about sexual identities, which likely contributed to some participants' lack of comfort. Additionally, a "queer generation gap" (Garner, 2004, p. 181) stemming from differences in social norms and experiences between the first and second generations also seemed to play a role. For example, some LGBTQ children and LGBTQ parents disagreed about how "out" to be in their communities, and also utilized different language (e.g., *queer* as opposed to *lesbian* or *gay*) to describe their own identities.

Lastly, participants in both Garner's (2004) and Kuvalanka and Goldberg's (2009) research discussed their disappointment upon disclosing their LGBTQ identities to their LGBTQ parents, especially when parents remained somewhat closeted themselves in regard to their own identities. Some LGBTQ parents voiced their fears about potential heterosexist discrimination their children might face or worried that others would "blame" them for their children's LGBTQ identity. Some of the gender variant (i.e., genderqueer, gender ambiguous) participants in Kuvalanka and Goldberg's study especially seemed unhappy with their mothers' reactions to their disclosures, as it seemed the mothers had difficulty comprehending gender variant identities. Thus, gender nonconforming second generation youth may face certain challenges and obstacles in that their gender identities may be stigmatized or misunderstood in the larger societal context (Wyss, 2004) and also, perhaps, within their own families.

Broadening and Deepening Our Understanding of Second Generation Youth

To further examine the experiences and perspectives of second generation individuals through the first empirical study focused solely on this population, I aimed to recruit a larger and more diverse sample than in Kuvalanka and Goldberg's (2009) secondary data analysis. Thirty second generation participants (ages 18–35 years; $M = 25.5$) were recruited via the COLAGE Second Generation listserv, as well as through LGBTQ offices on college/university campuses across the country. Although I sought to answer many questions in this study, in this chapter, I only focus on two: "Who are second generation youth?" and "What do they want us to know about them?"

A description of the study sample deepens what has been previously documented in regard to who second generation individuals are. Similar to the sample in Kuvalanka and Goldberg's (2009) secondary data analysis, the majority of participants ($n = 21$) identified as White, although 4 identified as bi- or multiracial (Native, Chicano, and White; Black/Native American and White; Black and White; African-American and White), 3 as White-Jewish, and 2 as Black/African-American. The majority of participants ($n = 17$) identified as female and 5 identified as male; however, the larger sample size allowed for a greater range of gender identifications, in that 8 participants utilized self-gender labels that fell outside the female/male binary (e.g., "transgenderqueer-fluid;" "male-bodied/genderqueer"). In terms of sexual orientation, the most common self-identification label was queer ($n = 16$), while 5 participants identified as gay, 3 as bisexual, 2 as lesbian, and 4 used "unique" labels, such as "gay-queer-homo" and "queer questioning." The majority of participants ($n = 21$) had one or more lesbian mothers, while 2 reported having a mother who was a "butch-dyke," and 1 participant had a mother described as "queer/gay." In addition, 3 participants had bisexual fathers, 1 had a gay father, 1 had a "female-to-male (FTM) transsexual" parent, and 1 had a "male-to-female transgender" parent. Finally, 11 participants grew up in the Northeast, 7 in the West, 7 in the South, and 5 in the Midwest. This sample begins to illustrate the diversity that exists among second generation individuals in regard to race and ethnicity, gender identity, sexual orientation, parent–child gender and sexual orientation identity combinations, and geographic locale.

This variation that exists in regard to social location undoubtedly contributes to a diverse range of experiences among the second generation—a point made by several participants when answering the question, "What do you want others to know about second generation youth?" One theme that emerged from the interview data was the notion that the second generation is a diverse group, such that no single participant could represent all second generation individuals. Many participants gave voice to this; it is not difficult to imagine that Maya, a White, queer woman who grew up on the West Coast with her bisexual and lesbian mothers, had a somewhat different second generation experience than Chris, a White, queer FTM transgender man who grew up with a straight FTM transsexual parent in the Midwest. For example, both Maya and Chris discussed how their parents played a role in their gender and sexual identity development and had very different perspectives in this regard. Maya felt that as a result of growing up with nonheterosexual mothers, it was more "natural" for her to also be with women. Maya explained:

In developing my own identity and reflecting on where I came from, it [having lesbian/bisexual mothers] definitely plays a part in it … . Growing up with so many women around me felt safe … . So, it seems only natural that being with a woman, and being in a women's community, feels safer. It feels, um, familiar. And … it certainly plays a part in my identity.

Chris, on the other hand, said he did not learn about being transgender or being non-heterosexual from his FTM transsexual father (i.e., his "egg" father), who identifies as heterosexual and is married to a woman. According to Chris,

I learned that gender was you were either a man or a woman, because it seemed like my egg father's transition was so fast that it was you're either male or female, and that's what was acceptable … .When it comes to sexual orientation, (it was) not ever talked about … .For the longest time I hated myself. I thought, why would god make a person that looks one way but feels another way, and whose sexual orientation is apparently an abomination? Why would he do that?

Maya and Chris provide just one of a myriad of examples of how experiences related to gender and sexual identity development can differ between members of the second generation—and many participants were aware of these variations. Jay, a White gay man, who grew up in the Northeast with a lesbian mother and her partner, explained,

A big thing that I would want people to know is that everyone's story is unique to those people, and what I'm saying to you now will likely be different from the other participants in your study. And I wouldn't ever want people to generalize based on my life story.

A second theme that emerged was the desire to have others realize and acknowledge that second generation individuals exist and deserve respect. For example, Jessica, a White lesbian woman who grew up with lesbian mothers in the Northeast, asserted: "We are here, and we're not going anywhere. We're part of the fabric of queer culture, we're a part of the fabric of American culture, and we're part of this world just as much as anyone else." Some of these participants felt that studies such as the one they were participating in could benefit other second generation youth who do not know other LGBTQ youth with LGBTQ parents, as well as all people who may grow to be more aware and accepting of LGBTQ-parent families. Tina, a White bisexual woman who grew up in the Midwest with a gay mother, explained how she, even now as an adult, knows few other second generation individuals and LGBTQ-parent families:

I've met a couple of different people, but like here in (my Midwestern state), I don't really know a whole lot of people my age. You know I know people who have younger children, but I don't know anybody my age, and you know people don't walk around and say, "Oh, hey guess what? My dad's gay." Or "My mom's a lesbian" … .You know, it's not usually advertised … .So, I think just the fact that someone's doing a study like this, you know, just to put it out there, whether it ends up in some book somewhere and some high school kid reads it or whatever, I think that's awesome—and, really, any information that's put out there publicly for people.

A final theme, voiced by several participants, was the desire for others to know that "Our queer parents did not cause us to be queer." These participants were concerned about and resisted this assumption. Interestingly, the vast majority of participants discussed the influence that having LGBTQ parents had on them; however, for most, this influence fell short of actually *causing* their "queerness." For example, Kelly, a White, queer woman who grew up with a queer dad in the Northeast, stated:

People are only influenced by their families up to a certain point. Our sexual orientation, sexuality, and gender identity and expression—while we may learn many things from our parents … we have our own experiences, and we are growing up in another time than when our parents did. It [our sexual orientation or gender identity] is not a prescribed path, and it's probably more complicated than many people think.

These complexities that influence gender and sexual orientation identity development are yet to be fully explored and understood. Examining the experiences of second generation individuals may provide greater insight into familial factors that influence all youth's gender and sexual socialization. Listening to what members of the second generation want others to know about them provides a solid base from which to begin future systematic study of this population.

Next Steps: What Might We Learn from Further Study of the Second Generation?

Researchers have just begun to explore the experiences of second generation individuals; thus, we still have much to learn from further study of this population. Social constructionism, as previously discussed, has been used to frame these initial investigations and could be useful for further inquiry. For example, a social constructionist perspective might lead one to ask: What factors and processes facilitate and/or impede the second generation's formation of their LGBTQ identities? More specifically, researchers could aim to better understand, describe, and explain how the sexual and gender identity development of LGBTQ youth is influenced by having LGBTQ parents in a heteronormative society. How does, for example, the presence of LGBTQ siblings and other extended family members, as well as affirming or rejecting attitudes from heterosexual and gender-conforming family and community members, play a role in the lives of these youth? Perhaps if heterosexuality is the "minority" identity in one's family or community, LGBTQ individuals would be able to negate the impact of societal homo- and trans-negativity.

Other theoretical perspectives, such as intersectionality (Anderson & McCormack, 2010), would be useful for examining the experiences of LGBTQ individuals with LGBTQ parents. An intersectionality perspective acknowledges the material ways in which people experience their multiple, socially constructed identities (Crawley, Foley, & Shehan, 2008). Thus, individuals' social locations pertaining to race, ethnicity, and social class—in addition to their nonheterosexual or gender nonconforming identities—are thought to be critical to understanding the full range of experiences of the second generation. This perspective would lead one to ask: How do race, ethnicity, and social class shape queer identity formation (Boykin, 2005) among second generation youth? How do second generation individuals navigate cultural differences in this regard? For example, one African-American female participant in my research reported using the sexual orientation self-identity label of "bisexual" when in the presence of other African-Americans and "queer" when talking with Caucasians. Further, consideration of the ramifications of multiple oppressions is a central tenet of intersectionality (Crawley et al., 2008). Thus, how do ethnic and racial minority families with second generation youth view and cope with racism in addition to, or in conjunction with, heteronormativity? What role does poverty play in the lives of second generation youth? Do economically poor second generation youth and their families have access to queer-supportive resources, such as Gay-Straight Alliances in schools, as well as all that the Internet has to offer, such as basic LGBTQ information and online support groups? Very little is known about LGBTQ people and families of lower socioeconomic status in general—and second generation youth and their families are no exception.

A life course perspective (Bengtson & Allen, 1993) might also be useful for future study of the second generation. This perspective highlights the importance of interpreting second generation individuals' experiences as linked to the lives of others who are close to them and in the context of historical time (Elder & Shanahan, 2006). A factor to be explored is the influence of the timing of parental coming out on children's sexual and gender identity formation and their experience of being a part of the LGBTQ community. Although it might be assumed that most LGBTQ parents serve as life-long LGBTQ role models for their children, a parent's disclosure of a nonheterosexual and/or gender nonconforming identity might happen later in life—perhaps during a child's questioning of her/his own identity, or even after a child has already come out as LGBTQ. Thus, when a parent comes out is likely to have an influence on second generation youth's exposure to queer identities and communities and, subsequently, on their LGBTQ identity formation (Goldberg, Kinkler, Richardson, & Downing, 2012). For example, having "out and proud" parents from a young age might encourage second generation youth to more readily accept their own queer identities. Having parents come out during their children's adolescence, when these youth may be questioning their own identities and also trying to establish independence from their parents, could perhaps cause some youth to postpone their own LGBTQ identity formation. Further, exploration into the "queer generation gap" as discussed by Garner (2004) could also be pursued. For example, second generation participants have stated that coming out—and being out—is very different now as compared to when their parents were young (Kuvalanka & Goldberg, 2009). How does this generation gap play a role in the first generation's role modeling and provision of support to the second generation? And does the gap remain, widen, or close throughout the life course? Thus, examination of relationships between the first and second (and third, fourth, etc.) generations may reveal intriguing changes over time.

Conclusion

Answers to the questions raised above would provide greater knowledge regarding the variation in experiences among the second generation. Subsequently, family practitioners might gain the necessary tools to better support *all* LGBTQ youth and their families—including heterosexual-parent families. Perhaps, then, a better understanding of *how* these parents provided acceptance, understanding, and broad conceptu-

alizations of gender and sexual orientation would help all parents better support their children. Based upon our findings that not all participants viewed their LGBTQ parents as sources of support (and, thus, being LGBTQ was not a "prerequisite" for parental support), it seems that there are supportive behaviors that all parents can embody (Kuvalanka & Goldberg, 2009).

In conclusion, despite the various factors that likely contribute to the diversity of experiences and perspectives among the second generation, several participants in my most recent study acknowledged that living in a heteronormative society with one or more LGBTQ parents is a commonality that they all shared. And, as one participant posited, this commonality has the potential to provide both unique benefits and challenges to all second generation youth:

> I think that our experience growing up and existing in the world is that much richer … and more difficult as well … . It's outside of the norm and outside of people's expectations and, in some cases, outside of what people find acceptable.

As scholars, we have a role to play in moving the conversation about second generation youth beyond the simplistic—and, often, homophobic—debate about whether or not "gay parents raise gay kids." Indeed, we have a responsibility to articulate the richness and diversity in experiences among this population with the aim of learning more about the second generation and their families, to improve understanding and, ideally, acceptance of all families.

References

Anderson, E., & McCormack, M. (2010). Intersectionality, critical race theory, and American sporting oppression: Examining Black and gay male athletes. *Journal of Homosexuality, 57*, 949–967. doi:10.1080/0091836 9.2010.503502

Bailey, J. M., Bobrow, D., Wolfe, M., & Mikach, S. (1995). Sexual orientation of adult sons of gay fathers. *Developmental Psychology, 31*, 124–129.

Bem, S. L. (1974). The measurement of psychological androgyny. *Journal of Consulting and Clinical Psychology, 42*, 155–162.

Bengtson, V. L., & Allen, K. R. (1993). The life course perspective applied to families over time. In P. G. Boss, W. J. Doherty, R. LaRossa, W. R. Schumm, &

S. K. Steinmetz (Eds.), *Sourcebook of family theories and methods: A contextual approach* (pp. 469–499). New York, NY: Plenum.

Biblarz, T. J., & Savci, E. (2010). Lesbian, gay, bisexual, and transgender families. *Journal of Marriage and Family, 72*, 480–497. doi:10.1111/j.1741-3737. 2010.00714.x

Boykin, K. (2005). *Beyond the down low; Sex, lies, and denial in Black America*. New York, NY: Carroll & Graf.

Brewaeys, A., Ponjaert, I., Hall, E. V., & Golombok, S. (1997). Donor insemination: Child development and family functioning in lesbian mother families. *Human Reproduction, 12*, 1349–1359. doi:10.1093/humrep/12.6.1349

Cohen, R., & Kuvalanka, K. A. (2011). Sexual socialization in Lesbian-Parent Families: An exploratory analysis. *American Journal of Orthopsychiatry, 81*, 293–305. doi:10.1111/j.1939-0025.2011.01098.x

COLAGE. (2010). 2nd Gen: FAQ. Retrieved from http://www.colage.org/programs/2ndgen/faq.htm

Costello, C. Y. (1997). Conceiving identity: Bisexual, lesbian, and gay parents consider their children's sexual orientations. *Journal of Sociology and Social Welfare, 24*(3), 63–89.

Crawley, S. L., Foley, L. J., & Shehan, C. L. (2008). *Gendering bodies*. Lanham, MD: Rowman & Littlefield.

Crotty, M. (1998). *The foundations of social research: Meaning and perspective in the research process*. London, England: Sage.

Dunne, G. (2000). Opting into motherhood: Lesbians blurring the boundaries and transforming the meaning of parenthood and kinship. *Gender and Society, 14*, 11–35.

Elder, G. H., Jr., & Shanahan, M. J. (2006). The life course and human development. In R. E. Lerner (Ed.), *Theoretical models of human development* (*The handbook of child psychology*, 6th ed., Vol. 1, pp. 665–715). New York, NY: Wiley.

Epstein, R. (Ed.). (2009). *Who's your daddy?: And other writings on queer parenting*. Toronto, ON: Sumac.

Fitzgerald, B. (1999). Children of lesbian and gay parents: A review of the literature. *Marriage and Family Review, 29*, 57–75.

Gabb, J. (2004). Sexuality education: How children of lesbian mothers 'learn' about sex/uality. *Sex Education, 4*(1), 19–34. doi:10.1080/1468181042000176515

Garner, A. (2004). *Families like mine: Children of gay parents tell it like it is*. New York, NY: Harper Collins.

Gartrell, N., Banks, A., Reed, N., Hamilton, J., Rodas, C., & Deck, A. (2000). The national lesbian family study: 3. Interviews with mothers of five-year-olds. *American Journal of Orthopsychiatry, 70*, 542–548. doi:10.1037/h0087823

Goldberg, A. E. (2007). Talking about family: Disclosure practices of adults raised by lesbian, gay, and bisexual parents. *Journal of Family Issues, 28*, 100–131. doi:10.1177/0192513X06293606

Goldberg, A. E., Kinkler, L. A., Richardson, H. B., & Downing, J. B. (2012). On the border: Young adults with LGBQ parents navigate LGBTQ communities. *Journal of Counseling Psychology, 59*, 71–85. doi:10.1037/a0024576

Golombok, S., Perry, B., Burston, A., Murray, C., Mooney-Somers, J., Stevens, M., & Golding, J. (2003). Children with lesbian parents: A community study. *Developmental Psychology, 39*, 20–33. doi:10.1037/0012-1649.39.1.20

Golombok, S., Spencer, A., & Rutter, M. (1983). Children in lesbian and single-parent households: Psychosexual and psychiatric appraisal. *Journal of Child Psychology and Psychiatry, 24*, 551–572. doi:10.1111/1469-7610.ep12366259

Gottman, J. S. (1990). Children of gay and lesbian parents. In F. W. Bozett & M. B. Sussman (Eds.), *Homosexuality and family relations* (pp. 177–196). New York, NY: Haworth Press.

Green, R., Mandel, J. B., Hotvedt, M. E., Gray, J., & Smith, L. (1986). Lesbian mothers and their children: A comparison with solo parent heterosexual mothers and their children. *Archives of Sexual Behavior, 15*, 167–184.

Heisler, J. M. (2005). Family communication about sex: Parents and college-aged offspring recall discussion topics, satisfaction, and parent involvement. *Journal of Family Communication, 5*, 295–312. doi:10.1207/s15327698jfc0504_4

Hines, M. (2004). *Brain gender*. New York, NY: Oxford University Press.

Horowitz, J. L., & Newcomb, M. D. (2001). A multidimensional approach to homosexual identity. *Journal of Homosexuality, 42*(2), 1–19. doi:10.1300/J082v42n02_01

Howey, N., & Samuels, E. J. (Eds.). (2000). *Out of the ordinary: Essays on growing up with gay, lesbian, and transgender parents*. New York, NY: St. Martin's Press.

Javaid, G. A. (1993). The children of homosexual and heterosexual single mothers. *Child Psychiatry and Human Development, 23*, 235–248.

Jensen, R. (2004). Homecoming: The relevance of radical feminism for gay men. *Journal of Homosexuality, 47*(3–4), 75–81. doi:10.1300/J082v47n03_05

Kirby, D. (1998, June 7). The second generation. *The New York Times*. Retrieved from http://query.nytimes.com/gst/fullpage.html?res=950CE1D91E3BF934A35755 C0A96E958260

Kitzinger, C. (1987). *The social construction of lesbianism*. London, England: Sage.

Kosciw, J. G., & Diaz, E. M. (2008). *Involved, invisible, ignored: The experiences of lesbian, gay, bisexual, and transgender parents and their children in our nation's K-12 schools*. New York, NY: GLSEN.

Kuvalanka, K., & Goldberg, A. (2009). "Second generation" voices: Queer youth with lesbian/bisexual mothers. *Journal of Youth and Adolescence, 38*, 904–919. doi:10.1007/s10964-008-9327-2

MacCallum, F., & Golombok, S. (2004). Children raised in fatherless families from infancy: A follow-up of children of lesbian and single heterosexual mothers at early adolescence. *Journal of Child Psychology and Psychiatry, 45,* 1407–1419. doi:10.1111/j.1469-7610.2004.00847.x

Martin, K. A. (2009). Normalizing heterosexuality: Mothers' assumptions, talk, and strategies with young children. *American Sociological Review, 74,* 190–207. doi:10.1177/000312240907400202

Mitchell, V. (1998). The birds, the bees…and the sperm banks: How lesbian mothers talk with their children about sex and reproduction. *American Journal of Orthopsychiatry, 68,* 400–409. doi:10.1037/h0080349

Mooney-Somers, J. (2006). What might the voices of the second generation tell us? *Lesbian & Gay Psychology Review, 7,* 66–69.

Morrow, D. F. (2004). Social work practice with gay, lesbian, bisexual, and transgender adolescents. *Families in Society, 85,* 91–99.

National Gay and Lesbian Task Force. (2011, April). *Anti-adoption laws in the U.S.* Retrieved from http://www.thetaskforce.org/reports_and_research/adoption_laws

Oswald, R. F., Blume, L. B., & Marks, S. (2005). Decentering heteronormativity: A model for family studies. In V. L. Bengtson, A. C. Acock, K. R. Allen, P. Dilworth-Anderson, & D. M. Klein (Eds.), *Sourcebook of family theory & research* (pp. 143–154). Thousand Oaks, CA: Sage.

Savin-Williams, R. C. (1996). Self-labeling and disclosure among gay, lesbian, and bisexual youths. In J. Laird & R. J. Green (Eds.), *Lesbians and gays in couples and families* (pp. 153–182). San Francisco, CA: Jossey-Bass.

Schwandt, T. (2000). Three epistemological stances for qualitative inquiry: Interpretivism, hermeneutics, and social constructionism. In N. K. Denzin & Y. S. Lincoln (Eds.), *Handbook of qualitative research* (2nd ed., pp. 189–214). Thousand Oaks, CA: Sage.

Sonnie, A. (Ed.). (2000). *Revolutionary voices: A multicultural queer youth anthology.* Los Angeles, CA: Alyson.

Stacey, J., & Biblarz, T. (2001). (How) does the sexual orientation of parents matter? *American Sociological Review, 66,* 159–183.

Sutfin, E. L., Fulcher, M., Bowles, R. P., & Patterson, C. J. (2008). How lesbian and heterosexual parents convey attitudes about gender to their children: The role of gendered environments. *Sex Roles, 58,* 501–513. doi:10.1007/s11199-007-9368-0

Tasker, F. L., & Golombok, S. (1997). *Growing up in a lesbian family: Effects on child development.* London, England: Guilford Press.

Wainright, J. L., Russell, S. T., & Patterson, C. J. (2004). Psychosocial adjustment, school outcomes, and romantic relationships of adolescents with same-sex parents. *Child Development, 75,* 1886–1898. doi:10.1111/j.1467-8624.2004.00823.x

Williams, T., Connolly, J., Pepler, D., & Craig, W. (2005). Peer victimization, social support, and psychological adjustment of sexual minority adolescents. *Journal of Youth and Adolescence, 34,* 471–482. doi:10.1007/s10964-005-7264-x

Wyss, S. E. (2004). 'This was my hell': The violence experiences by gender non-conforming youth in U.S. high schools. *International Journal of Qualitative Studies in Education, 17,* 709–730. doi:10.1080/0951839042000253676

Nancy A. Orel and Christine A. Fruhauf

Lesbian, Gay, Bisexual, and Transgender Grandparents

The most significant demographic trend during the past decade has been the "graying of America" (Shrestha & Heisler, 2011). The accelerated pace of the population aging is evident with the actuality that beginning January 1, 2011 approximately 10,000 Baby Boomers (i.e., those born between the years 1946 and 1964) will turn age 65 each day. Not only will there be a tremendous growth in the number of individuals who obtain "senior" status, but life expectancy has risen from 69.7 years in 1960 to 77.8 years in 2006 (Tootelian & Varshney, 2010). The dramatic increases in life expectancy has created a greater likelihood that individuals will be members of multigenerational families and that children will have extended relationships with their grandparents and possibly their great-grandparents. Because

N.A. Orel, Ph.D., L.P.C. (✉)
Gerontology Program, Department of Human Services, College of Health and Human Services, Bowling Green State University, 218 Health Center, Bowling Green, OH 43403-0148, USA
e-mail: norel@bgsu.edu

C.A. Fruhauf, Ph.D.
Department of Human Development and Family Studies, Colorado State University, 417 Behavioral Sciences Building, Campus 1570, Fort Collins, CO 80523-1570, USA
e-mail: Christine.Fruhauf@ColoState.edu

grandparenthood can begin well before age 65, with the average age of becoming a first time grandparent being 47, the majority of grandparents can expect to experience this family role for 30 or more years (Paul, 2002). Presently, 94% of older Americans with children are grandparents, and it is estimated that 50% of older adults with children will become great-grandparents (Smith & Drew, 2002). Further, it is estimated that 70 million people were grandparents in 2010 (U.S. News and World Report, 2011).

Historical and contemporary research has indicated that the grandparent–grandchild connection is of value, either directly or indirectly, for grandparents and grandchildren (Bengtson, 2001; Kemp, 2007; Kivett, 1991; Stelle, Fruhauf, Orel, & Landry-Meyer, 2010). The actual value derived from this relationship, however, will vary considerably depending on a multiplicity of factors that contribute to the quality and experience of the grandparent–grandchild relationship. Although researchers have empirically examined the grandparent–grandchild relationship for over 50 years, there has been a lack of attention given to understanding the diversity and contextual variation within this intergenerational relationship when grandparents self-identify as Lesbian, Gay, Bisexual, or Transgender (LGBT).

Accurate estimations of the current number of LGBT parents and grandparents are not available. However, using U.S. Census data, the Williams Institute estimated in 2011 that there are approximately nine million LGBT individuals in the USA, and same-sex couples were raising approximately 250,000 children under the age of 18 in 1999. Yet, these are conservative estimates (as many authors have previously discussed; Goldberg, 2010) given that LGBT individuals often do not lead openly lesbian, gay, or bisexual lives (Biblarz & Savci, 2010) and data are often miscounted (Gates & Cook, 2011). Optimistically, because the 2010 U.S. Census was the first time individuals were given the opportunity to report same-sex partners and same-sex spouses, more accurate and less conservative statistics will be available in the future about LGBT parenting and grandparenting. Additionally, with the increase in same-sex couples adopting children, finding surrogate mothers to bear children, and becoming pregnant through artificial insemination (Johnson & O'Connor, 2002), the number of same-sex parents is increasing (Goldberg, 2010). As a result, it is likely that the current and future aging LGBT population will experience grandparenthood in greater numbers than previous LGBT cohorts and, as a result, it is important to understand the grandparent–grandchild relationship within the context of LGBT families.

The purpose of this chapter is threefold. First, we provide a brief overview of a life course model on grandparent–grandchild relationships and the current literature on the grandparent–grandchild relationship. Second, we focus on areas where research is contributing to an emerging picture of the diversity of grandparent experiences within the grandparent–grandchild relationship, including the salience of sexual orientation to the grandparent role. Third, we present approaches and strategies that would enhance programs and services directed toward LGBT grandparents and grandchildren, as well as empower both LGBT grandparents and grandchildren. Lastly, we provide suggestions for further research.

Life Course Perspective on LGBT Grandparents' Relationship with Grandchildren

The life course perspective is a predominantly sociological perspective that focuses on familial relationships. The LGBT grandparent–grandchild relationship can best be elucidated from an application of major themes within a life course perspective on families (Bengtson & Allen, 1993; Elder, 2003). First, the temporal context refers to the appraisal of time as it is influenced by age within the relationship between the LGBT grandparent and grandchild, and can be viewed in three parts: ontogenetic, generational, and historical (Bengtson & Allen, 1993). Ontogenetic timing is the unique unfolding of each individual's development that is influenced by family unit changes, and LGBT grandparents may discover that they are apprehensive about being a grandparent because this role reminds them of their mortality. Generational timing is concerned with how individuals respond to the changing roles, role transitions, and role expectations that are placed on them in regard to their own generation within the family. An LGBT grandparent may welcome the role of being a mentor to a grandchild instead of being in the role of the parent. Historical timing refers to events within the broader social context and how these societal events influence individual development and relationship development. Today, LGBT grandparents may have greater ease in coming out to grandchildren than in prior years (Clunis, Fredriksen-Goldsen, Freeman, & Nystrom, 2005) when homosexuality was a forbidden topic as it was thought of as a mental illness, a crime, or threat to society (Kimmel, Rose, Orel, & Greene, 2006). An LGBT grandparent's personal history of disclosing her/his sexual orientation may also facilitate the process of coming out to her/his grandchildren (Fruhauf, Orel, & Jenkins, 2009).

Second, the social contexts between LGBT grandparents and their grandchildren include the social construction of meanings, cultural context, and the interplay of macro–micro levels of development. An exploration of the experiences of LGBT grandparents must take into consideration the similarities between the social construction of sexual orientation as a sexual minority status and the social construction of aging. Kimmel et al. (2006) indicate that both social categories are evaluated negatively, with flagrant acts of discrimination associated with them. Because it is possible to conceal sexual orientation and, even to some extent, chronological age, sexual orientation and age have similar social constructions. For example, within an ageist and heterosexist culture, the phrase (and former policy) "Don't ask, don't tell" is applicable and often applied to both older adults and LGBT persons by those who would prefer that *they* remain invisible. Yet, there are other structural statuses including race, class, gender, and (dis)ability that are not easily concealed and could complicate this issue even further (Institute of Medicine, 2011).

A third theme of the life course perspective, a diachronic perspective (Bengtson & Allen, 1993), involves the need to look at the dynamic aspects of roles and relationships and the examination of both continuity and change in the life course experience of LGBT grandparent–grandchild relationships. For example, LGBT grandparents may come out to their grandchildren when they determine that grandchildren are developmentally ready, or coming out to grandchildren may happen over a period of time. Conversely, LGBT grandparents may refrain from coming out to their grandchildren if adult children (parents) are disapproving of grandparents' sexual orientation or gender variance.

A fourth theme of the life course perspective that is important to understanding LGBT grandparenting is heterogeneity in structures and processes. This theme illustrates how individuals experience familial and societal relationships over time and proposes that the lives of one generation are linked to the lives of other generations. For example, a lesbian or bisexual grandmother may experience resiliency in the face of adversity, and as a result be able to show family members including grandchildren how to move forward during difficult times.

Historical Overview of Grandparenthood and the Grandparent–Grandchild Relationship

Prior to discussing the available literature on LGBT grandparents, it is imperative that a brief historical overview of grandparenthood and the grandparent–grandchild connection is presented

to illustrate the multidimensionality of the grandparent role and the diversity and contextual variation of intergenerational relationships. The majority of early conceptual articles on grandparenting presented grandmothers negatively and totally ignored grandfathers. For example, Abraham (1913/1955) labeled grandmothers in three generation families as "troublemakers," and Vollmer's (1937) article entitled *The grandmother: A problem in child rearing* described grandmothers as having an unfavorable and noxious influence on grandchildren. While these early psychoanalytic theorists emphasized the negative aspects of the grandparent role upon the psychological development of the child, ethnographic researchers in the 1950s presented a more favorable view of grandparenting (Apple, 1956). Social scientists have also recognized the importance of grandparents and were the first to define their specific roles and function. Van Hentig (1946) espoused the "vital role" that grandmothers played in the life of the family and concluded that a grandmother's role is a "primitive but effective mechanism of group survival" (p. 390). Grandparents were considered to be a source of wisdom, strength, and stability, and grandparents benefited from the high status and prestige that the role of grandparent was given. This favorable view of grandparenthood followed the Biblical prescription, which indicated that grandchildren would be a restorer of a grandparent's soul and sustain them in their old age (Ruth 4:14, Revised Standard Version).

During the 1960s and 1970s, researchers began investigating the varying roles of grandparents and the grandparent–grandchild relationship (e.g., Neugarten & Weinstein, 1964). Developmental theorists explored the changing meaning of grandparenthood according to the grandchild's level of cognitive development and found that the meaning of the grandparent role for a grandchild was dependent on the grandchild's level of cognitive maturity (Kahana & Kahana, 1971). However, Clavan (1978) conceptualized the grandparent role as being a roleless role because there exists a wide diversity of grandparenting behaviors coupled with an absence of sanctioned rights, obligations, and prescribed functions. Collectively, the research on the role of grandparenting has described this role in terms ranging from national guard or watch dog (Hagestad, 1985), arbitrator (Hagestad, 1985), stress buffer (Bengtson, 1985; Johnson, 1985), and roots (Hagestad, 1985). Grandparents have also been considered to be a resource person (Neugarten & Weinstein, 1964), valued elder (Kivnick, 1982), mentor (Kornhaber, 1996), conveyer of family legacy and culture (Bengtson, 1985), silent savior of children from faltering families (Creighton, 1991), surrogate parent (Neugarten & Weinstein, 1964), and the wardens of the culture (Guttman, 1985).

Unlike norms for other primary family roles, there are not explicit norms for grandparenting (Kemp, 2004), and most authors have highlighted the multidimensionality of the grandparent role and the issues of variability within the grandparent–grandchild relationship. Historical scholarly perspectives on the grandparent–grandchild relationship (see Szinovacz, 1998) indicate that this relationship is influenced by the age and gender of the grandparent and grandchild (Kivett, 1991); socioeconomic variables such as employment status, educational level, and economic resources (Cherlin & Furstenberg, 1986); geographical proximity and frequency of contact between grandparent and grandchild (Kemp, 2007); psychosocial compatibility (Kornhaber, 1996); personality characteristics (Kornhaber, 1996); disruptive life events (Connidis, 2003); and the mediating effects of parents (Barranti, 1985; Whitbeck, Hoyt, & Huck, 1993). Further, grandparenthood in African-American families, Latina/o families, and Asian families is minimally investigated. When grandparents of color are included in studies, researchers tend to examine crisis events (e.g., grandparents raising their grandchildren, divorce), particularly as these events relate to African-American grandparents. This research is often limited to comparisons with White families (Hunter & Taylor, 1998).

More recent and contemporary research on the grandparent–grandchild relationship has moved away from previous foci and has addressed the diverse nature of the grandparent–grandchild relationship (Stelle et al., 2010). For example,

recent grandparenting literature addresses issues concerning grandparents who are raising their grandchildren (Hayslip & Kaminski, 2005), taking into account racial and social class issues (Brown & Mars, 2000), international perspectives on grandparenting (Kenner, Ruby, Jessel, Gregory, & Arju, 2007), and grandparents who are recipients of primary care from their grandchildren (Fruhauf & Orel, 2008). Further, grandfathering (Roberto, Allen, & Blieszner, 2001), impact of divorce on grandparent–grandchild relationships (Bridges, Roe, Dunn, & O'Connor, 2007), adult grandchildren–grandchild relationships (Kemp, 2004), and grandparenting when grandchildren have special needs (Mitchell, 2007) have received attention in the literature, although limited. These foci take into account sensitivities to race, ethnicity, class, gender, and (dis)ability as they are salient to emerging grandparenting issues and provide insights into the continued diversity of grandparenthood.

Of all the aforementioned factors that influence the grandparent–grandchild relationship as well as the shift in grandparenting research away from a unitary focus on White, middle-class families (Stelle et al., 2010), the mediating role of the middle generation on the stability of the grandparent–grandchild relationship cannot be underestimated. While research continues to explore role expectations for grandparents and investigate relationships between grandparents and grandchildren, it is the parents who set the conditions by which the grandparent–grandchild relationship functions (Matthews & Sprey, 1985). The role parents play in the grandparent–grandchild relationship over the life course may be especially important to consider when grandparents are sexual minorities.

Definition of Families with an LGBT Emphasis

Although the vast majority of research on families has emphasized the experiences of family members from a heterosexual (heteronormative) perspective, it is apparent that LGBT persons are members of families and actively participate in their roles as sons, daughters, sisters, brothers, nieces, nephews, uncles, and aunts. A complete exploration of the historical understanding of LGBT family relationships is beyond the scope of this chapter, but it is important to address the changing American societal attitudes toward nonheterosexual orientations and behaviors during the past 50 years because this is the *lived history* of current LGBT grandparents.

Prior to the Stonewall Rebellion of 1969, LGBT persons were forced to live secretive lives in which their sexual orientation was "closeted" so that a public heterosexual identity could be managed (Seidman, 2002). Pervasive heterosexist attitudes created hardships for any family member who disclosed his/her sexual orientation. The Stonewall Rebellion of 1969 has been identified as the "turning point" for understanding gay and lesbian identities, and according to Seidman (2002), "never before had homosexuals openly declared their sexual identity as something good while criticizing American society for its intolerance" (p. 64). More than 40 years have elapsed from this cultural moment in which secrecy and closeting was nationally challenged [see Miller (2006) for a detailed account of gay historical information]. Contemporary events such as legalizing same-sex marriages and repealing "don't ask, don't tell" have currently created a disclosure imperative (McLean, 2007; Seidman, 2002), whereby LGBT individuals are expected to be open and honest about their sexual orientation with friends, family, and colleagues. However, problematic family relationships are still evident when LGBT persons assume the roles of mother, father, grandmother, or grandfather as little popular work along with mainstream society has addressed these topics. American society seems to deliver the most criticism, oppression, and intolerance to LGBT individuals who attempt to assume the roles that historically have been identified as key "family" milestones that only heterosexual individuals and couples experience. Historically, the terms *lesbian mother, gay father, lesbian grandmother, and gay grandfather* have been viewed as contradictions in terms (Clunis & Green, 1995; Orel & Fruhauf, 2006) because homosexuality was viewed as being inconsistent

with the ability to procreate and, as a result, become a parent and grandparent.

Although the research and scholarship on LGBT persons who are mothers, fathers, grandmothers, or grandfathers has rapidly increased within the past decade, to date, research on lesbian mothers dominates the research on LGBT families, with relatively little scholarship on bisexuals and transgender people as mothers, fathers, or grandparents (Biblarz & Savci, 2010). Therefore, we will begin the discussion on LGBT grandparents by presenting a brief discourse on the gendered experience of grandparenting.

Gendered Experience of Grandparenting

The literature on heterosexual grandparents documents that there are distinct similarities and differences between the experiences of grandmothers and grandfathers and these relate to how grandparenting has been historically conceptualized. Most notable is that generally when grandfathers have been examined within the literature there has been a tendency for grandfatherhood to be examined through a feminized conception of grandparenting (Mann, 2007). Because grandfatherhood has been examined from a perspective of how men are similar to and different from grandmothers, grandfathers are not only seen as different, but as less important, less active in intergenerational relations, offering less to grandchildren, and making a limited contribution to the grandparent–grandchild relationship compared to grandmothers.

Research has shown that grandmothers have closer relationships with grandchildren (Silverstein & Marenco, 2001) and that maternal grandparents have closer relationships with grandchildren than paternal grandparents (Chan & Elder, 2000; Eisenberg, 1988). The finding that maternal grandparents have closer relationships with grandchildren suggests that the gender of the parent also impacts the relationship between grandparent and grandchild. Likewise, the gender of the grandchild impacts the grandparent–grandchild relationship, with female grandchildren experiencing emotionally closer relationships with grandparents than male grandchildren (Eisenberg, 1988).

The literature on grandparenting highlights that being a grandparent is a gendered familial role and that grandparenting holds different expectations for behaviors and responsibilities for men and women (Stelle et al., 2010; Thomas, 1995). However, there is an inconsistency between the assumption and findings that the gender of the grandparental generation is an important factor to consider and the fact that there has been a complete "invisibility" of transgender grandparents within both the gerontological and LGBT literature. Likewise, the exploration of the ways in which gender *and* sexual orientation influences grandparenting remains largely unexplored.

Lesbian Motherhood and Lesbian Grandmotherhood

The most commonly reported number of lesbian mothers in the USA was estimated to be between 1 and 5 million in the late 1990s, with reports that the number of lesbian mothers has dramatically increased (Lambert, 2005). Current national estimates indicate that one in three lesbian couples are raising children (Gates & Ost, 2004). Accurate statistics are not available because national surveys omit questions on sexual orientation, single parenting, informal parenting, and caregiving arrangements (Tasker & Patterson, 2007). Likewise, statistics on whether children were born or adopted within the context of a heterosexual relationship before the mother identified as lesbian, and those in which self-identified lesbians adopted or bore children, is difficult to obtain because generally the classification of parents as lesbian, gay, or heterosexual is not available. However, the majority of research on lesbian mothers and their children tends to distinguish between these two broad types: those who gave birth to children within the context of a heterosexual relationship and those who chose to have a child or children through donor insemination (DI) or adoption (Goldberg, 2010).

Currently, more is known about lesbian motherhood than lesbian grandmothers despite the fact that statistically most lesbian mothers will become grandmothers since 94% of parents become grandparents (Smith & Drew, 2002). Biblarz and Savci (2010) indicated that "lesbian motherhood is a negotiated identity between the marginalized position of lesbianism and the mainstream and esteemed position of motherhood" (p. 483). Therefore, it is important to investigate how lesbian grandmothers conceptualize their identity knowing that they are both members of a marginalized sexual minority and yet hold a highly regarded and respected position as a grandmother. It is also important to investigate whether the experiences of lesbian grandmothers differ if they are the biological grandmother, co-grandmother, step grandmother, or social grandmother; to date no researcher has addressed this complex topic.

Since the 1980s, there has been discussion of lesbian grandmothers within popular magazines (e.g., *Lesbian Connection*) and anthologies. Some of these articles and stories highlighted lesbian grandmothers in an unfavorable manner. For example, in 1994 a Christian Fundamentalist magazine (e.g., *Alberta Report*) protested against a Vancouver judge who awarded custody of a child to her lesbian grandmother instead of to her biological father (Bray, 2008). However, on the popular 1990s situation comedy "Roseanne," one of the key characters played a lesbian grandmother. In the collected papers on *Lesbian Parenting, Living with Pride and Prejudice*, Jessica Walker wrote about her lesbian grandmother's struggles with her sexual orientation and her inability to be with her lesbian partner. Jessica wrote that she personally "cried over the tragic way that the lovers had been forced apart" (Walker & Walker, 1995, p. 165). Three additional anthologies that included chapters on lesbian grandmothers were *Women in Love: Portraits of Lesbian Mothers and Their Families* (Sevda & Herrera, 1998), *The Lesbian Parenting Book* (Clunis & Green, 2003), and *Lives of Lesbian Elders: Looking Back, Looking Forward* (Clunis et al., 2005). These anthologies shared the personal narratives of lesbian grandmothers and highlighted both their struggles and joys of being lesbian grandmothers.

Whalen, Bigner, and Barber (2000) published the first scholarly paper that examined the grandmother's role as experienced by lesbian women. The nine self-identified lesbian grandmothers were White, middle class, and well educated and thus not representative of the population of lesbian grandmothers. The lesbian grandmothers perceived their grandmother role as being multifaceted, with three primary roles (a) to provide emotional support to grandchildren, (b) to provide varied experiences to their grandchildren, and (c) to support the grandchildren's parents. The major reported benefit of enacting the grandparent role was receiving unconditional love from his/her grandchildren; this finding was consistent with previous grandparenting work (Hodgson, 1992). In fact, Whalen et al. (2000) indicated that "these women possibly would not have been distinguishable from those presumed to be heterosexual grandmothers had they been included in any of the previous studies on grandparenting or grandmotherhood" (p. 52). Unfortunately, Whalen et al. (2000) did not explore the effect of the grandmother's sexual orientation on the grandparent–grandchild relationship, and the grandmother's role was explored in a socially isolated manner.

In 2005, Serena Patterson conducted individual interviews with 14 lesbian grandmothers ranging in age from 41 to 73 who were living in the greater Vancouver or Toronto areas of Canada. Of the 14 grandmothers, 11 became grandmothers through their biological children and 3 became step grandmothers through the adult children of a lesbian partner. According to Patterson (2005a), the most significant finding was that a lesbian grandmother's identity as a lesbian occurred late in her life. The majority of lesbian grandmothers came out when their children were adults and/or their heterosexual marriages ended. These women viewed their lesbian identity formation as "an accomplishment or a gift of middle age" (Patterson, 2005b, p. 119) and then negotiated this new identity with their identities as mothers and grandmothers. The role of being a lesbian grandmother was celebrated and "affirms the rightness of their life's journey" (Patterson, 2005b).

Orel (2004, 2006), and Orel and Fruhauf (2006) were the first to specifically and systematically explore the effects of sexual orientation on the grandparent–grandchild relationship. Their qualitative research explored the perceptions, attitudes, and beliefs of lesbian and bisexual (LB) grandmothers by using the life course perspective as a guide (Bengtson & Allen, 1993). Applying the life course perspective to LB grandmothers, the authors indicated that the grandparent–grandchild relationship was embedded within the context of the grandmother's individual choices across the life span (e.g., decisions to disclose one's homosexuality), the structural contexts within which these decisions were made (e.g., level of homophobia within a culture), and the transitions that grandmothers experienced (e.g., previous heterosexual marriages and divorce).

Participants in the Orel (2004) study included 12 self-identified lesbian grandmothers and 4 self-identified bisexual grandmothers who ranged in age from 44 to 75 with a mean age of 60.9 years. Twelve of the participants were White, three were African-American, and one participant identified herself as "other" (Native American and Latino). During the face-to-face, semi-structured in-depth interviews with LB grandmothers, 4 of the 16 LB grandmothers were completely secretive about their sexual orientation, with neither their adult children nor grandchildren being aware of their self-identification as lesbian or bisexual women. An important finding was that LB grandmothers' descriptions of their relationships with their grandchildren were always placed within the context of their on-going relationship with their adult children (Orel & Fruhauf, 2006). LB grandmothers who had a strong, intimate relationship with their adult children were more likely to have a close relationship with their grandchildren. Adult children also determined the amount of access that they, or in some cases their partners, would have with their grandchildren. Therefore, adult children mediated the development of the relationship between LB grandmothers and their grandchildren. This research supports previous work suggesting parents are the gatekeepers to the grandparent–grandchild relationship, and they can facilitate or discourage the development of an emotionally intimate relationship between the grandparents and grandchildren (Matthews & Sprey, 1985).

Orel (2006) and Orel and Fruhauf (2006) also found that adult children's acceptance of the grandmother's sexual orientation determined LB grandmothers' opportunities to grandparent and that adult children's attitudes toward sexual orientation influenced the direction of the mediating effect (i.e., facilitating or discouraging) on the grandparent–grandchild relationship. The LB grandmothers were aware of the impact that their sexual orientation had on their relationships with their adult children and subsequently their grandchildren. For the four LB grandmothers who did not disclose their sexual orientation to their adult children or grandchildren, they expressed profound fear and anxiety concerning what would happen to their relationship with their grandchildren if their homosexuality/bisexuality was known. The LB grandmothers' level of concern was specifically related to assumptions that their adult children would not be able to accept their homosexuality/bisexuality and would then prevent them from seeing their grandchildren. Therefore, adult children are mediators in the grandparent–grandchild relationship, and they can also influence or inhibit disclosure. The decision-making process, and subsequently the ability to either remain secretive or disclose their sexual orientation to adult children and grandchildren, was a significant event for all 16 LB grandmothers. However, the actual process of coming out to adult children and grandchildren varied among the LB grandmothers.

Collectively, the limited research on LB grandmothers indicates that adult children not only influenced the formation and maintenance of the grandmother–grandchild relationship but also played a profound and significant role in the coming out process of LB grandmothers (Orel, 2006; Orel & Fruhauf, 2006; Patterson, 2005b). It is important to note that all LB grandmothers indicated that their sexual orientation per se was not significant in regard to their ability to assume the grandmother role and their subsequent relationships with their grandchildren. Rather, the significance of their sexual orientation was

related to their ability to have an open and honest relationship with adult children and grandchildren. Honesty and openness was severely compromised when LB grandmothers were fearful of disclosing an important personal dimension of their identity—their sexual orientation. This fear was created and fueled by the heterosexist and homophobic context over their life course (Clunis et al., 2005) in which the LB grandmother–grandchild relationship was embedded (Orel, 2006; Orel & Fruhauf, 2006; Patterson, 2005a). That is, LB grandmothers' past personal experiences with discrimination fostered intense fears of becoming alienated from their grandchildren if they were to disclose their sexual orientation. LB grandmothers feared that perhaps their adult children also held culturally sanctioned homophobic attitudes.

Focusing on the intersection of sexuality and gender, Orel and Fruhauf (2006) also found that the gender of adult children (parents) played a significant role in the coming out process of LB grandparents. Among adult children, it was women (mothers) who were more likely than men (fathers) to facilitate understanding of grandmothers' homosexuality in their children. A primary reason that women facilitated LB grandmothers' disclosure to their grandchildren was that generally it was women who were more likely to be aware of their mothers' sexual orientation. This finding is similar to general LGBT research that found that female family members are more likely to be aware of LGBT kin and more likely to be directly disclosed to than male family members (Ben-Ari, 1995; Savin-Williams, 2001).

Gay Grandfatherhood

Just as there are too few studies that have investigated the role of grandfathers in the grandparent–grandchild relationship, there are even fewer studies that have investigated grandparenting by gay grandfathers. Similar to what was previously reported for lesbian grandmothers, the first publications that highlighted the role of gay grandfathers appeared on LGBT elder Web sites (e.g., American Society on Aging's *Outword*) or in newspaper articles (e.g., *Philadelphia Inquirer*).

These articles highlighted gay grandfathers in a favorable manner and illustrated the diversity in the role of being a gay grandfather (Hochman, 2008). Gay grandfathers assumed a variety of roles with their grandchildren that were often specific to a particular grandchild and/or adult child, as well as being dependent on the developmental level of grandchildren. They served as a father figure, an active grandparent, reservoir of wisdom and culture, a friend, distant figure, and an absent figure. The majority of grandfathers expressed that their grandparenting role was not associated with being gay, but that their sexual orientation may have influenced the type of grandfather that they could be if adult children were not accepting of their homosexuality. Obviously, gay grandfathers who have appeared in newspaper articles were not hesitant about disclosing their sexual orientation to family members. Perhaps it is more socially acceptable for older men to be out to family members than older women as LGBT movements began with a focus on gay male rights (Miller, 2006) and slowly made visible the LBT population.

To better understand the sociocultural and sociopolitical context of gay grandfathers' lives, Fruhauf et al. (2009) specifically examined the experiences of gay grandfathers' coming out processes to their grandchildren. Participants in this study were 11 White gay grandfathers who ranged in age from 40 to 79 years. Semi-structured interviews were conducted and the participants were asked to describe themselves as gay grandfathers and to describe their coming out process. The interviews revealed that gay grandfathers took different approaches to disclosing their sexual orientation to their grandchildren, but all grandfathers indicated that adult children played a profound role in the coming out process. For example, adult children assisted by answering questions grandchildren asked about their grandfather's partner, where they slept, and if grandpa loved his partner. This finding illustrates that "in the coming out process, adult children serve as mediators between grandparents and grandchildren" (Fruhauf et al., 2009, p. 113) which converges with historical perspectives on the grandparent–grandchild relationship (Matthews

& Sprey, 1985) and LB grandmothering (Orel & Fruhauf, 2006). Consistently, the available research on LGB grandparents and the LGB grandparent–grandchild relationship illustrates the importance of the mediating role of adult children. Another consistent finding in the available LGB grandparent research is the emphasis that LGB grandparents give to being able to disclose their sexual orientation to their grandchildren. The strength of these findings warrants a more detailed description of the coming out process for LGB grandparents.

Disclosure of Sexual Orientation to Grandchildren

It is extremely important to explore, recognize, and acknowledge the societal expectations of grandparents and how these expectations play a role in the coming out process for LGBT grandparents and the grandparent–grandchild relationship. Generalized stereotypes about older adults include the expectations that they are emotionally and/or physically fragile, asexual, and cognitively incompetent or senile (Stelle et al., 2010). These stereotypes are not based in fact, but research indicates that when LGB grandparents come out to family members, they often face comments that reflect these beliefs/expectations (Fruhauf et al., 2009; Orel, 2006; Orel & Fruhauf, 2006). One grandmother in Orel (2006) said "when I told them (grandchildren) that I was a lesbian, the first thing they said is 'how can that be—you're not having sex, are you?' They probably also assumed that I was senile" (p. 185). Another grandfather in this study (Fruhauf et al., 2009) shared his story about telling his adult son that he was bisexual and was surprised by his son's response—"He says to me, well at your age it's not like you're going to be cruising the gay bars all night long so I guess it really doesn't matter." Conversely, the notion of physical frailty does not protect older gay men from being viewed as potential predators. One grandfather shared his sadness when after disclosing his sexual orientation to his daughter-in-law, she immediately said that he could no longer babysit for his granddaughter. He said, "She thought I was now a threat to my granddaughter. That was the most hurtful response I have ever received from anyone… about me being a gay man" (Fruhauf & Bigner, 2006).

In addition to the generalized negative stereotypes about older adults, there are also generalized positive stereotypes about older adults, specifically grandparents, which played a role in the coming out process of LGB grandparents. These positive stereotypes of grandparents include being providers of unconditional love and emotional and instrumental support and serving as a family guardian or protector. It is the common expectation that grandparents will provide unconditional love to their grandchildren. The gerontological literature clearly posits that grandparents are expected to be universally selfless, unconditionally love their grandchildren, and to be "unassuming and supportive in exchanges with their adult grandchildren" (Kemp, 2004, p. 507), as well as support grandchildren when parents are unwilling or unable to provide emotional support (Roberto et al., 2001). When LGBT grandparents disclose to their adult children and grandchildren, they are seeking both emotional support and understanding from them. LGBT grandparents are also asking for unconditional love. Because LGBT grandparents are asking for, and not providing, emotional support and unconditional love, this can be viewed as going against familial expectations and roles. Family members are being asked by their eldest family member to be supportive and willing to increase their knowledge and understanding and reduce their homophobic attitudes and beliefs. This expectation may pose too great a challenge in some families.

Research on the acceptance of children when a parent discloses his/her sexual orientation indicates that early adolescence (ages 13–16) is a more difficult time (Patterson, 1992) because those in early adolescence are working through their own emerging sexuality. Current research (Orel, 2006; Orel & Fruhauf, 2006) on the coming out process of LB grandmothers also revealed that children in earlier stages of development tend to experience less stress when their grandmothers come out to them. However, this is known from reports from LB grandmothers and not the grandchildren themselves. Although there is a significant amount of research attention paid to the children of lesbian and gay parents (Savin-Williams & Esterberg, 2000), there is limited research that has explored the experiences of grandchildren of LGBT grandparents (Perlesz et al., 2006).

The gerontological literature on the grandparent–grandchild relationship indicates that grandparents are expected to guard and protect their grandchild from both real and imagined foes (King, Russell, & Elder, 1998). Oftentimes, the foe is the parent (adult child). It has been commonly reported in the family counseling literature that grandparents and grandchildren get along so well because they have a common enemy—the adult child/parent (Walsh, 1989). It is also well documented that the grandparent–grandchild relationship is mediated by the parent(s), even after grandchildren reach adulthood (Matthews & Sprey, 1985). The available literature investigating the grandparent–grandchild relationship when grandchildren identify as LGBT shows that parents act as disclosers for their LGBT children (Herdt & Koff, 2000; Savin-Williams, 2001). Parents not only disclosed their LGBT children's sexual orientation to grandparents but also became strong advocates for their LGBT children by creating a climate of acceptance and demonstrating a loving stance. Conversely, parents can hinder the relationship between LGBT grandparents and their grandchildren through rejection of homosexuality and a climate of intolerance.

These findings on the coming out process of LGB grandparents speak to the diversity of expectations of grandparenthood and underscore the importance of examining grandparenthood and disclosure of sexual orientation within the context of the history of family relationships. Likewise, the intersections of race, ethnicity, sexuality, gender, and the family must be considered when discussing the coming out process and LGBT grandparents in general.

Research on the grandparent–grandchild relationship within communities of color has concluded that grandparents play a central role the lives of their grandchildren (Burton, 1996) and that the grandparenting role is highly revered for its ability to maintain ethnic identity and familial bonds between family members. Ethnic minority groups view grandparents as key to the preservation of family and minority communities. If homosexuality is viewed as being antithetical to issues of family and perpetuation of communities of color then LGBT grandparents of color would be less likely to disclose their sexual orientation than White LGBT grandparents. However, Orel (2006) found that the strong familial bonds within communities of color facilitated disclosure for African-American lesbian grandmothers. As one participant said, "When I first told them that I was a lesbian, there was this long silence. No one said anything. Then my son looks at me and says 'you're still my ma and grandma for my kids—that's all I need to know" (Orel, 2004).

Collectively, the research on LGB grandparents revealed that managing disclosure about sexual orientation was a primary issue for all LGB grandparents and that the decision to disclose or remain secretive was a reflection of familial and societal relationships over time. The decision to disclose one's sexual orientation was also dependent on the older adult's perceived level of homonegativity within the immediate family unit and within the culture (i.e., neighborhood, workplace). Although the ability to disclose one's sexual orientation to grandchildren was psychologically salient for LGB grandparents' identity, the level of homonegativity within their culture forced many LGB grandparents to maintain the illusion of heterosexuality. For example, LGB grandparents believed that their sexuality did not define who they were no more than one grandfather said his hair color defined him. LGB grandparents who did not disclose or remained secretive did so to prevent becoming estranged from their families of origin (Fruhauf et al., 2009; Orel & Fruhauf, 2006).

Programs and Practice Recognizing LGBT Grandparents and Their Grandchildren

While grandparenthood may be the "grand-generative aspect of old age" (Erikson, 1984, p. 164) that reflects the instrumental need for intergenerational relationships among all populations, the ability to enact this role intersects with a multitude of variables within multiple contexts, most salient of which is sexual orientation within a heterosexist environment. Clinicians, educators, counselors, researchers, and practitioners must be aware of the variance and diversity in intergenerational relationships. Those who are working directly with LGBT grandparents and their grandchildren should have the common goal of strengthening the existing intergenerational and interlocking family bonds to meet the individual needs of both LGBT grandparents and their grandchildren. Most importantly, programs and services aimed toward intergenerational relationships must move away from dominant assumptions and discourses of grandparents as exclusively heterosexual and without gender variation.

From a life course perspective, practitioners and programs need to recognize the variability in the experiences of both LGBT grandparents and grandchildren based on the continued aging of the grandparent and developmental level of the grandchild. Programs and practice also need to address the different experiences of LGBT grandparents dependent upon age of the initial transition to grandparenthood, the duration of grandparenthood, and most importantly their disclosure patterns (i.e., do grandparents use the assistance of adult children in coming out or do they take on an approach of coming out alone?). Attention is also needed for the cultural messages about sexual orientation within specific cohorts.

Because practitioners typically assume that grandparents are heterosexual, practitioners working with LGBT grandparents may overlook the saliency of grandparents' sexual orientation on the grandparent–grandchild relationship. Practitioners must listen for subtle messages to learn about an elder's sexual identity and orientation. Otherwise, practitioners who assume heterosexuality will overlook the unique challenges, issues, and concerns of LGBT grandparents. Unfortunately, for most LGBT grandparents, the "invisibility" of their status as a grandparent mirrors and perhaps compounds their general sense of invisibility as an LGBT elder. LGBT grandparents (and their partners) must receive the social support and recognition that is naturally granted to heterosexual grandparents within all cultures. Practitioners must also recognize that because LGBT grandparents have developed creative and resourceful ways to function within a heterosexist culture as LGBT *persons*, LGBT grandparents can provide creative and flexible definitions of grandparenting and grandparenthood. However, service providers must be ever mindful that societal and personal barriers may exist that require some LGBT grandparents to be closeted to family members. Research on LGB grandparents clearly indicates that "coming out" or disclosing one's sexual orientation is a life-long process with varying passages and multiple results.

Implications for Future Research and Concluding Remarks

Despite the fact that the literature on grandparenting and LGBT families has come a long way, researchers are only scratching at the surface. As a result, further research is still needed on LGBT grandparenthood. The LGBT grandparenting literature requires a closer examination of the gendered nature of familial relationships and the role and expectations of LGBT grandparents. There must be an understanding of how the role of an LGBT grandparent builds on previous roles and meanings of being a gay man, lesbian woman, and bisexual/transgender persons. In addition to gender, the intersection of race, social class, ethnicity, and (dis)ability needs to be addressed in future research.

Research on families where the eldest matriarchal or patriarchal figure is gay, lesbian, bisexual, or transgender must refrain from making comparisons between LGBT grandparents and heterosexual grandparents—this comparison only perpetuates heterocentrism. Future research must conduct independent studies on the B and T in LGBT. Likewise, further research is needed on LGBT grandparents from "de novo" families, or families in which LGBT grandparents conceived children within the context of LGBT relationships, rather than in previous heterosexual relationships. Future research needs to focus on understanding the implications of differences in race, ethnicity, cultural environments, socioeconomic status, and age among LGBT grandparents utilizing the

intersectionality perspective that examines multiple identities and the ways in which they interact (Crenshaw, 1989; Institute of Medicine, 2011). This will require the development and distribution of a large-scale national survey that focuses on LGBT grandparents. The authors have developed this survey, with distribution beginning in 2012.

Further research is needed on LGBT grandparenting particularly in relation to the intersectionality of grandchildren's gender, parental sexual orientation, class, race, ethnicity, and sociological context. Specifically, key research questions include (a) How do LGBT grandparents simultaneously construct sexual identities and grandparenting identities? (b) How does the LGBT grandparent–grandchild relationship change over time? and (c) How do LGBT grandparents negotiate the institutions that grandparenting and aging bring to them, such as schools and senior centers? This research would include an investigation of the experiences surrounding grandchildren's relationships with the "co-grandparent" or partners of LGBT grandparents. Most importantly, research is needed to explore the perceptions, attitudes, beliefs, and experiences of grandchildren of LGBT grandparents. Finally, LGBT grandparents, generally, have not received sufficient attention in research on LGBT family relationships. While our review specifically focused on two subgroups of grandparents (lesbian/bisexual grandmothers and gay grandfathers), there are other subgroups of LGBT grandparents who warrant attention. These include LGBT grandparents who suffer from cognitive disorders (e.g., Alzheimer's disease) and LGBT grandparents who reside in long-term care facilities. Further, with the increase in the grandparenting literature toward examining grandparents raising grandchildren it is important to this body of work to specifically include LGBT grandparents who are raising grandchildren. Likewise, more research is needed to explore the unique experiences of bisexual and transgender grandparents.

Based on the review of literature on the grandparent–grandchild relationship when a grandparent identifies as LGBT, a primary conclusion can be offered: namely, that one must consider the diversity and context in which the grandparent–grandchild relationship is embedded. Additionally, lifelong patterns of family experiences, exchanges, and attachment patterns must be taken into consideration to fully understand current intergenerational relationships.

The tenets of the life course perspective guided the discussion on the relationship between LGBT grandparents and their grandchildren. This required a focus on roles entrenched within the social/historical life course and an examination of individual differences to relationships in later-life families. The life course perspective reminds us of the linked lives of intergenerational relationships and the diversity and heterogeneity within intergenerational relationships. Likewise, we must be cognizant of the multiple pathways that these intergenerational relationships follow across time.

Research collectively indicates that managing disclosure about sexual orientation was the primary issue for LGB grandparents and that the ability to disclose sexual orientation to family members was salient for LGB grandparents' identity development. LGB grandparents' decision to disclose or remain closeted was influenced by their perceptions of the level of sexism, heterosexism, and homonegativity within their particular setting and context, as well as reflecting their familial relationships over time. Although one could argue that all LGBT people struggle with decisions related to coming out, LGBT grandparents are unique in that their decisions are influenced by their adult children. Therefore, any research that explores the LGBT grandparent–grandchild relationship must include the perceptions and experiences of *all* members of the family to better illuminate our understanding of contemporary LGBT grandparent–grandchild relationships.

References

Abraham, K. (1913/1955). Some remarks on the role of grandparents in the psychology of neuroses. In H. C. Abraham (Ed.), *Selected papers of Karl Abraham* (Vol. 2, pp. 44–48). New York, NY: Basic Books.

Apple, D. (1956). The social structure of grandparenthood. *American Anthropologist, 58,* 656–663. doi:10.1525/aa.1956.58.4.02a00060

Barranti, C. C. (1985). The grandparent-grandchild relationship: Family resource in an era of voluntary bond. *Family Relations, 34,* 343–352.

Ben-Ari, A. (1995). The discovery that an offspring is gay: Parents', gay men's, and lesbian's perspectives. *Journal of Homosexuality, 30,* 89–111. doi:10.1300/j082v30n01_05

Bengston, V. L. (1985). Diversity and symbolism in grandparents' role. In V. L. Bengston & J. F. Robertson (Eds.), *Grandparenthood* (pp. 11–27). Beverly Hills, CA: Sage.

Bengston, V. (2001). Beyond the nuclear family: The increasing importance of multigenerational bonds. *Journal of Marriage and the Family, 63,* 1–16.

Bengtson, V. L., & Allen, K. R. (1993). The life course perspective applied to families over time. In P. G. Boss, W. Doherty, R. LaRossa, W. Schumm, & S. Steinmetz (Eds.), *Sourcebook of family theories and methods: A contextual approach* (pp. 469–499). New York, NY: Plenum Press.

Biblarz, T. J., & Savci, E. (2010). Lesbian, gay, bisexual, and transgender families. *Journal of Marriage and Family, 72,* 480–497. doi:10.1111/j.1741-3737.2010.00714.x

Bray, C. (2008, June). *Making space for lesbian grandmothers: A review of Canadian research on gender and family work.* Paper presented at the 43rd Annual Meeting of the Canadian Sociological Association, Vancouver, BC.

Bridges, L. J., Roe, A. E. C., Dunn, J., & O'Connor, T. G. (2007). Children's perspectives on their relationship with grandparents following parental separation: A longitudinal study. *Social Development, 16,* 539–554. doi:10.1111j.1467-9507.2007.00395.x

Brown, D. R., & Mars, J. (2000). Profile of contemporary grandparenting in African-American families. In C. B. Cox (Ed.), *To grandmother's house we go and stay: Perspectives on custodial grandparents* (pp. 203–217). New York, NY: Springer.

Burton, L. M. (1996). The timing of childbearing, family structure, and the role responsibilities of aging Black women. In E. M. Hetherington & E. Blechman (Eds.), *Stress, coping, and resiliency in children and families* (pp. 155–172). Hillsdale, NJ: Lawrence Erlbaum Associates.

Chan, C., & Elder, G. (2000). Matrilineal advantage in grandchild-grandparent relations. *The Gerontologist, 40,* 179–190. doi:10.1093/geront/40.2.179

Cherlin, A. J., & Furstenberg, F. F. (1986). *The new American grandparent.* New York, NY: Basic Books.

Clavan, S. (1978). The impact of social class and social trends on the role of the grandparent. *The Family Coordinator, 10,* 351–357.

Clunis, D., & Green, G. (1995). *The lesbian parenting book: A guide to creating families and raising children.* New York, NY: Seal Press.

Clunis, D. M., & Green, G. D. (2003). *The lesbian parenting book: A guide to creating families and raising children* (2nd edition). New York: Sage.

Clunis, D., Fredriksen-Goldsen, K., Freeman, P., & Nystrom, N. (2005). *Lives of lesbian elders: Looking back, looking forward.* Binghamton, NY: Haworth Press.

Connidis, I. A. (2003). Divorce and union dissolution: Reverberations over three generations. *Canadian Journal on Aging, 22*, 353–368.

Creighton, L. (1991, December 16). Grandparents: The silent saviors. *U. S. News and World Report*, 80–89

Crenshaw, K. (1989). *Demarginalizing the intersection of race and sex: A black feminist critique of antidiscrimination doctrine, feminist theory, and antiracist politics.* Chicago, IL: University of Chicago Legal Forum.

Eisenberg, A. R. (1988). Grandchildren's perspectives on relationships with grandparents: The influence of gender across generations. *Sex Roles, 19*, 205–217. doi:10.1007/bf00290155

Elder, G. H., Jr. (2003). The life course in time and place. In W. R. Heinz & V. W. Marshall (Eds.), *Sequences, institutions and interrelations over the life course* (pp. 57–71). New York, NY: Aldine de Gruyter.

Erikson, E. (1984). Reflections on the last stage and the first. *Psychoanalytic Study of the Child, 39*, 155–165.

Fruhauf, C. A., & Bigner, J. J. (2006, November). The coming out process to grandchildren: Grandfathers' perceptions of their adult children's influence. In N. A. Orel (Chair), *Lesbian, gay, and bisexual grandparents: Overcoming societal obstacles.* Symposium conducted at the annual meeting of the Gerontological Society of America, Dallas, TX.

Fruhauf, C., & Orel, N. (2008). Developmental issues of grandchildren who provide care to grandparents. *International Journal of Aging and Human Development, 67*, 209–230. doi:10.2190/ag.67.3b

Fruhauf, C., Orel, N., & Jenkins, D. (2009). The coming out process of gay grandfathers: Perceptions of their adult children's influence. *Journal of GLBT Family Studies, 5*, 99–118. doi:10.1080/15504280802595402

Gates, G. J., & Cook, A. M. (2011). *Colorado Census snapshot: 2010.* Retrieved from http://www3.law.ucla.edu/williamsinstitute/pdf/Census2010Snapshot_Colorado.pdf

Gates, G., & Ost, J. (2004). *The gay and lesbian atlas.* Washington, DC: The Urban Institute.

Goldberg, A. E. (2010). *Lesbian and gay parents and their children: Research on the family life cycle.* Washington, DC: American Psychological Association.

Guttman, D. L. (1985). Deculturation and the American grandparent. In V. L. Bengtson & J. F. Robertson (Eds.), *Grandparenthood* (pp. 173–183). Beverly Hills, CA: Sage.

Hagestad, G. (1985). Continuity and connectedness. In V. L. Bengtson & J. F. Robertson (Eds.), *Grandparenthood* (pp. 31–48). Beverly Hills, CA: Sage.

Hayslip, B., Jr., & Kaminski, P. L. (2005). Grandparents raising their grandchildren: A review of literature and suggestions for practice. *The Gerontologist, 45*, 262–269. doi:10.1093/geront/45.2.262

Herdt, G., & Koff, B. (2000). *Something to tell you: The road families travel when a child is gay.* New York, NY: Columbia University Press.

Hochman, A. (2008). The grandparents are out: Gays and lesbians who married decades ago and had children now enjoy grandkids who know their story. *Philadelphia Inquirer* – 02/03/08. Philly Online, LLC.

Hodgson, L. G. (1992). Adult grandchildren and their grandparents: The enduring bond. *Intergenerational Journal of Aging and Human Development, 34*, 209–225. doi:10.2190/pu9m-96xd-cfyq-a8uk

Hunter, A. G., & Taylor, R. J. (1998). Grandparenthood in African American families. In M. E. Szinovacz (Ed.), *Handbook on grandparenthood* (pp. 70–86). Westport, CT: Greenwood Press.

Institute of Medicine. (2011). *The health of lesbian, gay, bisexual, and transgender people: Building a foundation for better understanding.* Washington, DC: National Academy of Science.

Johnson, C. L. (1985). A cultural analysis of the grandmother. *Research on Aging, 5*, 547–567. doi:10.1177/0164027583005004007

Johnson, S., & O'Connor, E. (2002). *The gay baby boom: The psychology of gay parenthood.* New York, NY: New York University Press.

Kahana, B., & Kahana, E. (1971). Grandparenthood from the perspective of the developing child. *Developmental Psychology, 3*, 98–105. doi:10.1037/h0029423

Kemp, C. L. (2004). "Grand" expectations: The experiences of grandparents and adult grandchildren. *Canadian Journal of Sociology, 29*, 499–525.

Kemp, C. L. (2007). Grandparent-grandchild ties: Reflections on continuity and change across three generations. *Journal of Family Issues, 28*, 855–881. doi:10.1177/0192513x07299599

Kenner, C., Ruby, M., Jessel, J., Gregory, E., & Arju, T. (2007). Intergenerational learning between children and grandparents in east London. *Journal of Early Childhood Research, 5*, 219–243. doi:10.1177/1476718x07080471

Kimmel, D., Rose, T., Orel, N., & Greene, B. (2006). Historical context for research on lesbian, gay, bisexual, and transgender aging. In D. Kimmel, T. Rose, & S. David (Eds.), *Lesbian, gay, bisexual, and transgender aging: Research and clinical perspectives* (pp. 1–19). New York, NY: Columbia University Press.

King, V., Russell, S. T., & Elder, G. H., Jr. (1998). Grandparenting in family systems: An ecological perspective. In M. Szinovacz (Ed.), *Handbook on grandparenthood* (pp. 53–69). Westport, CT: Greenwood.

Kivett, V. (1991). The grandparent-grandchild connection. *Marriage and Family Review, 16*, 267–290. doi:10.1300/j002v16n03_04

Kivnick, H. (1982). Grandparenthood: An overview of meaning and mental health. *Gerontologist, 22*, 59–66. doi:10.1093/geront/22.1.59

Kornhaber, A. (1996). *Contemporary grandparenting.* Thousand Oaks, CA: Sage.

Lambert, S. (2005). Gay and lesbian families: What we know and where to go from here. *The Family Journal: Counseling and Therapy for Couples and Families, 13*(1), 43–51. doi:10.1177/1066480704270150

Mann, R. (2007). Out of the shadows? Grandfatherhood, age and masculinities. *Journal of Aging Studies, 21*, 281–291. doi:10.1016/j.jaging.2007.05.008

Matthews, S. H., & Sprey, J. (1985). Adolescents' relationships with grandparents: An empirical contribution to conceptual clarification. *Journal of Gerontology, 40*, 621–626. doi:10.1093/geronj/40.5.621

McLean, K. (2007). Hiding in the closet? Bisexuality, coming out and the disclosure imperative. *Journal of Sociology, 43*, 151–166.

Miller, N. (2006). *Out of the past: Gay and lesbian history from 1869 to the present*. New York, NY: Alyson Books.

Mitchell, W. (2007). The role of grandparents in intergenerational support for families with disabled children: A review of the literature. *Child & Family Social Work, 12*, 94–101. doi:10.1111j.1365-2206.2006.00421.x

Neugarten, B. L., & Weinstein, K. (1964). The changing American grandparents. *Journal of Marriage and the Family, 26*, 199–204.

Orel, N. (2004, November). *Lesbian and bisexual women as grandmothers: The centrality of sexual orientation on the grandparent-grandchild relationship*. Paper presented at 57th Annual Scientific Meeting of Gerontological Society of America, Washington, DC.

Orel, N. (2006). Lesbian and bisexual women as grandparents: The centrality of sexual orientation on the grandparent-grandchild relationship. In D. Kimmel, T. Rose, & S. David (Eds.), *Lesbian, gay, bisexual, and transgender aging: Research and clinical perspectives* (pp. 248–274). New York, NY: Columbia University Press.

Orel, N., & Fruhauf, C. (2006). Lesbian and bisexual grandmothers' perceptions of the grandparent-grandchild relationship. *Journal of GLBT Family Studies, 2*, 42–70. doi:10.1300/j461v02n01_03

Orel, N., Fruhauf, C., Bigner, J., & Jenkins, D. (2006, November). *Lesbian, gay, and bisexual grandparents: Overcoming societal obstacles*. Paper presented at 59th Annual Scientific Meeting of the Gerontological Society of America, Dallas, TX.

Patterson, C. J. (1992). Children of lesbian and gay parents. *Child Development, 63*, 1025–1042.

Patterson, S. (2005a). This is so you know you have options: Lesbian grandmothers and the mixed legacies of nonconformity. *Journal of the Association for Research on Mothering, 7*(2), 38–48.

Patterson, S. (2005b). Better one's own path: The experiences of lesbian grandmothers in Canada. *Canadian Woman Studies, 24*, 118–122.

Paul, P. (2002). Make room for granddaddy. *American Demographics, 24*, 1–6.

Perlesz, A., Brown, R., Lindsay, J., McNair, R. De, Vaus, D., & Pitts, M. (2006). Families in transition: Parents, children and grandparents in lesbian families give meaning to 'doing family'. *Journal of Family Therapy, 28*, 175–199.

Roberto, K. A., Allen, K. R., & Blieszner, R. (2001). Grandfather's perceptions and expectations of relationships with their adult grandchildren. *Journal of Family Issues, 22*, 407–426.

Savin-Williams, R. C. (2001). *Mom, dad, I'm gay: How families negotiate coming out*. Washington, DC: American Psychological Association.

Savin-Williams, R. C., & Esterberg, K. C. (2000). Lesbian, gay, and bisexual families. In D. Demo, K. Allen, & M. Fine (Eds.), *Handbook of family diversity* (pp. 197–215). New York, NY: Oxford University Press.

Seidman, S. (2002). *Beyond the closet: The transformation of gay and lesbian life*. New York, NY: Routledge.

Sevda, B., & Herrera, D. (1998). *Women in love: Portraits of lesbian mothers and their families*. New York, NY: Bullfinch.

Shrestha, L. B., & Heisler, E. J. (2011, March). *The changing demographic profile of the United States* (Report No. 7–5700). Washington, DC: Congressional Research Service.

Silverstein, M., & Marenco, A. (2001). How Americans enact the grandparent role across the family life course. *Journal of Family Issues, 22*, 493–522. doi:10.1177/019251301022004006

Smith, P. K., & Drew, L. (2002). Grandparenthood. In M. Bernstein (Ed.), *Handbook of parenting, Vol. 3: Being and becoming a parent* (2nd ed., pp. 141–172). Mahwah, NJ: Lawrence Erlbaum Associates.

Stelle, C., Fruhauf, C., Orel, N., & Landry-Meyer, L. (2010). Grandparenting in the 21st century: Issues of diversity in grandparent-grandchild relationships. *Journal of Gerontological Social Work, 53*, 682–701. doi:10.1080/01634372.2010.516804

Szinovacz, M. E. (Ed.). (1998). *Handbook on grandparenthood*. Westport, CT: Greenwood Press.

Tasker, F., & Patterson, C. J. (2007). Research on gay and lesbian parenting: Retrospect and prospect. *Journal of GLBT Family Studies, 3*(2/3), 9–34.

Thomas, J. L. (1995). Gender and perceptions of grandparenthood. In J. Hendricks (Ed.), *The ties of later life* (pp. 181–193). Amityville, NY: Baywood.

Tootelian, D., & Varshney, S. B. (2010). The grandparent consumer: A financial "goldmine" with gray hair? *Journal of Consumer Marketing, 27*(1), 57–63. doi:10.1108/07363761011012958

U.S. News and World Report (2011, July). *The American grandparent: 3 in 10 adults in the U.S. have grandkids*. Retrieved from http://www.usnews.com/opinion/articles/2009/04/22/the-american-grandparent-3-in-10-adults-in-the-us-have-grandkids

Van Hentig, H. (1946). The social function of the grandmother. *Social Forces, 24*, 389–392.

Vollmer, H. (1937). The grandmother: A problem in child-drearing. *American Journal of Orthopsychiatry, 7*, 378–382. doi:10.1111/j.1939-0025.1937.tb06371.x

Walker, K., & Walker, J. (1995). Still family after all these years. In K. Arnup (Ed.), *Lesbian parenting: Living with pride and prejudice* (pp. 160–166). Toronto, ON: Canadian Scholars' Press and Women's Press.

Walsh, F. (1989). The family in later life. In B. Carter & M. McGoldrick (Eds.), *The changing family life cycle* (2nd ed., pp. 311–332). Boston, MA: Allyn and Bacon.

Whalen, D., Bigner, J., & Barber, C. (2000). The grandmother role as experienced by lesbian women. *Journal of Women and Aging, 12,* 39–57. doi:10.1300/j074v12n03_04

Whitbeck, L. B., Hoyt, D. R., & Huck, S. M. (1993). Family relationship history, contemporary parent-grandparent relationship quality, and the grandparent-grandchild relationship. *Journal of Marriage and Family, 55,* 1025–1035. doi:10.2307/352782

Williams Institute. (2011). *New research answers question: How many LGBT people are there in the United States?* Los Angeles, CA: Author. Press Release.

Ramona Faith Oswald and Elizabeth Grace Holman

Place Matters: LGB Families in Community Context

Lesbian, gay, and bisexual (LGB) individuals and their families are often presumed to live in urban "gay Meccas" rather than nonmetropolitan and more rural parts of the USA (Oswald & Culton, 2003). However, this urban stereotype is simply not true, particularly for LGB-parented families (Gates & Ost, 2004). LGB parents and their children live in a diversity of community settings, and these communities vary in their levels of support for LGB families. The purpose of this chapter is to document what is known about how the daily lives of LGB families are differentially impacted by where they live. Furthermore, we will discuss how communities can change to be more LGB affirming.

Geographical Diversity of LGB Families

In this chapter, the term "community" is used in two ways. First, "residential community" refers to the municipalities or unincorporated places where

R.F. Oswald, Ph.D. (✉) • E.G. Holman, M.S., M.S.W.
Department of Human and Community Development,
University of Illinois at Urbana-Champaign,
263 Bevier Hall, MC-180, 905 South Goodwin Avenue,
Urbana, IL 61801, USA
e-mail: roswald@illinois.edu; eholman@illinois.edu

LGB families live. Residential communities vary by degree of rurality/urbanicity and are nested within counties and states. Second, "LGB community" refers to the configuration of LGB organizations and social networks that exist in a specific place and that promote a sexual minority group identity as well as LGB-affirming values (Lockard, 1985). Our place-based approach is distinct from those who define communities as face-to-face and virtual social networks (e.g., Wellman, 2002). This is because we are concerned with linking LGB families to social conditions that are specific to particular places.

Same-sex couples with children tend to live in places with relatively low concentrations of same-sex couples and relatively high concentrations of households with children (Gates & Ost, 2004). For example, the east southcentral region of the USA (Alabama, Kentucky, Mississippi, and Tennessee) has the highest proportion of same-sex couple households with children (Gary Gates, personal communication, January 20, 2011; see also Tavernise, 2011). These states have lower numbers of same-sex couples than would be expected if the population was randomly distributed (Gates & Ost) and nationally average proportions of households with minor children (American Fact Finder, n.d.). Caution should be taken to avoid generalizing these trends to single-parent or polyamorous households, as U.S. Census data operationalizes LGB families as same-sex partner households with minor children. Germane to this chapter is the implication that LGB families live in places that may lack

LGB communities and/or that may lack public support for sexual minorities. For example, Mississippi has the highest rate of same-sex partner households with children (41.3% of all same-sex households) but the lowest gay/lesbian supportive laws ranking (shared with three other states) (Gates & Ost).

The existence of local LGB communities may partly depend upon the degree to which a place is urbanized. Urbanization refers to population density [urban areas have at least 1,000 people per square mile; Economic Research Service (ERS, 2007)] and is correlated with greater civic and economic infrastructure. Because less urban areas have fewer people and resources, it may be more difficult to sustain a local LGB community. For example, Oswald and Culton (2003) found that LGB life in central and southern Illinois tends to be organized around informal social networks that typically do not own, rent, or otherwise control actual physical meeting spaces or other cultural centers and are thus dependent upon permission to borrow space from others. The relatively private nature of these groups makes them difficult to enter; you may have to know someone who knows someone. Further, they can be difficult to maintain given conflicting personalities, interests, and geographical dispersion of members (Oswald & Culton). For example, members of three different LGB-parenting groups in this region struggled with the fact that being an LGB parent was not reason enough for members to travel far distances to meetings, or overcome personal and social class differences among parents and cohort differences among children (Holman & Oswald, 2011). These nonmetropolitan constraints contrast with highly urbanized places such as New York City, where the LGB Community Center has paid staff responsible for family programming, which includes at least monthly social events in addition to support groups and other services (http://www.gaycenter.org/families). If an LGB person in New York City felt that this Center did not meet his or her needs, numerous other local supports could be pursued. We do not suggest that formal supports are more important than informal ones, nor do we discount the empowerment and solidarity that can come from organizing rather than simply accessing

services (see Russell, Bohan, McCarroll, & Smith, 2010). Further, we recognize the importance of online resources for LGB families (Lev, Dean, De Filippis, McLaughlin, & Phillips, 2005). Our point is that LGB families in less urbanized communities may find it more difficult to access locally available LGB-affirming supports.

Researchers should avoid presuming that LGB families are involved with a local LGB community. Indeed, Gates and Ost (2004) estimate that one in four same-sex partner households with children live in communities without other same-sex couples. When a local LGB community is accessible, however, then it can play an important role in providing support (McLaren, 2009; McLaren, Jude, & McLachlan, 2008; Oswald & Culton, 2003). For example, LGB people who are "coming out" find important validation through identifying and involving themselves in activities with other LGB people (Rosario, Hunter, Maguen, Gwadz, & Smith, 2001). Further, children with lesbian mothers have been found to cope with stigma more effectively when they have contact with other children who have lesbian mothers, and when their mothers are in contact with other lesbians (Bos, Gartrell, Peyser, & van Balen, 2008).

Researchers should also consider gender, race, and class differences among LGB-parented families and how they relate to where these families live. For example, analyses using 2000 Census data indicate that female same-sex partner households are more likely than male same-sex partner households to include minor children (Baumle, Compton, & Poston, 2009). Further, although both female and male same-sex partner households are concentrated in similar areas, males seem to prefer locations that might be considered "gay identified" (e.g., San Francisco) whereas the national distribution of female households is more dispersed (Baumle et al.). Although these data are limited by their inclusion of only self-reported same-sex partner households, the findings suggest that the location of female households is less segregated by sexual orientation than that of male households. Baumle et al. surmise that this gender difference is due to economic and family considerations: Because female households are more likely to have children while also having lower incomes, female same-sex couples have less residential choice and more interest in child-related amenities found outside of gay enclaves. One implication of this is that single and partnered lesbian and bisexual female-headed families may be less visible as "LGB families" to members of their residential communities; others may perceive them as "mothers" more than as sexual minority women (see Sullivan, 2004). This may be especially true in residential communities where mothering outside of heterosexual marriage is normative. Gay and bisexual fathers, on the other hand, may be more visible because they are primary caregivers of children and therefore may be read by others as gender transgressive (Berkowitz, 2008). Being seen in this way could lead to gay and bisexual fathers either being overpraised for their father involvement, or stigmatized for violating masculinity norms.

Analyses using 2000 Census data have also documented racial differences among same-sex partner households. First, African-American, Hispanic/Latino, and Asian-American same-sex partner households tend to be located in areas with high concentrations of racially similar households. For example, African-American same-sex partner households are most concentrated in the south (Dang & Frazer, 2005), and Hispanic/Latino same-sex partner households are most concentrated in the southwest (Cianciotto, 2005). Second, racial minority same-sex partner households are more likely than their White counterparts to include minor children (Asian American Federation of New York, 2004; Cianciotto; Dang & Frazer). Third, although most children in these families are the offspring of one partner, those in African-American same-sex partner households are more likely than their counterparts in White households to be adopted, fostered, grandchildren, nieces, or nephews (Dang & Frazer). More research on ethnic minority LGB families is needed (Bennett & Battle, 2001), and this research should attend to differences related to living within a racial majority or racial minority context. The experience, for example, of an African American lesbian couple raising children in Burlington, VT (where 1% of the same-sex couples households include at least one African-American partner and 25% have children; Gates & Ost, 2004), is surely different than a similar couple raising children in Pine Bluff, AR where the majority of same-sex couples are African-American and presumably most are parents (Dang & Frazer).

There are also social class differences among same-sex partner households that intersect with gender and race. Again according to analyses using Census 2000 data, same-sex partner households are stratified such that male households have higher incomes than female (O'Connell & Lofquist, 2009). White couple households earn more than racial minority households (Asian American Federation of New York, 2004; Cianciotto, 2005; Dang & Frazer, 2005), and urban households earn more than rural (Albelda, Badgett, Gates, & Schneebaum, 2009). Furthermore, compared to heterosexually married couple households with children, both male and female same-sex partner households with children are more likely to live in poverty (Prokos & Keene, 2010). With the exception of higher poverty among LGB parents and their children, the above-mentioned economic trends mirror those for the general US population (ERS, 2004; Wheaton & Tashi, 2004).

Situating LGB families in community context encourages examination of family member attachments to their local communities. Residential place attachment is the sense that one belongs to, and is invested in, where one lives (Altman & Low, 1992), and it is associated with greater psychological well-being (McLaren, 2009; McLaren et al., 2008). Oswald and Lazarevic's (2011) study of 77 lesbian mothers living in nonmetropolitan Illinois found that they were more attached to their residential communities when they were in more frequent contact with their families of origin, when there was a local LGB organization, and when the mothers were less religious. These findings imply that place attachment is related to a local integration of both family of origin and the LGB community. Given the prevalence of religiously based anti-LGB sentiment in the region studied by Oswald and Lazarevic, it may be that less religious mothers are more immune to the effects of local religious hostility. Levels and predictors of attachment may vary in other LGB subpopulations, however. For example, lesbians and gay men have higher rates of residential migration than the general population, and this is associated with higher educational attainment (Baumle et al., 2009). It follows that more mobile LGB parents and their children may experience lower place attachment, and this may have effects on the quality of their family and community relationships. For example, a lesbian mother in Holman and Oswald's (2011) qualitative research on LGB families in nonmetropolitan contexts reported that she and her family were rejected by local church members, not because they were lesbians with children, but because the congregation did not like outsiders.

Future research should attend to how LGB parents negotiate visibility within their residential contexts. For example, Holman and Oswald (2011) interviewed a rural lesbian couple where one partner presented as more masculine. They reported being perceived by others as a husband and wife with children. In fact, the more feminine partner conducted all checkbook transactions in local businesses so that the more masculine partner would not be asked to produce identification. A different participant in the same study described how the fact that she was a single White mother with an African-American child meant that (a) people assumed she was heterosexual because she did not have a female partner and (b) issues of race were far more salient than sexuality when negotiating public spaces (see also Goldberg, 2009).

In sum, contextual research on LGB families should attend to complexities of geography, gender, race, class, place attachment, and visibility. The intersectionality approach (De Reus, Few, & Blume, 2005) that we are advocating will move the field toward an understanding of LGB diversity that is produced through both social structure and individual subjectivity.

Residential Community Climate

In addition to identifying residential and LGB trends related to geographical location and diversity, situating LGB families in community context requires us to theorize the link between macro and micro levels. For this we expand upon Meyer's (2003) minority stress theory that identifies minority stress processes (e.g., anti-LGB victimization, expectations of rejection, closeting, internalized homophobia) as the mechanisms through which health disparities (e.g., higher depression rates among sexual minorities) occur. In Meyer's model, the link between minority stress processes and outcomes is moderated by social support, coping, and LGB identity salience, integration, and valence. Minority stress processes are made possible by "general environmental circumstances" (p. 678). Meyer briefly describes these circumstances as macrosocial inequalities that lead to minority statuses and identities, but does not further develop the construct.

We expand upon Meyer's (2003) model by operationalizing circumstances in the environment as "residential community climate." Community climate is defined as the level of support for sexual minorities within a residential community (Oswald, Cuthbertson, Lazarevic, & Goldberg, 2010). This level of support is manifest within both distal and proximal institutions, norms, and social networks. Distal community manifestations of climate include the state and municipal legal codes, political affiliations, economic and social service infrastructure, and religious/moral tone. More proximal manifestations include workplaces, schools, healthcare settings, religious congregations, political activism, and friendship networks. The climate that is apparent within these institutions, norms, and networks allows or inhibits minority stress processes, which leads to outcomes for LGB individuals and their families.

Research provides support for our hypothesis that community climate enables minority stress processes, specifically perceived stigma. For example, the majority of Herek's (2009) nationally representative LGB sample ($N=662$) partly or fully believed that "most people where I live think less of a person who is LGB." The same endorsement pattern was found for "most people where I live would not want someone who is openly LGB to take care of their children." Research also links perceived stigma to the behavior of lesbian mothers and their children. For example, a study from the Netherlands found that mothers who reported higher levels of stigmatizing interactions within their communities were more likely to say that they felt they had to defend their position as a mother, and were more likely to report that their children had behavior problems (Bos, van Balen, van den Boom, & Sandfort, 2004).

In addition to research on perceived stigma, there is a growing body of evidence demonstrating that elements of community climate promote or inhibit the health and well-being of LGB individuals and their families as specified by minority stress theory (Meyer, 2003). Below we briefly describe different elements of community climate and then summarize and evaluate the research showing that it has an effect on LGB people and their loved ones. Much of this research uses samples of LGB adults and not specifically parents or their children. These distinctions are highlighted throughout so it is clear when we are extrapolating to LGB families.

Legal Climate

Residential communities vary in the legal rights and protections that they provide to LGB individuals and their families (Oswald & Kuvalanka, 2008). For instance, state and/or local laws may be in place to protect LGB people from discrimination in housing, employment, credit, public accommodation, and in educational settings. Further, state laws may provide or deny rights to LGB adults regarding marriage, adoption, fosterage, custody, and visitation. For example, if you live in Iowa, you are protected from discrimination on the basis of both sexual orientation and gender identity/expression [National Gay and Lesbian Task Force (NGLTF, 2009a)]. If you are criminally victimized for being LGB, Iowa can prosecute under their hate crimes statute (NGLTF, 2009b). Same-sex couples are allowed to marry in Iowa (NGLTF, 2010). If someone is abused by the same-sex dating partner, spouse, or roommate in Iowa, he/she is protected under the state's domestic violence laws (NGLTF, 2005).

Furthermore, Iowa allows LGB individuals and same-sex couples to adopt (including second-parent adoptions; NGLTF, 2008a, 2008b) and foster children (NGLTF, 2009c).

By contrast, compare Iowa to the adjacent state of Nebraska. Nebraska allows discrimination in housing, employment, credit, and public accommodation on the basis of sexual orientation (NGLTF, 2009a), but includes sexual orientation as a protected category in their hate crimes statute (NGLTF, 2009b). Regarding couple relationships, Nebraska has a constitutional amendment that bans not only marriage for same-sex couples but also any recognition of domestic partnerships or civil unions (NGLTF, 2009d). Despite the lack of same-sex relationship rights in Nebraska, victims of same-sex domestic violence are afforded the same rights and protections as heterosexual victims (NGLTF, 2005). Regarding parenting, Nebraska bans LGB individuals and same-sex couples from adopting or fostering children (NGLTF, 2008b, 2009c), including second-parent adoption (NGLTF, 2008a). This comparison illustrates the profound differences in legal climate that can be experienced simply by crossing from one state into another. In Iowa, LGB families are fully recognized. In Nebraska, LGB families are denied and the citizenship of LGB individuals is only recognized if they report criminal victimization. Thus, the legal climate for LGB families varies dramatically across the USA.

Legal Climate Outcomes

The denial of legal recognition or protection has a deleterious effect on LGB individuals' mental health, as well as the relationship quality within couples and families. The strongest empirical evidence for this claim comes from three longitudinal studies; supporting evidence can also be found in a body of cross-sectional research.

The first longitudinal study (Hatzenbuehler, McLaughlin, Keyes, & Hasin, 2010) used two waves of the population-based National Epidemiologic Survey on Alcohol and Related Conditions to examine whether institutional discrimination led to increased psychiatric disorders among 577 LGB adults (parental status not specified); 34,076 heterosexual respondents were used as a comparison group. They found that in states that passed constitutional amendments banning same-sex marriage, the mood disorder symptoms of LGB respondents rose by more than 30% from T1 (preelection) to T2 (postelection), but decreased more than 20% among LGB respondents living in states without such laws. Furthermore, generalized anxiety disorder increased more than 200% among LGB respondents living in states that implemented amendments; no significant change was found for those living in states without amendments. Comorbidity (the co-occurrence of two or more disorders) also significantly increased for those living in amendment states. Heterosexual respondents living in states with amendments did not have an increase in mood disorders; when heterosexuals living in these states did report an increase in a specific disorder (e.g., generalized anxiety) then the magnitude of change was much smaller than that evidenced by the LGB group (61% vs. 248%, respectively).

Rostosky, Riggle, Horne, and Miller (2009) also conducted a longitudinal study of this election. Despite the limitation of using a nonrepresentative Internet-based convenience sample ($N = 1,552$), they also found increased depressive symptoms, stress, and negative affect among LGB adults after the election. A limitation of both of these studies is that neither examined minority stress processes as mediators linking the election to mental health symptoms. Further, these studies did not control for parental status. These weaknesses are improved upon in the third longitudinal study described below.

In a study that explicitly tested how legal context impacts LGB parents, Goldberg and Smith (2011) examined the effects of both stigma and social support on depression and anxiety symptoms among 52 lesbian and 38 gay couples over a 1-year transition to adoptive parenthood. Data were collected from each partner at three time points: pre-adoption (T1), several months' post-adoptive placement (T2), and 1 year post-placement (T3). The authors found that depression significantly increased from T1 to T3, and this change was predicted by an interaction between state legal climate and internalized homophobia. Specifically, lesbian and gay adoptive parents who reported low levels of internalized homophobia at T1 showed little change in their depressive symptoms regardless of their state's legal climate for adoption. Strikingly though, lesbian and gay adoptive parents who reported high levels of internalized homophobia at T1 showed a significant increase in depressive symptoms at T3 when they lived in a state with a negative legal climate, and a significant decrease from T1 to T3 when their state was more legally supportive. A similar pattern was found for anxiety: All participants reported an increase in anxiety over time, but the change was significant only among those with both high levels of internalized homophobia and a less supportive legal climate. This study suggests that living in a hostile legal context increases both depression and anxiety among LGB parents, especially if the parents struggle with internalized homophobia.

Complementing these longitudinal studies, cross-sectional research (using geographically dispersed but predominately White, middle-class samples) has found that legal rights and protections are beneficial for LGB individuals, couples, and families. Specifically, LGB adults with a legally recognized same-sex relationship reported fewer depressive symptoms and stress, and higher well-being, compared to those in committed but nonlegal relationships (Riggle, Rostosky, & Horne, 2010). In a qualitative study of married same-sex couples in Massachusetts, Shecter, Tracy, Page, and Luong (2008) found that marriage was described by participants as bringing increased couple commitment, acknowledgment of their relationship from family and colleagues, a sense of societal legitimacy, and a reduction of homophobia within self and others. Also, Canadian lesbian mothers (who were defined by the authors as living in a nonheterosexist legal context because they have full legal rights under Canadian law) were found to have significantly fewer stigma-related worries than their American counterparts (Shapiro, Peterson, & Stewart, 2009). Furthermore, the presence of nondiscrimination laws has been associated with higher levels of disclosure and social support, and lower levels of internalized homophobia, among LGB individuals (Riggle et al., 2010; see also Hatzenbuehler, Keyes, & Hasin, 2009).

In sum, research is beginning to document a link between legal climate and the health and well-being of LGB people and their families. Although the strongest evidence comes from longitudinal research, these studies were short term and therefore we do not know the long-term effects of legal climate on LGB individuals or their families. Both qualitative and quantitative designs could be used in long-term longitudinal research. Further, with one exception (Goldberg & Smith, 2011), evidence is limited by the lack of attention to minority stress processes. When measured (e.g., internalized homophobia in Riggle et al., 2010), these variables are treated as outcomes rather than linking mechanisms.

Political Climate

The legal climate in a given residential community interacts with the political climate. Indeed, political processes are the vehicle for legislative decisions, and communities with more conservative-leaning residents are likely to be less supportive of LGB families. For example, people with more conservative values are less likely to support LGB rights (Wood & Bartkowski, 2004), and more likely to have negative attitudes toward LGB people (Herek, 2002).

Local political climates are also influenced by the local racial and economic composition. Latino communities, for example, tend to highly stigmatize homosexuality (Marín, 2003), perhaps due to a strong support for traditional gender roles (Herek & Gonzalez-Rivera, 2006). African-Americans are also more likely than Whites to condemn homosexuality as immoral, but at the same time, are more likely than Whites to support gay rights (Lewis, 2003). Increased education, a privilege of the middle and upper classes, also seems to lead to more liberal political attitudes and acceptance of gay rights (Ellison & Musick, 1993).

Political Climate Outcomes

Rostosky, Riggle, Horne, Denton, and Huellemeier's (2010) content analysis of open-ended responses from 300 LGB adults (72 of whom were parents) to a national online survey found that state-level anti-gay politics had a negative psychological impact on LGB adults regardless of whether or not the respondents lived in states that had amendments banning same-sex marriage. Other studies, however, suggest that the salience of political climate may be heightened when gay rights are on the local ballot. For example, an online survey of 2,511 LGB adults found that those who lived in states considering a constitutional amendment to ban same-sex marriage were exposed to higher levels of messages regarding gay rights (Riggle, Rostosky, & Horne, 2009).

Local political activism that flows from the political climate can have both negative and positive effects on LGB individuals and their families. Regarding negative effects, Russell and Richards (2003) surveyed 316 LGB adults involved in the fight against Colorado's Amendment Two (see Romer v. Evans, 1996). These participants reported stressors that they believed were the result of the Amendment Two battle, including encountering homophobia from a multitude of sources, perceiving divisions within the local LGB community, managing a sense of danger, failed witnessing (others do not believe your experience), and internalized homophobia. Although the parental status of these respondents was not documented, it is reasonable to infer that these stressors would make the daily hassles of parenting more difficult, thereby impacting parent–child relationships. For example, in the Riggle et al. (2009) study of the impact on LGB individuals when same-sex marriage amendments are on the state's ballot, LGB parents expressed worry about protecting their children from harm. Also, it is possible that children during the Amendment Two battle in Colorado (or any other LGB-rights struggle) were aware of the conflict, which could lead them to worry about the safety and legitimacy of their families. Extended family members also may be negatively impacted. For example, Arm, Horne and Leavitt (2009) interviewed 10 relatives of

LGB people regarding their experience of anti-LGB politics and found that relatives were distressed when they realized that such politics were having an effect on their loved ones and frustrated when people they expected to be supportive of gay rights were not. These studies lend support to the notion that anti-LGB political activism impacts not only LGB adults but their children and extended family members as well.

Positive effects of LGB activism also have been documented. Civic engagement has been associated with higher global and psychological health (Lindstrom, 2004), and thus participating in the struggle for LGB rights may strengthen individuals and families. In fact, LGB adults who lived in states with an anti-same-sex marriage amendment on the ballot in 2006 were more involved in LGB activism, and voted in the 2006 election at higher levels, than those who lived in other states (Riggle et al., 2009). Although Riggle and colleagues did not link civic involvement with psychological or social outcomes, evidence for this link can be found in the Russell and Richards (2003) study of LGB adults involved in the Amendment Two battle. As a result of their engagement, these respondents developed a point of view whereby they linked their personal struggles as LGB individuals to the larger political struggles represented by Amendment Two. Furthermore, they increased their LGB community involvement, developed the confidence to confront others' anti-gay attitudes, and provided emotional support to fellow activists. These changes suggest improved social and psychological well-being, which may translate into more positive relationships with children or other family members. In Arm et al. (2009), relatives of LGB adults who were involved in LGB activism reported reconfiguring their social networks to increase support. Also, Short's (2007) qualitative study of 68 lesbian mothers showed that involvement in activism helped them cope with homophobia and heterosexism.

Religious Climate

The local religious tone contributes to the overall climate for sexual minorities in itself, and also by interacting with legal and political systems (Oswald et al., 2010). Most religious denominations have an official stance toward the morality of same-sex desire and behavior, and the legitimacy of LGB identities (Siker, 2007). The official theological stance of a denomination regarding homosexuality may not be shared by all congregations or adherents (e.g., the Baptist Peace Fellowship of North America is LGB affirming; Baptist Peace Fellowship, 2010), but it does shape what is said and done within religious organizations as well as other community settings in which adherents are involved (Yip, 1997). Thus, variations in religious climate are important to understand.

Of the 149 denominations counted in the American Religious Identification Survey (the decennial census of American religious life), only 6 are officially and unambiguously affirming of LGB people: Episcopalian, Metropolitan Community Church (MCC), Reform Judaism, Unitarian-Universalist, Quaker, and United Church of Christ (Oswald et al., 2010). Nationwide, these affirming denominations account for 6% of all congregations (16,684 of 268,240) and 41% of all religious adherents in the USA (5,755,258 of 141,364,420) [Association of Religion Data Archives (ARDA, 2000a); Reform Judaism estimated at 25% of Jewish aggregate].

Where an LGB family resides partly determines their access to religious affirmation. For example, LGB-affirming adherents are most likely to live in the northeast (ARDA, 2000b). The northeast also has a high concentration of states that provide legal recognition for same-sex couples and LGB parenting; this may reflect an intersection between the religious, legal, and political climates. Also notable is that fact that MCC adherents are most likely found in Washington, DC, Texas, Florida, Colorado, and Nevada (ARDA, 2000b). Texas and Florida are ranked 1 and 5, respectively, in total number of evangelical congregations (ARDA, 2000c). Further, Washington, DC has a majority African-American population (McKinnon, 2001) and no African-American denomination is officially affirming of LGB people (Siker, 2007). The high number of MCC adherents in these locales may reflect the fact that LGB people living in these places were raised religious and are seeking religious affirmation as adults. Although the MCC is classified as mainline Protestant, it promotes church independence and worship styles that vary widely across congregations. Thus, members may be finding a worship style that fits their upbringing. Colorado and Nevada are more difficult to explain. However, the Fort Collins, Colorado MCC was founded in 1992 (MCC Family in Christ, 2010), the same year that Amendment Two passed, further suggesting links among religious, legal, and political climate.

Religious Climate Outcomes

LGB individuals are affected by religious messages regarding homosexuality (Rodriguez, 2010), especially if they consider themselves to be highly religious and/or identify with a particular denomination (Oswald, 2001). One study ($N=90$ same-sex couples) found that this perception compromised participants' ability to practice their religion (Rostosky, Otis, Riggle, Brumett, & Brodnicki, 2008). In another LGB survey sample, nearly two-thirds (42 of 66) of participants reported conflict between their religion and sexual identity and, as a result, reported feeling depressed, judged by their congregation, and ashamed of their sexual orientation (Schuck & Liddle, 2001).

Being faced with religious hostility can also motivate LGB people to organize within their denominations to promote LGB-affirming change (Comstock, 1993). Affirming congregations can serve as resources and as a source of empowerment for LGB individuals by including them in their services and providing a place to belong (Rodriguez, 2010). A study of 82 Midwestern LGB adults indicated that one's sense of support from a religious group was related to higher levels of self-esteem in individuals who were religiously oriented (Yakushko, 2005).

Although there are no studies that directly examine the religious involvement of LGB parents and their children, or religious climate effects on these families, it is clear that religion is important to some LGB parents. For example, in Oswald, Goldberg, Kuvalanka, and Clausell's

(2008) study of relationship commitment among same-sex couples ($N=190$), highly religious parents were the most likely respondents to have both legalized and ritualized their relationship. Further, qualitative research on children raised by LGB parents describes their struggles with other people's religious-based hatred for their parents (Goldberg, 2007).

Workplace Climate

The economic structure of a given residential community influences community climate through workplace climate. For example, Florida (2002) found that communities with more jobs in the "creative" and/or "bohemian" sectors (i.e., professional fields with a focus on knowledge production, diversity, creativity, and the arts) had higher rates of same-sex couples in residence. A different study (Klawitter & Flatt, 1998) found that communities with higher rates of same-sex couples in residence were also communities with more employers who include sexual orientation in their nondiscrimination policies. This link between economic sector, workplace climate, and density of same-sex partner households is theorized to occur because employers and community leaders see their economic future as dependent upon being able to attract top workers regardless of sexual orientation, and therefore invest in creating LGB-affirming workplaces and communities (Florida, 2010; Florida & Gates, 2002).

Creative and bohemian class employment is not evenly distributed across the USA (Florida, 2010). Even if it were, only about a third of US workers are employed in these sectors (Florida). Further, employment discrimination on the basis of sexual orientation is legal in 30 states [Human Rights Campaign (HRC, 2008)]. However, the majority (66%) of Fortune 1,000 companies that are headquartered in states that allow discrimination do in fact have workplace policies prohibiting discrimination and/or providing domestic partner benefits (HRC, 2008). For example, Texas allows sexual orientation discrimination, but is also home to 113 Fortune 1,000 companies, most of which (65%) have company policies forbidding discrimination

(HRC). These company policies have been found to have a greater effect than state or municipal laws on employee perceptions of workplace climate (Ragins & Cornwell, 2001). Thus, even though Texas bans state-level recognition of same-sex couples (NGLTF, 2009a), those couples may access support and benefits through their workplace and may feel that their employer is affirming. Situating LGB families in community context requires attention to the locally available workplace climates, benefits, and protections.

Workplace Climate Outcomes

Research on LGB adult workers has found a link between workplace climate and well-being. For example, a survey of 379 gays and lesbians found that a company's written nondiscrimination policies contributed to less job discrimination and more accepting coworkers; this more supportive climate was in turn related to increased job satisfaction (Griffith & Hebl, 2002). Workplace nondiscrimination policies have also been associated with higher disclosure of sexual orientation at work (Rostosky & Riggle, 2002), more positive relationships with supervisors, and increased organizational citizenship behaviors (Tejeda, 2006), and decreased levels of perceived discrimination (Ragins & Cornwell, 2001). Additionally, a positive association has been found between workplace heterosexism—the frequency of experiencing certain behaviors, such as being called a derogatory term in reference to one's sexual orientation—and depression (as measured by the Center for Epidemiologic Studies Depression Scale CES-D) among LGB employees (Smith & Ingram, 2004). In sum, workplace policies that affirm the existence of LGB employees communicate a message of acceptance and belonging that lead to more optimal outcomes (Button, 2001). A limitation of these studies is that they rely heavily on professional samples and do not include job type as a variable in their analyses.

School Climate

Given the fact that school-age children spend the majority of their waking hours in educational and extracurricular settings, and that LGB parents are involved in PTAs and other school affairs (Kosciw & Diaz, 2008), the supportiveness of a given classroom, school, or district surely impacts the quality of life for LGB families. Anti-LGB bullying and harassment are significant problems in US schools. For example, a national survey of middle and high school-aged children with LGB parents ($N=154$) and LGB parents with school-aged children ($N=558$) found that many students reported being mistreated by peers and staff; for example, some students recalled being reprimanded after disclosing their family structure or excluded from school events or class projects because they have an LGB parent (Kosciw & Diaz). Another report from the Gay, Lesbian, Straight Education Network (GLSEN, 2001) that surveyed LGBTQ students indicated that 83% reported verbal assault, 68% felt unsafe in their schools, and 41% were pushed or shoved.

School Climate Outcomes

Stigmatizing experiences at school have a negative effect on children's psychological health (Bos et al., 2008). Furthermore, although a homophobic school climate may not deter parents from being involved, it has been found to increase parental discomfort when attending parent–teacher meetings (Kosciw & Diaz, 2008). Similarly, a qualitative Australian study examining interactions between schools and lesbian-parented families found that mothers and children were more private when they perceived the school climate as more homophobic, and more "out and proud" when the school climate was affirming (Lindsay et al., 2006). When the family's approach did not match the school climate, parental discomfort prompted parents to either change their disclosure strategy (e.g., become more private) or actively challenge school policies (not always successfully).[1] Although the Lindsay et al. study was based upon a small nonrepresentative sample, it suggests that parents who are

---

[1] In a different publication, this research team reported parallel results for lesbian mothers' interactions with healthcare providers (McNair et al., 2008).

uncomfortable, and thus more private about their family situation, may not speak openly and honestly about their children, and may not be as effective in advocating for their children's needs. Parents who are vocal in their resistance to school homophobia may reap the benefits if they are successful, but they may also feel further ostracized if the school refuses to change.

Bos et al. (2008) found that children with lesbian mothers were more resilient in the face of stigma when they attended a school that included LGB issues in the curriculum. Unfortunately, LGB families do not necessarily have access to these schools. For example, in 2003 only 6% of public high schools in the USA (approximately 1,200) had a gay–straight alliance (GSA) (Fetner & Kush, 2008). The existence of GSAs appears to be linked to the general community climate. For example, in their national study using publically available data, Fetner and Kush found that GSAs were more likely to exist in urban or suburban schools serving more affluent communities (compared to rural or impoverished communities). The authors note that in less affluent school districts, all extracurricular activities suffer, including those that serve LGB individuals and families; perhaps too, smaller schools in more rural communities lack the critical mass to support specialized programming. A school was also more likely to adopt a GSA if there was another LGB organization visible in the community (Fetner & Kush), a resource often missing in rural communities. Furthermore, the 21 states which prohibit discrimination based on sexual orientation (see NGLTF, 2009a) had a higher percentage of schools with GSAs (Fetner & Kush, 2008).

Advocating for Community Change

As described above, residential contexts vary, and each aspect of a community's climate for sexual minorities can impact LGB parents and their families in significant ways. Religious affirmation, supportive legislation, a visible LGB community, and recognition and support from more proximal contexts such as schools and workplaces can all strengthen LGB families by promoting mental health and a sense of social inclusion. Conversely, a variety of studies that we have reviewed here demonstrate that LGB parents report increased depression, anxiety, stress, defensiveness, sense of vulnerability, and decreased support and disclosure in the face of negative contexts. A few studies that we reviewed also provided evidence that the children and relatives of LGB parents are also impacted by community climate.

Although most of the above discussed research examined the family–community interface at one time point, it is important to remember that communities change over time. Attitudes, beliefs, policies, and legislation are all variable. Illinois, for example, has a law forbidding the recognition of same-sex marriage (NGLTF, 2009d), and yet recently passed a civil union bill allowing same-sex couples to file for licenses (Huffington Post, 2011). Community support for LGB families reflects the successful mobilization of citizens who, over time, create community infrastructures that are LGB affirming. These movements stem from LGB individuals and their allies who experience stigma and discrimination and decide to resist and advocate for change. Thus, a negative community climate can contribute to empowerment when those affected mobilize themselves to make positive change. Indeed, the family members of LGB individuals in Horne, Rostosky, Riggle, and Martens' (2010) interview study were more likely to be political activists when they were more knowledgeable about, and affirming of, LGB personal and political struggles (see also Arm et al., 2009). Furthermore, LGB people confronted by hostile religious beliefs have organized to promote LGB-affirmation within their congregations and denominations (Comstock, 1993). LGB adults who lived in states that voted to constitutionally prohibit same-sex marriage in 2006 were more involved in LGB activism and more likely to vote in that election—despite concurrent reports of increased depression and stress (Riggle et al., 2009). In the fight against Amendment Two in Colorado, new structures were created, such as a safe schools coalition, and heterosexual allies became more active and visible (Russell et al., 2010).

Relying on negative pressure to stimulate organizing for change can, however, result in dissolution of the movement once success is achieved. In Colorado, for example, LGB community cohesion and mobilization fizzled after Amendment Two was struck down, probably because there was no longer an imminent threat against which to organize (Russell et al., 2010). Some LGB activists in Colorado considered it a success that the LGB community was less visible and that LGB concerns had been integrated into local non-LGB organizations. However, the reduced LGB community visibility and cohesion felt like a failing to people who valued having a sovereign LGB community (Russell et al.). This conundrum was also observed by Holman and Oswald (2011) in their qualitative study of how nonmetropolitan lesbian and gay parents negotiate sexual orientation in public settings. On the one hand, parents did not want their sexual orientation to matter; on the other hand, they wanted their children to have contact with other LGB families. This desire for both fitting in and being different made it difficult to organize LGB-specific resources.

Future Directions

The interaction between LGB families and their local communities is a new area of study; much of the literature reviewed in this chapter utilized adult nonparent samples and we inferred relevance to LGB families. Hence we encourage researchers to incorporate a community lens in their investigations of LGB-parented families. In particular we encourage studies that identify how community climate impacts children with LGB parents, and how communities can change to reduce the stigmatization of these families. Three community features that promote child well-being in the face of such stigma have been identified: (a) a visible presence of LGB-parented families so that they can be in touch with each other; (b) schools that include LGB issues in the curriculum or after school activities; and (c) the presence of a local LGB community that includes lesbian mothers (Van Gelderen, Gartrell, Bos, &

Hermanns, 2009). As the above discussion indicates, these resources are not available in all communities. What factors predict their existence, and how can they be developed and sustained?

In addition, given that LGB-affirming communities are good for LGB families, is it also true that this affirmation promotes heterosexual people's health and well-being, and/or the economic viability of residential communities? Hatzenbuehler et al. (2010) found that heterosexual people were psychologically unaffected by anti-gay politics; however, their analysis did not control for the degree to which heterosexual people identified with LGB political struggles. Research on the heterosexual family members of LGB people does suggest that learning to identify with LGB concerns promotes both individual and family well-being (Arm et al., 2009; see also Horne et al., 2010). In the community development realm, pro-LGB policies have been linked to community viability (Florida & Gates, 2002). Researchers should operationalize community climate as it changes over time and investigate the social and economic impact that increasing LGB affirmation has on families and communities in general, not just those that are LGB identified.

References

Albelda, R., Badgett, M.V. L., Gates, G., & Schneebaum, A. (2009). *Poverty in the lesbian, gay, and bisexual community*. UCLA: Williams Institute. Retrieved from http://www2.law.ucla.edu/williamsinstitute/pdf/LGBPovertyReport.pdf

Altman, I., & Low, S. (Eds.). (1992). *Place attachment*. New York, NY: Plenum.

American Fact Finder (n.d.). *Selected social characteristics in the United States: 2005–2009*. Retrieved from http://factfinder.census.gov/servlet/ADPTable?_bm=y&-geo_id=01000US&-qr_name=ACS_2009_5YR_G00_DP5YR2&-ds_name=ACS_2009_5YR_G00_&-_lang=en&-_sse=on

Arm, J. R., Horne, S. G., & Leavitt, H. M. (2009). Negotiating connection to GLBT experience: Family members' experience of anti-GLBT movements and policies. *Journal of Counseling Psychology, 56*, 82–96. doi:10.1037/a0012813

Asian American Federation of New York. (2004). *Asian Pacific American same-sex households: A census report on New York, San Francisco, and Los Angeles.*

New York: C. J. Huang Foundation. Retrieved from http://www.hawaii.edu/hivandaids/Asian_Pacific_Am_Same-Sex_Households__A_Census_Report_On_NY,_SF_LA.pdf

Association of Religion Data Archives. (2000a). *US membership report*. Retrieved from http://www.thearda.com/mapsReports/reports/US_2000.asp

Association of Religion Data Archives. (2000b). *American denominations: Profiles*. Retrieved from http://www.thearda.com/Denoms/Families/

Association of Religion Data Archives. (2000c). *Evangelical denominations: Total number of congregations (2000)*. Retrieved from http://www.thearda.com/mapsReports/maps/map.asp?state=101&variable=7

Baptist Peace Fellowship. (2010). *Statement on justice and sexual orientation*. Retrieved from http://www.bpfna.org/sxorient#Baptist_Peace_Fellowship_Statement_on_Justice_and_Sexual_Orientation

Baumle, A. K., Compton, D. R., & Poston, D. L. (2009). *Same-sex partners: The demography of sexual orientation*. New York: SUNY Press.

Bennett, M., & Battle, J. (2001). "We can see them but we can't hear them": LGBT members of African American families. In M. Bernstein & R. Reimann (Eds.), *Queer families queer politics: Challenging culture and the state* (pp. 53–67). New York: Columbia University Press.

Berkowitz, D. (2008, November). *Schools, parks, and playgrounds: Gay fathers negotiate public and private spaces*. Paper presented at the National Council on Family Relations in Little Rock, AK.

Bos, H. M. W., Gartrell, N. K., Peyser, H., & van Balen, F. (2008). The USA National Longitudinal Lesbian Family Study (NFFLS): Homophobia, psychological adjustment, and protective factors. *Journal of Lesbian Studies, 12*, 455–471. doi:10.1080/10894160802278630

Bos, H. M. W., van Balen, F., van den Boom, D. C., & Sandfort, T. G. M. (2004). Minority stress, experience of parenthood and child adjustment in lesbian families. *Journal of Reproductive and Infant Psychology, 22*, 291–304. doi:10.1080/02646830412331298350

Button, S. B. (2001). Organizational efforts to affirm sexual diversity: A cross-level examination. *Journal of Applied Psychology, 86*, 17–28. doi:10.1037/0021-9010.86.1.17

Cianciotto, J. (2005). *Hispanic and Latino same-sex households in the United States: A report from the 2000 Census*. Washington, D.C.: NGLTF Policy Institute and the National Latino/a Coalition for Justice. Retrieved from http://www.thetaskforce.org/downloads/reports/reports/HispanicLatinoHouseholdsUS.pdf

Comstock, G. D. (1993). *Gay theology without apology*. Cleveland, OH: Pilgrim Press.

Dang, A., & Frazer, S. (2005). *Black same-sex households in the United States (2nd edition): A report from the 2000 Census*. Washington, D.C.: NGLTF Policy Institute and the National Black Justice Coalition. Retrieved from http://www.thetaskforce.org/downloads/reports/reports/2000BlackSameSexHouseholds.pdf

De Reus, L. A., Few, A. L., & Blume, L. B. (2005). Multicultural and critical race feminisms: Theorizing families in the third wave. In V. L. Bengtson, A. C. Acock, K. R. Allen, P. Dilworth-Anderson, & D. M. Klein (Eds.), *Sourcebook of family theory and research* (pp. 447–460). Thousand Oaks, CA: Sage.

Economic Research Service (2007). *Measuring rurality: Urban influence codes*. United States Department of Agriculture. Retrieved from http://www.ers.usda.gov/Briefing/Rurality/UrbanInf/

Economic Research Service. (2004). *Rural America at a glance, 2004*. Retrieved from http://webarchives.cdlib.org/sw15d8pg7m/http://ers.usda.gov/publications/AIB793/AIB793_lowres.pdf

Ellison, C. G., & Musick, M. A. (1993). Southern intolerance: A fundamentalist effect? *Social Forces, 72*, 379–398. doi:10.2307/2579853

Fetner, T., & Kush, K. (2008). Gay-straight alliances in high schools: Social predictors of early adoption. *Youth and Society, 40*, 114–130. doi:10.1177/0044118X07308073

Florida, R. (2010, August 25). Where the creative jobs will be. *The Atlantic*. Retrieved from http://www.theatlantic.com/business/archive/2010/08/where-the-creative-class-jobs-will-be/61468/

Florida, R., & Gates, G. (2002). *Technology and tolerance: The importance of diversity to high-technology growth*. Washington, DC: The Brookings Institution.

Gates, G. J., & Ost, J. (2004). *The gay and lesbian atlas*. Washington, DC: The Urban Institute Press.

Gay, Lesbian, Straight Education Network. (2001). *National school climate survey*. New York: Author.

Goldberg, A. E. (2007). Talking about family: Disclosure practices of adults raised by lesbian, gay, and bisexual parents. *Journal of Family Issues, 28*, 100–131. doi:10.1177/0192513X06293606

Goldberg, A. E. (2009). Lesbian and heterosexual pre-adoptive couples' openness to transracial adoption. *American Journal of Orthopsychiatry, 79*, 103–117. doi:10.1037/a0015354

Goldberg, A. E., & Smith, J. Z. (2011). Stigma, social context, and mental health: lesbian and gay couples across the transition to adoptive parenthood. *Journal of Counseling Psychology, 58*, 139–150. doi:10.1037/a0021684

Griffith, K. H., & Hebl, M. R. (2002). The disclosure dilemma for gay men and lesbians: "Coming out" at work. *Journal of Applied Psychology, 87*, 1191–1199. doi:10.1037/0021-9010.87.6.1191

Hatzenbuehler, M. L., Keyes, K. M., & Hasin, D. S. (2009). State-level policies and psychiatric morbidity in lesbian, gay, and bisexual populations. *American Journal of Public Health, 99*, 2275–2281. doi:10.2105/AJPH.2008.153510

Hatzenbuehler, M. L., McLaughlin, K. A., Keyes, K. M., & Hasin, D. S. (2010). The impact of institutional discrimination on psychiatric disorders in lesbian, gay, and bisexual populations: A prospective study. *American Journal of Public Health, 100*, 452–459. doi:10.2105/AJPH.2009.168815

Herek, G. M. (2002). Heterosexuals' attitudes toward bisexual men and women in the United States. *Journal of Sex Research, 39*, 264–274. doi:10.1080/00224490209552150

Herek, G. M., & Gonzalez-Rivera, M. (2006). Attitudes toward homosexuality among U.S. residents of Mexican descent. *Journal of Sex Research, 43*, 122–135. doi:10.1080/00224490609552307

Herek, G. M. (2009). Hate crimes and stigma-related experiences among sexual minority adults in the United States: Prevalence estimates from a national probability sample. *Journal of Interpersonal Violence, 24*, 54–74. doi:10.1177/0886260508316477

Holman, E. G., & Oswald, R. F. (2011). Nonmetropolitan GLBTQ Parents: When and where does their sexuality matter? *Journal of GLBT Family Studies, 7*(5), 436–456.

Horne, S. G., Rostosky, S. S., Riggle, E. D. B., & Martens, M. P. (2010). What was Stonewall? The role of GLB knowledge in marriage amendment-related affect and activism among family members of GLB individuals. *Journal of GLBT Family Studies, 6*, 349–364. doi:10.1080/1550428X.2010.511066

Huffington Post. (2011, January 31). *Illinois civil unions law: Governor Quinn will sign historic legislation today.* Retrieved from http://www.huffingtonpost.com/2011/01/31/illinois-civil-unions-law_n_816243.html

Human Rights Campaign. (2008). *State of the workplace 2007–2008.* Retrieved from http://www.hrc.org/documents/HRC_Foundation_State_of_the_Workplace_2007-2008.pdf

MCC Family in Christ (2010). *Metropolitan Community Church Family in Christ: Our history and purpose.* Retrieved from http://www.fortnet.org/mccfic/aboutus.htm

Klawitter, M. M. and Flatt, V. (1998), The effects of state and local antidiscrimination policies on earnings for gays and lesbians. *Journal of Policy Analysis and Management, 17*, 658–686.

Kosciw, J. C., & Diaz, E. M. (2008). *Involved, invisible, ignored: The experiences of lesbian, gay, bisexual, and transgender parents and their children in our nation's K—12 schools.* New York: GLSEN in partnership with COLAGE and the Family Equality Council.

Lev, A. I., Dean, G., De Filippis, L., Evernham, K., McLaughlin, L., & Phillips, C. (2005). Dykes and tykes: A virtual lesbian parenting community. *Journal of Lesbian Studies, 9*, 81–94. doi:10.1300/J155v09n01_08

Lewis, G. B. (2003). Black-white differences in attitudes toward homosexuality and gay rights. *Public Opinion Quarterly, 67*, 59–78. doi:10.1086/346009

Lindsay, J., Perlesz, A., Brown, R., McNair, R., de Vaus, D., & Pitts, M. (2006). Stigma or respect: Lesbian-parented families negotiat-

ing school settings. *Sociology, 40*, 1059–1077. doi:10.1177/0038038506069845

Lindstrom, M. (2004). Social capital, the miniaturization of community and self-reported global and psychological health. *Social Science & Medicine, 59*, 595–607. doi:10.1016/j.socscimed.2003.11.006

Lockard, D. (1985). The lesbian community: An anthropological approach. *Journal of Homosexuality, 11*(3/4), 83–95. doi:10.1300/J082v11n03_06

Marín, B. V. (2003). HIV prevention in the Hispanic community: Sex, culture, and empowerment. *Journal of Transcultural Nursing, 14*, 186–192. doi:10.1177/1043659603014003005

McKinnon, J. (2001). *Census 2000 brief: The Black population.* Retrieved from http://www.census.gov/prod/2001pubs/c2kbr01-5.pdf

McLaren, S. (2009). Sense of belonging to the general and lesbian communities as predictors of depression among lesbians. *Journal of Homosexuality, 56*, 1–13. doi:10.1080/00918360802551365

McLaren, S., Jude, B., & McLachlan, A. J. (2008). Sense of belonging to the general and gay communities as predictors of depression among gay men. *International Journal of Men's Health, 7*, 90–99. doi:10.3149/jmh.0701.90

McNair, R., Brown, R., Perlesz, A., Lindsay, J., De Vaus, D., & Pitts, M. (2008). Lesbian parents negotiating the health care system in Australia. *Health Care for Women International, 29*, 91–114. doi:10.1080/07399330701827094

Meyer, I. H. (2003). Prejudice, social stress, and mental health in lesbian, gay, and bisexual populations: Conceptual issues and research evidence. *Psychological Bulletin, 129*, 674–697. doi:10.1037/0033-2909.129.5.674

National Gay and Lesbian Task Force. (2008a). *Second-parent adoption in the U.S.* No longer available on line.

National Gay and Lesbian Task Force. (2008b). *Anti-adoption laws in the U.S.* No longer available on line.

National Gay and Lesbian Task Force. (2009a). *State non-discrimination laws in the U.S.* Retrieved from http://www.thetaskforce.org/downloads/reports/issue_maps/non_discrimination_7_09_color.pdf

National Gay and Lesbian Task Force. (2009b). *Hate crime laws in the U.S.* Retrieved from http://www.thetaskforce.org/downloads/reports/issue_maps/hate_crimes_7_09_color.pdf

National Gay and Lesbian Task Force. (2009c). *Foster care laws and regulations in the U.S.* Retrieved from http://www.thetaskforce.org/downloads/reports/issue_maps/foster_care_regs_7_09_color.pdf

National Gay and Lesbian Task Force. (2009d). *State laws prohibiting recognition of same-sex relationships.* Retrieved from http://www.thetaskforce.org/downloads/reports/issue_maps/samesex_relationships_7_09.pdf

National Gay and Lesbian Task Force. (2010). *Relationship recognition for same-sex couples in the U.S.* Retrieved from http://www.thetaskforce.org/downloads/reports/issue_maps/rel_recog_9_10_color.pdf

National Gay and Lesbian Task Force (NGLTF). (2005). *Domestic violence laws in the U.S.* No longer available on line.

O'Connell, M., & Lofquist, D. (2009, May). *Counting same-sex couples: Official estimates and unofficial guesses.* Paper presented at the Population Association of America, Detroit, Michigan. Retrieved from http://www.census.gov/population/www/socdemo/files/counting-paper.pdf

Oswald, R. F. (2001). Religion, family, and ritual: The production of gay, lesbian, bisexual, and transgendered outsiders-within. *Review of Religious Research, 43*, 39–50. doi:10.2307/3512242

Oswald, R. F., & Culton, L. (2003). Under the rainbow: Rural gay life and its relevance for family providers. *Family Relations, 52*, 72–79. doi:10.1111/j.1741-3729.2003.00072.x

Oswald, R. F., Cuthbertson, C., Lazarevic, V., & Goldberg, A. E. (2010). New developments in the field: Measuring community climate. *Journal of GLBT Family Studies, 6*, 214–228. doi:10.1080/15504281003709230

Oswald, R. F., Goldberg, A. E., Kuvalanka, K., & Clausell, E. (2008). Structural and moral commitment among same-sex couples: Relationship duration, religiosity, and parental status. *Journal of Family Psychology, 22*, 411–419. doi:10.1037/0893-3200.22.3.411

Oswald, R. & Kuvalanka, K. (2008). Same-sex couples: Legal complexities. *Journal of Family Issues, 29*, 1051–1066.

Oswald, R. F., & Lazarevic, V. (2011). You live *where*? Lesbian mothers' attachment to nonmetropolitan communities. *Family Relations, 60*, 373–386.

Prokos, A. H., & Keene, J. R. (2010). Poverty among cohabiting gay and lesbian, and married and cohabiting heterosexual families. *Journal of Family Issues, 31*, 934–959. doi:11.1177/0192513X09360176

Ragins, B. R., & Cornwell, J. M. (2001). Pink triangles: Antecedents and consequences of perceived workplace discrimination against gay and lesbian employees. *Journal of Applied Psychology, 86*, 1244–1261. doi:10.1037/0021-9010.86.6.1244

Riggle, E. D. B., Rostosky, S. S., & Horne, S. G. (2009). Marriage amendments and lesbian, gay, and bisexual individuals in the 2006 election. *Sexuality Research and Social Policy, 6*(1), 80–89. doi:10.1525/srsp.2009.6.1.80

Riggle, E. D. B., Rostosky, S. S., & Horne, S. G. (2010). Psychological distress, well-being, and legal recognition in same-sex couple relationships. *Journal of Family Psychology, 24*, 82–86.

Rodriguez, E. M. (2010). At the intersection of church and gay: A review of the psychological research on gay and lesbian Christians. *Journal of Homosexuality, 57*, 5–38. doi:10.1080/00918360903445806

Romer v. Evans, (1996). 517 U.S. 620 Retrieved from http://supreme.justia.com/us/517/620/case.html

Rosario, M., Hunter, J., Maguen, S., Gwadz, M., & Smith, R. (2001). The coming-out process and its adaptational and health-related associations among gay, lesbian, and bisexual youths: Stipulation and exploration of a model. *American Journal of Community Psychology, 29*, 133–160. doi:10.1023/A:1005205630978

Rostosky, S. S., Otis, M. D., Riggle, E. D. B., Brumett, S. K., & Brodnicki, C. (2008). An exploratory study of religiosity and same-sex couple relationships. *Journal of GLBT Family Studies, 4*(1), 17–36. doi:10.1080/15504280802084407

Rostosky, S. S., & Riggle, E. D. B. (2002). 'Out' at work: The relation of actor and partner workplace policy and internalized homophobia to disclosure status. *Journal of Counseling Psychology, 49*, 411–419. doi:10.1037/0022-0167.49.4.411

Rostosky, S. S., Riggle, E. D. B., Horne, S. G., Denton, F. N., & Huellemeier, J. D. (2010). Lesbian, gay, and bisexual individuals' psychological reactions to amendments denying access to civil marriage. *American Journal of Orthopsychiatry, 80*, 302–310. doi:10.1111/j.1939-0025.2010.01033.x

Rostosky, S. S., Riggle, E. D. B., Horne, S. G., & Miller, A. D. (2009). Marriage amendments and psychological distress in lesbian, gay, and bisexual adults. *Journal of Counseling Psychology, 56*, 56–66. doi:10.1037/a0013609

Russell, G. M., Bohan, J. S., McCarroll, M. C., & Smith, N. G. (2010). Trauma, recovery, and community: Perspectives on the long-term impact of anti-LGBT politics. *Traumatology.* doi:10.1177/1534765610362799 Advance online publication.

Russell, G. M., & Richards, J. A. (2003). Stressor and resilience factors for lesbians, gay men, and bisexuals confronting antigay politics. *American Journal of Community Psychology, 31*, 313–328. doi:10.1023/A:1023919022811

Schuck, K. D., & Liddle, B. J. (2001). Religious conflicts experienced by lesbian, gay, and bisexual individuals. *Journal of Gay and Lesbian Psychotherapy, 5*(2), 63–82. doi:10.1300/J236v05n02_07

Shapiro, D. N., Peterson, C., & Stewart, A. J. (2009). Legal and social contexts and mental health among lesbian and heterosexual mothers. *Journal of Family Psychology, 23*, 255–262. doi:10.1037/a0014973

Shecter, E., Tracy, A. J., Page, K. V., & Luong, G. (2008). Shall we marry? Legal marriage as a commitment event in same-sex relationships. *Journal of Homosexuality, 54*, 400–422. doi:10.1080/00918360801991422

Short, L. (2007). Lesbian mothers living well in the context of heterosexism and discrimination: Resources, strategies, and legislative change. *Feminism and Psychology, 17*, 57–74. doi:10.1177/0959353507072912

Siker, J. S. (2007). *Homosexuality and religion: An encyclopedia.* Westport, CT: Greenwood Press.

Smith, N. G., & Ingram, K. M. (2004). Workplace heterosexism and adjustment among lesbian, gay, and bisexual individuals: The role of unsupportive social interactions. *Journal of Counseling Psychology, 51*, 57–67. doi:10.1037/0022-0167.51.1.57

Sullivan, M. (2004). *The family of woman: Lesbian mothers, their children, and the undoing of gender.* Berkeley, CA: University of California Press.

Tavernise, S. (2011, January 18). Parenting by gays more common in the South, Census shows. *The New York Times.* Retrieved from http://www.nytimes.com/2011/01/19/us/19gays.html?_r=1&ref=sabrinatavernise

Tejeda, M. J. (2006). Nondiscrimination policies and sexual identity disclosure: Do they make a difference in employee outcomes? *Employee Responsibilities and Rights Journal, 18*(1), 45–59. doi:10.1007/s10672-005-9004-5

Van Gelderen, L., Gartrell, N., Bos, H., & Hermanns, J. (2009). Stigmatization and resilience in adolescent children of lesbian mothers. *Journal of GLBT Family Studies, 5,* 268–279. doi:10.1080/15504280903035761

Wellman, B. (2002). Physical place and cyberplace: The rise of personalized networking. *International Journal of Urban and Regional Research, 25,* 227–252. 10.1111/1468-2427.00309.

Wheaton, L., & Tashi, J. (2004). *Poverty Facts 2004.* Washington, DC: The Urban Institute. Retrieved from http://www.urban.org/publications/411654.html

Wood, P. B., & Bartkowski, J. P. (2004). Attribution style and public policy attitudes toward gay rights. *Social Science Quarterly, 85,* 58–73. doi:10.1111/j.0038-4941.2004.08501005.x

Yakushko, O. (2005). Influence of social support, existential well-being, and stress over sexual orientation on self-esteem of gay, lesbian, and bisexual individuals. *International Journal for the Advancement of Counseling, 27,* 131–143. doi:10.1007/s10447-005-2259-6

Yip, A. (1997). Dare to differ: Gay and lesbian Catholics' assessment of official Catholic positions on sexuality. *Sociology of Religion, 58,* 165–180. doi:10.2307/3711875

LGBT Parents and Their Children: Non-Western Research and Perspectives

Carien Lubbe

Current knowledge about lesbian, gay, bisexual, and transgender (LGBT) families has developed mainly in a Euro-American (Westernized) cultural context, which, although characterized by diversity, represents a fairly monocultural perspective on LGBT families. When examining research from a non-Western perspective, factors such as globalization, geographical location, social and cultural frameworks regarding race, language, and religion, and localized understandings of gender, sex, and sexuality need to be recognized.

Accordingly, against a backdrop of major global change and conflict, postmodern worlds and traditional patriarchal societies come into conflict, highlighting inequalities in class, gender, race, culture, ethnic group, and religion that create patterns of exclusion and marginalization. Therefore, in exploring non-Western perspectives, can the Westernized terms of homosexuality, gay, lesbian, queer, and so forth be applied when trying to comprehend and understand what is taking place in local cultures? Can the existence of forms of same-sex practices in non-Western cultures be seen as evidence of or similar to same-sex practices viewed from a Western perspective?

Consequently, a cross-cultural theoretical framework might assist in interpreting the available research, allowing for the appreciation of widely diverse and previously unfamiliar cultures' indigenous knowledge. In this respect, cross-cultural approaches study the variations in human behavior, taking into account the cultural environment in which the behavior occurs. Gilbert Herdt (1997) observes that the "cultural study in non-Western societies stresses the importance of examining not only the environment in which same-gendered relations occur, but also the symbolic systems of beliefs, rules, norms and social exchanges surrounding sexuality" (p. 19). Similarly, Kiluva-Ndunda (2005) emphasizes the complexity of sexual and gender identities in the sense that different societies or contexts produce different sexualities based on cultural ideas about how these should be expressed.

This chapter briefly explores the historical background of same-sex-oriented people within non-Westernized cultures, to account for the possible presence and existence of LGBT-parent families, as well as to provide a background against which the diversity and complexities of same-sex practices in various cultures influence the way LGBT families should be considered. After this overview, research from five regions is explored along significant signposts of gender, heteronormativity, the legal and political framework, and religious influences.

C. Lubbe, Ph.D. (✉)
Department of Educational Psychology, University of Pretoria, Aldoel Building Room 2-54, Groenkloof campus, Pretoria, South Africa, 0002
e-mail: Carien.Lubbe@up.ac.za

A.E. Goldberg and K.R. Allen (eds.), *LGBT-Parent Families: Innovations in Research and Implications for Practice*, DOI 10.1007/978-1-4614-4556-2_14, © Springer Science+Business Media New York 2013

A Brief History of Same-Sex-Oriented People in Non-Western Cultures

How do the possible presence and practices of same-sex relationships in non-Westernized cultures relate to global movements and a Westernized understanding of same-sex practices? Every country exists within a particular historical and social context; therefore Westernized defined terms should be used cautiously and critically (Khamasi & Maina-Chinkuya, 2005). Nel (2007) argues that it is even potentially offensive to use Westernized gender and sexuality categories in different countries; that even in the Westernized world the categories are not self-evident, and there is an even greater need for localized questions as to what it means to the people in a specific country. Similarly, in terms of the concept of sexuality, Mkhize, Bennett, Reddy, and Moletsane (2010) argue that "there are no widely accepted, positive, non-colonial terms for a celebrated and chosen, non-conventional sexual identity" (p. 12). It would seem that Western theories and/or terminologies of sexualities cannot capture what is meant by, or is taking place in, local cultures (Herdt, 1997; Khamasi & Maina-Chinkuya, 2005; Nel, 2007), and the need arises to discuss broader considerations before addressing non-Western families, such as sex, gender, sexual identity, sexual practices, and sexual orientation.

The same-sex practices reported in the literature provide a contextual background against which lesbian- and gay-parent families can be understood in specific cultural and localized contexts. The examples given below indicate the presence and existence of same-sex practices, but also illustrate the complexity of taking into account cultural distinctions. For example, in Thailand, *Tom and Dee* same-sex relationships between females have been documented. Throughout Mexico, Central America, and South America, *travestis* may dress and to some extent live as women, adapting their clothing, hair, and bodies in line with their intent. Some have prominent roles in their local community as entertainers, hairdressers, beauticians, and even politicians (Aggleton, 2009). Similarly, in West Africa, feminized men have an important role to play in traditional dance troupes. For example, in Burkina Faso, such men play an important role in baptisms and marriages. In Senegal, researchers have described the existence of *ibbi* (the receptive partner) and *yoo* (the penetrative partner) relationships between men (Aggleton, 2009). Similarly, Nel (2007) mentions the male *Azande* warriors in northern Congo who routinely married male youths who functioned as temporary wives.

Furthermore, Graham (2003) mentions her fieldwork in South Sulawesi, Indonesia, where she never met or heard of *women* involved in romantic relationships with women, but encountered *females* involved in romantic relationships with women. This example illustrates the cultural factors involved in understanding sexuality and gender in a specific country. In this case, the feminine partner continues to identify herself as a woman, while the masculine partner identifies as a *calalai*, a female-bodied individual who is attracted to women, and whose behavior and attitude are more masculine-like. The feminine partner is also referred to as *linas*. In South Saluwesi, these couples occupy a place in their society where they are accepted, and even adopt children from close relatives, for example. However, there is no public acknowledgement of their status, and one partner is expected to be masculine and actively develop a masculine identity. The women Graham encountered in her fieldwork stated that the pressure to become mothers via marriage is strong. However, they were very creative in negotiating this, either by adopting or marrying, until they become pregnant and then they choose to find a *linas*.

Some authors point to certain words in different cultures and languages that refer to the concept of homosexuality. Epprecht (2008) mentions *skesana, matanyola, istabane,* and so forth. Likewise, GALZ (Gays and Lesbians of Zimbabwe) (2008) refers to *hungochani* in Shona and *ubunkotshani* in Ndebele among others. Mkhize et al. (2010) mention the derogatory terms such as *Nongayindoda* in isiZulu that stigmatize women who live beyond accepted heterosexual norms of dress, behavior, or desire, and the terms in Afrikaans *moffie* and in isiZulu *isitabane* that refer to effeminate young men. The authors highlight the fact that these words suggest a strong stigma or social disapproval. However, the mere fact that such words exist and some can be traced back over hundreds of years might indicate to a Westernized reader that forms of same-sex sexuality do exist.

Taking into account that in 82 countries same-sex sexuality is considered a crime and even the death penalty awaits (Ottosson, 2010), accessing information on LGBT families becomes a complicated affair. In countries such as Bangladesh, the Maldives, Singapore, and Uganda, people involved in same-sex practices can be imprisoned for years or even for life. In countries such as Iran, Yemen, Mauritania, Saudi Arabia, Sudan, and the United Arab Emirates, people involved in such practices can be sentenced to death for their sexual orientation (Vaggione, 2010). In much of sub-Saharan Africa for example, homosexuality is firstly interpreted as "foreign," and is portrayed as "un-African" and a "White import" (Nel, 2007, p. 101). According to some traditional African beliefs, people of a same-sex sexual orientation are considered cursed or bewitched by the forefathers. In Malawi, a country hostile to LGBT people, individuals with same-sex sexual orientations are currently imprisoned, blackmailed, or experience hostile reactions within their communities, and most live in secret (Watson, 2008). Thoreson and Cook (2011) also describe personal narratives of people with same-sex sexual orientations subjected to blackmailing and extortion practices in countries such as Zimbabwe, Malawi, Nigeria, Ghana, and Cameroon. The illegality and stigmatization of LGBT people foster victimization in extreme forms. The practice of same-sex sexuality therefore becomes either so rare or hidden in many of these countries that it becomes almost unnoticeable.

LGBT-Parent Families in a Non-Western Context

Sociocultural change and the blending of different influences such as the fusion of different cultures since the advent of colonialism, globalization, and urbanization have all influenced the way families are shaped (Khamasi & Maina-Chinkuya, 2005). Like many sociolo-

gists and feminists, Karraker (2011) argues for an inclusive definition of what constitutes a family, defining the family as a "collection of people related by blood, marriage, adoption, or other intimate bond, who often but not always share a common residence over a significant span of time" (p. 304), and allowing for the incorporation of the complexities of blended families, single parents, and the unions of LGBT persons. The concept of LGBT families is complex and variations exist within the LGBT community. In this chapter, the focus is on lesbian- and gay-parent families; thus, I address research findings that address either a single parent or two gay or lesbian individuals together who are acting as parents to children. A significant exclusion is any discussion on families with the presence of a bisexual or transgendered parent, which at this stage represents a huge silence in the current available research.

To identify studies on this topic, I conducted a literature search using English keywords such as "homosexuality," "lesbian," "gay," "parents," "adoption," "queer," "homosexual/transgender/bisexual parents," "families," "non-Western," "Africa," and so forth in PsycInfo, Social Work Abstracts, Sociological Abstracts, ERIC (Proquest), Social Sciences Citation Index, Sabinet, and EbscoHost. A wealth of information in the field of sexuality and especially HIV/AIDS research was uncovered, but with most emphasis on individuals, and fewer references to couples, with LGBT-parent families or LGBT parenting being almost nonexistent. As mentioned, the research presented is largely limited to research published in recognized scholarly journals in the English language. I acknowledge that more research certainly exists, but with the exceptions of a few articles that colleagues could translate from Portuguese and Spanish, only works in English were consulted.

Non-Western Research on Lesbian- and Gay-Parent Families

Working within a cross-cultural perspective, the following section is organized according to geographic region, to capture the contextual specifics of each country. However, certain similarities emerge, which will be addressed within each region. The first similarity that emerges from each region is the way gender and the roles of women and men are framed within traditional and normative discourses on the family, illuminating the intersection among gender, parenting, and sexuality. Second, heteronormativity and the cultural nuances involved in interpreting homosexuality within a specific country reveal deeper complexities, indicative of the presence of prejudice, discrimination, and stigma. Third, the legal and political policies and framework of each country also play an important role, with regard to LGBT rights but also in informing specific parental practices such as adoption or the right to reproductive health. Fourth, the role of religion is also paramount in a cross-cultural perspective. Although these four commonalities are used as guideposts for presenting key information, it should be noted that definite and complex intersections and interconnections exist across the four contexts.

South America and Latin America

The Influence of Religion

In this region, the heteronormative assumptions that result in stigmatization and discrimination are informed by a religious discourse. Vaggione (2010) observes that resistance to nonheterosexual parenthood is greatly influenced by the Catholic Church. The immense historical and sociopolitical influence of the church can be seen in the fact that the state bases its legislation on Catholic doctrine, and any attempt to resist Catholic principles is considered by various sectors as an attack against the state. The patriarchy and heteronormativity of the church is seen as natural and legitimate. Furthermore, many characteristics of motherhood are embedded in the Virgin Mary's Catholic model of motherhood; for example, that a mother sacrifices on behalf of her children and shows sensitivity and care for her children (Sardá-Chandiramani, 2010; Vaggione, 2010).

Legal and Political Frameworks

Sardá-Chandiramani (2010) states that same-sex sexualities in Latin America seem to be experiencing more social, institutional, and legal recognition. What is interesting is that in most Latin American countries, non-procreative/same-sex consensual relationships have never been illegal. The few countries that maintained such legislation (Chile and Ecuador) repealed it without problem in the early 1990s. The exception to this rule is Nicaragua, which passed a sodomy law in 1992 and only repealed it in 2007 (Ottosson, 2010). The only country where civil unions for same-sex couples exist at the national level is Uruguay (Sardá-Chandiramani, 2010). In addition, same-sex unions have been recognized on local and state levels in the big cities of Argentina, Brazil, and Mexico (Ottosson, 2010; Sardá-Chandiramani, 2010). Legal advances, as well as the presence of individuals and relationships (including families), confirm that the silence on the existence of same-sex desires and practices, and the identities built around them, has long been broken. However, inequality still exists at many levels, including the economic, class, race, and social levels (Herrera, 2009; Sardá-Chandiramani, 2010). Furthermore, the legal advances should still be viewed against the backdrop of cultural forces that shape Latin-American societies, as Uziel (2001) notes that even though the union of same-sex couples is tolerated, the family is perceived as the basis of society and receives special protection from the State. The essential concept of family still refers to the traditional family; same-sex partners who wish to adopt are seen as a threat to the family, and even single parenthood is still perceived unfavorably. It can therefore be deduced that a specific moral order of types of family exists.

The Intersection Between Religion and Legal/Political Frameworks: The Case of Adoption

The intersection between the above-mentioned legal advances and the role of religion can especially be seen when it comes to adoption rights.

The Catholic Church on both a national and an international level argues that adoption by homosexuals is immoral and in violation of the rights of the child, and can even be seen as an "act of violence against minors as their normal development would be obstructed" (Vaggione, 2010, p. 218) without the presence of both sexes. Sardá-Chandiramani (2010) mentions that apart from the Catholic Church, some Christian evangelical churches and right-wing conservative parties also offer strong resistance to marriage and adoption rights especially for same-sex couples. Feminist activism and the movement for sexual diversity have brought the debate on regulating the family into the public arena, an inevitable issue in establishing legitimacy and legality for LGBTQ rights.

Uziel (2001) provides an overview of the judiciary process of adoption in Brazil and, against the background of a case study, discusses various reasons for how the law is applied, first in terms of how masculinity is constructed in Brazil and second the relationship between homosexuality and the way the justice system perceives what constitutes a family. Her data consisted of court records from 1995 to 2000 in Rio de Janeiro, and interviews with two judges, five psychologists, and four social workers involved in evaluations for adoptions. Uziel's work shows the gendered belief in Brazil that the female identity is tied to motherhood, as women are seen as caretakers of children. Consequently, men are seen as being unable to perform such a function, whether for biological, social, cultural, or judicial reasons. Therefore, the idea of wanting to be a single father, and even more so if that man is homosexual, becomes almost unimaginable. This example highlights the intersection among gender, sexuality, parenthood, and societal beliefs embedded in a legal framework.

Herrera (2009) describes with regards to Chile that legislative frameworks and public policies do not protect lesbian partnerships, nor are adoption and reproductive technologies available to lesbians. Chilean society is strongly heteronormative, and same-sex partners face discrimination on a daily basis. As recently as 2004, the Supreme Court ruled that custody be given to the biological father, because Karen Atala, who happened to be a judge, lived with a female partner. The Court ruled that Atala was not able "to provide them [the children] with a proper social environment" (Herrera, 2009, p. 36). Most of the lesbian mothers in Herrera's ethnographic study (in which she interviewed 29 lesbians, 10 of whom were mothers) had children from a previous marriage. She found that the lesbian mothers hid their sexual identity to protect their relationship with their children, out of fear for custody battles and being labeled as incompetent mothers. This dilemma is similar to current Westernized societies where legal protection does not yet exist, or resembles earlier findings where legal protection does not yet favor lesbian or gay couples and their families.

Traditionalist Discourses on Motherhood and the Family

Traditionalist discourses on motherhood and gender are intertwined with heteronormative ideals on what constitutes a family constitutes and the roles that mothers and fathers ought to play. Álvarez and Álvares-Gayou Jurgenson (2003) reiterate the strong relationship between motherhood and families in Mexico, and refer to the heteronormative assumption that motherhood is only associated with heterosexual women: "Lesbian women who are interested, desire, aspire or actually exercise maternity are not only not understood, but persecuted, criticized or stigmatized" (p. 66). They studied 10 heterosexual and 10 lesbian women who were equivalent in age, educational level, number of children, years living with a partner, and socioeconomic status. Their findings revealed that heterosexual and lesbian mothers perceived maternity and being a mother in similar ways.

Herrera (2009) discusses the gendered identity of families in Chile, namely the heteronormative assumptions that place great emphasis on motherhood. Much of what it means to be a Chilean woman (identity) centers on one's children, and a woman achieves a sense of purpose in her life by becoming a mother. Furthermore, society expects a mother to be feminine, sensitive, caring, and always giving of herself.

As mentioned earlier in the section on religion, these characteristics of motherhood are strongly influenced by religious frameworks. Some of the women Herrera interviewed associated motherhood with heterosexuality and had difficulty associating motherhood with homosexuality, while others commented on homophobia as being the biggest obstacle, thinking of the potential influence it could have on their children.

Therefore, Herrera (2009) argues that traditional and transgressive elements coexist in the experiences and perceptions of motherhood in the narratives of the Chilean lesbians that she interviewed. This argument is congruent with Ellen Lewin's (1993) observation, based on her sample of mostly White lesbian mothers in the USA, that motherhood legitimates a lesbian's experiences. However, Herrera contends that, for Chilean lesbian couples, the traditional notions of motherhood are important, as they hope to gain legitimacy and social acceptance for their families. She argues that traditional discourses continue to have power over how people comprehend and create families. By embracing tradition and following a path of assimilation rather than differentiation, the families want to be included in the milieu of what is accepted. Chilean lesbians therefore do not differentiate themselves from the heterosexual model of parenthood, but adjust the existing model to normalize their families. They embrace tradition as much as they can, and follow the traditional expectations of family life. Herrera concludes that Chile has not yet consolidated alternative models of family and motherhood. However, she asserts that, with or without realizing it, the lesbian couples in her study are challenging the traditional family model by "(a) eliminating the father as parent, (b) the equality of gender roles within the couple, and (c) the centrality of care and affection in kinship" (Herrera, 2009, p. 50).

However, the various factors in negotiating parenthood are considered against the specific cultural background of Chile, where lineage and a secure bloodline are of importance. For example, as in a Western context, artificial insemination is the preferred option, as the children have some resemblance to the birth mother. In Chile, however, lesbian women cannot opt for assistance in hospitals and clinics and must use their own networks

for obtaining donors, whether known or unknown. Since self-insemination is the only option, the partner also plays a significant role. The involvement of both women as a couple correlates with the emphasis that Chilean society places on the significance of parenthood as a couple. The "other mother," her role as well as her place in the structure of the family, becomes important. However, the other mother is neither legally nor, in many instances, socially recognized, placing her in a vulnerable and fragile position (Herrera, 2009).

Another important issue that Sardá-Chandiramani (2010) raises is that the commonality in terms of the Spanish language in Latin American countries has led to strong research and advocacy being generated in this region, but has also "made the region somewhat insular" (p. 201). An informal search on Google, Google translate, and Google Scholar confirms the presence of scientific articles written in Spanish and Portuguese. Forging cross-cultural ties between Latin America and other world regions might advance our understanding of local culture. However, a perusal of the bibliographies of the articles reviewed confirmed that a great deal of research from the USA, UK, and Western Europe has been used, especially, to inform the theoretical underpinnings of gender, sexuality, identity, and parenting. Still, closer ties with the Latin American region might reveal ways in which different cultures and perspectives have been blended to advance our current knowledge on what family life holds for LGBT parents and their children.

In conclusion, heteronormative assumptions of traditional family life are strongly embedded within a religious discourse in South America and Latin America, where the legal and political frameworks are also strongly influenced by religion. These intersecting influences certainly present challenges for lesbian- and gay-parent families to establish legitimate and fully recognized families.

Israel

From the literature it would seem that two main forces are present in Israel, modernization and Westernization (Lavee & Katz, 2003; Shechner,

Slone, Meir, & Kalish, 2010). Simultaneously, the centrality of the traditional nuclear family dominates as a distinctive feature (Lavee & Katz, 2003; Shechner et al., 2010).

In examining research findings from Israel, the legal/political framework creates certain features that allow the emergence of lesbian- and gay-parent families. However, strong traditionalism where the stability of the family is highly valued provides an interesting backdrop against which the legal changes can be viewed.

Legal/Political Framework

Israel is a country where same-sex couples have been offered some rights of marriage since 1995, and joint adoption of children has been legal since 2008 (Ottosson, 2010). Lavee and Katz (2003) describe Israel as a child-oriented society, where children are highly valued by their parents and by society as a whole. Women receive a birth allowance, and families continue to receive allowances and tax deductions based on the number of children they have. Free medical care is provided for all mothers and children up to the age of three.

Ben-Ari and Livni (2006), however, caution that the liberal perspective of the courts does not necessarily reflect the public's attitude. What is interesting is that at the time when early articles on lesbian and gay parenting were written, Israeli law viewed the biological mother as a single mother, and the partner did not have any parental rights. The couples, however, perceived themselves as equal in status. Of note is that Shechner et al. (2010), who examined fatherless families in Israel by interviewing 30 women from two-mother lesbian families, 30 single heterosexual mothers by choice, and 30 mothers from two-parent heterosexual families, confirmed this in the fact found that lesbian mothers did not differ from heterosexual mothers in their psychological and parental adjustment.

Ben-Ari and Livni (2006) explored the subjective experiences of eight Israeli lesbian mothers. The age of the children ranged from 2 months to 13 years. All the pregnancies were planned, with seven of the eight couples opting for anonymous donor insemination. Ben-Ari and Livni's research provides insight into the establishment of equality in a lesbian couple relationship prior to and following the birth of a child, influenced by the legal status of same-sex relations in Israel. They found that a significant strategy to attempt to regain equality was in the couple's pursuit to access all possible legal rights and is significant since adoption rights were only granted in 2008, 2 years after the research findings have been published. In addition to the above, the couples also used other strategies, such as having both partners become pregnant and give birth and deciding that both parents will raise the children. The quest to establish equality should also be seen against the backdrop of the strong traditionalist discourse on motherhood present in Israel.

Traditionalist Discourses on Motherhood and the Family

Lavee and Katz (2003) maintain that strong traditionalism is present especially with regard to the family in Israel, as they argue that the family is "stronger and more stable than in other industrialized nations" (p. 213). Within this strong family, a vast diversity of family patterns exist in terms of family values, attitudes toward gender roles, and lifestyle choices. Lavee and Katz reject the notion of a clear, monolithic Israeli family. The blend of predominantly Jews (about 80%) and non-Jews of mainly Arabic descent also brings the cultural orientation of individualism versus collectivism to the fore. Despite these two different orientations, Ben-Ari and Lavee (2004) maintain that the centrality of family dominates. A finding that emerged that is especially relevant to the Israeli context is the high value that is placed on motherhood and the family. Ben-Ari and Livni (2006) assert that, after becoming mothers, the lesbian women in their sample reported feeling more accepted and less marginalized by both members of the community and their families of origin. Participants mentioned that their families of origin supported their decision to become pregnant, even if they did not approve of a lesbian lifestyle. Lesbian couples reported a change in attitude, including the partner, with the birth of a biological grandchild. This change reflects the Israeli culture where womanhood is equated to motherhood, and giving birth outside the traditional framework of a family is quite acceptable and even encouraged. The mainstream identity of motherhood overshadows the marginalized identity of being a lesbian, and therefore supports the legitimization of the lesbian couple.

Shechner et al. (2010) found that family processes such as satisfaction with the relationship and parental and couple adjustment shaped the well-being of families, regardless of sexual orientation. Another finding, which is well established in the literature, was that lesbian couples shared more equally in their parental duties. Furthermore, single heterosexual mothers were the most vulnerable group, as they received less positive social support from their families and friends, indicating that their single status marks their deviation away from the normative family and gives them minority membership. The traditional heterosexual married mothers received the highest level of positive family support, but lesbian mothers also attained high levels of positive family support, as motherhood provides an avenue to become part of the normative ideal of establishing a family.

Eastern Europe

Eastern Europe is such a diverse region, and it would be arrogant to create the impression that a comprehensive overview of this region is represented here. Research in the Czech Republic as well as Slovenia could be obtained and is discussed in terms of the legal frameworks and heteronormativity.

Legal/Political Framework

In 2006, the Registered Partnership Act of Same-Sex Persons was passed, granting gay and lesbian couples legal security. However, the law does not include provisions of any adoption arrangements;

it explicitly excludes any individual with the registered status from adopting a child. The Czech Family Act enables both married couples and single individuals to adopt children, given that a proper environment for the child is provided. According to Polášková (2007), her research using interpretative phenomenological analysis is the first project on lesbian and gay families to be conducted in the Czech Republic. Polášková (2007) interviewed 10 lesbian families (20 female parents and 13 children), focusing mainly on parenting experiences. Three couples had children from previous heterosexual marriages, four couples had undergone anonymous donor insemination at foreign clinics, and one couple had used donor insemination themselves with a known donor. In addition, two couples were in co-parenting agreements with gay male couples. Polášková (2007) mentions that some single lesbian women have managed to adopt a child, but they hid their sexual orientation and therefore their sexual orientation is not reflected in official records. Furthermore, Czech legislation does not allow for women without a male partner to apply for donor insemination and, although not explicitly stated, women either use a foreign clinic or manage to navigate past the standard procedures.

Heteronormativity and Parenthood

In Polášková's (2007) research, subtle indicators of heteronormativity were expressed through the concerns raised by some parents about their children's healthy development in terms of future sexual orientation, gender identity, and gender role behaviors. Some parents also ensured that their children had sufficient exposure to gender role models via their families or social networks, while others also made an effort to break away from gender stereotypes in raising their children, exposing their children to a wide variety of toys. In common with findings from Western-based research, the mothers negotiated the choice of children's surnames, either adopting the biological mother's surname or the social mother changed hers as a demonstration of her commitment to the family and as a way to gain public recognition. Children born from previous marriages kept their fathers' surnames so as not to stigmatize the children, or mothers obtained permission from the fathers to change the child's surname. Some families even created new surnames to establish a new identity. The issue of what to call the two mothers was also raised, whereby, for example, children referred to both women as "parents," or referred to the social mother as "aunt" or calling her by her name. With regard to the negotiation of the gender roles assigned to parenting, women valued the equal distribution of power within their relationship and explicitly moved away from traditional role expectations (Polášková, 2007).

Similarly, Švab (2007) reiterates the heteronormativity present in Slovenian society, in which LGBT parenthood becomes almost unthinkable for the gay men and lesbians whom she interviewed. She established that 42% of her respondents wanted to have a child, while 20% were undecided. Even though they wanted children, they mentioned that they did not think it was possible and expressed anxiety over the potentially negative consequences of homophobia for the children.

Švab and Kuhar (2005) report that Slovenia is marked by homophobia, and violence against gay men and lesbians is common. In Slovenia, gay and lesbian couples cannot adopt children, and reproductive technology, such as artificial insemination, is not an option for women without male partners. In this context, same-sex parenthood is both legally impossible and socially unacceptable. Moreover, the social and political climate of the country creates a barrier where thoughts of parenting are silenced. Participants suppressed their desire to have children and rationalized it as unwanted, mentioning that children need two gendered role models, while others made use of more positive forms of coping, such as taking over social roles for nieces and nephews, or becoming part of the social networks of other gay men and lesbians who had children (Švab, 2007; Švab & Kuhar, 2005). By engaging in these repressive thoughts, gay men and lesbians subtly reinforce the heteronormative ideals and reproduce discriminatory beliefs.

South Africa

A multitude of family formations have evolved in South Africa, as a consequence of the cultural, political, and economic conditions as well as personal choice. Simultaneously, what needs to be understood about South Africa is its diversity, the tension between a developed and developing economy, and the life worlds of its people.

Even the deployment of the terms "Black" and "White" in South Africa is not simple. As collective terms, they reflect the diversity present in issues such as class, ancestry, language, educational experience, the stories of their families under apartheid, and so forth. Nevertheless, they can be useful as, generally speaking, Black women represent the most vulnerable group in South Africa in terms of poverty, class stratification, and gender inequality (Mkhize et al., 2010).

Furthermore, lesbians, most notably Black lesbians, are subjected to violence in townships and other urban settings. Between 2006 and 2009, 10 cases of rape and murder of lesbian women were reported in South Africa (Gunkel, 2010; Mkhize et al., 2010). Such incidents are informed by culturally sanctioned homophobia and hate speech, based on perceptions that homosexuality is un-African, that gay men and lesbian cannot be afforded the same constitutional protections and rights, and that homosexuality should be criminalized and condemned from a religious point of view. In addition, the cultural intolerance emanating from varied notions of what is correct and proper gender behavior and what is not also affects different perceptions of people (Mkhize et al., 2010). Such intolerance occurs in spite of the current legal climate in which the Constitution guarantees the protection of all citizens, irrespective of sexual orientation.

In the almost 20 years since the new Constitution was written in 1994, there has been little research on LGBT families in general, and lesbian- or gay-parent families in particular. Potgieter's (1997) doctoral study was the first in-depth study addressing issues related to Black lesbians; although families are not the main focus of her research, she did explore discourses on motherhood from the perspective of Black South African lesbians (Potgieter, 2003).

Localized Discourses on Motherhood

Potgieter's (2003) groundbreaking work in South Africa illustrates the complexity of working in a non-Western environment, as well as the richness that can be obtained when research is undertaken to understand experiences and discourses from a local context in particular. Potgieter conducted six individual interviews and 10 focus groups (63 women in total). She observed that Black women in South Africa, as in other non-Western contexts, do not necessarily use labels familiar to Westernized societies to define themselves as lesbian. Since she conducted her interviews in the informal settlement of Khayelitsha near Cape Town, the languages of English and Xhosa (an official yet indigenous language) were used, and many women labeled themselves "*nongayindoda*, the Xhosa word for gay" (Potgieter, 2003, p. 138). However, many chose to speak in English, as one participant said, "We do not talk about this 'secret' in Xhosa" (Potgieter, 2003, p. 142). This comment alludes to the speculation that some forms of gayness do exist in African culture, although the difference between practices and identities should be treated with care.

The findings emphasized the essentialist notion that it is important and a natural instinct to have children; indeed, many of the women shared that they had heterosexual sex to have a baby. In my opinion, this way of conceiving a child might either be because other forms, such as artificial insemination, have not been explored or that access to this service is limited, or it might even be too expensive. Alternatively this practice resonates with reports that in African and other non-Western societies women who have same-sex relationships are assisted by men who fulfill certain functions, such as helping women reproduce (Chacha, 2003; GALZ, 2008; Potgieter, 2003).

Motherhood also assisted the participants in achieving "adult status" in the eyes of the community (Potgieter, 2003, p. 144). Potgieter (2003) explored the contradiction and tension between the normalizing discourse of being similar to heterosexual women, while also positioning themselves as lesbians and challenging certain traditional roles. However, doing routine household tasks and having a baby gave them "a comfortable space to 'be' lesbian" (Potgieter, 2003, p. 148).

Research Findings from Lesbian- and Gay-Parent Families Similar to Westernized Societies

Pockets of research are starting to appear in South Africa, mainly from postgraduate studies that include lesbian and gay parents who are willing to participate; most often, these participants come from more affluent sectors in society. Six research-based studies could be found focusing specifically on LGBT families via official search engines and informal networking across South Africa. A synopsis of the main findings of the above six studies can be summarized in two themes, namely children's experiences and parenting experiences against the backdrop of heteronormativity.

Children's Experiences Embedded in Heteronormativity

Lubbe (2005) focused on the experiences of children growing up in lesbian-parent families. Nine children in total from five households were interviewed, ages ranging from 9 to 18 years. In four of the five families the children were born in a previous heterosexual marriage, while the other family's children were adopted. In this study, the main findings suggest that the children experienced different levels of "okayness" in having lesbians parents, they were aware of others' open-mindedness or not, and they expressed the need for openness in their relationships with others. The findings are consistent with Annandale's (2008) research, which explored the experiences of adolescents with gay parents. In-depth case studies were carried out with three adolescents, each of whom had a gay father. Annandale found that the participants were affected by the discovery of their father's homosexuality; however, they chose to eventually accept their father's sexual orientation and expressed the wish to establish open and trustworthy relationships with their fathers.

Similarly, Lubbe and Kruger (2012) explored the disclosure practices of a South African-born adolescent raised in a lesbian-parent family in the

USA. Dominant discourses that influenced disclosure were identified, namely religion, school, friends, acquaintances, and society at large, as well as individual emotional well-being. Protective factors against heterosexism were support from parents, friends, and significant others (Annandale, 2008; Lubbe & Kruger, 2012; Lubbe, 2008), as well as schools with an accepting and open-minded atmosphere (Judge, Manion, & De Waal, 2008; Lubbe & Kruger, 2012; Lubbe, 2007; Pon, 2008). Judge et al. (2008) shared an anecdote of a lesbian couple of color (a particular race category in South Africa) who adopted two daughters to give both parents equal status. They shared their experiences of adoption before the Civil Union Act (prior to 2006), as one partner had to adopt the child as a single mother, while with the second adoption the legal changes created by the Act made it much easier. They also shared that the school was very supportive when they told members of the school system about their changed marital status.

Parenting Experiences and Heteronormativity

Two qualitative studies have explored the parenting experiences of lesbian couples who chose to have children through assisted reproductive technology, namely artificial insemination and in vitro fertilization (Suckling, 2009; Swain, 2009). Furthermore, Pon (2008) conducted the first study of adoptive gay parents and their experiences with the preschool system. Key themes on parenting centered on the experiences of general heterosexism through social interactions, as well as significant institutional challenges, most notably from the medical, legal, and religious domains. Religion emerged as the most homophobic and exclusionary discourse toward parents in Pon's study. This subtheme of religion is also present in the studies of Lubbe (2005) and Lubbe and Kruger (2012). Lack of social support from friends and family resulting in feelings of isolation were evident in Suckling's (2009) research. Other themes included concerns about providing male role models or a "father" figure, as well as equipping their children to come to terms with their family unit and their conception.

The participants in Pon's study also prepared their children with social and emotional skills to handle possible prejudice and discrimination from their peers and teachers, indicative of the heteronormativity of society. Being proactive in the schools facilitated the process of acceptance and acted as a discourse of empowerment (Pon, 2008). All three studies are indicative of the highly reflective skills of negotiating what it means to become and be a parent.

What can be deduced from research being done in South Africa? Members of the middle to upper classes are adopting and having children with the help of assisted reproductive technologies, and previously married LGBT individuals are keeping custody of their children in the current more liberating legal environment. There are a variety of experiences within and between families, as is the case in other Westernized countries. Also, true of any family irrespective of the parent's sexual orientation, there is a continuum of experiences from highly functioning families that encounter the occasional homophobic incident here and there, with children being well adjusted, "okay," open and proud; to couples struggling with intense rejection, nonacceptance, and internalized homophobia. Most findings cohere with what is known in Westernized societies, mainly because research is done in partnership with White, middle-class participants. What remains silenced and invisible in research is that when race, ethnicity, and lower socioeconomic factors are explored, research becomes almost nonexistent, as is perhaps also the case in most other Westernized societies. Furthermore, even though South Africa has a very advanced constitution and legal arena, living as a family in a heteronormative patriarchal society, where differences, distrust, fear, and hatred are on the rise, can be a totally different story.

Imagining Lesbian- and Gay-Parent Families in Traditionalist Cultures

Other small vignettes found in scholarly work on same-sex practices reveal the presence of LGBT families, although their focus is not on parenting or LGBT families per se. The occurrence of woman–woman marriage in Southern African countries is not ordinarily seen as lesbian, even if occasional sexual exchange may occur, but has always taken place in African societies with varying degrees and for different reasons (Matebeni, 2008). Instances of these marriages are found among the Venda, Balobedu (Lovedu), Pedi, Zulu, and Narene peoples. Such marriages are performed for two main reasons: (a) because the woman marrying is in a powerful position as a result of owning land and property, and (b) because she is childless. The female husband remains the most important "father figure" for children born to women marriages, and sons continue her lineage (Chacha, 2003; Matebeni, 2008; Morgan & Wieringa, 2005; Nel, 2007). Chacha (2003) argues that woman–woman marriages are predominantly a precapitalist tradition on the African continent and flourished in the nineteenth century. This highlights the intersection among sexuality, gender, marriage, and cultural traditions, such as the economics of production, resource control, and social security.

Women marriage also happens among *sangomas* (traditional healers), although not all *sangomas* explicitly self-identify as lesbians (Mbali, 2009; Munro, 2009; Nel, 2007). One example is the narration of the relationship between the female husband and the ancestral wife by Nkabinde (2008), where she shares the story of Hlengiwe, who came to be married to Ntombikhona. In Hlengiwe's words, she mentions that she had been in love with Ntombikhona for more than 12 years, and the children loved her as their mother. The sexual relationship between them is secret though. Hlengiwe says that "she is 100% a lady" and they are "just two women loving each other" (Nkabinde, 2008, p. 116). This story illustrates the presence of children living with two mothers, but whether we can equate their family structure and identify it as a lesbian-parent family remains questionable.

In another example, GALZ (2008) describes the phenomenon of mine marriages in South Africa, focusing on the Basotho people (people from Lesotho), where new mine workers choose a husband who will look after him and his

interests, called *Komba-E-Kehle* or *mteto ka sokisi*. A case study is presented by Epprecht (2008) about a man who had a wife in Lesotho, taking on a male husband and living in an apartment in town. The man is referred to as the second wife and is accepted by the family and the wife in Lesotho, who is quoted as saying "I'm very lucky that my husband is going out with a gay" (Epprecht, 2008, p. 169). Epprecht states "Hlohoangwane adopted the dress and manners of a respectable modern, middle-class housewife and adopted children to complete the marriage" (p. 170). This statement also alludes to the presence of children and the existence of another variety of a gay-parent family.

The various forms and variety within South Africa are found in another example from the Sesotho culture where limited and discreet female–female physical intimacy is allowed: Co-wives of one husband are allowed to express physical affection for one another that includes kissing and snuggling. In common with a Kenyan example, a widow can take a young woman in marriage if she has the resources to pay *bohali* (cattle as price or token of agreement for a marriage to take place). The wife in this type of marriage is supposed to get pregnant by a discreet arrangement with a man who would have no claims to the offspring. The female *ntate* (father, Sir, or Mister) is entitled to show affection for her wife as well. Another form that is allowed is female–female *setsoalle*, which has no material benefits or costs, but the emotional benefits are widely accepted and admired. This *setsoalle* friendship is supported by men as they claim that it makes their wives more loyal and loving (GALZ, 2008).

Africa

The complexity of finding and doing research in the rest of Africa becomes daunting. Epprecht (2008) confirms the presence in Africa of men who have sex with men, and women who have sex with women. However, he cautions that they do not necessarily identify this as lesbian or gay behavior, nor do they necessarily take on such a specific identity. Heterosexual marriage and reproduction are highly valued in most African societies. In instances where same sex or "pseudo-homosexualities" are allowed, it occurs within the confined spaces of specific rituals or designated social roles. Furthermore, the laws criminalizing homosexuality were imposed by colonialism, and African leaders adopted the colonial laws post independence. Another challenge is the invisibility of lesbian women, bisexual women, and transgender persons, due to the fragility of human rights on the African continent (Gunkel, 2010; Nel, 2007; Ottosson, 2010).

Morgan and Wieringa (2005) give an example of a self-identified lesbian couple in Kenya who started the process of adopting two children, but foresaw that they would immigrate to the USA given the stigmatization of LGBT people in Kenya. The authors mention two other examples of lesbians considering motherhood, indicating that the presence of lesbian- and gay-parent families might become a possibility in the future.

In Tanzania and Uganda same-sex practices are so forbidden that there is no or little evidence of lesbians or gay men having children. Narratives from Namibia reveal opposition to motherhood from lesbian women, as they relate it to having sex with a man before you can have children. Some self-identified lesbians from Namibia do have children which they now raise with their partners, having had sexual relationships with men when they were younger or having been raped. Morgan and Wieringa (2005) also explore the position of *lesbian men* who are mothers to their own biological children, but also fathers to the children of their partner.

The literature emerging from Africa, such as the untold stories on blackmail, stigmatization, and imprisonment in Malawi (Watson, 2008), and blackmail and extortion of LGBT people in sub-Saharan Africa (Thoreson & Cook, 2011), reveals the confrontation of stigma, discrimination, hate crimes, and violation of basic human rights on an individual level. These violations force me to ask how, if individuals are silenced, is it possible for families to not be almost absent and invisible as well.

Concluding Remarks

Institutional, social, and cultural forces shape and regulate same-sex sexualities globally. Laws and government policies, as well as religious practices, undeniably have an impact on same-sex sexualities and, consequently, on LGBT-parent families. Before more families can be open and dare to venture into a heteronormative world, basic human rights need to be secured.

From the research that has emerged over the last few years, the claim that LGBT families *do* exist out there can be made; whether they themselves identify as LGBT though might be a totally different matter. Much more research is needed within an indigenous framework where partnerships between researchers and participants are fostered to acknowledge, value, and produce local knowledge. If questions related to same-sex identity are never asked, claims that LGBT-parent families do not exist will continue to go unchallenged. Non-Western perspectives on LGBT-parent families bring to light a world of fragile rights and vulnerable families.

References

Aggleton, P. (2009). Researching same-sex sexuality and HIV prevention. In V. Reddy, T. Sandfort, & L. Rispel (Eds.), *From social silence to social science: Same-sex sexuality, HIV & AIDS and gender in South Africa* (pp. 2–13). Cape Town, South Africa: HSRC Press.

Álvarez, P. M., & Álvares-Gayou Jurgenson, J. L. (2003). Experience and meaning of maternity in lesbian and heterosexual women. *Archivos Hispanoamericanos de Sexología, IX* (1), 65–80.

Annandale, G. C. (2008). *The experiential world of adolescent learners with homosexual parents* (Unpublished master's thesis). University of South Africa, Pretoria, South Africa.

Ben-Ari, A., & Lavee, Y. (2004). Cultural orientation, ethnic affiliation, and negative daily occurrences: A multidimensional cross-cultural analysis. *American Journal of Orthopsychiatry, 74*, 102–111. doi:10.1037/0002-9432.74.2.102

Ben-Ari, A., & Livni, T. (2006). Motherhood is not a given thing: Experiences and constructed meaning of biological and nonbiological lesbian mothers. *Sex Roles, 54*, 521–531. doi:10.1007/s11199-006-9016-0

Chacha, B. K. (2003, June). *Does a woman who marries a woman become a man? Real desires in woman to woman marriages in Africa, a historical perspective.* Paper presented at the Sex & Secrecy Conference, Johannesburg, South Africa.

Epprecht, M. (2008). *Heterosexual Africa? The history of an idea from the age of exploration to the age of AIDS.* Athens, OH: Ohio University Press.

GALZ (Gays and Lesbians of Zimbabwe). (2008). *Unspoken facts: A history of homosexualities in Africa.* Harare, Zimbabwe: Gays and Lesbians of Zimbabwe.

Graham, S. (2003, June). *Giving love and affection: Female-Female romantic relationships in South Saluwesi, Indonesia.* Paper presented at the Sex & Secrecy Conference, Johannesburg, South Africa.

Gunkel, H. (2010). *The cultural politics of female sexuality in South Africa.* New York, NY: Routledge.

Herdt, G. (1997). *Same sex, different cultures: Exploring gay and lesbian lives.* Boulder, CO: Westview Press.

Herrera, F. (2009). Tradition and transgression: Lesbian motherhood in Chile. *Sexuality Research and Social Policy, 6*(2), 35–51.

Judge, M., Manion, A., & De Waal, S. (2008). "Saying to our children we are a unit" (Interview with Lael Bethlehem and Emilia Potenza). In M. Judge, A. Manion, & S. de Waal (Eds.), *To have and to hold: The making of same-sex marriages in South Africa* (pp. 324–328). Johannesburg, South Africa: Fanele Press, Jacana Media.

Karraker, M. W. (2011). Families worldwide. In J. Lee & S. M. Shaw (Eds.), *Women worldwide: Transnational feminist perspective on women* (pp. 303–313). New York, NY: McGraw-Hill.

Khamasi, J. W., & Maina-Chinkuya, S. N. (2005). Introduction. In J. W. Khamasi & S. N. Maina-Chinkuyu (Eds.), *Sexuality: An African perspective: The politics of self and cultural beliefs* (pp. 1–20). Eldoret, Kenya: Moi University Press.

Kiluva-Ndunda, M. M. (2005). Reflecting on the construction of sexuality: A Mkamba woman's perspective. In J. W. Khamasi & S. N. Maina-Chinkuyu (Eds.), *Sexuality: An African perspective: The politics of self and cultural beliefs* (pp. 21–36). Eldoret, Kenya: Moi University Press.

Lavee, Y., & Katz, R. (2003). The family in Israel: Between tradition and modernity. *Marriage & Family Review, 35*(1/2), 193–217. doi:10.1300/J002v35n01_11

Lewin, E. (1993). *Lesbian mothers: Accounts of gender in American culture.* Ithaca, NY: Cornell University Press.

Lubbe, C. & Kruger, L. (2012). The disclosure practices of a South African born adolescent raised in an American lesbian parent family. *Journal of GLBT Family Studies, 8*, 385–402. doi: 10.1080/1550428X.2012.705622

Lubbe, C. (2005). *The experiences of children growing up in same-gendered families* (Unpublished doctoral dissertation). University of Pretoria, Pretoria, South Africa.

Lubbe, C. (2007). To tell or not to tell: How children of same-gender parents negotiate their lives at school.

Education as Change, 11(2), 45–65. doi:10.1080/16823200709487165

Lubbe, C. (2008). The experiences of children growing up in lesbian-headed families in South Africa. *Journal of GLBT Family Studies, 4*, 325–359. doi:10.1080/15504280802177540

Matebeni, Z. (2008). Blissful complexities: Black lesbians reflect on same-sex marriage and the Civil Union Act. In M. Judge, A. Manion, & S. de Waal (Eds.), *To have and to hold: The making of same-sex marriages in South Africa* (pp. 249–257). Johannesburg, South Africa: Fanele Press, Jacana Media.

Mbali, M. (2009). Gay AIDS activism in South Africa prior to 1994. In V. Reddy, T. Sandfort, & L. Rispel (Eds.), *From social silence to social science: Same-sex sexuality, HIV & AIDS and gender in South Africa* (pp. 80–99). Cape Town, South Africa: HSRC Press.

Mkhize, N., Bennett, J., Reddy, V., & Moletsane, R. (2010). *The country we want to live in: Hate crimes and homophobia in the lives of black lesbian South Africans.* Cape Town, South Africa: HSRC Press.

Morgan, R., & Wieringa, S. (2005). *Tommy boys, lesbian men and ancestral wives: Female same-sex practices in Africa.* Johannesburg, South Africa: Jacana Media.

Munro, B. M. (2009). Queer family romance: Writing the "new" South Africa in the 1990s. *GLQ: A Journal of Lesbian and Gay Studies, 15*, 397–439. doi:10.1215/10642684-2008-030

Nel, J. A. (2007). *Towards the "good society": Healthcare provision for victims of hate crime from periphery to centre stage* (Unpublished doctoral dissertation). University of South Africa, Pretoria, South Africa.

Nkabinde, N. Z. (2008). *Black bull, ancestors and me: My life as a lesbian Sangoma.* Johannesburg, South Africa: Fanele Press, Jacana Media.

Ottosson, D. (2010). *State-sponsored Homophobia: A world survey of laws prohibiting same sex activity between consenting adults* (ILGA report). Retrieved from http://old.ilga.org/Statehomophobia/ILGA_State_Sponsored_Homophobia_2010.pdf

Polášková, E. (2007). The Czech lesbian family study: Investigating family practices. In R. Kuhar & J. Takács (Eds.), *Beyond the pink curtain: Everyday life of LGBT people in Eastern Europe* (pp. 201–215). Ljubljana, Slovenia: Peace Institute.

Pon, Q. L. S. (2008). *The stories of adoptive gay parents about acceptance and discrimination in the pre-school of their child or children* (Unpublished master's thesis). University of Johannesburg, Johannesburg, South Africa.

Potgieter, C. (1997). *Black, South African, lesbian: Discourses of invisible lives* (Unpublished doctoral dissertation). University of the Western Cape, Cape Town, South Africa.

Potgieter, C. (2003). Black South African lesbians: Discourses on motherhood and women's roles. *Journal of Lesbian Studies, 7*, 135–151. doi:10.1300/J155v07n03_10

Sardá-Chandiramani, A. (2010). Sexualities in the 21st century. In I. Dubel & A. Hielkema (Eds.), *Urgency required: Gay and lesbian rights are human rights* (pp. 194–203). The Netherlands: Humanist Institute for Cooperation with Developing Countries (Hivos). Retrieved from http://www.hivos.net/Hivos-Knowledge-Programme/Themes/Urgency-Required/News/Urgency-Required-Out-Now

Shechner, T., Slone, M., Meir, Y., & Kalish, Y. (2010). Relations between social support and psychological and parental distress for lesbian, single heterosexual by choice, and two-parent heterosexual mothers. *American Journal of Orthopsychiatry, 80*, 283–292. doi:10.1111/j.1939-0025.2010.01031.x

Suckling, C. (2009). *Donor insemination families: A qualitative exploration of being lesbian parents raising sperm donor children in South Africa.* Unpublished master's thesis, University of KwaZulu Natal, KwaZulu Natal, South Africa.

Švab, A. (2007). Do they have a choice? Reproductive preferences among lesbians and gay people in Slovenia. In R. Kuhar & J. Takács (Eds.), *Beyond the pink curtain: Everyday life of LGBT people in Eastern Europe* (pp. 217–230). Ljubljana, Slovenia: Peace Institute.

Švab, A., & Kuhar, R. (2005). *The unbearable comfort of privacy: The everyday lives of gays and lesbians* [Adobe Digital Editions version]. Retrieved from http://www2.arnes.si/~ljmiri1s/eng_html/publications/pdf/MI_gay_eng.pdf

Swain, K. (2009). *Becoming a same-gendered family and being a "parent": A qualitative exploration of the experiences of a South African lesbian couple who chose to become parents through assisted reproductive technology* (Unpublished master's thesis). University of KwaZulu Natal, KwaZulu Natal, South Africa.

Thoreson, R., & Cook, S. (2011). *Nowhere to turn: Blackmail and extortion of LGBT people in Sub-Saharan Africa.* New York, NY: International Gay and Lesbian Human Rights Commission. Retrieved from http://www.iglhrc.org/binary-data/ATTACHMENT/file/000/000/484-1.pdf

Uziel, A. P. (2001). Homosexuality and adoption in Brazil. *Reproductive Health Matters, 9*(18), 34–42.

Vaggione, J. M. (2010). Non-heterosexual parenthood in Latin America. In I. Dubel & A. Hielkema (Eds.), *Urgency required: Gay and lesbian rights are human rights* (pp. 218–222). The Netherlands: Humanist Institute for Cooperation with Developing Countries (Hivos). Retrieved from http://www.hivos.net/Hivos-Knowledge-Programme/Themes/Urgency-Required/News/Urgency-Required-Out-Now

Watson, P. (2008). *Queer Malawi, untold stories.* Johannesburg, South Africa: Gay and Lesbian Memory in Action (GALA) and the Centre for the Development of People (CEDEP).

LGBT Parents and the Workplace

15

Eden B. King, Ann H. Huffman, and Chad I. Peddie

The workplace is a critical context in which to understand the experiences of lesbian, gay, bisexual, and transgendered (LGBT) parents. A growing body of research emerging from the disciplines of organizational and counseling psychology provides important evidence regarding LGBT workers. In her comprehensive review of the literature on LGBT people in the workplace, management scholar Belle Ragins (2004) described three dominant challenges faced by LGBT people. First, Ragins reflected on the issues that arise as a function of the fact that the invisibility of an LGBT identity often leads to assumptions of heterosexuality. LGBT workers who have not disclosed their sexual or gender identity may be subject to indirect discrimination as their coworkers disparage gay or lesbian people or make "gay" jokes. In contrast, LGBT workers who have disclosed their identity face different issues, such as

15

E.B. King, Ph.D.(✉)
Department of Psychology, George Mason University, 4400 University Drive, MSN 3f5, Fairfax, VA 22030, USA
e-mail: eking6@gmu.edu

A.H. Huffman, Ph.D.
Department of Psychology and W. A. Franke College of Business, Northern Arizona University, Box 15106, Flagstaff, AZ 86011, USA
e-mail: ann.huffman@nau.edu

C.I. Peddie, M.A.
Human Resources Research Organization, 66 Canal Center Plaza, Suite 700, Alexandria, VA 22314, USA
e-mail: ianscorp@aol.com

backlash and discrimination as a result of their disclosure (King, Reilly, & Hebl, 2008). These outcomes illustrate a disclosure dilemma wherein many LGBT workers encounter negative outcomes regardless of the disclosure decision they make. This dilemma can result in psychologically demanding and constant efforts to manage an LGBT identity at work (Button, 2001) to avoid discrimination.

Indeed, the second challenge Ragins (2004) described is negative coworker reactions. Ragins argued that LGBT workers likely face negative coworker reactions due to the perceived controllability of sexual orientation and to the threats that some coworkers experience in response to LGBT people. These threats include a tangible threat (fear of health and safety), a symbolic threat (defensiveness of moral or political views), and personal threats (questions regarding one's own sexual identity). This framework is consistent with experimental evidence that heterosexual job applicants are rated (Horvath & Ryan, 2003) and treated (Hebl, Foster, Mannix, & Dovidio, 2002) more positively than gay and lesbian applicants. In addition, Ragins' ideas about negative reactions are also consistent with survey data which demonstrate that as much as 66% of LGBT people report experiencing discrimination (Croteau, 1996) and more than a third of gay and lesbian professionals indicate encountering sexuality-related physical or verbal harassment at work (Ragins & Cornwell, 2001).

The third and final challenge Ragins (2004) highlighted is the lack of social support that

A.E. Goldberg and K.R. Allen (eds.), *LGBT-Parent Families: Innovations in Research and Implications for Practice*, DOI 10.1007/978-1-4614-4556-2_15, © Springer Science+Business Media New York 2013

LGBT people likely find inside and outside of the workplace. Because of their minority status and the concealability of their identity, LGBT workers may find it difficult to identify other LGBT people at work. This lack of connection may make it difficult for LGBT employees to access both tangible and psychosocial resources (King et al., 2008). For example, LGBT people might not know who it is safe to ask about accessing same-sex partner benefits, or who to talk to about experiences of heterosexism. At an institutional level, some of the structures (families, schools, churches) that support members of other stigmatized groups (such as women and ethnic minorities) are not always as welcoming of or helpful to LGBT people (Ragins, 2004). This lack of support, both internal and external to their workplaces, can lead to feelings of isolation. In sum, research has demonstrated that LGBT people encounter numerous challenges in the workplace.

However, very little empirical evidence has considered the unique challenges that may emerge when LGBT people balance the demands of work with the responsibilities of family (i.e., work–family conflict). Although a substantial body of psychological research on the work–family interface has explored antecedents and consequences associated with work–family conflict among heterosexual workers (see Eby, Casper, Lockwood, Bordeaux, & Brinley, 2005), little is known about the ways in which the work–family interface is experienced by LGBT people. Thus, the goal of this chapter is to integrate the growing body of research on LGBT workplace issues with primarily heterocentric research on the work–family interface. We will begin by briefly discussing the major conclusions of work–family interface research. Next, we will synthesize research on LGBT workplace and family issues to highlight the concerns of LGBT parents and the ways in which these experiences might be improved. We will conclude by offering potential next steps for research and practice with the hope of building understanding related to potential barriers and opportunities for LGBT parents at work.

The Work–Family Interface

Research on the intersection of the work and family domains has burgeoned in the past two decades, dismantling the expectation that the balance of these two domains could be achieved through the enactment of traditional gender roles. These traditional gender roles frame men as "breadwinners," whose sole responsibility is in the workplace, and women as "homemakers," whose sole responsibility is child and household labor (Eagly, 1987). Surges of women entering the workforce beginning with the second wave of the feminist movement of the 1960s created family settings where traditional gender roles were no longer functional (Bond, Thompson, Galinsky, & Prottas, 2002). Today, most parents, regardless of family structure, are balancing multiple roles that blend work and family responsibilities.

Importantly, as implied by the heterocentric description of the evolution of the work–family interface above, very little of this rapidly growing area of research has focused on the ways in which LGBT people balance work and family. A recent methodological review of work–family research in organizational psychology and management identified no studies on LGBT families (Casper, Eby, Bordeaux, Lockwood, & Lambert, 2007). Instead, existing organizational/management research (including that of this chapter's authors) tends to take a heterocentric approach wherein parents are implicitly defined as opposite-gender, married, cohabiting couples (see Dunne, 2000). This presumption is particularly problematic in light of the fact that research on LGBT families in other disciplines (such as family psychology and sociology) generally does not directly address the *work* experiences of LGBT people. Here we will briefly review organizational scholarship on the work–family interface as a basis for building understanding of the ways in which simultaneous involvement in family and work is experienced by employees. Next, we describe the ways that parents, scholars, and employers might be informed by fully integrating LGBT parents in conceptualizations of the work–family interface.

Theoretical Models of the Work–Family Interface

The term "work–family interface" refers to the experiences that occur at the intersection between work and family domains. Common perspectives that address this interface include work–family conflict (Kahn, Wolfe, Quinn, Snoek, & Rosenthal, 1964) and work–family enrichment (Greenhaus & Powell, 2006). A common theme underlying each of these perspectives is their reliance on *role theory* (Katz & Kahn, 1978), which posits that people are involved in multiple roles that can affect one another. A "work" role is defined as the engagement in activities that result in the provision of monetary goods and services which sustain living (Piotrkowski, Rapoport, & Rapoport, 1987). "Family" roles entail involvement, obligation, or responsibility to collections of individuals related by marriage, biology, or adoption (Piotrkowski et al., 1987). Activities related to the family domain involve contributions to the sustaining of family well-being such as child care or food preparation.

Whereas many researchers initially conceptualized the work–family interface as a unidirectional phenomenon whereby experiences at work were observed to impact those of the family, researchers now realize that this interface is actually bidirectional (Frone, Russell, & Cooper, 1992). The most common term used to capture the negative aspects of the work–family interface is work–family conflict. The concept of work–family conflict hinges on the scarcity hypothesis, which posits that the treatment of roles in the work and family domains are incompatible to a certain extent (Kahn et al., 1964). *Role conflict* emerges when the demands of one role make it difficult to fulfill the demands of another role. Greenhaus and Beutell (1985) defined three distinct forms of work–family interrole conflict: time-based conflict, strain-based conflict, and behavior-based conflict. Time-based conflict captures situations where participation in either work or family events is prevented by simultaneously occurring responsibilities in the other domain. As an example, a parent might miss a parent–teacher conference due to a meeting at work. Strain-based conflict involves the affective experiences—such as anxiety, stress, and tension—that arise due to demands in both domains. Finally, behavior-based conflict stems from a discrepancy between styles of behavior in both roles. For example, a partner may be expected to be loving and supportive at home, while assertive and authoritative as a supervisor at work.

Although much of the research devoted to the work and family interface focuses on the negative effects of one domain on the other, it is important to realize that under certain conditions the interaction of work and family can have positive effects (Barnett & Hyde, 2001; Greenhaus & Powell, 2006). Researchers investigating positive work–family interactions suggest that participating in multiple roles may be beneficial, such that one's participation in one role can enhance performance in another role (e.g., work–family enrichment; Barnett & Hyde, 2001).

Consequences of the Work–Family Interface

A growing body of research (limited to heterosexual workers, most of whom have children) has established that work–family conflict is linked with important outcomes in work settings as well as in other areas of life (e.g., Greenhaus & Beutell, 1985). For example, with regard to work, meta-analytic work has uncovered a strong negative relationship between work–family conflict and job satisfaction (Allen, Herst, Bruck, & Sutton, 2000). Additionally, Allen et al. (2000) identified unfavorable relationships between work–family conflict and affective organizational commitment, turnover, and job performance. Similarly unfavorable relationships emerge between work–family conflict and other aspects of life. Again, meta-analyses found a strong negative relationship between work–family conflict and life satisfaction (Allen et al., 2000). Allen et al. (2000) also identified negative relationships between work–family conflict and both marital and family satisfaction. These findings were found to hold among professionals working in a wide variety of occupational settings.

A relatively small set of studies has considered the positive outcomes of work–family enrichment. Positive work–family interactions have been found to hold favorable relationships with work outcomes including job satisfaction and organizational commitment (Van Steenbergen, Ellemers, & Mooijaart, 2007). Similarly, work–family enrichment is positively associated with individual outcomes such as well-being and satisfaction (Van Steenbergen et al., 2007).

Factors that Influence the Work–Family Interface

In addition to investigating important outcomes of work–family conflict and enrichment, researchers have also explored the factors that might facilitate a positive work–family interface (almost exclusively among opposite-sex couples with children). Eby et al. (2005) reviewed predictors of the work–family interface including family characteristics, job attributes, organizational characteristics, spouse variables, and individual differences. This review demonstrated strong relationships between elements of the work domain and work–family conflict such as work demands (e.g., work hours; Grzywacz & Marks, 2000), involvement in work (Carlson & Perrewé, 1999), and an unsupportive organizational culture or supervisor (Nielson, Carlson, & Lankau, 2001). Similarly, empirical research has demonstrated that family characteristics such as concerns about child care (Buffardi & Erdwins, 1997) and the degree to which individuals identify psychologically with their family role (Carlson & Perrewé, 1999) can increase work–family conflict. There have been fewer studies on predictors of work–family enrichment. Research has shown that characteristics such as self-esteem, family support, job characteristics, and supervisor support and family-related characteristics such as family member support are all positively related to work–family enrichment (Grzywacz & Marks, 2000).

One individual difference variable that has been shown to influence the work–family interface of heterosexual employees is gender. Gender plays an important role in the work–family

interface in part because of the ideology of gender roles described at the outset of this section. In the work domain, men are perceived to be fulfilling the ideals of masculinity by focusing on their careers, whereas women are seen as eschewing the feminine gender role by engaging in the same behavior (Eagly, 1987). Equally problematic is the parallel process in the home domain: women who focus on their families are seen as embodying femininity, whereas men sometimes receive social penalties for heavy involvement in their families (such as working part-time; Eagly & Steffen, 1984). Ultimately, in line with Eagly (1987), social expectations about the roles of men and women are perpetuated through gendered behaviors.

Indeed, women in heterosexual relationships tend to be responsible for the majority of household and child-care labor irrespective of their employment status (see Coltrane, 2000). Importantly, however, evidence regarding gender differences in work–family conflict is mixed, with some studies suggesting women experience more conflict than men (Behson, 2002) and others suggesting comparable levels of conflict (Duxbury & Higgins, 1991). More nuanced analyses of gender differences in the factors that give rise to work–family conflict point to the variable impact of specific conditions; for example, in their study of 131 men and 109 women, Duxbury and Higgins (1991) found that being oriented toward work was a stronger predictor of conflict for women than men, whereas being oriented toward family was a stronger predictor of conflict for men than women. One generally consistent finding is that becoming a parent tends to have more detrimental effects on the careers of women than men. In one survey study of nearly 100 supervisor–subordinate dyads (King, 2008), heterosexual men and women with children reported equivalent levels of commitment to work and desire for development and advancement, but their supervisors perceived the fathers to be more committed to work and interested in development and advancement than mothers. Moreover, these inaccurate perceptions accounted for gender discrepancies in pay and promotions, whereby men were paid more than women and were more likely to be promoted. Such findings are consistent with the notion that women's workplace advancement is often blocked by a "motherhood penalty" or a "maternal wall" (Williams, 2004).

In summary, there is a large and growing body of evidence on predictors and outcomes of the work–family interface for opposite-sex, cohabitating, married couples (Casper et al., 2007). But what of families of LGBT people?

The Work–Family Interface of LGBT Parents

Empirical data regarding the work–family interface for people in same-sex relationships are scarce. In fact, it has only been since 1990 that the U.S. Census has collected data regarding unmarried partners. Researchers have begun to explore the experiences of LGBT parents in part by inferring an LGBT identity for individuals who indicate that they have an "unmarried partner" of the same sex (Prokos & Keene, 2010). Evidence from the Census suggests that these couples tend to be more highly educated and more inclined to hold two incomes than heterosexual families (Black, Sanders, & Taylor, 2007). Additionally, the Census estimates that 22% of male same-sex couples and 33% of female same-sex couples have children, whereas approximately 45% of heterosexual couples have children (Simmons & O'Connell, 2003).

It is not yet clear whether empirical findings on the work–family interface of heterosexual parents can be generalized to LGBT parents. On the one hand, O'Ryan and McFarland's (2010) interview-based study of five lesbian and four gay couples found that LGBT parents use strategies that are not unlike those of heterosexual parents to balance work and family (e.g., carefully weighing work decisions and creating positive social networks). In addition, Mercier's (2006) interview-based study of 21 lesbian parents suggested that workplace flexibility was considered a benefit for family in much the same way as it is for heterosexual parents. Tuten and August (2006) studied 58 lesbian mothers and found that work characteristics such as job role autonomy, fewer hours worked, and supportive work–family

culture and policies reduced work–family conflict in a manner consistent with the research on heterosexual couples. On the other hand, however, it should be noted that the extent to which these women were "out" at work predicted work–family conflict over and beyond these typical variables (Tuten & August, 2006). These findings suggest that there are unique characteristics of the workplace (such as the extent to which coworkers and supervisors are supportive of LGBT workers) that might need to be taken into account for LGBT employees.

Some research points to other potential work–family differences between heterosexual and LGBT employees. For example, in a longitudinal study of 29 lesbian couples (58 women) who were becoming parents, it was predicted that work characteristics typically affecting heterosexual couples' relationships, such as hours worked and organizational support, would similarly affect lesbian parents. However, contrary to hypotheses, these variables were not related to the partners' relationship conflict (Goldberg & Sayer, 2006). One of the explanations for differences in the experience of work–family conflict between LGBT and non-LGBT individuals may relate to gender dynamics; LGBT-parent families experiences of work–life conflict and balance may inevitably differ from those of heterosexual-parent families because the partners are of the same gender. Indeed, in support of this notion, studies of families involving lesbian parents have often found that work, household, and child-care labor are often shared more equally in lesbian couples than in heterosexual couples (e.g., Patterson, Sutfin, & Fulcher, 2004). Given the mixed nature of these findings, it is important to consider the theoretical perspectives that might help to explain the experiences of LGBT parents at the intersection of work and family domains.

Applying and Extending Existing Theories to LGBT Parents

The limited body of research directly focusing on how LGBT parents experience and manage work–family conflict points to the need to develop a deeper understanding of the work–family inter-face of LGBT parents. To achieve this deeper understanding, a critical next step is to examine the ways in which existing theories of the work–family interface and of LGBT workplace experi-ences can be useful in understanding the work–family interface of LGBT people.

Role Theory

As the dominant model used to understand the work–family interface in heterosexual parents, role theory (Katz & Kahn, 1978) has the capacity to provide insights about LGBT parents. Specifically, in recognizing that people sustain multiple roles—each of which is accompanied by pressure, expectations, forces, and behaviors—that can be mutually conflicting, role theory high-lights the importance of considering *all* of the roles individuals occupy. Like their heterosexual counterparts, working LGBT parents are engaged in the roles of work and family. However, unlike their counterparts, LGBT parents may experience expectations, forces, and pressures from their social identity group. That is, being LGBT may constitute an additional role for some people that can potentially enhance or conflict with their other roles.

On the conflict side, being LGBT may some-times make it difficult to fulfill the demands of work and parent roles. For example, LGBT peo-ple who work in jobs in which their identity is particularly stigmatized may face feelings of inauthenticity (if they do not disclose their iden-tity) or discrimination (if they do disclose) that could interfere with their work-role behaviors. As another example, because many Americans endorse a traditional view of family as consisting of opposite-sex parents and children (Collins, 1998), LGBT parents may also occasionally experience conflict between their LGBT and par-ent identities. For example, LGBT parents likely want to express their sexual identity openly in their communities while also wanting to protect their children from the negative consequences of bigotry. Indeed, one semi-structured interview-based study with six daughters of lesbian parents found that lesbian mothers had carefully prepared

their children for heterosexism by openly defining and discussing sexual orientation and warning them about the possibility of future incidents (Litovich & Langhout, 2004). On the enhance-ment side, being a parent might help LGBT peo-ple in ways that are similar to heterosexual people. According to an expansionist perspective (Barnett & Hyde, 2001), people can gain positive views of the self, additional avenues of social support, and even stress relief through involvement in parent-ing. It is possible that becoming a parent could help LGBT people connect with their coworkers and supervisors through shared experiences. In addition, parenthood may act as unique informa-tion that distances LGBT people from negative stereotypes (see Singletary & Hebl, 2009).

Stigma Theory

Grounded in Erving Goffman's (1963) influential book, *Stigma: Notes on the Management of Spoiled Identity*, stigma theory suggests that par-ticular characteristics are imbued with social meaning. A *stigma*, which originally referred to a mark burned into the skin of thieves in ancient Greece, is a characteristic that is devalued in a particular context. Holders of stigmas are typi-cally subject to economic disadvantage, stereo-typing, and discrimination (Crocker, Major, & Steele, 1998). Stigmas vary along several dimen-sions, two of the most meaningful of which are *concealability* and perceived *controllability* (Crocker et al., 1998). According to Goffman, individuals with stigmas that are concealable, like LGBT people, must uniquely decide whether, how, when, and to whom to disclose their iden-tity. Individuals with stigmas that are perceived to be controllable, like LGBT people, are likely to be blamed for their identity or condition and thus might face particularly negative reactions (Goffman, 1963).

Research on LGBT people from the perspec-tive of stigma theory has demonstrated that people with nonheterosexual sexual identities are targets of stereotyping and discrimination that is emblem-atic of stigma. For example, one experimental field study demonstrated that job applicants were treated more negatively when they wore a hat that said "gay and proud" than when they wore a hat that said "Texan and proud" (Hebl et al., 2002). The stigma perspective has also yielded insights about the dilemmas that LGBT people face in their decisions regarding disclosure of their sexual identity to their coworkers, supervisors, and clients. As an example, using an experience sampling methodology with 50 LGBT workers, King, Mohr, Peddie, Jones, and Kendra (2010) found that LGBT people felt like they had to make a decision about whether or not to reveal their sexual identity while at work an average of nine times over a 3-week period. In addition, stigma theory has been used to help explain persistent negative beliefs about and attitudes toward LGBT people; the extent to which people believe homosexuality to be a choice (and therefore a "controllable condition") is associated with more negative stereotypes and prejudice about LGBT people (Haider-Markel & Joslyn, 2008).

In stigma theory, the emphasis on the concealable nature of an LGBT identity has important implications for LGBT parents in two primary areas: (a) disclosure disconnects, and (b) access to resources. In her discussion of concealable stigmas, Ragins (2008) described the processes involved with disclosing a stigmatized identity across work and nonwork domains. Her theoretical paper highlighted the interface between work and nonwork disclosures, and argued that the level of disclosure across these domains could be indicative of identity denial ("out" in neither domain), identity disconnects ("out" in one domain but not the other), or identity integration ("out" in both domains). Because LGBT parents must balance their own personal concerns about disclosure as well as their concerns about their children, they may be vulnerable to identity disconnects, which, Ragins argued, creates psychological incongruence, stress, and anxiety.

Moreover, LGBT parents' disclosure dilemmas may make it difficult to access helpful resources in both work and nonwork domains. In the work domain, the availability of particular work–life policies may not result in positive gains for some employee groups including LGBT people (Ryan & Kossek, 2008). One of the reasons for this variability in utility of work–life benefits is that supervisors often serve as gatekeepers

with regard to work–family benefits such as family leave, flexible work schedules, and telecommuting. Thus, the interpersonal relationships between LGBT parents and their supervisors could pose challenges to managing the intersection of the work and family domains. In fact, evidence suggests that in all employees, the relationship between the supervisor and subordinate may be responsible for employees' reluctance to partake in such benefits due to fear of retribution (Bowen & Orthner, 1991). LGBT parents therefore likely face multiple barriers to accessing resources. First, they must disclose their parental status, which may also make them vulnerable to discussions of their sexual identity. In other words, LGBT people may have to "out" themselves at work when they become parents. Second, not all benefits available to heterosexual employees may be universally available to same-sex parents (Ryan & Kossek, 2008). Third, LGBT parents often must rely on their supervisor's equanimity to allow them to utilize benefits.

Similar barriers may be encountered by LGBT parents who have not disclosed their sexual identity widely outside of work. Many heterosexual parents manage care for their children by relying heavily on immediate family members such as grandmothers (Fuller-Thomson, Minkler, & Driver, 1996). When LGBT parents have not disclosed their sexual identity to their families, or when their families have not fully embraced their LGBT identity, LGBT parents may not have access to the potentially useful support of involved families. Fears about losing control over sexual identity disclosure may also make it harder for LGBT parents to gain the benefits of involvement in social organizations (e.g., "mommy's day out" groups or church organizations) that provide support. The disclosure dilemmas that are central to stigma theory imply several distinct issues that LGBT parents could face at the intersection of work and family.

Minority Stress

The second major theoretical lens that has been brought to bear on the experiences of LGBT workers is minority stress. Drawing from general views of stress as physical, mental, or emotional strain or pressure that can be due to conditions in the social environment, Meyer (2003) suggested that members of stigmatized groups experience a unique form of *minority stress*. LGBT people tend to live their lives, residing and working, in close proximity with heterosexuals and few other LGBT people (Waldo, 1999). According to Meyer (2003), LGBT people experience not only general stressors that are common to nonminority groups but also distal stressors (e.g., discrimination and violence) and proximal stressors (e.g., expectations of rejection, identity management efforts, and internalized homophobia). Consistent with general models of stress, the accumulation of stressors can ultimately affect mental health outcomes. In addition to its numerous applications in counseling psychology (see Meyer, 2003), the minority stress perspective has been used to help explain some of the workplace experiences of LGBT people. For example, fear of disclosing a nonheterosexual identity is a unique minority stressor that has been correlated with job attitudes and career outcomes (Ragins, Singh, & Cornwell, 2007).

A direct extension of this theory to LGBT parents might suggest that an LGBT identity may exacerbate the stress of the work–family interface. The implication is not only that LGBT people would generally experience more stressors than non-LGBT people but also that LGBT parents would experience more stressors than LGBT people who are not parents. In other words, because less than a third of same-sex couples have children (Simmons & O'Connell, 2003), LGBT parents may comprise a minority or subgroup within LGBT communities. Framed in this way, being an LGBT parent could be seen as a predictor of work–family conflict. It is also possible that the stressors experienced by LGBT people could exacerbate the consequences of work–family conflict. Take as an example a common experience of work–family conflict: a breakdown in child care. The stress of this breakdown might be worse for LGBT parents than for heterosexual parents because the latter group may have easier access to work- and nonwork resources (such as emergency care services

through work or familial care). Finally, an LGBT identity could in some cases buffer the consequences of work–family conflict; it is possible that LGBT parents have developed resilience and coping strategies that help them deal with such stressors (Meyer, 2010). More research is needed to address each of these important questions.

An Intersectionality Perspective

To this point, we have discussed the potential experiences of LGBT parents in general without describing the wide variability that exists within this population or the nuances that emerge at the intersection of sexual orientation, gender, ethnicity, or socioeconomic status. A theoretical paradigm that is applicable to both minority stress and stigma theories while attending to these important identities is the perspective of *intersectionality*. From the lens of critical race and feminist theories (Crenshaw, 1988), intersectionality underscores the notion that people who are members of multiple stigmatized social identity categories have unique experiences (Cole, 2009). For example, Crenshaw (1988) examined the intersection of gender and race in her exploration of African-American women. She found that discrimination associated with membership in one stigmatized identity group can be compounded when another stigmatized identity is also possessed. Consistent with this, survey research (Berdahl & Moore, 2006) indicated that ethnic minority women faced a "double jeopardy": not only did women report more sexual harassment than men but also minorities reported more ethnic harassment than did Whites; minority women experienced the greatest amount of harassment overall. Similarly, it has been argued that LGBT people of color may face more discrimination than LGBT people who are White (Moradi et al., 2010). In response to this, Meyer (2010) contended that although there may be an internal conflict between racial and sexual identities such that perceptions of oneself as a particular sexuality interfere with values associated with one's race, LGB people of color can have positive racial and sexual identities.

An intersectionality perspective might be particularly useful in considering the workplace experiences of LGBT parents, who may be stigmatized as a function of their sexual identity as well as their parental status (in addition to gender, race, and other characteristics). Research on heterosexual parents suggests that women (but not men) face stigmatization in the workplace when they become parents (e.g., Cuddy, Fiske, & Glick, 2004). Heterosexual women with children are perceived as less committed to work and less interested in advancement than are women without children or men (King, 2008). It is possible that (consistent with a "double jeopardy" perspective) these negative effects of maternal status are exacerbated among lesbian women, who possess the devalued characteristics of being women, mothers, and gay. However, there is some evidence that lesbians with children actually have higher income (Baumle, 2009) and perceived work commitment (Peplau & Fingerhut, 2004) than their gay male and heterosexual counterparts. More research is needed to reconcile these contradictory findings.

An intersectionality perspective might also help to frame efforts toward understanding how LGBT parents from different socioeconomic groups experience the work–family interface. The notion of work–family balance, a theoretical equilibrium among the time, affect, and behavior experienced across multiple domains, may be a luxury for many families whose jobs do not easily support the costs of food, shelter, and health care. The work–family interface for such people may be characterized by extremely long hours or a "patchwork" of multiple jobs, desperation and anxious moods, and a lack of access to high quality child care (Ford, 2011). LGBT parents in low-paying jobs may experience high levels of continuance commitment; in other words, they may prioritize keeping their jobs above all else (Meyer & Allen, 1993). As such, LGBT parents without substantial economic resources may feel particularly high levels of fear about disclosure and discrimination, or may feel stuck in environments that are unfriendly to gay people and families. Overall, existing theories on the experiences of LGBT people suggest that people who occupy

the intersection of a minority sexual identity and parenthood likely experience challenges in balancing their involvement in multiple roles, particularly with regard to disclosure disconnects, access to resources, and the frequency of stressors.

In her critique of feminist work on gender and the family, Ferree (2010) discussed differences between locational and relational intersectionalities. The former approach focuses on social identity categories and the perspectives of individuals who possess multiple marginalized identities (e.g., poor African-American women; Ferree, 2010). This is contrasted with a focus on processes (such as racializing particular ethnic groups) that arise from complex and unequal relations (Ferree, 2010). Thus, it is the latter approach that may be particularly helpful for understanding ongoing, interpersonal dynamics such as the work–family interface. In line with this, Shields (2008) stated that focusing on differences between categories of people is a "seductive oversimplification" (p. 303) that should be supplanted with a focus on explanation of processes. In the case of LGBT parents and the workplace, then, these arguments imply that attention should be devoted to the processes underlying systems of workplace inequality. Structures and processes that subordinate LGBT parents, such as the absence of domestic partnership benefits, workplace policies that are unfriendly to families (e.g., lack of flex time), and a lack of federal protection for employment discrimination for people with LGBT identities, perpetuate challenges faced by LGBT parents.

Future Directions

Our review of extant theory and research has revealed sizeable gaps in scholarly understanding of the workplace experiences of LGBT parents. It is clear that much more work is needed to fully describe, explain, and predict the conditions under and ways in which LGBT parents can create and sustain positive interfaces between their work, family, and LGBT roles and identities. In the consideration of future research we have identified critical areas that must be addressed, including comparisons between LGBT and heterosexual families, accessibility of family-oriented benefits, and the implementation of LGBT friendly benefits.

One important direction for future research is developing more fine-tuned comparisons between LGBT and heterosexual parents and between specific groups within LGBT parents (such as lesbians and gay men, bisexual parents, single gay parents, transgendered parents across transition stages, and LGBT parents across socioeconomic statuses) in relation to the work–family interface. Preliminary comparative research (e.g., Tuten & August, 2006) has suggested that there may indeed be important differences between these groups. Experiences might also vary as a function of the manner in which children came to be; LBT parents who physically carry a child throughout pregnancy likely have different needs than LGBT people who adopt children. It would be useful to understand the unique needs and stressors, as well as exacerbating and buffering factors, for each of these groups. A nuanced understanding of when and why such differences emerge may help identify strategies for LGBT individuals, counselors, human resource practitioners, and consultants to take toward improving the work–family interface of LGBT parents.

A fundamental issue in speculating upon differences in the management of the work–family interface between LGBT and heterosexual people is consideration of the availability and utilization of family-friendly organizational benefits. When requesting to access benefits related to work–family balance (e.g., domestic partner benefits, parental leave) it may become necessary for LGBT employees to "out" themselves. The requirement to disclose sexual identity in this manner may deter some LGBT parents from seeking such benefits even when they are available (see Ryan & Kossek, 2008). Indeed, the current discussion of disclosure dilemmas and double jeopardy points to the importance of identifying and assessing strategies for helping LGBT workers access resources. Existing research suggests that basic structures such as clear procedures regarding same-sex partner benefits, antidiscrimination policies that include LGBT people, and LGBT employee resource groups, diversity councils, and mentorship programs may improve the experiences of LGBT workers (for a review, see King & Cortina, 2010).

To fully support LGBT parents it may be necessary for organizations to implement procedures that allow employees to make use of family-friendly policies without providing detailed information about their family structures that may require disclosure of an LGBT identity. Importantly, however, research has also suggested that formal policies protecting LGBT workers may only be useful to the extent that they are enacted within informal organizational environments that are supportive of LGBT people (Huffman, Watrous, & King, 2008). It is possible that supportive supervisors, mentors, or social networks could help LGBT parents navigate disclosure decisions that facilitate better access to resources. More evidence is needed to clarify not only which policies are most helpful to LGBT parents but also how to implement procedures that allow for their utilization.

Conclusion

In summary, bodies of evidence on the work–family interface and on the workplace experiences of LGBT people are rich and growing. Unfortunately, however, these streams of research have developed in disconnected silos—very few studies have explored the work–family experiences of LGBT people. The limited existing research suggests that there are likely meaningful similarities and differences between the experiences of LGBT and heterosexual parents in balancing work and family. Thus, we argue that scholars have both an opportunity and an obligation to consider the integration of role conflict, stigma, minority stress, and intersectionality theories and research as they apply to LGBT parents.

References

Allen, T. D., Herst, D. E. L., Bruck, C. S., & Sutton, M. (2000). Consequences associated with work-to-family conflict: A review and agenda for future research. *Journal of Occupational Health Psychology, 5*, 278–308. doi:10.1037//1076-899B.5.2.278

Barnett, R. C., & Hyde, J. S. (2001). Women, men, work and family: An expansionist theory. *American Psychologist, 56*, 781–796. doi:10.1037/0003-066X.56.10.781.

Baumle, A. K. (2009). The cost of parenthood: Unraveling the effects of sexual orientation and gender on income. *Social Science Quarterly, 90*, 983–1002. doi:10.1111/j.1540-6237.2009.00673.x

Behson, S. J. (2002). Coping with family to work conflict: The role of informal work accommodations to family. *Journal of Occupational Health Psychology, 7*, 324–341. doi:10.1037/1076-8998.7.4.324

Berdahl, J. L., & Moore, C. (2006). Workplace harassment: Double jeopardy for minority women. *Journal of Applied Psychology, 91*, 426–436. doi:10.1037/0021-9010.91.2.426

Black, D., Sanders, S., & Taylor, L. (2007). The economics of lesbian and gay families. *Journal of Economic Perspectives, 21*, 53–70.

Bond, J. T., Thompson, C., Galinsky, E., & Prottas, D. (2002). *Highlights of the national study of the changing workforce.* New York, NY: Families and Work Institute.

Bowen, G. L, & Orthner, D. K. (1991). Effects of organizational culture on fatherhood. In F. W. Bozett & S. M. H. Hanson (Eds.), *Cultural variations in American fatherhood* (pp. 187–217). New York: Springer Publishing Company, Inc.

Buffardi, L. C., & Erdwins, C. J. (1997). Child-care satisfaction: Linkages to work attitudes, interrole conflict, and maternal separation anxiety. *Journal of Occupational Health Psychology, 2*, 84–96. doi:10.1037/1076-8998.2.1.84

Button, S. B. (2001). Organizational efforts to affirm sexual diversity: A cross-level examination. *Journal of Applied Psychology, 86*, 17–28. doi:10.1037/0021-9010.86.1.17

Carlson, D. S., & Perrewé, P. L. (1999). The role of social support in the stressor-strain relationship: An examination of work-family conflict. *Journal of Management, 25*, 513–540. doi:10.1177/014920639902500403

Casper, W. J., Eby, L. T., Bordeaux, C., Lockwood, A., & Lambert, D. (2007). A review of research methods in IO/OB work-family research. *Journal of Applied Psychology, 92*, 28–43. doi:10.1037/0021-9010.92.1.28

Cole, E. R. (2009). Intersectionality and research in psychology. *American Psychologist, 64*, 170–180. doi:10.1037/a0014564

Collins, P. H. (1998). It's all in the family: Intersections of gender, race, and nation. *Hypatia, 13*, 62–82.

Coltrane, S. (2000). Research on household labor: Modeling and measuring the social embeddedness of routine family work. *Journal of Marriage and Family, 62*, 1208–1233. doi:10.1111/j.1741-3737.2000.01208.x

Crenshaw, K. (1988). Race, reform and retrenchment: Transformation and legitimation in anti discrimination law. *Harvard Law Review, 101*, 1331–1387.

Crocker, J., Major, B., & Steele, C. (1998). Social stigma. In D. Gilbert, S. T. Fiske, & G. Lindzey (Eds.), *Handbook of social psychology* (4th ed., pp. 504–553). Boston, MA: McGraw-Hill.

Croteau, J. M. (1996). Research on the work experiences of lesbian, gay, and bisexual people: An integrative review of methodology and findings. *Journal of Vocational Behavior, 48*, 195–209. doi:10.1177/1059601108321828

Cuddy, A. J. C., Fiske, S. T., & Glick, P. (2004). When professionals become mothers, warmth doesn't cut the ice. *Journal of Social Issues, 60*, 701–718.

Dunne, G. (2000). Opting into motherhood: Lesbians blurring the boundaries and transforming the meaning of parenthood and kinship. *Gender and Society, 14*, 11–35. doi:10.1177/089124300014001003

Duxbury, L. E., & Higgins, C. A. (1991). Gender differences in work-family conflict. *Journal of Applied Psychology, 76*, 60–74. doi:10.1037/0021-9010.76.1.60

Eagly, A. H. (1987). *Sex differences in social behavior: A social-role interpretation.* Hillsdale, NJ: Lawrence Erlbaum Associates.

Eagly, A. H., & Steffen, V. J. (1984). Gender stereotypes stem from the distribution of women and men into social roles. *Journal of Personality and Social Psychology, 46*, 735–754. doi:10.1037/0022-3514.46.4.735

Eby, L. T., Casper, W., Lockwood, A., Bordeaux, C., & Brinley, A. (2005). Work and family research in IO/OB journals: Content analysis and review of the literature. *Journal of Vocational Behavior, 66*, 124–197. doi:10.1016/j.jvb.2003.11.003

Ferree, M. M. (2010). Filling the glass: Gender perspectives on families. *Journal of Marriage and Family, 72*, 420–439. doi:10.1111/j.1741-3737.2010.00711.x

Ford, M. T. (2011). Linking household income and work-family conflict: A moderated-mediation study. *Stress and Health, 27*, 144–162.

Frone, M. R., Russell, M., & Cooper, M. L. (1992). Antecedents and outcomes of work-family conflict: Testing a model of the work-family interface. *Journal of Applied Psychology, 77*, 65–78.

Fuller-Thomson, E., Minkler, M., & Driver, D. (1996). A profile of grandparents raising grandchildren in the United States. *The Gerontologist, 37*, 406–411.

Goffman, E. (1963). *Stigma: Notes on the management of spoiled identity.* Englewood Cliffs, NJ: Prentice Hall.

Goldberg, A. E., & Sayer, A. G. (2006). Lesbian couples' relationship quality across the transition to parenthood. *Journal of Marriage and Family, 68*, 87–100. doi:10.1111/j.1741-3737.2006.00235.x

Greenhaus, J. H., & Beutell, N. J. (1985). Sources of conflict between work and family roles. *Academy of Management Review, 10*, 76–88. doi:10.2307/258214

Greenhaus, J. H., & Powell, G. N. (2006). When work and family are allies: A theory of work-family enrichment. *Academy of Management Review, 31*, 72–92. doi:10.2307/20159186

Grzywacz, J. G., & Marks, N. F. (2000). Reconceptualizing the work-family interface: An ecological perspective on the correlates of positive and negative spillover between work and family. *Journal of Occupational Health Psychology, 5*, 111–126. doi:10.1037/1076-8998.5.1.111

Haider-Markel, D. P., & Joslyn, M. R. (2008). Beliefs about the origins of homosexuality and support for gay rights. *Public Opinion Quarterly, 72*, 291–310.

Hebl, M., Foster, J. M., Mannix, L. M., & Dovidio, J. F. (2002). Formal and interpersonal discrimination: A field study examination of applicant bias. *Personality and Social Psychological Bulletin, 28*, 815–825. doi:10.1177/0146167202289010

Horvath, M., & Ryan, A. M. (2003). Antecedents and potential moderators of the relationship between attitudes and hiring discrimination on the basis of sexual orientation. *Sex Roles, 48*, 115–131. doi:10.1023/A:1022499121222

Huffman, A., Watrous, K., & King, E. B. (2008). Diversity in the workplace: Support for lesbian, gay, and bisexual workers. *Human Resource Management, 47*, 237–253. doi:10.1002/hrm.20210

Kahn, R. L., Wolfe, D. M., Quinn, R., Snoek, J. D., & Rosenthal, R. A. (1964). *Organizational stress.* New York, NY: Wiley.

Katz, D., & Kahn, R. (1978). *The social psychology of organizations* (2nd ed.). New York, NY: Wiley.

King, E. B. (2008). The effect of bias on the advancement of working mothers: Disentangling legitimate concerns from inaccurate stereotypes as predictors of career success. *Human Relations, 61*, 1677–1711. doi:10.1177/0018726708098082

King, E. B., & Cortina, J. M. (2010). The social and economic imperative of LGBT-supportive organizations. *Industrial-Organizational Psychology: Perspectives of Science and Practice, 3*, 69–78. doi:10.1111/j.1754-9434.2009.01201.x

King, E. B., Mohr, J., Peddie, C., Jones, K., & Kendra, M. (2010). *Identity management experiences of LGB newcomers.* Unpublished manuscript, George Mason University.

King, E. B., Reilly, C., & Hebl, M. R. (2008). The best and worst of times: Dual perspectives of coming out in the workplace. *Group and Organization Management, 33*, 566–601. doi:10.1177/1059601108321834

Litovich, M. L., & Langhout, R. D. (2004). Framing heterosexism in lesbian families: A preliminary examination of resilient coping. *Journal of Community and Applied Social Psychology, 14*, 411–435.

Mercier, L. R. (2006). Lesbian parents and work: Stressors and supports for the work-family interface. *Journal of Gay & Lesbian Social Services: Issues in Practice, Policy & Research, 19*, 25–47. doi:10.1080/10538720802131675

Meyer, I. H. (2003). Prejudice, social stress, and mental health in lesbian, gay, and bisexual populations: Conceptual issues and research evidence. *Psychological Bulletin, 129*, 674–697. doi:10.1037/0033-2909.129.5.674

Meyer, I. H. (2010). Identity, stress, and resilience in lesbians, gay men, and bisexuals of color. *The Counseling Psychologist, 38*, 442–454. doi:10.1177/0011000009351601

Meyer, J. P., & Allen, N. J. (1993). Commitment to organizations and occupations: Extension and test of a three-component conceptualization. *Journal of Applied Psychology, 78*, 538–551. doi:10.1037/0021-9010.78.4.538

Moradi, B., Wiseman, M. C., DeBlaere, C., Goodman, M. B., Sarkees, A., Brewster, M. E., & Huang, Y. P. (2010). LGB of color and White individuals' perceptions of heterosexist stigma, internalized homophobia, and outness: Comparisons of levels and links. *The Counseling Psychologist, 38*, 397–424. doi:10.1177/0011000009335263

Nielson, T. R., Carlson, D. S., & Lankau, M. J. (2001). The supportive mentor as a means of reducing work-family conflict. *Journal of Vocational Behavior, 59*, 364–381. doi:10.1006/jvbe.2001.1806

O'Ryan, L. W., & McFarland, W. P. (2010). A phenomenological exploration of dual-career lesbian and gay couples. *Journal of Counseling and Development, 88*, 71–79.

Patterson, C. J., Sutfin, E. L., & Fulcher, M. (2004). Division of labor among lesbian and heterosexual parenting couples: Correlates of specified versus shared patterns. *Journal of Adult Development, 11*, 79–89. doi:1068-0667/04/0700-0179/0

Peplau, L. A., & Fingerhut, A. (2004). The paradox of the lesbian worker. *Journal of Social Issues, 60*, 719–735. doi:10.1111/j.0022-4537.2004.00382.x

Piotrkowski, C. S., Rapoport, R., & Rapoport, R. (1987). Families and work. In M. B. Sussman & S. K. Steinmetz (Eds.), *Handbook of marriage and the family* (pp. 251–283). New York, NY: Plenum Press.

Prokos, A. H., & Keene, J. R. (2010). Poverty among cohabiting gay and lesbian, and married and cohabiting heterosexual families. *Journal of Family Issues, 31*, 934–959. doi:10.1177/0192513X09360176

Ragins, B. R. (2004). Sexual orientation in the workplace: The unique work and career experiences of gay, lesbian and bisexual workers. In J. J. Martocchio (Ed.), *Research in personnel and human resources management.* (Vol. 23, pp. 35–129). doi:10.1016/S0742-7301(04)23002-X

Ragins, B. R. (2008). Disclosure disconnects: Antecedents and consequences of disclosing invisible stigmas across life domains. *Academy of Management Review, 33*, 194–215. doi:10.2307/20159383

Ragins, B. R., & Cornwell, J. M. (2001). Pink triangles: Antecedents and consequences of perceived workplace discrimination against gay and lesbian employees. *Journal of Applied Psychology, 86*, 1244–1261. doi:10.1037/0021-9010.86.6.1244

Ragins, B. R., Singh, R., & Cornwell, J. M. (2007). Making the invisible visible: Fear and disclosure of sexual orientation at work. *Journal of Applied Psychology, 92*, 1103–1118. doi:10.1037/0021-9010.92.4.1103

Ryan, A. M., & Kossek, E. E. (2008). Work-life policy implementation: Breaking down or creating barriers to inclusiveness? *Human Resource Management, 47*, 295–310. doi:10.1002/hrm.20213

Shields, S. A. (2008). Gender: An intersectionality perspective. *Sex Roles, 59*, 301–311.

Simmons, T., & O'Connell, M. (2003). *Married-couple and unmarried-partner households: 2000*. Washington, DC: U.S. Department of Commerce, Economics and Statistics Administration, U.S. Census Bureau.

Singletary, S. L., & Hebl, M. (2009). Compensatory strategies for reducing interpersonal discrimination: The effectiveness of acknowledgments, increased positivity, and individuating information. *Journal of Applied Psychology, 94*, 797–805. doi:10.1037/a0014185

Tuten, T. L., & August, R. A. (2006). Work-family conflict: A study of lesbian mothers. *Women in Management Review, 21*, 578–597. doi:10.1108/09649420610692525

Van Steenbergen, E. F., Ellemers, N., & Mooijaart, A. (2007). How work and family can facilitate each other: Distinct types of work-family facilitation and outcomes for women and men. *Journal of Occupational Health Psychology, 12*, 279–300. doi:10.1037/1076-8998.12.3.279

Waldo, C. R. (1999). Working in a majority context: A structural model of heterosexism as minority stress in the workplace. *Journal of Counseling Psychology, 46*, 218–232. doi:10.1037/0022-0167.46.2.218

Williams, J. C. (2004). The maternal wall. *Harvard Business Review, 82*, 26–40.

Part III

Applications: Clinical Work, Policy, and Advocacy

Clinical Work with LGBTQ Parents and Prospective Parents

16

Arlene Istar Lev and Shannon L. Sennott

In the past few decades, same-sex marriage and LGBTQ parenting have become embedded in the fabric of both the social discourse within the LGBTQ community as well as mainstream society. Across the nation—indeed crossing the boundaries of nation–states—same-sex coupling and child-rearing opportunities continue to expand despite contentious debates about the legal status for same-sex parented families and shifting social opinions about transgender identities. Although still vilified in many parts of the world, in most Western countries same-sex couples, with or without legal rights, are building families and raising children. Historically LGBTQ parents have been closeted and rearing children primarily from previous marriages. Currently an increasing number of LGBTQ-identified people are planning families and raising children "out and proud," thereby changing the nature of the discourse, and presenting with different clinical issues.

A.I. Lev, L.C.S.W-R., C.A.S.A.C. (✉)
School of Social Welfare, and Choices Counseling and Consulting, University at Albany, 523 Western Ave, Suite 2A, Albany, NY 12203-1617, USA
e-mail: Arlene.Lev@gmail.com

S.L. Sennott, L.I.C.S.W. (✉)
Translate Gender, Inc., 265 Westhampton Rd., Northampton, MA 01062, USA

The Institute for Dialogic Practice,
265 Westhampton Road, Northampton, MA 01062, USA
e-mail: Shannon@translategender.org;
shannon.sennott@gmail.com

Becoming parents for most LGBTQ people requires conscious preparation and complex decision making, and the needs and concerns presented by individuals vary across sexual identity status (Lev, 2004a). To conflate the issues and needs of gay men and lesbians, or bisexual women and transmen seeking to become parents under the LGBTQ umbrella, muddies multifaceted issues. Lesbian, gay, bisexual, and trans people face different biological possibilities, social imperatives, and public bias in making choices to become parents. They are also faced with different challenges regarding legal rights and financial security, not to mention unique individual choices. The acronym LGBTQ can conflate the important distinctions among individuals, especially regarding those who are bisexual, because people in heterosexual relationships are often assumed to be straight, and those in same-sex relationships are presumed to be gay or lesbian (Chap. 6). Ross and Dobinson identify the dearth of empirical investigations into the experience of bisexual parents, and it is only recently that bisexual research subjects have been separated out from lesbian and gay subjects. For LGBTQ people who are single there is the additional element of invisibility that for some may be welcome and for others may be very isolating. In this chapter, we will first discuss the LGBTQ family cycle and family-building strategies. We will then explore each group within the LGBTQ acronym and include case studies with analysis, utilizing an eclectic therapeutic framework based in feminist, transfeminist, narrative, relational, and systemic theoretical models.

A.E. Goldberg and K.R. Allen (eds.), *LGBT-Parent Families: Innovations in Research and Implications for Practice*, DOI 10.1007/978-1-4614-4556-2_16, © Springer Science+Business Media New York 2013

Clinical Competency in the Therapeutic Setting with LGBTQ Parents

Clinical approaches to working with LGBTQ parents ought to be informed by systemic, narrative, transfeminist (Sennott, 2011), and relational systems perspectives. The therapeutic utilization of an eclectic clinical framework that includes intersectional and contextual approaches (Lebow, 2005; McDowell, 2005; Nichols & Schwartz, 2009; Walsh, 2003) allows for a focus on the client's strengths through the exploration and emergence of the client's intersecting identities (i.e., race, class, ability, religion, education, size, citizenship, and age) (Sennott & Smith, 2011). The utilization of a transfeminist therapeutic approach in working with LGBTQ individuals incorporates an awareness that there does not exist a hierarchy of authentic lived experience for women and to privilege one type of womanhood over another is inherently antifeminist. A transfeminist perspective acknowledges that most trans and gender nonconforming individuals have had lived experiences, in the past or present, as a girl or woman and have suffered the direct repercussions of socially condoned misogyny and gender-based oppression (Sennott, 2011). Therapists who work with LGBTQ clients need training in basic family systems theory and should have knowledge of the multiple options for family building in LGBTQ communities (Goldberg, 2010; Lev, 2004a). This includes an understanding of the legal constraints on LGBTQ family security and stability. Clinicians also need to understand the coming out process and how this can affect the developmental life cycle of families, including families of origin, as well as the role of internalized homophobia in the development of believing one has the "right" to become parents (Ashton, 2010; Lev, 2004a). Parenting places LGBTQ people under a social microscope as they come into contact with the medical profession, adoption specialists, day care providers, and educational institutions; families often need support in how to manage presenting their families to outsiders, and addressing subtle, as well as blatant,

homophobia and transphobia from professionals (Lev, 2004b; Sennott, 2011). As LGBTQ parenting enters the twenty-first century, many queer parents and queer potential parents have moved far past the question of whether they have the right to become parents, raising the question of whether clinicians are prepared to examine the in-depth discourse these parents are bringing to therapy regarding values, legalities, gender, and unique family-building strategies (Lev, 2004a).

The LGBTQ Family Life Cycle

Working with LGBTQ people requires an understanding of both the "normative" life cycle issues all couples and families face, as well as the unique life cycle issues experienced by those with diverse sexual orientations and gender identities and expressions. Life cycle models in general have come under great scrutiny in the past few decades. Models of individual development (Erikson, 1956), as well as older ecological models (Bronfenbrenner, 1979), have been criticized for ignoring women's unique developmental process (Gilligan, 1993; Jordan, Kaplan, Miller, Stiver, & Surrey, 1991). Additionally, the complex multidimensionality of class, race, ethnicity, and religion has routinely been minimized and ignored within standard family life cycle models (McGoldrick & Hardy, 2008). Psychological theories of LGBTQ people have focused on individual coming out processes, and not on the ways that LGBTQ people engage in larger families and systems.

Numerous models have been developed to examine the specific coming out processes for lesbian and gay people (Cass, 1979; Coleman, 1982; Troiden, 1993), and with various adaptations, those of bisexual people as well (Weinberg, Williams, & Pryor, 1994; Brown, 2002). Transgender coming out stages have also been examined developmentally, identifying the specific processes of identity development (Devor, 1997; Lev, 2004b). There has been much criticism that these models are embedded within White, Western perspectives (Cass, 1998; Morales, 1996) and ignore the complex issues for people of color who are LGBTQ (Ashton, 2010; Bowleg,

Burkholder, Teti, & Craig, 2008). Additionally, these models generally emphasize the coming out and identity integration processes itself, but not the larger issues of couple and family building, or how sexual orientation issues and gender identity are integrated into general life cycle development (McDowell, 2005).

Slater (1999) examined a specific lesbian life cycle, and although she mentions the development of lesbian parenting, the focus of her model is on couple development, not on the complex issues of becoming parents in a heterosexist culture. Slater accurately recognizes that for many lesbians having children is not the primary focus of their relationship. Slater, as well as Weston (1991), emphasizes the ways that lesbian and gay people have built extended families within the queer community outside of their family of origin *and* without rearing a younger generation. From Slater's and Weston's perspectives, looking at LGBTQ families through a traditional family life cycle lens ignores the alternative family structures that have been built to nurture queer people. More recently, Christopher Carrington's (1999) research and observations about domesticity in what he terms "lesbigay families" point to a pattern of "accommodation to the predominate social structure" (p. 219). Carrington also notes that these patterns and accommodations are unrecognized, especially the seclusion and devaluation of domesticity within LGBT families, leading lesbigay families to share more experiences with heterosexual families than many previously believed them to share.

Moving away from heterosexist notions of family, and the rigid proscription of gender role expectations and parenting mandates, was one of the central features of the early days of the gay and lesbian-feminist liberation movements (Jay, 1994; Rich, 1993). Indeed, for many lesbian and gay men, the idea that one could actively choose to not have children and step outside of mainstream familial expectations was extremely liberating. However, this possibility left those who wanted to parent having to "choose" whether to be queer *or* be a parent, for queer parenting was an oxymoron (Lev, 2004a). Kelly McCormick, the Founder and Director of *Momazons*, one of the first national organizations for lesbian moth-

ers, recently passed away at the age of 51 after struggling for many years with a disabling health condition. She was an advocate and organizer for lesbian parents, providing opportunities for lesbians to explore parenting options, and with her partner Phyllis Gorman, often shared their journey of becoming parents to their son, Keegan. Phyllis recently said, "Kelly's legacy in creating *Momazons* is that now this generation is able to decide whether they want to parent, whereas before, we were simply grieving that we couldn't" (Personal communication, 2011).

If we start from the premise that some LGBTQ people *will* desire to have children, and that LGBTQ people build unique family structures and community affiliations, then we must assume that LGBTQ people also have unique life cycle experiences that "queer" the study of the family life cycle. Decentering heterosexuality allows us to look at some of the ways that LGBTQ parents "do family" (Hudak & Giammattei, 2010), and "become parent" (Riggs, 2007), that recognizes the evolution of new family forms, and honors emerging values and norms that differ from the heteronormative expectations (Lev, 2010).

McGoldrick, Carter, and Garcia-Preto (2010) have developed a family life cycle model that integrates LGBTQ people within the larger issues of family processes, highlighting the unique issues of sexual orientation and gender identity, as well as the complex matrix of race, ethnicity, class, dis/ability, and religion. They do this within a larger context of the historical, economic, and political influences embedded within a social justice perspective. Ashton (2010) utilizes McGoldrick and colleagues' work to specifically examine the LGBTQ life cycle in terms of both family of origin and families of choice. The life cycle stages are: (a) leaving home: emerging young adults; (b) joining of families through marriage/union; (c) families with young children; (d) families with adolescents; (e) launching children and moving on at midlife; (f) families in late middle age; and (g) families nearing the end of life (McGoldrick et al., 2010). On the surface, LGBTQ people move through the family life cycle in the same way as other people do. However, due to the nature of homophobia and transphobia, LGBTQ people are at a developmental disadvantage (Ashton, 2010). The first stage of development for young adults, leaving home, is affected by earlier developmental milestones, and the challenging coming out processes for LGBTQ youth.

When heterosexual youth are beginning to explore their sexual feelings in puberty, many remain closeted and fearful of their feelings for same-sex peers. Historically, this has meant that LGBTQ youth sometimes experience a lag developmentally (Rosario, Schrimshaw, & Hunter, 2004; Rotheram-Borus & Langabeer, 2001), where they do not experience life cycle socialization and dating patterns at the same age as their heterosexual, gender conforming peers. As social mores shift, youth are coming out younger and younger. There are increasing social supports in place for LGBTQ youth to explore dating and intimacy at developmentally appropriate ages, although this is impacted by geographic location, and the values of one's family of origin (LaSala, 2010).

For youth who are gender nonconforming—transgender, transsexual, or genderqueer—puberty can be a confusing and challenging time (Burgess, 1999). Often sexuality and exploration take a back burner to the pressing issues of body incongruence, and the search for gender affirming medical treatments. It is hard to imagine in the current climate a healthy normative adolescence for a gender nonconforming child, even in the most supportive families and communities (Cooper, 1999; Lev & Alie, 2012). Every aspect of dating, intimacy, and exploring sexual orientation is affected by living in a body that is betraying one's authentic gender expression.

LGBTQ young adulthood may start painfully early, because youth have had to prematurely become independent due to the effects of homophobia within their families (Ryan, Huebner, Diaz, & Sanchez, 2009). Adulthood may be delayed due to the need to "catch up" socially and developmentally; the earlier challenges of managing sexual orientation and gender identity issues as youth may also delay the process of coupling and partnering. Even after the difficulties of establishing oneself as an LGBTQ person,

finding partners can be daunting, especially for those living in more rural or less liberal communities. Once relationships have been initiated, same-sex couples must negotiate the same developmental tasks as heterosexual couples, but do so within the frame of a larger homophobic culture. Numerous legal constraints and the ability to find supportive social and/or religious communities can impede the ability to form permanent and secure partnerships (Ashton, 2010). For those transgressing gender norms, dating and establishing relationships are affected by shifting bodies and sexual orientations, as well as financial and legal constraints due to medical needs and oppressive laws.

Like all couples, LGBTQ couples experience the joining of two families of origin, who may be at different stages of accepting their LGBTQ child/relative (Lev, 2004a). Having family of origin support can greatly affect an LGBTQ couple's decision to become parents. This process must be negotiated developmentally, cognitively, and within a larger sociocultural and historical lens. The process of becoming parents is rarely as simple as it is for most heterosexual parents, and LGBTQ people must interface with medical personnel, as well as create expensive legal paperwork to protect their families (Lev, 2004a). Although LGBTQ parents have much in common with other parents rearing young children, or coping with the realities of growing teens, these normative stages are affected by unique issues, outlined later in the chapter when we look at the individual identities within the LGBTQ communities.

Family-Building Strategies in LGBTQ Communities

In addition to the diversity across identities, LGBTQ family-building strategies vary greatly across race/ethnicity, class, religion, disability, and age. Research on lesbian parenthood has historically tended to examine middle-class, White women and men, who become parents through donor insemination and adoption (Goldberg & Gianino, 2012; Patterson, 1995). Our clinical experience has shown that many working-class people and same-sex couples of color often become parents via previous heterosexual sexual encounters, and often view donor insemination, private adoption, and surrogacy as financially prohibitive (Moore, 2008). Social class often impacts prospective parents' relationships with the foster care system. For some working-class prospective parents, adoption through foster care may be their only viable option to become parents, and they may fear discrimination and bias in this system. Despite the positive advances in foster care policies regarding lesbian and gay parents (Evan B. Donaldson Adoption Institute, 2003), some couples may assume they will be rejected or highly scrutinized for being queer since their relationships with social institutions may not have been supportive in the past. Bisexual people in heterosexual relationships tend to hide these aspects of their identities from medical professionals and adoption agencies, and it is perhaps true for bisexual people in gay or lesbian relationships also, assuming that this information would only muddy the already complex bureaucratic process of becoming parents (Chap. 6).

Despite all the ways that LGBTQ parents are potentially different from heterosexuals, there are also similarities in the ways their families are formed. Many LGBTQ people, like heterosexuals, become stepparents after becoming involved with someone who already has children (Lynch, 2004); sometimes this is warmly welcomed and other times it is "the price" for falling in love. LGBTQ people who are stepparents must address all the same concerns as other stepparents, except they often do so without social or legal sanction for these relationships.

For those LGBTQ people who desire to become parents, there is a parallel to that of heterosexual people, in terms of the psychospiritual longing for parenthood, the financial strain associated with parenthood, and the need to reorganize one's life, work, and priorities to properly parent children. Like heterosexual couples, LGBTQ people may face infertility challenges and require the assistance of medical experts or adoption specialists (Goldberg, 2010; Goldberg, Downing, & Richardson, 2009; Lev, 2004a).

Additionally, like many heterosexual couples, some LGBTQ people are older when beginning their parenting journey, in part because of advances in reproductive technologies but also because of the changes in cultural acceptance of LGBTQ people in the past few decades. Beginning parenting in one's 40s or even 50s has become increasingly more common, and for LGBTQ people raised in more repressive times, they could never have seriously entertained the possibility of becoming parents until they were older.

It is also worth noting (Chap. 8) that not all couples (lesbian, gay, bisexual, trans, or heterosexual) are in exclusive monogamous partnerships, although LGBTQ couples who are polyamorous are likely to experience more scrutiny and judgment if their relationship configuration is revealed. Although both LGBTQ and heterosexual couples may be in open relationships, the more mainstream LGBTQ people *appear to be*, the less resistance they will experience in their attempts to build their families.

In our clinical experience, some LGBTQ people minimize the differences in their family structure in an effort to normalize their families, as evidenced in this clinical example: When a 10-year-old boy told his biological mother, "Everyone keeps asking me who Tammy is when she picks me up after school," his mother responded, "Tell them it's none of their business." Although this answer may be technically accurate, it is not particularly helpful for a young child seeking language to explain his family to his friends at school. It actually further reinforces silence and increases the social discomfort for the child, who is not only isolated in school but also does not have parents as allies in helping him negotiate the differences. Helping children speak openly about LGBTQ issues, in age-appropriate ways, is a parental duty specific to LGBTQ parents, but not all parents have the skills to initiate or structure the conversation.

Finally, it is important to note that many, if not most, LGBTQ parents seeking therapy are dealing with the same basic issues and concerns that all parents must address, including exhaustion managing a home and family, adult relationship struggles as co-parents as well as intimate partners, struggles with discipline strategies, and concerns for their children's well-being (real or imagined). As parents address issues such as a child's learning disability, mental health concerns, drug use, and academic problems, they may not be focused at all on LGBTQ-related concerns, but are simply seeking a supportive environment where their own sexuality and gender are respected.

Clinical Considerations for Parenting with Lesbian and Bisexual Women

Lesbians seeking to retain custody of their children following a heterosexual divorce were the first group of sexual minorities to challenge the legal system's bias against queer parenting (Goldberg, 2010). The societal bias against lesbian motherhood centered on the assumption that children needed both a mother and father to develop traditional sex role behavior, including an eventual heterosexual orientation (Tasker & Golombok, 1997). It took the results of a decade of psychological research (Patterson, 2006) to prove to the courts that children reared by lesbian mothers exhibited psychological stability and heteronormative identities. This research and the subsequent legal decisions allowing lesbian mothers to retain custody of their children paved the way for other sexual minorities (gay men, trans parents) to begin to challenge the courts on their right to remain parents, as well as seek out strategies to become parents (Goldberg, 2010).

Lesbians and bisexual women, because they are biologically capable of conceiving and carrying a child, arguably have the easiest path to becoming parents. Donor insemination through sperm banks is readily available and accessible to most women with middle-class salaries, and donor insemination performed at home, or through sex with a male friend or lover, is a possibility for many women (Lev, 2004a). Lesbians can also choose to adopt domestically, either privately or through the child welfare system (Goldberg, 2010). As cultural mores shift, lesbian motherhood is less frequently challenged in the courts, especially in urban environments, and

when custody is challenged, issues of lesbianism are rarely the focus. However, lesbian (and gay male) couples cannot adopt internationally as a couple, but must have one partner move through the legal system as a single parent—a process that can be emotionally challenging to partnerships that already lack legal sanction and societal support (Goldberg, 2010; Lev, 2004a).

Although there has been a plethora of research on lesbian parenting, much of it has focused on White, middle-class women, living in urban centers with access to affirmative communities (Goldberg, 2010; Lev, 2010). With few exceptions there is a lack of research on the familial dynamics within lesbian families who are working-class, racial or ethnic minorities, living with disabilities, or who are butch/femme identified, especially regarding their pathways to parenting. Clinical experience suggests that, although the literature reveals that lesbian couples tend toward egalitarian relationships, dividing chores and responsibilities evenly (Goldberg, 2010), it is possible that these are class-based privileges not available to working-class women, or disabled women. Housework is a classically gendered activity, yet some evidence suggests that in butch/femme couples and African-American lesbian couples, housekeeping duties were not divided along expected gender roles (Levitt, Gerrish, & Hiestand, 2003; Moore, 2008). Research has not yet explored the dynamics of butch/femme couples and how they negotiate decisions about pregnancy, breast feeding, or the division of labor, raising questions about how gender actually functions within same-sex parenting couples (Lev, 2008). Therapists should explore issues of class, culture, racial identity, and gender with LGBTQ couples and not assume that research on White LGBTQ individuals reflects the dynamics of those who are minorities within minorities.

Lesbians and bisexual women seek therapy for numerous reasons. Sometimes they are seeking information on family planning strategies, or struggling with the complexities of infertility. Lesbian couples may have differing views on donor insemination, use of known versus unknown donors, and the importance of biological fathers in their children's lives. Questions about adoption choices (domestic, international, foster care) are often salient. Most commonly, differences in parenting strategies, conflict and exhaustion caused by the demands of children, and struggles in parenting children with special needs are reasons lesbian couples seek out therapeutic guidance. Lesbian couples and individuals also seek out assistance when contemplating separation and divorce. The following vignette explores the intersection of gender and sexuality in a lesbian relationship and the tension that can arise when socially sanctioned gender roles are scripted into a same-sex partnership.

Case of Lily and Nicola

Lily, 32 and Nicola, 30, a White couple, came into therapy because they were contemplating a separation. They had been together for over a decade and had a commitment ceremony 8 years previously. They shared the parenting of two children, Noa, 6 years old, and Lucinda, 3 years old, both birthed by Lily, and conceived with donor sperm. Lily was a stay-at-home mom, who was homeschooling their children, and Nicola worked as a contractor with a construction company. Nicola and Lily were loving parents to their children, but their relationship had felt hollow for the past few years, while they struggled with typical issues that families with young children face. They had little time for their relationship due to their parental philosophy of extreme hands-on parenting: they were reluctant to hire babysitters, and they practiced attachment parenting, including extended breastfeeding and co-sleeping. Although both parents believed strongly in these values, the lion's share of the work fell on Lily, who was with the children every day, while Nicola worked long hours to singlehandedly support the family.

Separating presented unique challenges for this lesbian-parent family. Unable to marry in the state where they lived, and unable to afford the legal paperwork to secure their family, Nicola had no legal ties to her children. She was terrified Lily would not let her see the children if she moved out, and Lily admitted to using the power of her legal status to forestall Nicola from leaving. Lily had few employable skills, and was extremely resistant to working out of their house while her children were small. She was completely financially dependent on Nicola. The couple felt trapped in a relationship where they were no longer "in love," and unable to maintain a lifestyle they had carefully created unless they remained together.

They were both deeply committed to the needs of their children, yet couldn't see remaining together.

Lily and Nicola's decade-long relationship and shared commitment to their children were strengths for them as parents; however, breaking up required a massive shift in the foundation of their lives together. The stability and security of their home life was not only threatened by the separation, but suddenly they were confronted with legal ambiguities, forcing them to face complex ethical dilemmas. Nicola feared the loss of being a parent to her two children. She had no legal standing as a nonbiological mother, and depended on Lily's good will to maintain her parenting role. Lily was in a situation familiar to many heterosexual mothers, especially those who are stay-at-home parents. She feared the loss of the parenting lifestyle she was accustomed to, including full financial support from Nicola. The fact that Lily was aware of the power she held as the legal and biological parent of the two children and that she wielded this power in an attempt to keep Nicola from leaving the relationship was the crux of the relational mistrust between the two—an idea they both accepted, when the therapist presented it. It was a strength that they were aware of their unequal parental power, as there are many couples who do not want to admit that there are certain axes of privilege as a birth parent in a same-sex partnership. Lily felt powerless because Nicola wanted to leave, and understood that she would not be able to continue parenting, her primary job, in the way she had been. She was losing not only her dream of her family, and the relationship she shared with Nicola, but her entire way of life was threatened. Nicola felt powerless to maintain an equal parenting relationship with Lily, and feared she had no recourse; she was legally a stranger to her children.

The values and ethical stance of the therapist in a case like Lily and Nicola's can significantly impact the outcome for this family. The therapist must hold the fears of each partner, especially in light of these power differentials, and yet make a firm stance that, despite the lack of legal protections, both women are mothers to their children and must remain so in the eyes of their children as well as one another. The therapist must examine their own experiences and how that affects their values and opinions about this family. The therapist should consider whether and how their own status as a person in a committed relationship with or without legal protection; their parental status (i.e., nonparent, legal parent, nonlegal parent) may affect their values and perspectives about this family. It is essential that the therapist maintain a "holding environment" that provides a container for the couple and family, that disallows using the homophobic legal system to minimize Nicola's role as a parent. Although lesbian and gay couples often form their families outside of the legal system, they sometimes resort to that very system during separations. The judicial system, embedded in homophobic constructs about families, will rarely recognize the structure of queer families. When LGBTQ couples are separating, judges will often only honor the biological or legal partner; sadly, some LGBTQ people purposely seek out legal measures to wield power over their (ex)-partners (Shuster, 2002).

For Lily and Nicola, their commitment to the kind of life they wanted for their children was able to supersede their disappointment, anger, and fear of ending their marriage. Both women needed to grieve the loss of their marriage, and it was important for the therapist to acknowledge and name their relationship as a marriage regardless of the lack of legal recognition. Over time Lily was able to tell Nicola that she would not use her biological status to impede Nicola's right to her children or her contact with them. They were able to write a contract stating this, but more importantly they were able to create a separation ritual outlining the contract that served as a way of concretizing their separation even more than a legally binding document (Imber-Black & Roberts, 1998). Nicola was able to commit to not abandoning the children financially, although she was clear with Lily that she could not support her indefinitely. They began to engage in conversations about how Lily could return to school so she could become more employable, while still remaining home with the children while they were young. Nicola eventually found a small apartment, and they began to develop an equitable parenting

arrangement, with the children dividing time between their parents. The women continued to grieve, but their focus became helping their children cope with the changes in their family, rather than wielding domestic and judicial power over one another through the course of their separation.

Differences in parenting styles can emerge in the face of intersecting identities just as easily as they do in the context of a relationship separating. The following case outlines some of the complex issues when two women of different ethnic backgrounds partner, each having children from previous relationships. The multiple intersecting identities of age, race, religion, and previous parental and marital status all affect this couple's ability to communicate and support one another, as both of these women are parenting in midlife, and have children spanning more than 2 decades.

Case of Jeanette and Gladys

Jeanette and Gladys sought out therapy because their 5-year relationship was "in trouble." Jeanette, a White woman in her mid-40s, was the mother of four children. The oldest three were from a previous marriage to a White man, who had left when the children were small. Gladys, who was African-American and in her mid-50s, identified herself as "seriously Christian." She had two grown children, born in a heterosexual relationship. Her husband had died of a heart attack 20 years earlier, and she raised her children as a single mother, before coming out as a lesbian when they were teenagers. The youngest child, aged 4, was African-American and originally fostered by Jeannette who did emergency foster care work for the State, and was later adopted by both women.

Jeanette and Gladys were both assertive and verbal about their issues and needs, and often spoke animatedly over one another. They owned their own home and struggled to pay the bills. Gladys worked as a nurse and was very proud of her work at the hospital where she had been for over 30 years. Jeanette worked as a teacher's aide in a public school, which made it easy to pick the kids up after school, including the little one who was in a day care center across the street. They both agreed the house was a "disaster" though they had different opinions as to whose fault that was.

Gladys was very critical of Jeanette's parenting. She felt Jeannette was "weak" and that the children ran wild. She stated she would "never tolerate that behavior from her [now grown] boys." Jeanette felt that Gladys was "too hard" on the kids, who were "after all just kids." Gladys felt that Jeanette didn't support her when she disciplined the kids; Jeanette said, "I don't like when you talk to my kids that way."

There were numerous issues affecting the relationship between Jeanette and Gladys. Each had very different parenting styles, and had experience raising children before they were a couple. Their entire relationship revolved around their children; as a stepfamily, they had never had time together as a couple without children. Both women had extensive histories living as heterosexuals, and when the topic of lesbianism was introduced, both agreed that they did not like "that word" and both felt that "being gay was not really an issue." They had rarely discussed their relationship with their children, who referred to Jeannette as "Mommy" and Gladys as "Auntie," including their youngest who they had adopted together. The social worker who assisted them with adopting their foster child had never really explored their relationship dynamics. It was not clear whether Gladys really felt she was a full-fledged parent to this child, and her relationship with the older children they were parenting was even more ambivalent, creating unclear roles within the family.

Utilizing a genogram (McGoldrick, Gerson, & Petry 2008), the therapist was able to help map the family dynamics and history, allowing the couple to examine both of their previous marriages, as well as their relationships to their older children as single parents. This experience introduced a deeper conversation about what it meant for each of them to join together as a stepfamily, with two parents. With therapeutic guidance, they also explored both of their cultural, racial, and religious backgrounds, and how that informed their parenting philosophies and beliefs about their role as parents. The therapist employed a narrative approach, allowing the women to reveal their unique stories, grounded in an understanding of the complex intersectionalities in these women's lives.

Additionally, the couple began to explore what it meant to be in a relationship with another woman, how that was different than their previous relationships with men, and how that might impact their children, including whether they were comfortable being seen as a lesbian-parent family. Utilizing a feminist therapeutic understanding that was affirming of diverse orientations and experiences allowed Gladys to say that she thought she could "love either a man or a woman," and Jeanette revealed that perhaps she had been "gay her whole life but didn't know it until she fell in love with Gladys." Both women were visibly softened by this statement.

It is easy for therapists to assume that because a couple is "out" that they are comfortable with their relationship and have accepted and adapted to being lesbian or gay. However, there are many ways that people cope with their sexual orientation, and there are various steps in the process of integrating one's identity. Models developed in the 1980s still have some resonance in terms of the stages of coming out; however, coming out processes, as Cass (1998) has stressed, are a Western phenomenon, not a universal truth, or cross-cultural experience. Social mores regarding gay identity have shifted, and people can come out with greater ease, and are, therefore, less likely to feel confined by established social rules about their identity development or how they *should* experience it. Tolman and Diamond (2001) show that research on sexual identity categories has failed to represent the diversity of sexual and romantic feelings people can express or experience. It was important therapeutically that the therapist was able to support both Gladys and Jeanette in their unique experiences of their sexuality, historically and currently, and not assume that their sexual identities (i.e., labels and experiences) within their lesbian relationship were the same.

As Gladys began discussing her Christian beliefs in therapy, she became increasingly agitated. She revealed her fears that her grandmother, who had raised her, would feel strong disapproval knowing Gladys was "like that." For Gladys, being Christian and lesbian was a conflict that she had coped with through avoidance, or denial, rather than attempts at resolution, and the therapeutic context allowed for an exploration of these cognitive distortions. For Gladys to acknowledge the pain she felt in going to church and listening to her preacher criticize homosexuality was a powerful breakthrough. By creating a holding environment for Gladys's pain, therapy became a safe place to explore her relationship with God, Jesus, and religious tolerance. It was therapeutically important to honor the importance of Jesus and the role of the church in Gladys' life, not avoid these contentious and often tender topics with comments that were dismissive about religiosity, or revealed a politically charged call-to-arms regarding homophobia within the church. Gladys had to come into her sexuality knowing that her god approved of and loved her, a journey that a therapist can guide without necessarily sharing those values.

Within the context of therapy, the couple was able to explore what it meant to share parenting together and raise *their* child, an African-American child who was adopted, as well as the children who were stepchildren to Gladys. This created difficult conversations about race, with Gladys confronting Jeanette, "What do you know about raising a Black girl-child?" Previous to this discussion in therapy, Gladys and Jeanette had never discussed race, their interracial relationship, the adoption of an African-American child, or the blended racial configuration of their children. Additionally, they had never talked with their children—including Gladys' older children—about their relationship, their love, the nature of their families, or how the children should view their commitment to one another and to each of their six children. Forming a stepfamily is particularly challenging for gay and lesbian couples who are integrating not only a socially stigmatized identity (i.e., being gay) but also an identity that has historically been culturally invisible (i.e., stepparenting) (Lynch, 2004).

Having all of these issues out in the open did not make them vanish; yet, the couple no longer felt their relationship was "in trouble," but rather that they could begin to address their "troubles." Most significantly, the family began to attend a welcoming Christian congregation, which served to provide a spiritual home for their family, where

they were accepted as a family. Gladys and Jeanette are building a family that is coping with multiple, intersecting issues including being in a lesbian couple, having an interracial relationship, being adoptive parents, and forming a stepfamily. This process created numerous conflicts regarding household authority, especially the conflicting roles of having two mothers, with different parenting styles and histories, competing for the role of "the" mother, a role familiar to both of them in previous heterosexual marriages and as single parents (see Moore, 2008).

Clinical Considerations with Gay and Bisexual Men and Parenthood

Although societal prejudice about men raising children is fierce (Chap. 10), and the financial costs of becoming parents can be steep, gay fatherhood is increasingly common (Berkowitz & Marsiglio, 2007; Brown, Smalling, Groza, & Ryan, 2009; Downing, Richardson, Kinkler, & Goldberg, 2009; Gates, Badgett, Macomber, & Chambers, 2007; Gates & Ost, 2004) and research on their family-building process is increasing (Biblarz & Savci, 2010). Gay and bisexual men are building families through domestic adoption, surrogacy, and partnerships with women.

Historically, when gay men were coming out and leaving heterosexual marriages there was little chance of gaining custody of their children. The reasons for this were twofold: one was because of the prejudice toward fathers in general, and the second was the specific prejudice toward gay males (Bigner & Bozett, 1990). The courts have historically favored mothers in custody battles in general; gay men were levied the additional prejudice of being "homosexual" within a cultural milieu that assumed gay men were sexual predators of children. Therefore gay men often lost all rights to their children, sometimes even including visitation. In the past two decades, gay men are increasingly choosing to become parents after coming out (Berkowitz, 2007; Biblarz & Savci, 2010). As prejudice has lessened (though it is certainly still present) gay men have increasing opportunities to become parents (Berkowitz, 2007; Gianino, 2008). Compared to lesbians who are able to conceive and carry children with or without societal support, gay men are at an obvious disadvantage. However, as more adoption agencies become welcoming toward gay and lesbian potential parents (Brodzinsky, 2003), gay men are taking advantage of these new potentialities. Additionally, gay men who are financially able are seeking out opportunities to build families through surrogacy (Bergman, Rubio, Green, & Padron, 2010; Lev, 2006a). Of course, gay men can also become parents from a previous marriage or through stepparenting. It is important to note that gay men are often sperm donors for lesbian woman, and depending on the legal and social relationships that develop over time, they can be in parent-like relationships with these children (Lev, 2004a).

Gay men can seek clinical consultation early in their process of becoming parents for a number of reasons. Perhaps they are seeking reassurance that being gay will not negatively affect their children (Gianino, 2008); perhaps they want support in becoming a single dad. Sometimes the members of a couple have different opinions about how to become parents (adoption versus surrogacy), or different concerns (finances or joint custodial rights) (Berkowitz & Marsiglio, 2007). Additionally, gay men may seek out home study evaluations, which are a standard process for all adoption processes (Lev, 2006b; Mallon, 2007). The case below outlines Duncan and Mario's process of becoming parents and how they navigated multiple concerns regarding parenthood.

Case of Duncan and Mario

Duncan and Mario had been partnered for a decade when they sought out counseling because they were hoping to become parents. Duncan, a 37-year-old gay man of European descent, entered therapy excited about becoming a parent; he came from a large family and was an uncle to numerous nieces and nephews. Mario, a 43-year-old gay man, came from an immigrant family with strong Christian values. Although he too had a large family, they

were rejecting of his partnership with Duncan, and he feared that he would not have family support in choosing to become a parent. This concern raised complex issues for Mario, including his own confusion and shame about his homosexuality, and where his children would "fit" into his family. It was important to Mario that he pass his culture on to his children, but he could not imagine having his children exposed to his family of origin's homophobia. Although both men were solidly employed, Duncan came from a middle-class family, whereas Mario was raised in poverty. Duncan was open to various routes to parenting, including adoption and surrogacy, and did not see the finances as a major concern: "What else should we be spending money on that is more important than this?" Mario was concerned about the financial costs of having children, as well as rearing them. However, he also disclosed another concern, which was that "adopting children through foster care will mean we will have troubled children—I don't think I could do that."

Through the course of therapy, Mario was able to tell his parents that he was planning to have a child. To his surprise, although they had serious reservations, they also expressed (an odd kind of) support saying, "This will make your lifestyle more normal." Mario and Duncan decided to meet with a social worker to explore foster-to-adopt possibilities. After going through the program, they both felt that the children needing homes who were currently in the foster care system had needs beyond what they were able to provide. This decision was difficult for both men. Duncan expressed that he felt "guilty" that he was uncomfortable fostering children. He felt that he was "the kind of person" who "should" want to do this, yet he really didn't want to: "It just didn't feel right."

They then began to investigate possibilities for surrogacy. This process was difficult because of the extensive financial costs, complications with the laws regarding surrogacy, and the complex issues involving biological parentage. They eventually decided to use a donor egg, and a separate gestational surrogate. It was important for Mario that their child was of Latino decent, so they chose to use his sperm. To their surprise they ended up developing a warm relationship with their surrogate. They were present for their child's birth, and ended up maintaining an ongoing familial relationship with their surrogate.

Duncan and Mario came from extremely different families of origin and though they were both gay men, the extent to which their core beliefs and values differed was great. The first therapeutic task was to assist this couple in exploring their own definitions and configurations of parenthood, in an affirmative manner, and to also assist them in examining their parenting options including foster parenting, public adoption, private adoption, and surrogacy. It was important that the therapist be patient about the decision-making process, and validate each of the diverse options available to them, with the hope that eventually the couple would learn to trust their intuition about what was right for their family. It was especially salient in working with Duncan and Mario to acknowledge their reservations about adopting a child through foster care, without judgment or guilt. Gently, the couple was informed about the potentiality of any child to have "high needs," and that choosing another option would not eliminate that possibility. However, it was equally important that they not feel "guilty," honoring their right to make choices that were the best fit for the family. Although Duncan was comfortable having the child be biologically Mario's, it was obvious he had not thought much about the racial and cultural considerations that come with rearing a Latino child, which also became an important focus of therapy. Duncan's lack of conscious awareness of the racial identity of their future child highlighted the differences in their backgrounds, and the assumptions embedded in Duncan's White privilege. It also initiated a conversation about the home in which their child would be reared, including the cultural environment, religious, and ritualistic or moral aspects of family life.

Through the use of therapy Duncan and Mario began to formulate what their family would look like structurally, particularly how they would create a nurturing environment for their Latino child with racially mixed parents. This process included an exploration of both partners' ideas of masculinity and the roles each possessed, both domestically and professionally, within their family. As Duncan and Mario examined these roles, they realized that they had differing feelings about who would be the primary earner in the family and who would provide the primary caregiving to their children. Through discussion of this in therapy they were able to plan ahead for a more equitable parenting relationship.

Clinical Considerations with Gender Nonconforming and Transgender Parents

Trans people choosing to begin families can face complex medical challenges, as well as discrimination from service providers (Currah, Minter, & Green, 2009). Trans (i.e., transgender, genderqueer, cross-dressing, transsexual) people have been consciously becoming parents throughout the course of LGBTQ history (More, 1998; White & Ettner, 2004) although it has only recently come under the public microscope. Trans individuals are able to become parents more openly now than a decade ago; however, they are still vulnerable to scrutiny by social service providers when they seek assistance with adoption, surrogacy, and fertility issues (Lev, 2004a).

Increasing numbers of trans people are coming out and seeking services for gender dysphoria, including referrals for medical and surgical treatments (Ettner, Monstrey, & Eyler, 2007). Many of these people have been parenting children in heterosexual marriages (Brown & Rounsley, 1996; Erhardt, 2007); often their partners and children know nothing about their gender identity conflicts. When spouses are apprised of the gender issues, they often experience an intense betrayal, anger, and grief as Lev (2004b) has outlined. The family is thrown into a state of chaos, and even if the children do not know the cause of the marital distress they are affected by the ongoing discord in the family.

Gender Transition After Parenthood

Gender transitions before parenthood can be psychologically stressful as the biological processes of pregnancy can be in direct conflict with a person's gender identity and expression. Transmen who have retained their uterus and ovaries are capable of pregnancy, and many men have chosen to father their children they have birthed (Epstein, 2009). Although more prevalent in larger cities, Internet discussions on the topic reveal that transmen are exploring these options with both male and female partners. When transmen become pregnant they both challenge "patriarchal fatherhood" (Ryan, 2009, p. 147) and also transform the notion of motherhood. Additionally, transwomen are beginning to store semen before they begin transition so they can choose to have biological children with a female partner (De Sutter, 2001).

Historically, as with LGB people coming out after having married, the community response has been that one "must" or "should" divorce to live authentically. There is tremendous pressure from others (especially from support groups on the Internet) that disclosure foreshadows divorce, and within the current political and legal system, coming out will often mean loss of custody of children for trans people (Lev, 2004a). Options for trans parenting are increasing as society and families begin to understand that there are alternatives to cutting off all connections with a parent who comes out as trans.

A common presenting therapeutic concern a therapist may encounter while working with trans parents is when an individual in a heterosexual couple comes out to his/her partner as transgender, often after many years of marriage and parenting together. Working with trans people coming out later in life and with families is a delicate process. When a spouse comes out as trans it is often shocking and emotionally challenging for his/her partner. Couples work with trans partners is still in its infancy, though some clinical models are beginning to develop (Lev, 2004a; Malpas, 2006); work with trans parents and their children remains an unexplored area clinically. As seen in the case of Louis, the therapist's role is to help individuals and couples navigate when and how to tell their children about a parent's trans identity, and, to aid in the negotiation of different opinions and levels of acceptance of the news.

Case of Louis

When Louis sought out therapy the first thing he said was, "I've never spoken to anyone about this in my life." Louis was 35 years old, was married to his high school sweetheart, and they had three children, a 14 year old, a 9 year old, and a 3 year old.

He described his home life as generally happy, and he loved being a father. His work was stressful, but he was satisfied that he could support his family.

Louis presented with a classic presentation for transsexualism. This meant that his gender identity was based on a desire to medically transition fully into a woman and also included a lifelong sense of himself as being "a woman inside." He had hidden his cross-dressing from his wife, although he did not think she would "freak out." His sense of shame and isolation was extreme, but in his fantasy of transitioning, his reality testing was weak. On the one hand he could not imagine a life without moving forward to affirm his gender as a woman, and on the other hand, his lack of insight into how transitioning might affect his job, his wife, or his children was extreme. He saw himself having to make a choice to continue to live "as a man" (which meant continuing to be married to his wife and parenting his children), or to live "as a woman" (which meant leaving his wife and children); he saw no possibility for a middle ground—to live as a woman and continue to be a parent to "his" children.

The first step in working with Louis was to create a safe place to explore his gender, including his experiences in childhood, his current knowledge about transitioning, and his goals for the future. It was also necessary to examine his relationship with his wife, and why he had not shared this important part of himself with her before. As Louis became more secure and comfortable in his identity, the next steps were to begin the process of self-disclosure with his wife.

Once the disclosure with Louis's wife was made and a conversation could begin, his wife started the process of moving through established stages of shock, betrayal, turmoil, and (potential) acceptance (Lev, 2004b). Typically it is most therapeutically supportive for both partners to go through these stages together, with the guidance of the therapist to help normalize and validate the process and help the non-trans partner to understand that their feelings and emotions are appropriate. It is essential that they have time to process issues of betrayal and grief, before the transgender issues are discussed with children. The children are usually the primary concern for a wife when her husband first comes out as trans. Often the greatest concern for wives is how the revelation of the gender issues, or the parent's transition, will affect the children's own gender development and sexuality (Green, 1995; White & Ettner, 2004), although there is no evidence that having a trans parent will negatively affect a child's developing sexual orientation or gender identity. The issues facing children are more about social acceptance and embarrassment. The emerging literature reveals that the younger children are told of their parents' gender identification the easier it is to accept (White & Ettner, 2004). The therapist must create a supportive environment for the family through this difficult and challenging time; the more the therapist can normalize this life cycle transition, the easier it will be for the parents to support their children through the familial changes. It is also necessary to validate the children's pain, betrayal, confusion, and fear, and assist the transitioning adults to hear these fears without perceiving this as a rejection of their identity. The therapist is challenged to take a both/and view, supporting the person in authenticity, while also validating his/her parental role and ability to maintain close and loving relationships with their children (and hopefully their spouse as well).

When a mother comes out as transgender and decides to transition, it is often difficult because the socially constructed identities and roles of "motherhood" are some of the most prescribed in Western culture. Given the position of privilege and power that most husbands have over their female-bodied partners, socially and financially, great care must be taken regarding how a father could influence the future custody of children when a mother decides to transition to a male identity. In the case of Jared and Robert it is clear how vulnerable Jared becomes after his transition from female to male as he is forced to create a new identity as a parent as well as manage extreme prejudice and discrimination from his (ex) husband Robert.

Case of Jared and Robert

Jared and Robert met when Jared was female identified at age 18. Jared, named JoLynn at the time, saw Robert as a safe and protective escape from an abusive family of origin and married Robert only months after meeting him. Jared recounts the story of his first years with Robert, clear that he told Robert about how he felt "like a man on the inside" and that Robert said that he "didn't mind." Jared speculated that Robert was himself interested in men and thought that perhaps this was part of his attraction to Jared, even when he was living as JoLynn. They both wanted to be parents and so Jared agreed to live as JoLynn until they had their two children, Samantha and Lily. After giving birth to their second child, Lily, JoLynn became increasingly more depressed and anxious due to concerns related to her gender identity and expression. JoLynn told Robert that she needed to transition as soon as possible to be the most stable and effective parent to their two daughters.

Robert was not able to accept this, and he became cruel, stating that he was not a "fag" and would not be married to a "fake man." Robert filed for divorce and demanded that Jared give up all parental rights to their children. Jared fought and won joint custody of their two children but the verbal abuse continued, as Robert berated Jared in front of the children. Jared's depression and isolation increased as Robert further ostracized him from the family, continuing to call Jared "JoLynn" and using female pronouns to address him. He also insisted that their daughters keep calling Jared "Mommy" even though they had decided to call Jared "Maddy" in a family therapy session months earlier.

Legal advocacy and therapeutic work with Jared began with recognizing the complex matrix of both present and past traumas that inform Jared's self-esteem and trans identity development. Most importantly, Jared's ability to parent his two daughters was an empowering and connective force in his life, critical to his mental health and emotional stability. For Jared, neither his gender identity nor his transition was directly affecting his children's well-being; rather, it was the rupture in the family system caused by Robert's extremely rejecting reaction. When Jared's parenting was called into question due to Robert's transphobia and misogyny, it was critical that Jared's identity as "Maddy" be explored and cultivated within the therapeutic relationship as this was an unquestionable achievement for Jared and needed to be acknowledged and nurtured.

Often parents who are transitioning have difficulty envisioning themselves as parents in their newly gendered bodies. They have internalized the transphobia within the socially accepted norms that point to trans parents as an impossibility. Assisting newly transitioned clients in the exploration of their trans parenthood is critical to their identity development as a trans parent. Utilizing a transfeminist approach, the therapist's role is to create language and conversation around future possibilities and hopes that clients have for their children and for themselves in the role of parent. The Transfeminist Qualitative Assessment Tool (TQAT) (Sennott, 2011) was developed to help therapists, in the beginning stages of family assessments, ask questions that would aid trans clients in exploring their assumptions and expectations about parenthood through an examination of their own parent's gender roles and behaviors. The TQAT allows for a new language of parenthood to evolve, for each individual, and the possibilities of parenting roles to open up in the newly transitioned individual (Sennott, 2011).

There are a multitude of clinical challenges that can arise when working with parent partnerships where one or both of the members are gender nonconforming or trans. It is common for therapists to assume that when one or both partners identify as trans, that transition or gender identity issues are a primary concern or consideration for the prospective parents. This assumption is not always a reality, especially with younger queer-identified partnerships. In fact, it can be quite damaging to the therapeutic alliance if a therapist focuses on this aspect of a relationship in a pathologizing manner instead of understanding it as a supportive and empowering characteristic of the parents' connection. Therapists ought to be educated and aware of the possibilities for pregnancy and surrogacy in partnerships with trans individuals. As touched on earlier, some trans-masculine- and trans-feminine-identified individuals might wish to freeze their eggs or sperm and have them held for later in their adult life. Other trans-identified partners may wish to discontinue gender affirming hormone therapy to either get pregnant or to inseminate a partner. Therapists should watch for signs of emotional and physical stressors if a client decides to stop hormone treatments; these potential stressors should be carefully explored with a client both before and during the process.

This is especially true for trans-masculine individuals who stop testosterone and become pregnant because they might be experiencing physical changes and increased gender dysphoria as they carry a baby to term. On the other hand, there is a position of curiosity that the therapist must take. It is critical not to *assume* that a person who is trans-masculine identified who makes the choice to become pregnant is going to experience this dysphoria, because the desire to give birth at some point in his life could be a part of his personal narrative of what it means to transition.

The Next Generation of LGBTQ Parents

The new generation of LGBTQ parents are planning to become parents in collaboration with their coming out, their gender transitions, and their partnerships. Younger LGBTQ people no longer wonder if parenting is a possibility; now it is often an assumed reality and birthright. Therapeutic work with these clients is often more about making decisions and negotiating difference within a partnership, just as it would be in working with prospective parents who are not LGBTQ. It is not uncommon for LGBTQ family therapists to meet with a lesbian or gay couple who are specifically looking for a safe place to process their differing hopes and expectations for parenthood, or with a queer-identified polyamorous relationship that includes a number of prospective parents instead of just two. One might meet with a trans-masculine adolescent and his parents to discuss gender affirming hormone therapy and surgery, as well as how he may freeze his eggs before transition so that a future partner or surrogate, 10 years from now, can carry a baby that is genetically his. The parenting possibilities are endless if therapists allow themselves to think outside of the box with young LGBTQ prospective parents.

Even with this burgeoning fleet of new queer-identified parents there are many clinical considerations for therapists to be mindful of, most poignantly the collective trauma of stigma, gender oppression, and the history of children being ripped away from LGBTQ parents in the past when they have come out to partners and family members. Therapists have a delicate balance to reach, building and empowering the clients' identities as parents while making space to explore possible fears and resentments that clients may have about how their families of origin and society may react to their parenthood. One thing that therapists can usually count on with the new generation of LGBTQ parents is that they are freer to make parenting decisions than LGBTQ people a decade ago, and this increasing freedom makes the therapeutic work rewarding and enlightening as one moves with clients into uncharted territories of gender, sexuality, and identity politics. The following vignette, written by the first author, depicts a case in which the clinician utilizes the relational aspects of the therapeutic relationship, to both create connection with the couple and to slow down the therapeutic process.

Case of Grace and Karin

Loud, angry voices emanated from the waiting room, interrupting my current session. I awkwardly excused myself and walked to the other end of the long hallway to the waiting room, where two White women in their early 20s sat, engaged in a fierce argument. I introduced myself, and asked them to please lower their voices, and told them our session would start in about 15 minutes. One woman seemed embarrassed, but the other woman seemed annoyed that I would disturb their argument. I could hear them reengage, albeit in lower voices, as I walked back to my office.

When Grace and Karin came into my office, they immediately resumed their battle, barely acknowledging my presence. With pitched voices, Karin and Grace yelled over one another, making me wish I had a referee whistle in my clinical bag of tricks. I had to stand up and loudly insist that they stop arguing. After setting up basic communication rules (one person talks at a time), I introduced myself and asked them to do the same. Karin, with long wavy hair, black lipstick, and multiple piercings, told me she was a college student in political science, and Grace, with a short crew cut and visible tattoo sleeves, said she had recently graduated from college and was working as a medical assistant in a local hospital.

Quieter now, but no less intense, Karin explained why they were seeking help from a therapist. "We want to have a child," Karin explained,

adding, in a sarcastic tone, "at least I do." Grace quickly jumped in, "We both want the same thing. The issue is how to make it happen. You see, Karin wants to get pregnant, which I'm okay with, but it is *how* she wants to do it that worries me." For the first time, there was silence in the room.

Karin said, "I don't see what the big deal is." She turned to me with a look that was both pleading and challenging. "I want to have a child the natural way, you know? I don't want to use a sperm bank," she said, her voice acerbic. "I want my children, *our* children, to know their biological father… I mean it's only right. What's the big deal about having sex with a guy anyway?" she asked pointedly.

Grace looked at me with raised eyebrows, clearly expecting me to take her side on this issue. "Tell me that's not gross," she says. "I mean, I don't care if someone likes sex with boys, but to have sex with one just to make a baby, *my* baby, ugh!" I paused thoughtfully. "How long have you two been together," I asked, biding my time and trying to get a clearer image of their history. Without pause, they simultaneously answered, "3 weeks."

Karin and Grace represent an emerging generation of young LGBTQ prospective parents. Born 20 years after Stonewall, reaching adulthood in a world where gay marriage is discussed on the evening news, and having received college credits for discussing the relationship between queer theory and postcolonial racism, Grace and Karin came to their lesbian relationship secure in the knowledge that they could become parents. Unlike an older cohort of LGBTQ parents, Grace and Karin do not verbalize concerns about how being gay might affect their children's development, or if lesbian motherhood might be a handicap in rearing a male child. They appear to have no concerns about the social world—their families of origin, their LGBTQ community, their jobs; they are solid in their inalienable right to become queer parents.

That they are also young in both age and in relational status, and have not engaged in any detailed conversations about finances, childrearing philosophies, or relationship stability, mirrors the same immaturity and naiveté of their non-LGBTQ peer group; that is, they are experiencing these developmental milestones at the appropriate time in the life cycle (Sassler, 2010). The idea that a young lesbian couple would fantasize and plan for their family as part of their courtship, that they imagine children as part of their human birthright, and that they are (somewhat) educated about how to create a family, reflects a new era in LGBTQ family building. This new generation is not asking permission of the world, and could care less what the research says about their families; they simply believe that having children is what couples in love *do*. Perhaps the reader is oddly relieved to discover that unlike heterosexual couples, conception will take a bit of planning—maybe even another 3 or 4 weeks!

Although on the surface, Karin and Grace's issues are similar to other young couples considering parenting, their presenting problem illustrates the unique interpersonal and emotional struggles that queer and same-sex couples face when choosing to become parents. An additional concern is whether their relationship is legally sanctioned in the state in which they live and how that might affect their child's legal status, particularly if Karin were to become pregnant in what she viewed as the "natural way." Legal issues, including health insurance and paternity rights, financial responsibilities, extended family and community support, as well as the complex issues of parenting "style" and values, are all potential fodder for the clinical conversation.

It is common for clinical concerns about the use of known donors verses anonymous donors to arise within younger LGBTQ couples. Therapists can educate themselves about what possibilities are available to queer and trans prospective parents; however, it is also helpful to direct clients to fertility clinics that serve the LGBTQ community in their area because these clinics often provide counseling and services for people who are considering donor insemination. There are often therapeutic issues between partners related to known donor use ranging from disagreements about who each partner wants to approach for donation to how much involvement each partner wants the donor to have in the child's life, to negotiating feelings of disappointment and internalized homophobia when a prospective known donor says "no." It is for this reason that many queer couples decide to only use another queer-identified person as their donor, so that they can keep the identity of their baby and their

expanding family intact within their LGBTQ community.

Conclusion

Clinical work with LGBTQ parents and prospective parents can be a rewarding and enlightening experience when therapists have properly educated themselves regarding the multitude of parenting possibilities for LGBTQ people. It is helpful to utilize an eclectic therapeutic approach that is informed by systemic, narrative, transfeminist, and relational systems perspectives. There is a new generation of LGBTQ prospective parents who are looking for clinicians able to work competently with the matrix of intersecting identities that each parent may hold. The challenge for clinicians is no longer to help LGBTQ parents fit into a heteronormative construct of parenting and child rearing. The new charge for therapists is to nurture and foster the endless possibilities and choices that are becoming a reality for LGBTQ parents and prospective parents.

References

Ashton, D. (2010). Lesbian, gay, bisexual, and transgender individuals and the family life cycle. In M. McGoldrick, B. Carter, & N. Garcia-Preto (Eds.), *The expanded family life cycle* (pp. 115–132). Boston, MA: Allyn and Bacon.

Bergman, K., Rubio, R.-J., Green, R.-J., & Padron, E. (2010). Gay men who become fathers via surrogacy: The transition to parenthood. *Journal of GLBT Family Studies, 6,* 111–141. doi:10.1080/15504281003704942

Berkowitz, D. (2007). A sociohistorical analysis of gay men's procreative consciousness. *Journal of GLBT Family Studies, 3,* 157–190. doi:10.1300/J461v03n02_07

Berkowitz, D., & Marsiglio, W. (2007). Gay men: Negotiating procreative, father, and family identities. *Journal of Marriage and Family, 69,* 366–381. doi:10.1111/j.1741-3737.2007.00371.x

Biblarz, T. J., & Savci, E. (2010). Lesbian, gay, bisexual, and transgender families. *Journal of Marriage and Family, 72,* 480–497. doi:10.1111/j.1741-3737.2010.00714.x

Bigner, J. J., & Bozett, F. W. (1990). Parenting by gay fathers. In F. W. Bozett & M. B. Sussman (Eds.), *Homosexuality and family relations* (pp. 155–175). New York, NY: Harrington Park Press.

Bowleg, L., Burkholder, G., Teti, M., & Craig, M. L. (2008). The complexities of outness: Psychosocial predictors of coming out to others among black lesbian and bisexual women. *Journal of LGBT Health Research, 4*, 153–166. doi:10.1080/15574090903167422

Brodzinsky, D. M. (2003). *Adoption by lesbians and gay men: A national survey of adoption agency policies, practices and attitudes.* Retrieved from http://www. adoptioninstitute.org/whowe/Gay%20and%20 Lesbian%20Adoption1.html

Bronfenbrenner, U. (1979). *The ecology of human development: Experiments by nature and design.* Cambridge, MA: Harvard University Press.

Brown, T. (2002). A proposed model of bisexual identity development that elaborates on experiential differences of women and men. *Journal of Bisexuality, 2*, 67–91.

Brown, M. L., & Rounsley, C. A. (1996). *True selves understanding transsexualism- for families, friends, coworkers, and helping professionals.* San Francisco, CA: Jossey-Bass.

Brown, S., Smalling, S., Groza, V., & Ryan, S. (2009). The experience of gay men and lesbians in becoming and being adoptive parents. *Adoption Quarterly, 12*, 229–246. doi:10.1080/10926750903313294

Burgess, C. (1999). Internal and external stress factors associated with the identity development of transgendered youth. In G. P. Mallon (Ed.), *Social services with transgendered youth* (pp. 35–48). New York, NY: Routledge.

Carrington, C. (1999). *No place like home: Relationships and family life among lesbians and gay men.* Chicago, IL: University of Chicago Press.

Cass, V. C. (1979). Homosexuality identity formation: A theoretical model. *Journal of Homosexuality, 4*, 291–235. doi:10.1300/J082v04n03_01

Cass, V. C. (1998). Sexual orientation identity formation, a western phenomenon. In R. J. Cabaj & T. S. Stein (Eds.), *Textbook of homosexuality and mental health* (pp. 227–251). Washington, DC: American Psychiatric Association.

Coleman, E. (1981/1982). Developmental stages of the coming out process. *Journal of Homosexuality, 7*, 731–743. doi:10.1300/J082v07n02_06

Cooper, K. (1999). Practice with transgendered youth and their families. In G. P. Mallon (Ed.), *Social services with transgendered youth* (pp. 111–130). Binghamton, NY: Haworth Press.

Currah, P., Minter, S., & Green, J. (2009). *Transgender equality: A handbook for activists and policymakers.* Washington, DC: ALGBTIC Board.

De Sutter, P. (2001). Gender reassignment and assisted reproduction: Present and future reproductive options for transsexual people. *Human Reproduction, 16*, 612–614. doi:10.1093/humrep/16.4.612

Devor, H. (1997). *FTM: Female-to-male transsexuals in society.* Bloomington, IN: Indiana University Press.

Downing, J. B., Richardson, H. B., Kinkler, L. A., & Goldberg, A. E. (2009). Making the decision: Factors influencing gay men's choice of an adoption path.

Adoption Quarterly, 12, 247–271. doi:10.1080/ 10926750903313310

Epstein, R. (Ed.) (2009). *Who's your daddy? And other writings on queer parenting.* Toronto, ON: Sumach Press.

Erhardt, V. (2007). *Head over heels: Wives who stay with cross-dressers and transsexuals.* Binghamton, NY: Haworth Press.

Erikson, E. (1956). The problem of ego identity. *Journal of the American Psychoanalytic Association, 4*, 56–121.

Ettner, R., Monstrey, S., & Eyler, A. E. (Eds.). (2007). *Principles of transgender medicine and surgery.* New York, NY: The Haworth Press.

Evan B. Donaldson Adoption Institute. (2003). *Adoption by lesbians and gays: A national survey of adoption agency policies, practices, and attitudes.* Retrieved from http://www.adoptioninstitute.org/whowe/Gay% 20and%20Lesbian%20Adoption1.html

Gates, G., Badgett, M. V. L., Macomber, J. E., & Chambers, K. (2007). *Adoption and foster care by gay and lesbian parents in the United States.* Washington DC: The Urban Institute.

Gates, G., & Ost, J. (2004). *The gay and lesbian atlas.* Washington, DC: The Urban Institute.

Gianino, M. (2008). Adaptation and transformation: The transition to adoptive parenthood for gay male couples. *Journal of GLBT Family Studies, 4*, 205–243. doi:10.1080/15504280802096872

Gilligan, C. (1993). *In a different voice: Psychological theory and women's development.* New York, NY: Harvard University Press.

Goldberg, A. E. (2010). *Lesbian and gay parents and their children: Research on the family life cycle.* Washington DC: American Psychological Association.

Goldberg, A. E., Downing, J. B., & Richardson, H. B. (2009). The transition from infertility to adoption: Perceptions of lesbian and heterosexual preadoptive couples. *Journal of Social & Personal Relationships, 26*, 938–963. doi:10.1177/0265407509345652

Goldberg, A. E., & Gianino, M. (2012). Lesbian and gay adoptive parents: Assessment, clinical issues, and intervention. In D. Brodzinsky & A. Pertman (Eds.), *Lesbian and gay adoption: A new American reality* (pp. 204–232). New York, NY: Oxford University Press.

Green, R. (1995). Gender identity disorder in children. In G. O. Gabbard (Ed.), *Treatments of psychiatric disorders* (2nd ed., pp. 2001–2014). Washington, DC: American Psychiatric Press.

Hudak, J. M., & Giammattei, S. V. (2010). Doing family: Decentering heteronormativity in "marriage" and "family" therapy. *AFTA Monograph Series: Expanding Our Social Justice Practices: Advances in Theory and Training, 6*, 49–58.

Imber-Black, E., & Roberts, J. (1998). *Rituals for our times: Celebrating, healing, and changing our lives and our relationships.* Latham, MD: Jason Aronson, Inc.

Jay, K. (Ed.). (1994). *Lavender culture.* New York, NY: New York University Press.

Jordan, J. V., Kaplan, A. G., Miller, J. B., Stiver, I. P., & Surrey, J. L. (Eds.). (1991). *Women's growth in connection: Writings from the Stone Center.* New York, NY: Guilford Press.

LaSala, M. C. (2010). *Coming out, coming home: Helping families adjust to a gay or lesbian child.* New York, NY: Columbia University Press.

Lebow, J. L. (Ed.). (2005). *Handbook of clinical family therapy.* Hoboken, NJ: Wiley.

Lev, A. I. (2004a). *The complete lesbian and gay parenting guide.* New York, NY: Berkley.

Lev, A. I. (2004b). *Transgender emergence: Therapeutic guidelines for working with gender-variant people and their families.* New York, NY: Routledge.

Lev, A. I. (2006a). Gay dads: Choosing surrogacy. *The British Psychological Society Lesbian and Gay Psychology Review, 7,* 72–76.

Lev, A. I. (2006b). Scrutinizing would-be parents (Gay): Gays looking to adopt will have to endure rigorous home studies. *Washington Blade,* pp. 6b-7b.

Lev, A. I. (2008). More than surface tension: Femmes in families. *Journal of Lesbian Studies, 12,* 127–144. doi:10.1080/10894160802161299

Lev, A. I. (2010). How queer- the development of gender identity and sexual orientation in LGBTQ-headed families. *Family Process, 49,* 268–290.

Lev, A. I., & Alie, L. (2012). Addressing the needs of youth who are LGBT and their families: A system of care approach. In S. Fisher, G. Blau, & J. M. Poirier (Eds.), *Improving emotional and behavioral outcomes for LGBT youth: A guide for professionals* (pp. 43–66). Baltimore, MD: Brookes.

Levitt, H. M., Gerrish, E. A., & Hiestand, K. R. (2003). The misunderstood gender: A model of modern femme identity. *Sex Roles, 48,* 99–113.

Lynch, J. M. (2004). Identity transformation: Stepparents in lesbian/gay stepfamilies. *Journal of Homosexuality, 48,* 45–60. doi:10.1300/J082v47n02_06

Mallon, G. P. (2007). Assessing lesbian and gay prospective foster and adoptive families: A focus on the home study process. *Child Welfare, 86,* 67–86.

Malpas, J. (2006). From 'otherness' to alliance: Transgender couples in therapy. *Journal of GLBT Family Studies, 2,* 183–206. doi:10.1300/J461v02n03_10

McDowell, T. (2005). Practicing a relational therapy with a critical multicultural lens. Introduction to a special section. *Journal of Systemic Therapies, 24,* 1–4.

McGoldrick, M., Carter, B., & Garcia-Preto, N. (Eds.). (2010). *The expanded family life cycle.* Boston, MA: Allyn and Bacon.

McGoldrick, M., Gerson, R., & Sueli, P. (2008). *Genograms: Assessment and intervention* (3rd ed.). New York, NY: W. W. Norton.

McGoldrick, M., & Hardy, K. V. (Eds.). (2008). *Re-visioning family therapy: Race, culture, and gender in clinical practice.* New York, NY: Guilford Press.

Moore, M. R. (2008). Gendered power relations among women: A study of household decision making in black lesbian stepfamilies. *American Sociological Review, 73,* 335–356. doi:10.1177/000312240807300208

Morales, E. (1996). Gender roles among latino gay and bisexual men: Implications for family and couple relationships. In J. Laird & R. J. Green (Eds.), *Lesbians and gays in couples and families: A handbook for therapists* (pp. 272–297). San Francisco, CA: Jossey-Bass.

More, S. D. (1998). The pregnant man - an oxymoron? *Journal of Gender Studies, 7,* 319–325. doi:10.1080/0 9589236.1998.9960725

Nichols, M. P., & Schwartz, R. C. (Eds.). (2009). *Family therapy: Concepts and methods* (7th ed.). Boston, MA: Pearson/Allyn & Bacon.

Patterson, C. J. (1995). Lesbian mothers, gay fathers, and their children. In A. R. D'Augelli & C. J. Patterson (Eds.), *Lesbian, gay, bisexual identities over the lifespan: Psychological perspectives* (pp. 262–290). New York, NY: Oxford University Press.

Patterson, C. J. (2006). Children of lesbian and gay parents. *Current Directions in Psychological Science, 15,* 241–244.

Rich, A. (1993). Compulsory heterosexuality and lesbian existence. In H. Abelove, M. Barale, & D. Halperin (Eds.), *The lesbian and gay studies reader* (pp. 227–254). New York, NY: Routledge.

Riggs, D. (2007). *Becoming parent: Lesbians, gay men, and family.* Queensland: Post Pressed.

Rosario, M., Schrimshaw, E. W., & Hunter, J. (2004). Ethnic/racial differences in the coming-out process of lesbian, gay, and bisexual youths: A comparison of sexual identity development over time. *Cultural Diversity and Ethnic Minority Psychology, 10,* 215–228. doi:10.1037/1099-9809.10.3.215

Rotheram-Borus, M. J., & Langabeer, K. A. (2001). Developmental trajectories of gay, lesbian, and bisexual youth. In A. R. D'Augelli & C. J. Patterson (Eds.), *Lesbian, gay, and bisexual identities and youth: psychological perspectives* (pp. 97–124). New York, NY: Oxford University Press.

Ryan, C. (2009). *Supportive families, healthy children: Helping families with lesbian, gay, bisexual, and transgender children.* Retrieved from http://family-project.sfsu.edu/publications

Ryan, C., Huebner, D., Diaz, R. M., & Sanchez, J. (2009). Family rejection as a predictor or negative health outcomes in White and Latino lesbian, gay, and bisexual young adults. *Pediactrics, 123,* 346–352. doi:10.1542/peds.2007-3524

Sassler, S. (2010). Partnering across the life course: Sex, relationships, and mate selection. *Journal of Marriage and Family, 72,* 557–571. doi:10.1111/j.1741-3737. 2010.00718.x

Sennott, S. L. (2011). Gender disorder as gender oppression: A transfeminist approach to rethinking the pathologization of gender non-conformity. *Women & Therapy, 34,* 93–113. doi:10.1080/02703149.2010.53 2683

Sennott, S., & Smith, T. (2011). Translating the sex and gender continuums in mental health: A transfeminist approach to client and clinician fears. *Journal of Gay*

and Lesbian Mental Health, 15, 218–234. doi:10.1080
/19359705.2011.553779

Shuster, S. (2002). An ounce of prevention: Keeping couples out of court. *In the Family, 7*(3), 7–11.

Slater, C. (1999). *The lesbian family life cycle*. Chicago, IL: University of Illinois Press.

Tasker, F., & Golombok, S. (1997). *Growing up in a lesbian family*. New York, NY: Guilford Press.

Tolman, D. L., & Diamond, L. M. (2001). Desegregating sexuality research: Cultural and biological perspectives on gender and desire. *Annual Review of Sex Research, 12*, 33–74.

Troiden, R. R. (1993). The formation of homosexual identities. In L. D. Garnets & D. C. Kimmel (Eds.), *Psychological perspectives on lesbian and gay male*

experiences (pp. 191–217). New York, NY: Columbia University Press.

Walsh, F. (Ed.). (2003). *Normal family processes: Growing diversity and complexity*. New York, NY: Guilford Press.

Weinberg, M. S., Williams, C. J., & Pryor, D. W. (1994). *Dual attraction: Understanding bisexuality*. New York, NY: Oxford University Press.

Weston, K. (1991). *Families we choose: Lesbians, gays, kinship*. New York, NY: Columbia University Press.

White, T., & Ettner, R. (2004). Disclosure, risks and protective factors for children whose parents are undergoing a gender transition. *Journal of Gay & Lesbian Psychotherapy, 8*, 129–145. doi:10.1080/19359705.20 04.9962371

Clinical Work with Children and Adolescents Growing Up with Lesbian, Gay, and Bisexual Parents

Cynthia J. Telingator

Lesbian, gay, and bisexual people desire to parent for many of the same reasons as heterosexually oriented men and women. However, the process of considering parenting and then becoming a parent may be more complex for sexual minorities. It may involve "coming out" as a lesbian, gay, or bisexual parent at work and in the community, and dealing with familial and societal expectations and prohibitions. Also, it is difficult for parents to anticipate the unique issues their children may confront at different developmental stages. Although lesbian-, gay-, and bisexual-parent families are more visible and are increasingly accepted in today's society, they continue to be effected by societal bias on a multitude of levels. The potential impact of this bias may differ for each member of the family.

A therapist should consider both the psychological and the social issues that may have impacted the parent's development over their life course, and how those experiences may influence their parenting. Indeed, the transition to parenthood is a significant life transition and is informed by continuities and discontinuities from all previous stages of development (Engel, 1977; Halfon & Hochstein, 2002). A life course perspective emphasizes that development is lifelong and continuous. The interaction between one's life stages and experiences cannot be understood in isolation, but is influenced at each developmental stage by one's previous development, as well as the responses of the environment in which one is raised (Johnson, Crosnoe, & Elder, 2011). A life course developmental construct is used in this chapter to illuminate the importance of one's "coming out" process and how it may influence the dynamic in one's relationships with members of one's own generation, and across generations.

Growing up as a sexual minority can influence the strengths and vulnerabilities one brings to parenting. For example, based on their own experiences of discrimination and stigma, lesbian, gay, and bisexual parents may have a heightened level of anxiety around the safety and well-being of their children. This anxiety may blind them to a deeper understanding of the specific needs and feelings of their children. A therapist may be in a unique position to help the parent to understand where there may be misattunement between the feelings and needs of the parent(s) and the child(ren), and can help them to find a way to traverse those differences. The dynamics between parents and children in lesbian-, gay-, and bisexual-parent families can be understood by developing an appreciation of how their lives and life courses are interwoven, and how the narrative of their experiences may converge and diverge.

A therapist can help parents to increase their awareness of subtle issues that may be particular to children of lesbian, gay, and bisexual parents. Clinicians can also help the parents to appreciate

C.J. Telingator, M.D. (✉)
Child and Adolescent Psychiatry,
Cambridge Health Alliance, Harvard Medical School,
1493 Cambridge Street, Cambridge, MA 02138, USA
e-mail: cindy_telingator@hms.harvard.edu

A.E. Goldberg and K.R. Allen (eds.), *LGBT-Parent Families: Innovations in Research and Implications for Practice*, DOI 10.1007/978-1-4614-4556-2_17, © Springer Science+Business Media New York 2013

and distinguish between what issues may be normative developmental struggles for any child, and what may occur as a consequence of having lesbian, gay, or bisexual parents. A biopsychosocial understanding of development can help the clinician to formulate an understanding of the vulnerabilities and the strengths of each member of the family, and the family as a whole. Although research has shown that stressful life events and repeated or chronic environmental challenges can impact individual vulnerability to illness, it has also revealed that having a sense of psychological well-being and living within a supportive environment can be protective (Fava & Sonino, 2008; McEwen, 1998; Ryff & Singer, 1996).

A clinical vignette will be used to highlight how a therapist can help a family understand the influence of parents' life course on their children's lives in the context of treating an adolescent with same-sex parents.

Clinical Vignette: Melissa

Melissa is a 16-year-old Caucasian girl growing up in a city in Massachusetts. She is a little over five feet four inches, wears her brown hair down to her shoulders, and takes pride in her appearance. She loves sports and music and is a particularly gifted cross-country runner. She has many male and female friends and enjoys social activities as well as time spent alone. She volunteers for an organization that helps children who are living in poverty around the world, and she works for a community food bank once a month. She was referred to therapy due to concern about her sadness and a change in her behavior.

During the therapists' initial meeting with Melissa's parents the following information was elicited. Melissa has two mothers, Denise and Jill, who have raised her since birth. Her mothers are currently in their 40s. They first became a couple in their 20s and discussed their wish to have children early on. Their dream to each have a child was complicated by the fact that Jill was diagnosed with Lupus when she was 23 years old, and was intermittently treated with steroids

for this illness. Because of this, Jill felt she would not feel safe trying to conceive a child or carry a pregnancy. Denise, on the other hand, wanted to give birth to a child.

When they were in their early 30s they began to discuss having children more seriously and explored their options. One lingering question was whether to use a donor who would agree to be known when the child was 18, or to try to find a friend who would agree to donate sperm and be known to the child from birth. In the end, their desire to have their child know the person who donated sperm led them to consider the option of identifying a friend who would agree to be the donor.

Denise had a friend at work named Robert. Denise and Robert were in the field of technology and had become friends while working together. As Denise and Robert grew closer, she began to speak to him about her wish to have children. She told him of her ambivalence about using a sperm bank, and her wish to have her children know the identity of the sperm donor. Robert later spoke with Denise and told her that he and his partner Zack had discussed the possibility of donating sperm to Jill and Denise so they could have a child. Denise was moved by this offer and arranged a meeting with Jill and Zack for the four of them to discuss in greater detail this possible means of conceiving a child. Together and separately, the two couples tried to anticipate issues that could arise.

After completing an initial evaluation, Melissa's therapist requested to meet with each couple (Denise and Jill, Robert and Zack) to get a better history of their relationships, both with Melissa and with each other. She inquired about the concerns that each couple had regarding this decision prior to Melissa's conception, their feelings about each other after she was born, and what worries still existed about their relationship with the other couple with regard to Melissa. Both couples expressed that they had felt anxiety about this arrangement throughout the process. Some of their anxieties were articulated to the other couple prior to deciding to conceive, but others were not shared, both for conscious reasons, but also because they had not been anticipated. One early discussion Jill and Denise had with Robert and Zack was to clarify who would be the "parents" to the child. They all agreed that Denise and Jill would be the parents and that Robert and Zack would be involved in the child's life. Initially, the four of them did not deepen this discussion to include defined roles for Robert and Zack, or how the men's roles would be constructed by the child.

None of the adults knew exactly how this arrangement would take shape, but agreed that they would work it out over time and that the child would know that Robert was the sperm donor. Robert and Zack would spend time with Melissa, but the details of this were not considered at this early stage. Denise and Jill were fortunate to live in a state that allowed for second-parent adoption. They did not want to use a "known" donor unless the donor agreed to give up parental rights. Robert agreed to this stipulation. As a result, Jill would be allowed to be the second parent on the birth certificate, permitting her to have the legal rights of a second parent. It was agreed that Jill and Denise would have full legal and physical custody, and they would make all financial, physical, and school-related decisions. No specifics were written into the contract about how much time the child would spend with Robert and Zack, but all agreed that the decision to conceive with a "known" donor was intended to give the child an opportunity to know Robert, the sperm donor, and to have a relationship with him and Zack.

Denise conceived after switching from home-based insemination to a clinic for intrauterine insemination in which a doctor used a catheter to place the sperm directly into the uterus. The couple's daughter, Melissa, was born without complications. Although Robert had given up parental rights after Melissa's birth, both Denise and Jill became increasingly anxious that he would change his mind. If he did, it would mean that Jill would not be allowed to adopt Melissa and become her legal parent. While Denise and Jill tried to anticipate issues their child might face in her life due to having lesbian parents, they never considered that they would become fearful of their child being "taken away" by the men who

helped to conceive her. They did not feel comfortable discussing this fear with Robert and Zack and began to pull away from them as the due date approached. When Melissa was born, all four of them were at the hospital, although only Jill was present during the delivery. Immediately after her birth Robert and Zack spent some time with Melissa, but Jill asked them to leave so she and Denise could have alone time to "bond" with Melissa. Denise and Jill's fears had begun to create a boundary between Robert, Zack, and Melissa, which Melissa would experience as a small child, but not understand until much later.

Before they began to think about how they would conceive, Denise and Jill had discussed their concern that their child might experience discrimination secondary to their sexual orientation. They knew that they wanted to raise a child in a community that was diverse with regard to race, class, and ethnicity. They had hoped that the public school their child would attend would have other lesbian- and gay-parent families, but had no way to ensure this would happen. They were very aware of the potential difficulties due to stigmatization that their child might face coming from a "different" family, but did not know how this would manifest in a school setting day to day, or if their child or others in the community would communicate with them about these incidents.

Throughout grade school and middle school, Melissa's parents listened for any difficulties she might be having with peers or with teachers as a result of having two mothers. They tried to not overemphasize this difference, but they also wanted to create a space where Melissa could talk about struggles she might encounter for any reason, including having lesbian parents. She was open with them, and other than an occasional disagreement with a friend that had nothing to do with her parent's sexuality, Melissa did not share any experiences of rejection or discrimination that they could directly relate to having two mothers. Melissa had never experienced any bullying directed toward her or her family, but she was acutely aware of, and hurt by, the comments her peers made with regards to "gay" people.

Prior to entering high school, Melissa began to share less of her day-to-day experiences with them, and although Denise and Jill continued to be concerned, they wanted to give her the space to bring issues to them when they arose. Melissa did well socially and academically, and, as was true throughout grade school and middle school, her teachers continued to comment on her capacity as a leader. Her sensitivity and awareness of how other children were treated based on race, class, and disabilities were beyond what her teachers normally encountered in her age group.

Unbeknownst to her parents, going to high school was a difficult transition for Melissa, and slowly over time she became more withdrawn and socially isolated. Initially, she was very popular and socially active in school, and she was involved in after-school activities and community projects. She was attracted to both men and women, and as her sexual feelings intensified toward a female friend, she began to feel conflict around an unspoken pressure she felt to be a "normal" child of lesbian parents. She did not want to betray the sense of loyalty she had to both her parents and to the community to prove that children who were raised with gay or lesbian parents were just as "healthy" as children raised in heterosexual homes. She understood that mainstream society defined "healthy" as heterosexual and behaving in a way that embraced "typical" gender role expressions. She inherently rejected the notion that there was a typical way to express herself either in terms of gender or her sexuality. She, by virtue of being raised in her family and in her community, came to appreciate the spectrum of gender and sexuality that can exist across and within individuals, and she felt that she did not yet know what all of this meant to her.

As her freshman year progressed, Melissa had increasing difficulty focusing on her schoolwork, and her grades began to drop. She stopped bringing friends to her house and participating in after-school activities. When her school counselor approached her to talk to her about her deteriorating grades, she began to open up about the fact that she was struggling. Melissa agreed with the counselor that she should let her parents know that she was not doing well.

Melissa's parents called her pediatrician to get a referral. The pediatrician recommended a thera-pist whom she knew was comfortable doing both individual and family therapy. The therapist initially met with Melissa a couple of times and then met separately with her mothers to get a family history. Melissa told the therapist that she had two mothers, and when the therapist asked what she knew about her conception, the family's story unfolded. The therapist recognized that although she had two parents, there were other significant adults in Melissa's life. She asked to meet with Melissa's mothers as well as with Zack and Robert separately as couples, and then all together over several sessions to get a history. The therapist wanted to hear both the individual and collective narratives about the process of the decision to have Melissa, and about the roles and relationships that each of them had had with Melissa since she was born.

Melissa liked this therapist because she asked about Melissa's "family," and included questions that allowed Melissa to speak about Zack and Robert. She did not normally talk about them with her mothers, or with her friends. During the initial phase of therapy, Melissa primarily focused on her feelings of disappointment with her friends, and with a relationship she had with a boy at school that had recently ended. Issues around having a "different" family were not addressed during this phase. The therapist felt that it was important to learn from Melissa about how she perceived her relationship with her mothers, as well as with Robert and Zack before making assumptions about the significance that each one had in her life, and her relationship with each of them. The therapist did not assume that her family structure was the reason for therapy.

The therapist believed that Melissa's symptoms would likely resolve with both individual and family therapy. This therapy would include work with Melissa's parents as well as Zack and Robert as separate couples and then together. Some of these meetings would include Melissa, and others would not. The therapist referred the family to a family therapist she felt would be a good match to do this work, and continued to do individual therapy with Melissa. During the course of her individual psychotherapy, Melissa came to understand that some of the disappointment she felt toward others for not meeting her needs was related to her resistance to expressing those needs for fear of not having them fulfilled. She also recognized her tendency to take care of others rather than herself. She felt that she "needed" a boyfriend rather than feeling that she wanted to have one. Although she felt close with friends, she had never been particularly close with anyone she had dated. She realized that it was this feeling of isolation and loneliness that was making her feel sad. She was not able to allow herself to be intimate with others in a way that fulfilled her needs. As she discussed these issues in therapy she began to feel less sad and anxious, and reengaged with her peers and school.

Over time she began, tentatively, to express her disappointment in her "family" to her therapist. In the context of her therapy, she referred to her mothers as well as Robert and Zack as her family. Her mothers were her parents, but all four of them were a part of her family. This inclusion was true of all of their parents, her parents' siblings, and her cousins, to varying degrees. She felt disappointed and angry when she thought about how her mothers, Zack, and Robert had not been particularly helpful in figuring out these relationships. She was angry with her mothers at times, but was primarily angry with both of her "dads." She was not able to articulate what prompted this anger, but she was able to say that it was not something she wanted to talk about. Over the period of almost a year she began to open up more about her feelings about growing up in her family.

She felt very close to both of her mothers. She had always referred to Denise as "mommy," and Jill as "mama." Denise and Jill had chosen those names before Melissa was born, and since she was an infant they had referred to each other as "mommy" and "mama." When friends or other adults asked her who her "real mother" was, Melissa felt intense anger and sadness. Both Denise and Jill were her "real mothers," and she felt this deeply. She could not understand the ignorance of others who felt that a biological connection made one of her mothers more "real" than the other.

Since she was young, Melissa had a sense that she needed to protect her parents' lifestyle and was frustrated that her parents' concerns were often focused on her experience of having "gay" parents. Most of the time she felt this was a nonissue in her day-to-day life. In contrast to her friends who had different-sex parents, she felt that adults, and at times her peers, were overly curious and intrusive with regards to her family. She believed that this was solely based on her parents' sexual orientation. For Melissa, her personal relationship with each of her parents was her main concern, not their sexual orientation.

She was angry and sad that she was not the one who had any say in how the relationships between the significant adults in her life were constructed. She had spent much of her life to this point confused about who was defining how she related to each of her mothers, and Robert and Zack. Her hopes that it would be spoken about more overtly were never realized. Therefore, she always tried to interpret what she was supposed to do and did not have the opportunity to explore what she wanted to do. She did not feel that her parents understood what she wanted, or that they asked her about what she needed from each of them. She felt that her parents had made assumptions about how much time she wanted to spend with whom, and she was frustrated with herself for letting her parents take the lead in defining her relationships.

Through her work in therapy, she had begun to recognize that she could allow herself to think about the question of what her wishes were for her relationship with Robert and Zack. Melissa had first been told about Robert helping Denise "make a baby" when she was five. As she got older, her mothers offered more details about "how" babies are created. It was not until she was much older that she questioned how the decision to use Robert's sperm and Denise's egg had been made. As a child, Melissa would spend several hours a couple of times a month with Robert and Zack. From an early age, she understood that they were important people but they were referred to as "Robert" and "Zack." Melissa described to her therapist what it was like for her when all four of them were together. As a small child, Melissa could sense their anxiety but could not name it. As she got older and learned that Robert was her biological father, she began to understand more about Robert's and Zack's desire to spend time with her, but she still did not understand why her mothers seemed different when they were around. She loved her mothers, but this did not dispel her fantasies about having more time with Robert and Zack. When she was around 7 or 8 years old she would fantasize that Robert and Denise would get married and Zack and Jill would get married. She imagined that then they could all live together.

As she got older this marriage fantasy waned, but her longing to be closer to Zack and Robert continued. Robert and Zack seemed to want Melissa to initiate their time together, but her mothers did not specifically encourage her to do so. In turn, her fears that her moms would be angry if she wanted to spend time with them kept her silent. She was left feeling sad and disappointed that none of the adults were helping her to navigate this complicated family structure. She had close friends but did not share this pain with them. She was angry that Zack and Robert were not more involved in her life, and they addressed her as "Melissa." She could never recall hearing them describe her as "my daughter." She referred to Robert and Zack by their proper names but did not feel comfortable doing so. It made her feel more distant from them, and she was upset that she had never been asked what she wanted to call them. She interpreted the fact that no one spoke to her about her wishes as a statement that they had all agreed that calling them anything other than Robert and Zack was not acceptable.

Since she was young she had always thought of them as "sort of dads," and she developed secret names for them. Starting when she was seven or eight she secretly referred to Robert as "dad" and Zack as "daddy." To her they were part of her family. Melissa did not see them as often as she wished, and they were not often spoken about in the context of day-to-day family issues. She often tried to imagine ways in which she could eliminate the awkwardness between her mothers and them, but she didn't know how to accomplish this. When she was younger she made up reasons why they were not closer, and most of the fantasies included something that she had done to create this tension. Now that she was older she understood that she was not fully responsible for the tension, but she still felt in part that it was her fault. She did not have any friends who had a family that closely approximated the complexity of her family and felt as a result that none of her friends could help her with this issue; in fact, she never talked about it with them.

Over the course of therapy, Melissa began to express her sadness about Robert and Zack's limited involvement in her life. Concurrent to Melissa's individual therapy a family therapist was working with her and her family. Her mothers had agreed to work with Robert and Zack in family work to revisit their early history together. With Melissa's permission, her individual therapist worked closely with the family therapist to help guide family treatment. In family therapy, Jill, Denise, Robert, and Zack expressed appreciation for the insight Melissa had given them into how the communication—or lack thereof—among the four of them had led to misunderstandings and distortions. Denise and Jill were able to tell Robert and Zack that although their wish was to use a known donor they did not anticipate that they would be fearful that Robert and Zack would try to take Melissa away from them. They shared that these feelings had dissipated over the years as they became more comfortable with parenting and more secure in their relationship with Melissa and as a family. They realized that some of the anxiety that they felt about Robert and Zack were a projection of their early experiences coming out, and their anxiety of not knowing who might cause them or their child harm. The therapist recognized that for Melissa, the very people who could have been helpful were the same ones who were seen as potentially harmful.

Zack and Robert were able to speak to the family therapist about their deep sense of rejection and experience of anger and disappointment when Melissa was first born and they were sent away. They felt an immediate connection to Melissa that they did not anticipate when they agreed to donate sperm. As she got older and interacted with them, they were struck by how much they wanted to spend more time with her, and spend time alone with her to build their own relationships. They then became anxious that they would be cut off from having any contact with Melissa if they requested to have more of a relationship with her and subsequently limited the time they spent with her. It appeared to the therapist that a consequence of this was that Melissa felt rejected by them, as this dynamic was never explicitly communicated to her mothers or to her prior to her therapy.

A meeting was held with Melissa's therapist, Melissa, the family therapist, her mothers, and Robert and Zack. In this meeting Melissa was able to tell Robert and Zack that she wanted them to spend more time with her. She also expressed her wish that she didn't have to refer to them solely as "Zack" and "Robert." Denise, Jill, Robert, and Zack were all responsive to this request. In a series of family meetings, the family therapist was able to help both couples and Melissa to understand the origin of some of the tensions that existed between the couples and help them to work together to renegotiate their relationships. Both couples were able to speak to their fears and wishes with Melissa, and this increased ability to openly communicate allowed them in a unified way to allow Melissa to pursue relationships with Zack and Robert in a way that met her needs.

The work that Melissa, Denise, Jill, Robert, and Zack were able to do in individual and family therapy helped Melissa to get developmentally back on track. Her inability to articulate her experience of her relationships in her family led to her sadness and anger that brought her to treatment, and that her work in individual and family therapy helped her to understand. The family therapy allowed her to engage and reengage with her family in ways that felt more satisfying for her and helped to improve her mood. Following this work with her family they terminated family therapy, but Melissa continued with individual therapy for another 6 months. She was able to focus her individual therapy on working to separate from her parents, gain a better understanding of her own identity, and reengage with her peer group. Her mood improved as did her grades. Over time she terminated with her therapist with the understanding that she could return to do individual and family work at other points in her life in which it might be useful to her and her family.

Clinical Relevance of the Intersection of Parents and Their Childrens' Life Course

To better understand lesbian-, gay-, and bisexual-parent families, it is helpful to first understand the parents' history developmentally both in the context of their family of origin and throughout their life course. When taking a history, the clinician should include biological, social, and psychological vulnerabilities and strengths of each member of the family. This information can be incorporated into the formulation of the family dynamics and the symptoms that have brought the identified patient and their family to therapy. The clinician's understanding of the issues may be reformulated as one works with the family over time. In addition to the parent's biological, psychological, and social history, the parent's developmental history should include the parents' experience of "coming out," and their decision-making process around having children.

Understanding the parent's life course in terms of the historical, social, and cultural context of each parent's path to self-identifying as a lesbian, gay, or bisexual individual will help the therapist to appreciate the parent's own developmental experiences, and how these experiences may influence his or her parenting. Some lesbian, gay, and bisexual individuals were raised in families and communities who were accepting of their sexual orientation and gender expression. But, it is not unusual to work with parents who as children and adolescents experienced emotional distancing from parents, peers, and their community due to being "different" starting at a young age. Through verbal and nonverbal communications of anger and disappointment which may have included verbal and physical harassment from parents, peers, or other members of the community, individuals may have experienced rejection and discrimination in a multitude of ways at each stage of their lives starting in childhood.

Throughout development, individuals may have experienced and understood this rejection in a variety of ways, but ultimately it may have been internalized as a rejection of their core self. It is not uncommon to work with sexual minorities who from an early age attempt to "cover" to manage the stigma of being a sexual minority and try to keep it from "looming large" (Goffman, 1963). This process of rejection may lead to a shame-based identity and result in the individual living with internalized homophobia. This internalized sense of fear and shame can have a long-term impact on individual self-esteem and may consciously or unconsciously influence one's parenting (Kaufman & Raphael, 1996).

Thinking about becoming a parent may provoke anxiety as the individual faces the possibility that his or her children may experience rejection and discrimination solely based on the sexual orientation of their parent(s). A study by Bos and van Balen (2008) revealed that one of the primary concerns of lesbians considering parenthood is the possibility of their child having negative experiences as a consequence of being raised in a nontraditional family in a heterosexist and homophobic society. The children of lesbian, gay, and bisexual parents have "membership by association of a stigmatized minority group" (Goldberg, 2007, p. 550).

Children who are born into a "different" family constellation may not feel "different" even though their parents are "different" from other parents. The children of lesbian, gay, and bisexual parents do not necessarily experience the same minority group identity as their parents. Although children and adolescents may feel protective of the LGBTQ community, and feel a part of this community by virtue of being a child with a lesbian, gay, or bisexual parent, this aspect of their lives may or may not be pivotal to their identity (Goldberg, Kinkler, Richardson, & Downing, 2012). Parents may unwittingly over-emphasize this aspect of their own identity in an effort to communicate their concerns about the discrimination their child may face. The constant reference to a parent's sexual orientation may be confusing for the child who does not understand why it is an ongoing topic of conversation.

Lesbian, gay, and bisexual parents' desire to foresee struggles and protect their children from the stigma of having lesbian, gay, or bisexual parent can be consciously and unconsciously consuming. Previous experiences of their own rejection, discrimination, and verbal/physical assaults for being lesbian, gay, or bisexual may heighten their fear for their child's safety and well-being. In a study conducted in the Netherlands on lesbian mothers, Bos, van Balen, van den Boom, and Sandfort (2004) found that mothers with increased levels of perceived stigma, internalized homophobia, and higher levels of perceived rejection felt a greater need to justify their position as mother. This response to real and perceived stigmatization may impact the children as well. Bos and van Balen (2008) found that children with lesbian mothers who perceived higher levels of stigmatization for having lesbian parents had a lower sense of well-being. Girls who perceived high levels of stigma reported low self-esteem, and boys who perceived high levels of stigma were rated by their parents as being more hyperactive, which may have been a reflection of increased levels of anxiety.

The negative effects of homophobic stigmatization on children's self-esteem and behavior have been shown to be counteracted by frequent contact with other offspring of same-sex parents, being in a school that teaches tolerance, and having mothers who perceive themselves as active members of the lesbian community (Bos & van Balen, 2008). Bos, Gartrell, Peyser, and van Balen (2008) compared planned lesbian-mother families in the USA with families in the Netherlands and found that in both countries, there was a negative effect of homophobia on children's psychosocial adjustment. The extent to which socioeconomic status and stigmatization are interrelated is underexamined in research; however, one study by Tasker and Golombok (1997) did suggest that children from lesbian-mother families with lower socioeconomic status were more likely to experience peer stigma because of their mothers' sexual orientation than those from middle-class lesbian-mother families. This finding highlights the importance of considering social class in clinical work with lesbian-, gay-, and bisexual-parent families in addition to other aspects of their identity which place them in a minority group.

The stress that lesbian, gay, and bisexual individuals experience due to being a member of a sexual minority has been understood as a type of "minority stress." Minority stress theory posits that people from stigmatized social categories experience negative life events and additional stress due to their minority status (Meyer, 1995, 2003). Meyer (2003) further described four different minority stress processes in lesbian, gay, and bisexual adults: experiences of prejudice; expectations of rejection or discrimination; hiding and concealing one's sexual orientation; and internalized homophobia, which is the process of turning societal negative attitudes toward oneself.

A secondary process that has been described is one of "microaggressions." Microaggressions are social or environmental, verbal and nonverbal, and intentional and unintentional brief assaults on minority individuals (Balsam, Molina, Beadnell, Simoni, & Walters, 2011; Sue et al., 2007). These microaggressions can take the form of microassaults, microinsults, and microinvalidation (Balsam et al., 2011). Whether or not they are intended as an aggression, children may witness or experience these types of transgressions toward lesbian, gay, and bisexual people as an assault on their parents, and secondarily on them.

Experiences of microaggressions may occur in a variety of settings and be very confusing for children and adolescents. They may experience anxiety for the safety and well-being of their parents, and subsequently for themselves. Parents in turn may have their own anxiety concerning the safety and well-being of their children. This anxiety may be expressed by maintaining a kind of hypervigilance around the child's interactions with adults and peers at school and in the community, with the hope of protecting them. It may be difficult for family members to consciously identify these microaggressions and therefore impede the ability of the family to discuss the overt and covert stress it creates for the family system.

An ongoing dialogue between parents and children that is developmentally attuned is important to help the communication between them

around the child's experience of being raised in a "different" family structure than many of their peers, and the homophobia that may be misdirected toward them based on their parents' sexual orientation. Indeed, Gartrell, Deck, Rodas, Peyser, and Banks's (2005) longitudinal study of 78 lesbian-parent families with 10-year-old children found that 43% of the children in this study reported that they had experienced stigmatization due to their mother's sexual orientation.

Grade school and middle school years may be the hardest for children of lesbian, gay, and bisexual parents (Goldberg, 2010; Ray & Gregory, 2001). Children of lesbian, gay, and bisexual parents often lack a "group" at school who share a similar family structure and with whom they can identify, and for that reason, they may feel "different" themselves. During grade school, it is not unusual for children to be exposed to the stigma directed toward people who are identified as lesbian, gay, or bisexual. Children with lesbian, gay, or bisexual parents may be bullied due to the sexual orientation of their parents, and they may experience comments and jokes about nonheterosexual people as a personal affront, even when they are not directed specifically toward them or their families. Children of lesbian, gay, and bisexual parents may or may not share these comments or their experiences with their parents in order to protect their parents. Children often develop an early awareness of homophobia and the impact of stigmatization and discrimination on individuals, families, and communities (Goldberg, 2007).

In some cases, children are taught overtly or covertly either by their families, or from their experiences in school and with friends, or both, that it is not safe to talk openly to others about their family. Parents may choose to not "come out" at work, at their children's school, or in the community in which they are raising their children (Stein, Perrin, & Potter, 2002). Depending on the community in which they are raised, children may need to closely monitor what they say to friends and other adults about their lives. They learn that their safety may be dependent on the need to "hide" aspects of their family. This need to maintain secrecy can impact children's capacity to form trusting relationships where they can openly explore different parts of themselves, and use these relationships to begin to separate from their parents.

Both family and friends can be important sources of support to buffer the children's experience of heterosexism. Based on her review of the literature, Goldberg (2010) concluded that both living in a community that was supportive, as well as having relationships with other children of lesbian, gay, and bisexual parents, can help children to feel "less vulnerable and alone" (p. 161). Goldberg (2010) also concluded what was helpful to adult children of lesbian, gay, and bisexual parents to cope effectively with heterosexism while they were growing up was open communication between parents and their children.

For lesbian, gay, and bisexual parents, having a close, positive, and meaningful connection with their children is associated with better mental health outcomes for the children (Golombok, 2000). For example, Bos and Gartrell (2010) found that although homophobic stigmatization can have a negative impact on the psychological well-being of lesbian-mother families, being raised by "loving, nurturing, supportive parents can counteract these detrimental effects" (p. 569). This finding is consistent with earlier data that showed that warm and supportive relationships between parents and their children, as well as children and their peers, may be protective for children, and may buffer them from the negative psychological consequences of real or perceived stigmatization (Bos & van Balen, 2008; Frosch & Mangelsdorf, 2001; Golombok, 2000). Close and loving relationship with one's parents through adolescence continues to have a positive influence on the well-being and healthy psychosocial development of children (Udell, Sandfort, Reitz, Bos, & Dekovic, 2010). It is also important to appreciate that undergoing stress can sometimes be a positive learning experience and lead to personal growth (Cox, Dewaele, van Houtte, & Vincke, 2011; Savin-Williams, 2008).

The developmental tasks of adolescence may bring new challenges for the children of lesbian, gay, and bisexual parents. Adolescents are often duly aware that their parents have been stigmatized for being a sexual minority, and that their own sexuality may reflect back on their parents. Based on societal prejudices, children of lesbian, gay, and bisexual parents may fear coming out as nonheterosexual themselves (Goldberg, 2010). Due to societal, peer, and developmental pressures and their desire to appear "normal," adolescents with lesbian, gay, and bisexual parents may remain more secretive with their peers about the nature of their family constellation (Perlesz et al., 2006). This secretiveness may cause them to isolate their parents away from their social worlds.

The parents' own experiences of coming out may make them more sensitive to openly discussing issues around gender and sexuality with their children and more supportive of their children's questions about sexuality (Mitchell, 1998). Although the parents may be open and accepting of their children exploring their sexuality, parents' anxiety and desire to protect their children from the stigmatization they had to deal with in their lives may complicate the messages they give their children about sexual orientation and gender expression (Bos & Gartrell, 2010).

As adults, children of lesbian, gay, and bisexual parents describe themselves as being more tolerant and open minded as a direct consequence of being raised by parents who were sexual minorities, and who socialized their children to appreciate differences (Goldberg, 2007). Additionally, they often feel that a consequence of being in a home where the parent's sexual orientation was openly discussed allowed them to think more deeply about their sexuality, and understand it more complexly (Goldberg, 2010). Further, as adolescents and adults, they often view themselves as more comfortable than children who were raised in heterosexual-parent homes to resist for themselves and others heteronormative expectations around gender and sexuality (Goldberg, 2007). An awareness of the factors that have contributed to the resilience and vulnerability in the lives of both the parents and their children will help the therapist to contextualize the issues they face and formulate a biopsychosocial treatment that takes into consideration their life course.

Core Considerations for Therapy

Each family will be unique, and the perspective of each adult and child should be taken into consideration by the therapist as one listens to the family narrative, and the narrative of each member of the family. A clinical evaluation should incorporate a standard method of assessment, formulation, and treatment planning. Since lesbian-, gay-, and bisexual-parent families are constructed in a multitude of ways, a family history should take this complexity into consideration. A developmental history of the child should include a history of conception, and the history of the individual's and couple's decision-making process around having a child, or how a new family constellation was constructed that differed from the child's family of origin.

Understanding what the child knows about his or her conception and how the family defines relationships within the nuclear family and the extended family, as well as understanding the relationship with an egg donor, sperm donor, or a gestational carrier, is important. Understanding the role of other significant adults involved in the life of the child is essential. All of these issues should be further contextualized if the child was adopted. The therapist should stay mindful of the fact that the definition of these relationships may not begin to capture the real or fantasized meaning of these relationships both for the child and for the parent(s).

Over time the therapist should inquire about how the child thinks about these varying relationships as well as the meaning of each of them to the child (Corbett, 2001). Whether the child is adopted or born with known or unknown donors into a lesbian-, gay-, or bisexual-parent family, the child's fantasies and yearnings about these people with whom they have biological ties may evolve and impact their relationships with those closest to them. It is not a reflection of the love the children have for the parents who are raising them, or their loyalty and devotion to them, but is rather a desire to know more about the people with whom they have biological ties. This desire will be different for every child and every family, but the clinician's awareness of this dynamic is important.

If transparency and the permission to talk about their biological origins does not exist between children and their parents, children may suppress their curiosity and desire to know more about these people. Foreclosing on the possibility of exploring this part of their heritage may impact both the child and the parents. In his description of a clinical case where this issue was relevant, Ken Corbett (2001) wrote:

> As opposed to their (parents') fears that their (child's) fantasies would prove over stimulating or separate them as a family, they were able to entertain the opposite—the possibility of minds opening onto and into their collective fantasies in such as a way as to bring them together in a family. (p. 610)

Helping the child speak to questions and feelings that emerge at different developmental stages about their biological origins can help the child to traverse normal developmental challenges without closing off access to real or imagined relationships. The ability of the family to openly discuss these complicated relationships may be helpful in the child's process of identity development (Ehrensaft, 2008).

Creating a therapeutic space which is safe for both the parent(s) and the child(ren) to share their individual narrative and the narrative of the family is essential. Each voice is important to understand how an individual's experience may be similar to and different from that of the other. The historical experiences of the parents, as well as the current experiences of the parents and the children in the community in which they live, should be considered during the evaluation and during the course of the treatment. The impact of internalized homophobia, stigma, shame, and heterosexism and microaggressions before, during, and after their "coming out" as lesbian, gay, or bisexual individuals may have implications for their parenting style.

The children's experiences of microaggressions, and overt and subtle experiences of homophobia and stigmatization at each developmental stage, may have implications for their ability to negotiate relationships inside the family with relationships outside of the family. The therapist should inquire about experiences of stigmatization and heterosexism and offer support and psychoeducation. The therapist can help to separate out the parent's feelings and experiences from that of the child, and model for the parents how to discuss difficult issues with their children in a developmentally appropriate manner.

If the parents are able to manage their anxiety around heterosexism and stigma, the children are likely to feel more secure. They will be more likely to sense that the parents are willing and able to discuss experiences they are having both in the home and outside the home. By extension, if parents have difficulty with managing this anxiety, it may result in the children being more fearful and feeling that it is not permissible to discuss their worries with their parents or with others.

Young children may pick up on parents' feelings of anxiety but not have a context or the developmental capacity to understand the complex societal issues contributing to such anxiety (Telingator & Patterson, 2008). They may internalize the anxiety as being a communication of something negative about themselves, and as they get older it may result in feelings of shame and stigma similar to their parents and may impact the child's self-esteem (Fisher, Wallace, & Fenton, 2000). A child or adolescent's capacity and ability to discuss their experiences with others may be an important variable in maintaining self-esteem when dealing with some of these issues. Gershon, Tschann, and Jemerin (1999) found that adolescents with lesbian mothers who used social supports to help them to deal with homophobic stigmatization scored higher on self-esteem than adolescents who did not use such strategies. In this study, adolescents who practiced more disclosure about the sexual orientation of their parents even with high levels of perceived stigma had higher self-esteem about their ability to form close friendships.

Although parents may feel that discussing issues of homophobia and heterosexism that the child may face may not be in the child's best interest, the opposite may be true. Corbett (2001) wrote about the treatment of the son of a lesbian couple:

> We (therapist and parents) worked toward the understanding that, while we wish to protect our children from pain, anxiety, and hate, we are in fact helpless to stop those feelings from entering into

our child's lives, and furthermore a life without pain and loss would be an impossibly distorted one. (p. 607)

The lesbian, gay, or bisexual parents may have experienced "hate" directed toward them or their community during the course of their lives. They may now need to help their children to live in a world where they may experience hate directed toward their parents, and may themselves experience discrimination.

It is important to gain an understanding of the community in which the family resides and appreciate the stressors the family faces. The therapist should identify individual relationships and places where the family members can talk freely about their lives and their family, and in what environments they feel that they must maintain secrecy due to fears for themselves and their family (Telingator & Patterson, 2008). An appreciation of how and where each member of the family has found support and experienced stigma is essential.

In the case of Melissa, she was born into a family with privilege, who were able to choose the school and community in which she was raised. Melissa was both comfortable with her parents' sexuality and was living in a community in which it was safe to be an adolescent with lesbian parents. Although it was a difficult process for Melissa to sort out her own sexuality from that of her parents, she was able to use her therapy to work through what she thought and felt were both parental and societal expectations of her sexuality, and to identify what her own attractions were to begin to explore this aspect of her identity.

Further, although Melissa's parents experienced anxiety about her well-being, they were living as "out" lesbians, and Robert and Zack were "out" to family, friends, at work, and in their community. They had support in the school, and were friends with other lesbian and gay families and in the community. Although the vignette did not highlight issues they had confronted in their own coming out processes, each of them had access to supportive communities, friends, and families to varying degrees from the time they were children. Each of them was able to access therapy to help with emotional distress which was interfering with functioning at different points in each of their lives. Although they had not been able to address the anxiety and conflicts that had resulted in Melissa and her family to seek therapy, they were able to use the individual and family treatments to get back on track developmentally both as individuals and as a family. The level of family, school, and community support in this case was unusual. It is important for the clinician to stay mindful of the individual circumstances of each family they encounter, and to formulate a treatment plan that incorporates both their immediate and long term needs. Assessing the both the children's and the parent's safety in their community, and in work and school settings is essential.

The life of every family is embedded in a sociocultural framework that informs both the developmental life cycle of the parents, and the child. The societal constructs of what is "normal" and what is "not normal" are dictated by the majority. As our culture evolves and the impact of this evolution influences societal norms, we as a society will need to continue to learn how to incorporate people who are diverse in their gender expression and sexual orientation. This change over time is likely to have a positive impact on those who are part of a minority group, as well as the family members who may or may not be a part of that minority group. In the meantime, the freedom to discuss the impact of homophobia, stigma, and shame within one's family may help to improve their communication, strengthen family bonds, and ultimately strengthen the resilience of the child and the family. For the families who run into developmental challenges, therapists can ideally create a safe space in which to freely discuss these complex matters.

References

Balsam, K. F., Molina, Y., Beadnell, B., Simoni, J., & Walters, K. (2011). Measuring multiple minority stress: The LGBT people of color microaggressions scale. *Cultural Diversity & Ethnic Minority Psychology, 17*, 163–174. doi:10.1037/a0023244

Bos, H. M., & Gartrell, N. K. (2010). Adolescents of the USA National Longitudinal Lesbian Family Study: Can family characteristics counteract the negative effects of stigmatization? *Family Process, 49,* 559–572. doi:10.1111/j.1545-5300.2010.01340.x

Bos, H. K., Gartrell, N. M., Peyser, H., & van Balen, F. (2008). The USA National Longitudinal Lesbian Family Study (NLLFS): Homophobia, psychological adjustment, and protective factors. *Journal of Lesbian Studies, 12,* 455–471. doi:10.1080/10894160802278630

Bos, H. M., & van Balen, F. (2008). Children in planned lesbian families: Stigmatization, psychological adjustment and protective factors. *Culture, Health & Sexuality, 10,* 221–236. doi:10.1080/13691050701601702

Bos, H. M., van Balen, F., van den Boom, D., & Sandfort, T. G. (2004). Minority stress, experience of parenthood and child adjustment on lesbian families. *Journal of Reproductive and Infant Psychology, 22,* 291–304. doi:10.1080/02646830412331298350

Corbett, K. (2001). Nontraditional family romance. *The Psychoanalytic Quarterly, 70,* 599–624.

Cox, N., Dewaele, A., van Houtte, M., & Vincke, J. (2011). Stress-related growth, coming out, and internalized homonegativity in lesbian, gay, and bisexual youth. An examination of stress-related growth within the minority stress model. *Journal of Homosexuality, 58,* 117–137. doi:10.1080/00918369.2011.533631

Ehrensaft, D. (2008). When baby makes three or four or more: Attachment, individuation, and identity in assisted-conception families. *The Psychoanalytic Study of the Child, 63,* 3–23.

Engel, G. L. (1977). The need for a new medical model: A challenge for biomedicine. *Science, 196,* 129–136. doi:10.1126/science.847460

Fava, G., & Sonino, N. (2008). The biopsychosocial model thirty years later. *Psychotherapy and Psychosomatics, 77,* 1–2. doi:10.1159/000110052

Fisher, C. B., Wallace, S. A., & Fenton, R. A. (2000). Discrimination distress during adolescence. *Journal of Youth and Adolescence, 29,* 679–695. doi:10.1023/A:1026455906512

Frosch, C. A., & Mangelsdorf, S. C. (2001). Marital behavior, parenting behavior, and multiple reports of preschoolers' behavior problems: Mediation or moderation? *Developmental Psychology, 37,* 502–519. doi:10.1037/0012-1649.37.4.502

Gartrell, N. K., Deck, A., Rodas, C., Peyser, H., & Banks, A. (2005). The National Lesbian Family Study: 4. Interviews with the 10-year-old children. *American Journal of Orthopsychiatry, 75,* 518–524. doi:10.1037/0002-9432.75.4.518

Gershon, T. D., Tschann, J. M., & Jemerin, J. M. (1999). Stigmatization, self-esteem, and coping among the adolescent children of lesbian mothers. *Journal of Adolescent Health, 24,* 437–445. doi:10.1016/S1054-139X(98)00154-2

Goffman, E. (1963). *Stigma: Notes on the management of spoiled identity*. New York, NY: Simon & Schuster.

Goldberg, A. E. (2007). (How) does it make a difference? Perspectives of adults with lesbian, gay, and bisexual parents. *American Journal of Orthopsychiatry, 77,* 550–562. doi:10.1037/0002-9432.77.4.550

Goldberg, A. E. (2010). *Lesbian and gay parents and their children: Research on the family life cycle*. Washington, DC: American Psychological Association.

Goldberg, A. E., Kinkler, L. A., Richardson, H. B., & Downing, J. B. (2012). On the border: Young adults with LGBQ parents navigate LGBTQ communities. *Journal of Counseling Psychology, 59*, 71–85. doi:10.1037/a0024576

Golombok, S. (2000). *Parenting: What really counts?* London, UK: Routledge.

Halfon, N., & Hochstein, M. (2002). Life course health development: An integrated framework for developing health, policy, and research. *The Milbank Quarterly, 80*, 433–479.

Johnson, M. K., Crosnoe, R., & Elder, G. H., Jr. (2011). Insights on adolescence from a life course perspective. *Journal of Research on Adolescence, 21*, 273–280. doi:10.1111/j.1532-7795.2010.00728.x

Kaufman, G., & Raphael, L. (1996). *Coming out of shame: Transforming gay and lesbian lives*. New York, NY: Doubleday.

McEwen, B. S. (1998). Protective and damaging effects of stress mediators. *New England Journal of Medicine, 338*, 171–179.

Meyer, I. H. (1995). Minority stress and mental health in gay men. *Journal of Health and Social Behavior, 36*, 38–56. doi:10.2307/2137286

Meyer, I. H. (2003). Prejudice, social stress, and mental health in lesbian, gay, and bisexual populations: Conceptual issues and research evidence. *Psychological Bulletin, 129*, 674–697. doi:10.1037/0033-2909.129.5.674

Mitchell, V. (1998). The birds, the bees … and the sperm banks: How lesbian mothers talk with their children about sex and reproduction. *American Journal of Orthopsychiatry, 68*, 400–409. doi:10.1037/h0080349

Perlesz, A., Brown, R., Lindsay, J., McNair, R., deVaus, D., & Pitts, M. (2006). Family in transition: Parents, children and grandparents in lesbian families give meaning to 'doing family'. *Journal of Family Therapy, 28*, 175–199. doi:10.1111/j.1467-6427.2006.00345.x

Ray, V., & Gregory, R. (2001). School experiences of the children of lesbian and gay parents. *Family Matters, 59*, 28–34.

Ryff, C., & Singer, B. (1996). Psychological well-being: Meaning, measurement, and implications for psychotherapy research. *Psychotherapy and Psychosomatics, 65*, 14–23. doi:10.1159/000289026

Savin-Williams, R. C. (2008). Then and now: Recruitment, definition, diversity, and positive attributes of same-sex populations. *Developmental Psychology, 44*, 135–138. doi:10.1037/0012-1649.44.1.135

Stein, M., Perrin, E., & Potter, J. (2002). A difficult adjustment to school: The importance of family constellation. *Journal of Developmental and Behavioral Pediatrics, 23*, 171–174.

Sue, D. W., Capodilupo, C. M., Torino, G. C., Bucceri, J. M., Holder, A. M., Nadal, K. L., & Esquilin, M. (2007). Racial microaggressions in everyday life: Implications for clinical practice. *American Psychologist, 62*, 271–286. doi:10.1037/0003-066X.62.4.271

Tasker, F. L., & Golombok, S. (1997). *Growing up in a lesbian family: Effects on child development*. London, UK: Guilford Press.

Telingator, C. J., & Patterson, C. J. (2008). Children and adolescents of lesbian and gay parents. *Journal of the American Academy of Child and Adolescent Psychiatry, 47*, 1364–1368. doi:10.1097/CHI.0b013e31818960bc

Udell, W., Sandfort, T., Reitz, E., Bos, H. M., & Dekovic, M. (2010). The relationship between early sexual debut and psychosocial outcomes: A longitudinal study of Dutch adolescents. *Archives of Sexual Behavior, 39*, 1133–1145. doi:10.1007/s10508-009-9590-7

Schools and LGBT-Parent Families: Creating Change Through Programming and Advocacy

18

Eliza Byard, Joseph Kosciw, and Mark Bartkiewicz

Over the past three decades, a growing number of lesbian, gay, bisexual, and transgender (LGBT) parents have joined school communities nationwide as their children reached school age. In the 1990s, a new wave of children with LGBT parents began elementary school, their parents among the first to have chosen to have children in the context of a same-sex relationship (Goldberg, 2010). As documented in the films of pioneering lesbian filmmaker Debra Chasnoff, the lesbian moms depicted in the 1984 film, *Choosing Children,* began to interact with and interrogate the practices of the schools profiled in the 1996 film, *It's Elementary: Talking About Gay Issues in Schools.* Meanwhile, a continuing "gayby boom" in the 1990s led to sharply increased visibility of LGBT parents in schools from 2000 on (Goldberg, 2010).

Current estimates suggest that there are between two and nine million children being raised by LGBT parents in the USA, and it is likely that these numbers have been increasing in recent years (Cahill, Ellen, & Tobias 2003; Gates, 2011; Movement Advancement Project, Family Equality Council, & Center for American Progress, 2011). Today, the experiences of the children of LGBT parents pose a growing challenge for schools and families and represent an emerging issue for advocates working on ending discrimination and violence directed at LGBT people in K-12 education. For the past two decades, the "Safe Schools movement" in the USA has focused on improving the school experiences of LGBT youth and mitigating the impact of homophobia and transphobia on school climate and youth development overall. The growing number of school-age children with LGBT parents requires educators and advocates to examine the ways anti-LGBT bias and behavior play out in schools from a new angle.

Despite the growing urgency of these issues, little is known about the school-related experiences of LGBT parents and their children. Much of the existing research on LGBT-parent families has focused on comparing children of LGBT parents with those raised by heterosexual parents in terms of their psychological well-being, gender identity and gender role behavior, and sexual orientation, in order to determine whether the children of straight parents are "better off" (Biblarz & Savci, 2010; Goldberg, 2010). These studies have paid little attention to the social context of family life, such as school experience, or to family processes, such as family communication, that might account for any differences among children across family types (Stacey & Biblarz, 2001). These studies have also largely included only gay or lesbian parents and have not been inclusive of parents who identify as bisexual or transgender. Although some prior research has

E. Byard, Ph.D. (✉) • J. Kosciw, Ph.D.
• M. Bartkiewicz, Ph.D.
GLSEN (the Gay, Lesbian and Straight Education Network), 90 Broad Street, 2nd Floor,
New York, NY 10004, USA
e-mail: ebyard@glsen.org; jkosciw@glsen.org;
mbartkiewicz@glsen.org

A.E. Goldberg and K.R. Allen (eds.), *LGBT-Parent Families: Innovations in Research and Implications for Practice*, DOI 10.1007/978-1-4614-4556-2_18, © Springer Science+Business Media New York 2013

examined whether children with same-sex parents are different from other children with respect to school-related outcomes, there is limited research that explores the family–school relationship, school climate, and other school-related experiences for LGBT parents as well as their children. This chapter summarizes research findings on the school-related experiences of LGBT parent-headed families and presents the key challenges faced by LGBT parents with respect to their children's schools. We examine resources and programming for K-12 schools specific to LGBT parent-headed families, address advocacy issues pertaining to crucial resources and supports related to K-12 education, and delineate specific steps that key stakeholders can take to improve school climate for LGBT-parent families, both students and parents. A list of resources for parents, educators, and students is provided at the end of the chapter.

Prevalent Anti-LGBT Bias and Behavior in Schools and Its Impact on Parents and Students

Ensuring that one's child gets the best possible education can be daunting enough for any parent. LGBT parents and their children face an added layer of difficulty and challenge in this regard. LGBT parent-headed families that join school communities enter environments that are largely hostile to LGBT people and with respect to LGBT issues. In the past decade, a growing body of literature focused on the school experiences of LGBT students has revealed a bleak picture— K-12 schools across the USA are hostile environments for LGBT students and with regard to LGBT issues in general. For example, middle and high school students report that sexual orientation and gender expression are among the top three reasons students in their schools are bullied or harassed (GLSEN & Harris Interactive, 2005). Further, there is strong evidence that LGBT students are more likely to be bullied and harassed than other students (Centers for Disease Control and Prevention, 2011; GLSEN & Harris Interactive, 2005). More than 90% of LGBT students report hearing anti-LGBT language "frequently or often" in their schools (Kosciw, Greytak, Diaz, & Bartkiewicz, 2010). Harassment and victimization based on sexual orientation or gender identity/expression are commonplace in schools and can hinder access to quality education and diminish educational aspirations (Kosciw et al., 2010).

This scenario is hardly welcoming for LGBT parents and their children. Children must negotiate hallways where LGBT people like their parents are denigrated, and parents themselves may face discrimination or harassment in relation to their sexual orientation or gender identity, difficulties which non-LGBT parents do not encounter. Studies suggest that the moment when the children of LGBT parents enter school for the first time is a critical moment of reckoning for the family. For example, Casper, Schultz, and Wickens (1992) conducted qualitative interviews with 17 gay and lesbian parents with children in daycare through fifth grade. They found that when children of gay or lesbian parents entered school for the first time, they became cognizant of how their family configuration countered the norm. Further, these children had to contend with the fact that their family constellation was either not represented at school or represented as deviant. For their part, parents are painfully aware of the homophobia in their communities and schools and may therefore take steps to address these issues with their children in advance in an effort to prepare them for the experience. In a qualitative study of lesbian mothers of children aged 7–16, Litovich and Langhout (2004) found that most mothers spoke with their children about the possibility of experiencing homophobia because of their family's constellation.

Existing studies detail the extent to which anti-LGBT bias and behavior in schools affects LGBT-headed families, an impact visible to other members of the school community. Findings from a national study of 1,580 K-12 public school principals found that three-quarters of secondary school principals and four in ten elementary school principals reported that students at their school have been harassed because they have an LGBT parent or family member (GLSEN &

Harris Interactive, 2008). In fact, this same study found that only about half of secondary school principals and 60% of elementary school principals reported that a student with an LGBT parent would feel very safe at their school. Further, many of the principals surveyed in this study believed that a gay or lesbian parent might feel uncomfortable attending a school function—with one in six principals reporting that a lesbian or gay parent would feel less than comfortable participating in the following activities at their school: joining the PTA or PTO (15%), helping out in the classroom (15%), or chaperoning a field trip (16%). Similarly, Russell, McGuire, Lee, Larriva, and Laub (2008) found that LGBT students in 6th through 12th grade were likely to report that their school environments were less safe for students with LGBT parents than for other students.

Involved, Invisible, Ignored (Kosciw & Diaz, 2008), a report by the Gay, Lesbian and Straight Education Network (GLSEN) in partnership with two national LGBT family organizations (Children of Lesbians and Gays Everywhere (COLAGE)) and the Family Equality Council (FEC), reported on the school experiences of LGBT parents of children in K-12 schools and students who have LGBT parents. This study (which we will subsequently refer to as the GLSEN family study) captured the experience of 588 parents and 154 youth between the ages of 13 and 20. The study's sample was more likely to be White than the general population of LGBT parents. Compared to the 59% of the same-sex parents who identified as White in the 2000 US Census data (Dang & Frazer, 2005), 88% of the same-sex parents in the GLSEN sample identified as White. Among the students, 64% of the GLSEN family study sample was White versus 55% in the estimates derived from census data (Dang & Frazer, 2005). The vast majority of the students (81%) and parents (78%) in the GLSEN family study were enrolled or had a child enrolled in a public school, with about 15% of public school parents and 41% of public school students reporting that they or their child attended a charter or magnet school. Respondents lived in all areas of the country, though predominantly in the Northeast and West, and in urban, suburban, and rural or small town communities.

A number of parents in the study reported that they did not feel acknowledged or accepted by school personnel. Many parents described the ways in which they were made to feel excluded, like one mother who said that "The teacher's assistant most always ignores my partner or is short with her, especially if she picks up my daughter without me." Almost a fifth of parents in the GLSEN family study reported that they felt that school personnel failed to acknowledge their type of family (15%) or felt that they could not fully participate in their child's school community because they were an LGBT parent (16%). Respondents described various forms of exclusion—both overt and covert—including being excluded or prevented from fully participating in school activities and events, being excluded by school policies and procedures, and being ignored and feeling invisible. Parents described situations in which they, their partner or significant other, and/or their child were not able to participate in school activities because they were an LGBT parent, such as when their child was not allowed to make two Mother's Day gifts for the child's two mothers or when they were not permitted to display a family collage on the wall with the other students' work because it showed two lesbian mothers.

These slights, whether intentional or out of ignorance, are detrimental to the family–school relationship. For some LGBT parents, the relationship may be further damaged by overt forms of mistreatment by other members of the school community, such as other parents and their children's peers. In a longitudinal study of lesbian mother-headed families (150 mothers of 85 children), Gartrell et al. (2000) found that 18% of these mothers reported that their school-age children had had homophobic interactions with peers or teachers. Morris, Balsam, and Rothblum (2002) found in a large sample of lesbian mothers that 16% of their sample reported that they had experienced harassment, threats, or discrimination at their children's school or by other parents. In research by Kosciw (2003), 16% of the parents surveyed reported having been mistreated or received negative reactions by their child's teacher or daycare provider. Finally, in the GLSEN family study (Kosciw & Diaz, 2008), parents reported a relatively low incidence of negative experiences from school personnel. This finding is due perhaps in part to the fact that these parents may have chosen the school specifically because it was thought to be a positive, affirming environment, or because of the work the parents have done in proactively talking with school personnel about their families. LGBT parents were more likely to report that they had been mistreated by other members of the school community. Namely, 26% of parents in GLSEN's family study reported mistreatment by other parents, and 20% reported hearing negative comments about being LGBT from other students at their child's school. Parents described events in which they were subjected to hostile behaviors from school staff and other parents, had to deal with general discomfort and ignorance, or had their parenting skills called into question because they were LGBT.

The experiences of the children in the GLSEN family study provide additional texture to this picture of a hostile school climate (Kosciw & Diaz, 2008). The most commonly reported reason that these students feel unsafe in school was because of their family constellation—that is, having LGBT parents (23%)—or because of their actual or perceived sexual orientation (21%). Among students with LGBT parents, 40% reported being verbally harassed in school because of their family. Although the vast majority of students in the study identified as heterosexual, 38% reported being verbally harassed in school because of their actual or perceived sexual orientation. As with the parents, students' mistreatment did not always come from other students, but also from adult members of the school community. Nearly a quarter of students had been mistreated by or received negative comments from the parents of other students specifically because they had an LGBT parent (25% for both). A small percentage of students reported being directly mistreated by or receiving negative comments from a teacher because of their family (11% and 15%, respectively), also mirroring the parents' experience.

Other research further highlights the in-school victimization that children of LGBT parents face. In a qualitative study of 46 adult children of LGB parents, Goldberg (2007) found that some of these adult children of LGB parents recalled experiencing bullying during their youth related to their family constellation. Further, Tasker and Golombok (1997) interviewed young adults with lesbian mothers and found that 36% of the participants reported that they had been teased by peers sometime during their school years because of their mother's sexual orientation, and 44% reported that they had been teased during their school years about their own sexual orientation or "inappropriate" gender role behavior.

Such negative school experiences have consequences for both LGBT parents and their children. Among parents, feeling excluded from the school community reduces their sense of connection to the school and makes them less likely to take part in school life. In the GLSEN family study, LGBT parents who felt excluded from the school community were less likely than other LGBT parents to have been involved in a parent–teacher organization (44% vs. 63%), to volunteer at school (47% vs. 72%), and to belong to other community groups (e.g., neighborhood associations) with parents from their child's school (25% vs. 40%) (Kosciw & Diaz, 2008). Because parent engagement can both enhance a student's learning and improve family–school communication regarding any negative experiences a student may have, this reduced parental involvement with school life could have significant consequences for student achievement and well-being.

For the children of LGBT parents, bullying and harassment may affect their in-school relationships and their ability to learn and be part of the school community. Compared to a national sample of secondary school students, students with LGBT parents in the GLSEN family study were more than twice as likely to have skipped a class in the past year because of feeling unsafe (15% vs. 6%) and to have missed at least one entire day of school also because of feeling unsafe (17% vs. 5%) (Kosciw & Diaz, 2008). Other research further suggests that this hostile school climate has a concrete negative impact on the well-being of children of LGBT parents. For example, in a study of 100 planned lesbian families in the Netherlands, Bos, van Balen, van den Boom, and Sandfort (2004) found that lesbian mothers who experienced greater rejection in their community were more likely to report behavioral problems in their children.

Proactive Strategies for Parents and Schools

Despite the daunting reality of school life for LGBT parents and their children, there are signs of hope, including indications that in-school resources and supports may act as a buffer against a hostile school climate. For example, in Russell et al.'s (2008) study of student experience in California, students who had access to LGBT resources and supports were more likely to report that their school environments were safer for students with LGBT parents. There are steps that both parents and schools can take to improve school climate and educational opportunity for these students, and research indicates that LGBT parents are alert to these measures, engaging with schools in order to pave the way for a positive school experience.

Parental Strategies: School Choice, Engagement, and Advocacy

One of the most common strategies among LGBT parents for dealing with the challenges of school climate is exercising whatever forms of school choice may be available to them. Parents in the USA have the option of sending their children to public (zoned, charter, or magnet) schools, or to private (nonreligious or religious-affiliated) schools, though these choices can be seriously limited by issues of proximity, access, and ability to pay. Parental decision-making regarding school selection may be based on any number of factors, including practicality (finding the closest school to their home), the academic approach of the school (e.g., the Montessori method), or a school's

academic reputation. Research demonstrates that in addition to these considerations, LGBT parents often weigh a number of other factors when making a decision about school enrollment and seem to be more likely to choose an alternative to their neighborhood public school than their straight peers, when such choice is accessible to them. The GLSEN family study found that although the majority of LGBT parents sent their child to a public school, the percentage was significantly lower than available statistics on the general population of parents (78% vs. 89%) (Kosciw & Diaz, 2008). As noted above, a significant percentage of both parents and students in the study indicated that they attended a charter or magnet public school, a form of school choice that may require significant advocacy and some means of travel to and from school each day, but not necessarily additional financial resources.

Parents' options regarding school enrollment are heavily dependent on what choices are available in their communities, on how actively they can advocate for their child within a public school system, or on their ability to pay private school tuition or access financial aid. What we know about the demography of LGBT parent-headed families indicates that these constraints may pose a very significant challenge for the LGBT-parent population as a whole. Children of same-sex couples are twice as likely to live in poverty than the children of married heterosexual couples, and their parents are more racially and ethnically diverse than the married heterosexual parent population (Albelda, Badgett, Schneebaum, & Gates, 2009; Dang & Frazer, 2005). A study of data from the 2000 US Census found that 96% of US counties housed at least one same-sex couple raising children, with the highest concentrations found in New York City, Los Angeles, and the San Francisco Bay Area, but other families were found in less hospitable areas like Mississippi, Wyoming, Alaska, Arkansas, Texas, Louisiana, and Oklahoma (Sears, Gates, & Rubenstein, 2005). It is critical that school systems everywhere take steps to improve school climate; indeed, the burdens of advocacy (sometimes difficult because of community climate) or choice (which is not always an option) should not be left on the shoulders of LGBT parents.

When in a position to choose what school their child will attend, many LGBT parents consider the diversity of the school and the reputation of the school regarding diversity. When asked about their decision-making, parents in the GLSEN family study most commonly reported that they chose to send their children to the local or neighborhood school (54%) or a school with a strong academic reputation (54%). Yet nearly one-third of parents (31%) also reported that they considered the diversity of the school population (Kosciw & Diaz, 2008). Notably, the GLSEN family study also found that LGBT parents who chose a private, nonreligious school were more focused on the diversity of the school population than other LGBT parents in the study. Nearly half (46%) of the LGBT private school parents in this study reported that the school's reputation for being welcoming of LGBT-parent families was a key consideration in their school decision-making, and this percentage was much higher than the parents of children in religious private schools and the parents of children in public schools (15% and 11%, respectively). In addition, a sizeable percentage of parents reported seeking out schools that have experience with diverse family forms—about a quarter of public school parents and private religious school parents (29% and 23%, respectively) and nearly half of private school parents (45%). Even among parents whose child attended their local public school, about a quarter reported that they chose their school, in part, because of reasons related to diversity. This finding suggests that LGBT parents may not only seek out what schools would be most accepting but also seek to live in communities that would be more tolerant of families like their own. This research is corroborated by a qualitative study of lesbian mothers conducted by Mercier and Harold (2003), which found that in order to minimize any potential for problems, parents often selected their child's school because it was known for its openness and multiculturalism.

For LGBT parents of elementary-aged children, school demographics are particularly important for their decision-making process. In the GLSEN family study, elementary school parents were more likely than middle school or high

school parents to base their school selection on knowing that the school included other LGBT-parent families, had a reputation for a diverse population, and had a reputation for welcoming LGBT-parent families. Concerns about school diversity may be even greater among LGBT multiracial families and families of color. Likewise, in the GLSEN family study, families with a student of color were more likely to choose a school based on its diverse population than families with a White student regardless of the race/ethnicity of the parent or parents (43% vs. 25%). Of course, as noted above, parents who do not have the means to pay tuition may not have any choices to make, if they live in a district with only one zoned school available. Similarly, parents who base their school selection on the family's religion or who wish their child to receive religious instruction in school may also have fewer options available to them.

As they consider school choices and in preparation for initial enrollment, LGBT parents often approach schools proactively to discuss their family constellation in an effort to lay the foundation for a more positive school experience. In the GLSEN family study, private school parents were most likely to have approached the school ahead of time, but it was not uncommon for public and religious school parents to do so (Kosciw & Diaz, 2008). Overall, about half of all parents (45%) said that they had specifically sought out information from the schools pertaining to how they would be with LGBT issues before enrolling their child. Of these parents, the vast majority (78%) reported that the information gained was very important in making a decision to enroll their child.

Once a child is enrolled in school, LGBT parents are very likely to reach out to the school to try to set the stage for a good school year. This outreach is an effort these parents may well need to make again and again, as their child has new teachers, for example. In the GLSEN family study, about half of the parents (48%) reported that they had gone to the school at the start of the school year to talk about their family (Kosciw & Diaz, 2008). About two-thirds of parents reported that they had spoken with teachers at their child's school about being an LGBT parent and 45% had such discussions with the principal during the school year.

There is also evidence that LGBT parents may be more likely than heterosexual parents to remain actively engaged with their child's school through volunteering and other forms of parental involvement. Nearly all parents (94%) in the GLSEN family study reported that they had attended a parent–teacher conference or Back-to-School night, and two-thirds had volunteered at the school (Kosciw & Diaz, 2008). About half of the parents reported that they belonged to the school's parent–teacher organization (e.g., PTA or PTO) and an even higher percentage reported that they had taken part in activities of this organization in the past year (regardless of belonging to the organization). These rates of school participation are higher than the general population of K-12 parents—for example, LGBT parents were significantly more likely than a national sample of parents to be members of the school's parent–teacher organization (41% vs. 26%). There may be a number of reasons for this heightened engagement with a school: LGBT parents may be particularly concerned about averting potential problems for their children or getting engaged with the school after negative incidents, as well as simply trying to support their child's educational experience.

Organizations serving LGBT parents, their children, and the schools they attend have produced resources to assist parents in assessing a school's climate with respect to LGBT-parent families and LGBT issues in general. These resources can help parents select among schools or identify areas for improvement in the school in which a child is enrolled. Some also help parents figure out how best to approach a school about their family and think about the ways to be engaged in their children's education. GLSEN's *Is This the Right School For Us?* is designed to help parents with children in kindergarten through sixth grade judge whether or not a school will be a good place for their family (see resource list). For parents with children already in school, this resource also offers information about improving school climate, for example, addressing issues

such as inclusion of LGBT resources in a school library and staff training on LGBT issues. The FEC offers a resource called *Opening Doors: Lesbian, Gay, Bisexual and Transgender (LGBT) Parents and Schools*, which includes a wide array of information for LGBT parents and educators, supporting parents' proactive approach and encouraging ongoing dialogue between family and school (see resource list). For parents, the resource includes information about how to go about becoming involved in their children's education, such as suggesting being as open as possible about their family constellation. For educators, the booklet provides guidance as to how school staff can best support children of LGBT parents, such as working with school administrators to make school forms and other documents inclusive. *Opening Doors* also offers suggested questions and answers that parents and educators can ask one another in an effort to create a safe and respectful learning environment (see resource list). Also available from FEC is an abbreviated version of the resource, called *Back to School Tool: Building Family Equality in Every Classroom*, and a "Rainbow Report Card," which is an online-based, interactive tool that has LGBT parents answer questions about their children's school and then generates a report for them with custom recommendations (see resource list).

School-Based Interventions that Improve LGBT-Parent Families' Experiences

There are a number of in-school programs, approaches, and interventions that have a positive impact on LGBT-headed families' experiences, mitigating the homophobia and transphobia that can create barriers to full inclusion and a great educational experience. These in-school changes are an important focus for parental—and general—advocacy, as they can have a beneficial effect on improving school climate for a wide range of students. Ultimately, improvements in school climate that reduce homophobia and transphobia can contribute to greater individual well-being, improved academic achievement, and greater educational attainment among the students most affected by these forms of bias and violence.

Anti-Bullying/Harassment Policies and Laws

Bullying and harassment based on sexual orientation and gender identity/expression are commonplace in America's secondary schools (Kosciw et al., 2010). One of the several ways that GLSEN has attempted to address this problem is through the passage of comprehensive anti-bullying/harassment laws and policies that prohibit bullying and harassment of all students, regardless of their sexual orientation or gender identity/expression. Laws and policies that enumerate categories of protections, such as sexual orientation and gender identity/expression, may provide students with greater protection against bullying and harassment in that they offer explicit protections. These laws and policies often have associational language that follows an enumerated list (e.g., "any student or students associated with any individual with any of the listed characteristics"). Such language protects the child of an LGBT person. In the GLSEN family study, three-quarters of parents (75%) and students (73%) reported that their school had some type of policy for dealing with incidents of harassment and assault (Kosciw & Diaz, 2008). However, far fewer reported that the school's policy explicitly mentioned sexual orientation and/or gender identity/expression (42% of parents and 35% of students). Notably, students with LGBT parents whose school had an LGBT-inclusive anti-bullying/harassment school policy reported fewer negative experiences in school, particularly with regard to being mistreated by teachers and other students at school because of their family constellation. Parents who reported that their child's school had a comprehensive policy were more likely to report that addressing their child's harassment was an effective intervention (89%), compared to parents who said their child's school had a generic policy (72%) or no policy at all (62%). Parents themselves reported a lower frequency of mistreatment in school when the school had a comprehensive policy and were less likely

to feel unacknowledged as an LGBT-parent family. Thus, policies may act as a buffer against a hostile school climate for students of LGBT parents and also create a more welcoming school environment for parents themselves. When researching schools for their children, LGBT parents may want to pay particular attention to each prospective school's policy on bullying and harassment and determine if there are clear and effective systems in place for reporting and addressing incidents that students experience so that all students, including those with LGBT parents, feel safe at school.

A growing number of states across the country have added explicit protections for LGBT students in their state education antidiscrimination and harassment statutes, including, notably, states such as Arkansas and North Carolina. Such laws have primary importance for protecting students from bullying and harassment and may also afford protection to the children of LGBT parents with regard to harassment related to their actual or perceived sexual orientation and harassment related to their family constellation. As with school policies, these laws often include association language that would protect the child of an LGBT person. Recent research suggests that same-sex couples raising children in states with favorable LGBT laws have greater psychological well-being than parents who live in states with less favorable legal climates (Goldberg & Smith, 2011).

Currently, only 15 states plus the District of Columbia have comprehensive anti-bullying/harassment laws that include sexual orientation and/or gender identity/expression. The GLSEN family study found that—above and beyond the laws' impact on LGBT student experience—state-level comprehensive anti-bullying/harassment legislation was associated with better school climate for LGBT-parent families in a range of ways (Kosciw & Diaz, 2008). For example, students in these states were less likely than students in states with generic "anti-bullying" laws or no laws at all to hear certain types of biased language in school, such as homophobic remarks (73% vs. 92% and 95%, respectively). Parents from states with comprehensive legislation were least likely to report not feeling acknowledged by the school community as an LGBT-parent family and were most likely to report that the school was inclusive of LGBT-parent families (9% vs. 15% and 20%, respectively). There was no evidence that generic bullying-prevention legislation has any benefits for LGBT-headed families over having no legislation at all.

Although there may be many contributing factors that might result in differences across states by type of anti-bullying/harassment law, these findings nevertheless lend evidence to the claim that comprehensive laws that include sexual orientation and/or gender identity/expression may be more effective than generic laws or no law at all in creating safer schools for LGBT students and families. Comprehensive anti-bullying/harassment and antidiscrimination legislation at the state and federal level that specifically enumerates sexual orientation and gender identity/expression as protected categories alongside others such as race, faith, and age, and that includes association language that would encompass students with LGBT parents, is an important focus of advocacy in order to improve the experiences of LGBT-parent families in school and to create a safe learning environment for all students.

As part of our work to ensure safe schools for all students, GLSEN has worked with local, state, and national coalitions as well as elected officials to pass legislation and policies that are comprehensive (requires policy development, reporting mechanisms, and educator and student training) and enumerate the categories of students protected (including actual or perceived sexual orientation and gender identity). (Tools available from GLSEN on these issues are included in the Resource List at the end of this chapter.)

Supportive School Staff and Staff Training

For students, having a supportive adult at school can benefit their academic experience and may be particularly important for those who encounter negative reactions from other members of the school community because of their family. For LGBT parents, as for any parents, positive family–school communication is also beneficial for the child's educational attainment. In the GLSEN family study, the majority of LGBT parents

(67%) reported that there were at least a few supportive teachers or school staff at their child's school (Kosciw & Diaz, 2008). More than half (55%) of the students with LGBT parents in this study could identify many (six or more) supportive school staff people. For these students, the presence of supportive school staff was related to their academic achievement. For example, students with LGBT parents who could identify many supportive staff at their school reported a GPA half a grade higher than those students with LGBT parents who did not have any supportive school staff (3.4 vs. 2.9). Identification of a greater number of supportive educators was also related to fewer missed days of school due to safety concerns (Kosciw & Diaz, 2008).

Unfortunately, most school personnel do not receive professional development that encompasses LGBT-related issues and can lead to a more supportive school environment. In a study of public school principals, only 33 out of 1,010 principals whose schools provided professional development on bullying or harassment reported that it included specific content on students' sexual orientation (30%), the sexual orientation or gender identity/expression of students' family members (26%), or students' gender identity/expression (24%) (GLSEN & Harris Interactive, 2008). Perhaps not surprisingly, secondary school principals were more likely than elementary school principals to report that their school provides professional development inclusive of sexual orientation and or gender identity/expression content (29% of secondary school principals vs. 15% of elementary school principals; GLSEN & Harris Interactive, 2008). Elementary school principals were more likely than secondary school principals to report that their professional development on bullying/harassment was general and did not specify sexual orientation and/or gender identity/expression (42% vs. 29%; GLSEN & Harris Interactive, 2008).

Based on the GLSEN family study, we know that few LGBT parents (10%) reported being aware that school personnel had any training on LGBT issues (Kosciw & Diaz, 2008). Yet, parents who said their child's school had trainings on LGBT-related issues for school personnel were less likely than other parents to report that their child had been bullied or harassed in school, both in general (14% vs. 31%) and specifically related to their family (7% vs. 20%). In addition, parental reports of educator trainings were associated with a more positive response from school personnel when parents addressed their child's harassment. These parents were also less likely to report that they themselves had experienced mistreatment in school related to being LGBT.

Overall, trainings on LGBT issues directed at education professionals may be easier for a school to implement than some other LGBT-inclusion measures. Resistance is generally highest to programming, information, or training directed at students. School- or district-wide implementation of educator trainings on issues related to LGBT issues (including LGBT-parent families) and bias-based bullying and harassment may help to give teachers and administrators the tools they need to create an inclusive environment in which all students feel respected and a part of the school community. In addition, such trainings may help educators become more cognizant and sensitive of LGBT family issues and be more likely to include LGBT-inclusive curricular resources in their classrooms. Above and beyond the inclusive curricular resources, school personnel should work on ensuring that administrative items, such as field trip permission forms, are more inclusive (e.g., using the general and neutral "parent1" and "parent2" as opposed to "mother" and "father").

Inclusive Curricular Resources

An LGBT-inclusive curriculum provides positive representations of LGBT people, history, and events and helps to create a tone of acceptance of LGBT people and increased awareness of LGBT-related issues. An LGBT-inclusive curriculum should be age-appropriate and carried out differently in an elementary school as opposed to a secondary school. In an elementary school, a school library might include books that represent different types of families, including LGBT-parent families, while a history class in secondary school might include LGBT historical figures or a discussion of the beginnings of the contemporary Gay Liberation Movement in the late 1960s. As seen in the experiences of LGBT students, inclusive curricula help promote respect for all and can improve an individual LGBT student's school experiences and increase their sense of school connectedness (Kosciw et al., 2010). GLSEN's 2009 National School Climate Survey, a study of the school experiences of 7,261 LGBT students between the ages of 13 and 21, found that LGBT students in schools with an inclusive curriculum were less likely to report hearing homophobic remarks and experience less victimization at school based on their sexual orientation or gender expression (Kosciw et al., 2010). However, with regard to access to information about LGBT-parent families and other LGBT-related topics, less than a third of both students (27%) and parents (29%) in the GLSEN family study reported that the school curriculum included representations of LGBT people, history, or events in the past school year (Kosciw & Diaz, 2008). When asked specifically about the inclusion of representations of LGBT-parent families in classroom activities, less than a third (31%) of all students said that representations of LGBT-parent families were included when the topic of families came up during class activities (Kosciw & Diaz, 2008).

Curricular inclusion is in some ways the "next frontier" in LGBT issues in K-12 education, and the use of LGBT-inclusive curricular materials can be difficult in the absence of strong community support. However, to the extent that curriculum in the early grades focuses on family studies, the presence of LGBT-parent families in schools nationwide forces the issue in elementary school settings in a significant new way. For those teachers and schools in a position to include these materials, and for those families in a position to advocate for greater representation of LGBT people in class materials, there are resources available to assist schools in including positive representations of LGBT people, history, and events in their curriculum:

Include Diverse Families

Whenever possible, educators should include examples of diverse families, including same-sex couples and LGBT parents, while referencing families in the classroom. Providing students with these examples can help LGBT students and students with LGBT family members feel included in the classroom. For example, educators can be more inclusive in their language when addressing issues pertaining to families. Instead of always saying "mom and dad" when referring to parents, educators can be more inclusive by saying "parents."

Include LGBT History

Educators can raise the visibility of LGBT people and communities by providing students with concrete examples of LGBT people in history and LGBT-related historical events. For example, when teaching about the Holocaust or about civil rights movements, educators can include the persecution, struggles, and successes of the LGBT community. Educators can also show documentary films, such as *Out of the Past: The Struggle for Gay and Lesbian Rights in America* (1998) or *Gay Pioneers* (2003), that highlight different eras in the LGBT rights movement (see resource list). There are also lesson plans such as GLSEN's *When Did It Happen: LGBT History Lesson* (2001) to teach about important leaders and events in LGBT history, or *Unheard Voices* (2011), an LGBT oral history resource with lesson plans, created by GLSEN, the Anti-Defamation League, and StoryCorps.

Use LGBT-Inclusive Literature

Using LGBT-inclusive literature helps to create a welcoming space for students with LGBT parents, as well as promote respect and acceptance among all students. Several organizations provide resource lists of books that feature positive and diverse representations of LGBT characters that educators can use in the classroom, including GLSEN's BookLink, an online resource featuring LGBT-themed and LGBT-inclusive books organized by grade level, to find appropriate books for their curriculum (see resource list). For example, it offers information about resources such as *And Baby Makes four* (Benjamin & Freeman, 2009), a book about the experiences of a young child of a two-mom household whose

family is about to expand with the addition of a new baby.

Films such as *It's Elementary—Talking About Gay Issues in Schools* (referenced above) afford educators the opportunity to help young people address prejudice of all kinds and the techniques to help them do so. COLAGE, a national organization that serves individuals with a LGBTQ parent, offers a youth-produced documentary film by and about youth with LGBTQ parents called *In My Shoes: Stories of Youth with LGBTQ Parents*. Both films have accompanying discussion and action guides (see resource list).

Celebrate LGBT Events

Celebrating LGBT events can help LGBT students feel included in the school. Educators can promote LGBT events throughout the schools as educators would any other cultural celebration. Educators can celebrate LGBT History Month in October or LGBT Pride Month in June by displaying signs, alerting students, and recognizing the struggles, contributions, and victories of the LGBT community.

Supportive Student Clubs

Student clubs that provide support to LGBT students, such as Gay–Straight Alliances (GSAs), may also be a resource and source of support for secondary school youth for LGBT-parent families. Research has shown that GSAs can provide safe, affirming spaces and critical support for LGBT students and also contribute to creating a more welcoming school environment (GLSEN & Harris Interactive, 2005; Goodenow, Szalacha, & Westhimer, 2006; Kosciw et al., 2010; Szalacha, 2003). The presence of a GSA or similar supportive student club may be beneficial for LGBT-parent families. For example, these types of clubs may provide a safe space in which students with LGBT parents can talk openly about their experience, regardless of their own sexual orientation or gender identity. They may also contribute to creating a more welcoming school environment and provide children of LGBT parents a sense that their school community is supportive of LGBT people. However, no research has been conducted to examine potential benefits of GSAs for children of LGBT parents specifically. Only about a third (34%) of the students in the GLSEN family study reported that their school had a GSA or other kind of student club that provided support to LGBT students and their allies (Kosciw & Diaz, 2008). Compared to the general population of students, students with LGBT parents in the GLSEN family study were more likely to report that their school had a student club that addresses LGBT issues (34% vs. 22%).

GLSEN's *Jump-Start Guide* is a resource designed for students to help with new and already established Gay–Straight Alliances (GSAs) or similar clubs at schools (see resource list). The guide consists of eight self-contained sections and takes students through the process of establishing or reestablishing a supportive student club such as a GSA, identifying the club's mission and goals, and provides information on assessing school climate.

Conclusion

The growing numbers of children of LGBT parents enrolled in schools nationwide are forcing critical issues into the open in school communities. Even those schools that are interested in creating a more inclusive school community face challenges that are not completely under their control and that could require them to take a much more proactive stance on LGBT issues than they ever imagined. Findings from the GLSEN family study show that LGBT parents are more likely to report having problems with students in the school or parents of other students than they were to report having problems with school personnel. It is important for school personnel to understand that harassment by students of anyone in the school community, whether it be a student or a parent of a student, should not be tolerated. Schools should provide training for school staff to deal effectively with a student being bullied or harassed because they are or are perceived to be LGBT, or because they have an LGBT family member. Further, professional development for educators should include multicultural diversity training that includes information about LGBT-parent families.

Results from GLSEN's family study also highlight the important role that institutional supports can play in making schools safer for students of LGBT parents. Given that students with LGBT parents in this study were more than twice as likely to have skipped a class in the past year because of feeling unsafe as compared to a national sample, it is important to consider the steps that schools can take to improve school climate and improve youth's educational outcomes. Supportive student clubs, such as GSAs, that address LGBT issues in education may be beneficial for LGBT-parent families in that these types of clubs may provide a safe space in which students with LGBT parents can talk openly about their experience, regardless of their own sexual orientation or gender identity. Beyond supportive student clubs, schools should also increase access to age-appropriate and accurate information regarding LGBT people, history, and events. An LGBT-inclusive curriculum can help to create a tone of acceptance of LGBT people and increase awareness of LGBT-related issues.

In the GLSEN family study, students of LGBT parents whose school had a comprehensive safe school policy were less likely to report mistreatment because of having LGBT parents. Additionally, parents who reported that their child's school had a comprehensive policy reported a lower frequency of mistreatment in school when the school had a comprehensive policy. These findings highlight the need for schools to adopt and implement comprehensive anti-bullying/harassment policies with clear and effective systems for reporting and addressing incidents that students experience so that all students, including those with LGBT parents, feel safe at school. As with school-level policies, the GLSEN family study shows that state-level comprehensive safe school legislation was associated with better school climate for LGBT-parent families. Students in states with comprehensive legislation were less likely to hear homophobic remarks in their schools and LGBT parents in these states were more likely to feel included in the school community. This finding highlights the dire need to pass comprehensive anti-bullying/harassment and antidiscrimination legislation at the state and federal level that specifically enumerates sexual orientation and gender identity/expression as protected categories alongside others such as race, faith, and age in an effort to create safe learning environments for all students and their families. Taken together, the resources and supports outlined in this chapter can enhance the family–school relationship and create a school environment that is positive and respectful.

Resource List

Resources for Parents

Is This the Right School For Us?

GLSEN's *Is This the Right School For Us?* is a guide to assess school climates for LGBT parents of elementary-aged children (K-6). http://www.glsen.org/cgi-bin/iowa/all/news/record/1674.html.

Opening Doors: Lesbian, Gay, Bisexual, and Transgender (LGBT) Parents and Schools

The Family Equality Council's *Opening Doors* resource includes a wide array of information for both LGBT parents and educators. An abbreviated version is also available, called *Back to School Tool: Building Family Equality in Every Classroom.* http://www.familyequality.org/site/PageServer?pagename=resources_publications.

Rainbow Report Card

The Family Equality Council's Rainbow Report Card is an online-based, interactive tool that has LGBT parents answer questions about their children's school and then generates a report with custom recommendations. http://www.familyequality.org/site/PageServer?pagename=resources_publications.

Resources for Policy and Legislative Advocacy

GLSEN's Policy and Legislative Resources

These tools are designed to provide the kinds of information necessary to launch and sustain effective campaigns for safer schools laws and policies, and are available at http://www.glsen.org/policy.

Enumeration: A tool for advocates explains some of the major reasons why anti-bullying and anti-harassment laws and rules that use enumerated categories are better at protecting students, educators, and school systems.

Model District Anti-Bullying & Harassment Policy highlights key points regarding enumeration, complaint procedure, professional development, and student training.

Model State Anti-Bullying and Harassment Legislation explains the policy objectives for each section of the Model, and presents some key points and alternatives to consider. There is also commentary throughout that will help stakeholders tailor the model language to the specific needs of their state, while keeping the original intent of the legislation intact.

Model District Policy on Transgender and Gender Nonconforming Students contains a model policy with explanatory notes on the range of issues schools may face related to transgender and gender nonconforming students. This resource was created by GLSEN in partnership with the National Center for Transgender Equality (NCTE).

Resources for Educators

Lessons and Curricula

GLSEN's Education Department offers free curricula and lesson plans for educators to use with elementary, middle, and high school students. These resources provide a framework for facilitating classroom discussions and engaging students in creating safer schools for all, regardless of sexual orientation, gender identity, or gender expression: http://www.glsen.org/educator.

Ready, Set, Respect! GLSEN's Elementary School Toolkit

The GLSEN toolkit was developed in partnership with the National Association of Elementary School Principals and the National Association for the Education of Young Children (NAEYC).

Ready, Set, Respect! contains suggested lesson plans that focus on name-calling, bullying and bias, LGBT-inclusive family diversity, and gender roles and diversity. The templates are designed for teachers to use as either stand-alone lessons or for integration into existing curriculum content or school-wide anti-bullying programs. The toolkit also contains helpful tips for teaching more inclusively and intervening in bullying and promoting respectful recess playtime and physical education.

Safe Space Kit

GLSEN's *Safe Space Kit* is designed to help educators create a safe space for LGBT youth in school. This guide provides concrete strategies for supporting LGBT students, educating about anti-LGBT bias, and advocating for changes in your school. The Kit also shows how to assess the school's climate, policies, and practices and outlines ways to advocate for change inside the school.

No Name-Calling Week

No Name-Calling Week (NNCW) is an annual week of educational and creative activities focused on ending name-calling in K-12 schools. The NNCW site provides educators with LGBT-inclusive lesson plans and extensive bibliographies (divided by school level). http://www.nonamecallingweek.org.

BookLink

Organized by grade level, GLSEN's BookLink makes it easy to find LGBT-themed/inclusive books and videos to use in the classroom. http://www.glsen.org/booklink.

For example: Benjamin, J., & Freeman, J. (2009). *And baby makes four.* Motek Press.

Resources for Students

Jump-Start Guide for Gay–Straight Alliances

This guide consists of eight self-contained sections designed to help students bring fresh and creative energy to leading their student club. The resources take you through the process of establishing or reestablishing a Gay–Straight Alliance, identifying the student club's mission and goals, and assessing your school's climate. http://www.glsen.org/jumpstart.

Day of Silence

On the National Day of Silence hundreds of thousands of students nationwide take a vow of silence to bring attention to anti-LGBT name-calling, bullying, and harassment in their schools. http://www.dayofsilence.org/.

Additional Resources

General Books and Information

COLAGE Bookstore. http://www.colage.org/bookstore/.

Research

GLSEN's Research Department supports the organization's mission by conducting original research, evaluating GLSEN programs and initiatives, and creating resources that document anti-LGBT bias in education (K-12 schools). GLSEN Research reports include the following:

2009 National School Climate Survey: The Experiences of LGBT Youth in Our Nation's Schools

Playgrounds and Prejudice: Elementary School Climate in the United States, A Survey of Students and Teachers

Year One Evaluation of the New York City Department of Education Respect for All Training Program

From Teasing to Torment: School Climate in America, A Survey of Students and Teachers

Shared Differences: The Experiences of LGBT Students of Color in Our Nation's Schools

Harsh Realities: The Experiences of Transgender Youth in Our Nation's Schools

The Principal's Perspective: School Safety, Bullying and Harassment

Involved, Invisible, Ignored: The Experiences of Lesbian, Gay, Bisexual and Transgender Parents and Their Children in Our Nation's K-12 Schools

GLSEN Research Briefs

All available at: http://www.glsen.org/research.

Films

Chasnoff, D., & Klausner, K. (Directors). (1984). *Choosing children* (film). Cambridge Documentary Films.

Chasnoff, D., & Cohen, H. (Directors). (1996). *It's elementary: Talking about gay issues in schools.* New Day Films.

Dupre, J. (Director). (1998). *Out of the past: The struggle for gay and lesbian rights in America.* Allumination.

Gilomen, J. (Director). (2008). *In my shoes: Stories of youth with LGBTQ parents.* COLAGE.

Holsten, G. (Director). (2003). *Gay pioneers.* Glennfilms.

References

Albelda, R., Badgett, M. V. L., Schneebaum, A., & Gates, G. (2009). *Poverty in the lesbian, gay and bisexual community.* Los Angeles, CA: The Williams Institute.

Biblarz, T. J., & Savci, E. (2010). Lesbian, gay, bisexual, and transgender families. *Journal of Marriage and Family, 72,* 480–497. doi:10.1111/j.1741-3737.2010.00714.x

Bos, H. M. W., van Balen, F., van den Boom, D. C., & Sandfort, T. G. M. (2004). Minority stress, experience of parenthood and child adjustment in lesbian families. *Journal of Reproductive and Infant Psychology, 22,* 1–14. doi:10.1080/02646830412331298350

Cahill, S., Ellen, M., & Tobias, S. (2003). *Family policy: Issues affecting gay, lesbian, bisexual and transgender families.* New York, NY: National Gay and Lesbian Task Force Policy Institute.

Casper, V., Schultz, S., & Wickens, E. (1992). Breaking the silences: Lesbian and gay parents and the schools. *Teachers College Record, 94,* 109–137.

Centers for Disease Control and Prevention. (2011). *Sexual identity, sex of sexual contacts, and health-risk behaviors among students in grades 9–12: Youth risk behavior surveillance, selected sites, United States, 2001–2009* (Vol. 60). Atlanta, GA: MMWR.

Dang, A., & Frazer, S. (2005). *Black same-sex households in the United States: A report from the 2000 Census* (2nd ed.). New York, NY: National Gay and Lesbian Task Force Policy Institute.

Gartrell, N., Banks, A., Reed, N., Hamilton, J., Rodas, C., & Deck, A. (2000). The US National Lesbian Family Study: 3. Interviews with mothers of five-year-olds. *American Journal of Orthopsychiatry, 70,* 542–548. doi:10.1037/h0087823

Gates, G. (2011). *How many people are lesbian, gay, bisexual and transgender?* Los Angeles, CA: The Williams Institute.

GLSEN & Harris Interactive. (2005). *From teasing to torment: School climate in America, a survey of students and teachers.* New York, NY: Gay, Lesbian and Straight Education Network.

GLSEN & Harris Interactive. (2008). *The principal's perspective: School safety, bullying and harassment. A survey of public school principals.* New York: Gay, Lesbian and Straight Education Network.

Goldberg, A. E. (2007). (How) does it make a difference? Perspectives of adults with lesbian, gay, and bisexual parents. *American Journal of Orthopsychiatry, 77,* 550–562. doi:10.1037/0002-9432.77.4.550

Goldberg, A. E. (2010). *Lesbian and gay parents and their children: Research on the family life cycle.* Washington, DC: American Psychological Association.

Goldberg, A. E., & Smith, J. Z. (2011). Stigma, social context, and mental health: Lesbian and gay couples across the transition to adoptive parenthood. *Journal of Counseling Psychology, 58,* 139–150. doi:10.1037/a0021684

Goodenow, C., Szalacha, L., & Westheimer, K. (2006). School support groups, other school factors, and the safety of sexual minority adolescents. *Psychology in the Schools, 43,* 573–589. doi:10.1002/pits.20173

Kosciw, J. G. (2003). *The relationship of homophobic harassment and discrimination to family processes, parenting and children's well-being in families with lesbian and gay parents* (Unpublished doctoral dissertation). New York University, New York.

Kosciw, J. G., & Diaz, E. M. (2008). *Involved, invisible, ignored: The experiences of lesbian, gay, bisexual and transgender parents and their children in our nation's K-12 schools.* New York, NY: Gay, Lesbian and Straight Education Network.

Kosciw, J. G., Greytak, E. A., Diaz, E. M., & Bartkiewicz, M. J. (2010). *The 2009 National School Climate Survey: The experiences of lesbian, gay, bisexual and transgender youth in our nation's schools.* New York, NY: Gay, Lesbian and Straight Education Network.

Litovich, M. L., & Langhout, R. D. (2004). Framing heterosexism in lesbian families: A preliminary examination of resilient coping. *Journal of Community and Applied Social Psychology, 14,* 411–435. doi:10.1002/casp. 780

Mercier, L. M., & Harold, R. D. (2003). At the interface: Lesbian-parent families and their children's schools. *Children and Schools, 25,* 35–47.

Morris, J. F., Balsam, K. F., & Rothblum, E. D. (2002). Lesbian and bisexual mothers and nonmothers: Demographics and the coming-out process. *Journal of Family Psychology, 16,* 144–156. doi:10.1037/0893-3200.16.2.144

Movement Advancement Project, Family Equality Council, & Center for American Progress. (2011). *All children matter: How legal and social inequalities hurt LGBT families*. Denver, CO: Movement Advancement Project.

Russell, S. T., McGuire, J. K., Lee, S.-A., Larriva, J. C., & Laub, C. (2008). Adolescent perceptions of school safety for students with lesbian, gay, bisexual, and transgender parents. *Journal of LGBT Youth, 5*, 11–27. doi:10.1080/19361650802222880

Sears, R. B., Gates, G., & Rubenstein, W. B. (2005). *Same-sex couples and same-sex couples raising children in the United States: Data from census 2000*. Los Angeles, CA: The Williams Institute.

Stacey, J., & Biblarz, T. J. (2001). (How) does the sexual orientation of parents matter? *American Sociological Review, 66*, 159–183. doi:10.2307/2657413

Szalacha, L. A. (2003). Safer sexual diversity climates: Lessons learned from an evaluation of Massachusetts safe schools program for gay and lesbian students. *American Journal of Education, 110*, 58–88. doi:10.1086/377673

Tasker, F. L., & Golombok, S. (1997). *Growing up in a lesbian family: Effects on child development*. New York, NY: Guilford Press.

The Law Governing LGBT-Parent Families

Julie Shapiro

Many LGBT people, alone or in couples, want to add children to their families. There are a variety of ways this can be done, and individuals or couples may explore several paths before settling on a plan (Goldberg, 2010). One initial choice is often whether to pursue adoption or some form of assisted reproduction. Either of these choices will lead to more choices. For example, if one chooses adoption, does one pursue domestic or foreign adoption? Can a couple adopt a child together? Choosing assisted reproduction leads to other questions, and generally different ones for women (who typically have access to ova and need sperm) and men (who generally have access to sperm but need both ova and a woman to gestate the child). LGBT couples becoming parents will face yet more questions: For example, whatever the method by which one person attains legal parentage, will the other person's parental rights also be secure? If not, can steps be taken to secure them?

As complicated and layered as these choices are, it is essential to understand that each choice brings with it its own set of legal considerations. Failure to consider the legal ramifications of the various courses of action being considered can result in future difficulties for the individuals and families involved. Understanding the basic outlines of the law of parentage as it pertains to LGBT people can assist individuals in understanding their options and in assessing their legal positions and also help them understand why attention to legal status issues is so critical.

Because there is so much variation in the law as well as near constant change in law, it is practically impossible to accurately summarize the current state of the law at any given moment. Even if it were possible to do so at any given moment, the summary would quickly become unreliable and outdated, as the law in this area changes rapidly just as social attitudes are changing. The goal of this chapter is therefore not to provide a specific account of the law as it stands today. Instead, this chapter provides a brief introduction to the major legal principles that shape the law. For more specific and concrete analysis of individual situations, one would be well advised to consult a lawyer familiar with the relevant law in the relevant jurisdiction.[1]

J. Shapiro, J.D. (✉)
Fred T. Korematsu Center for Law and Equality,
Seattle University School Of Law, 901, 12th Avenue,
Sullivan Hall, PO Box 222000, Seattle,
WA 98122-1090, USA
e-mail: shapiro@seattleu.edu

[1]National legal organizations that focus on lesbian, gay, and transgender rights may be helpful in locating a knowledgeable local attorney. The websites of both the Lambda Legal Defense and Education Fund (http://www.lambdalegal.org/) and The National Center for Lesbian Rights (http://www.nclrights.org/) offer legal help desks. A recent publication provides guidance for queer couples who are engaged in co-parenting disputes. *Protecting Families: Standards for LGBT Families* is jointly produced by GLAD (Gay and Lesbian Advocates and Defenders) and NCLR. The standards can be reviewed at http://www.glad.org/protecting-families.

A.E. Goldberg and K.R. Allen (eds.), *LGBT-Parent Families: Innovations in Research and Implications for Practice*, DOI 10.1007/978-1-4614-4556-2_19, © Springer Science+Business Media New York 2013

From a legal perspective, the process by which LGBT adults become parents (adoption or assisted reproduction) is critical. During this process one or both adults (if there are two adults) may gain recognition as a legal parent. Different legal outcomes will result as a function of both on the process used and the law of the relevant states.

Once recognition as a legal parent is attained, subsequent legal issues become significantly less complicated. The rights of legal parents are well understood and do not vary based on the sexual identity of the parents. For instance, resolution of a custody dispute for an LGBT couple where both parties are legal parents is legally indistinguishable from a heterosexual child custody case: The individual facts of the case will be critical, but the two adults stand on equal legal footing. The deciding factor will be the best interests of the particular child or children involved. By contrast, if one member of the couple is not a legal parent, she or he will be at a nearly insurmountable legal disadvantage. This chapter uses the initial question of recognition as a legal parent as the organizing structure for a larger discussion of the legal issues facing LGBT parents and prospective parents.

Overview: The General Structure of Family Law in the United States

Nearly all family law in the USA is state (as opposed to federal) law. This means that as a general rule, family law is made by state legislatures or state courts rather than by the United States Congress or federal courts. While it is easy to point to broad commonalities (e.g., every jurisdiction has marriage, all have recognized parent/child relationships, all legally recognized parents have strong rights and obligations vis-à-vis their children) the specifics of the law (e.g., who can get married, when is a person recognized as a parent) vary significantly state to state. Each of the 50 states as well as the District of Columbia and the US territories has its own body of law (Crockin & Jones, 2010).

For married heterosexual-parent families, the most important aspects of family law (marriage and the recognition of parent/child relationships) are well established and reasonably uniform. While there are some state-to-state differences in the finer points of marriage eligibility (minimum age for marriage varies, for instance), unrelated adult heterosexuals who are not already married are generally eligible to marry in all states. Additionally, states readily accord respect to marriages performed in other states, so if a heterosexual couple marries in New York, they can travel freely around the USA, knowing that all other states will recognize their marriage. Thus, the state-law nature of family law is rarely a source of difficulty or even comment for these couples. If a heterosexual couple marries and has children in one state, they will automatically be recognized as married parents in every other state.

By contrast, the laws that protect or affect LGBT-parent families vary widely state to state. These variations have been the subject of substantial political turmoil in the last decades. There is much less uniformity concerning the terms for recognition of either adult relationships or parent/child relationships, and the general approaches of the states vary widely (Herek, 2006). Some states allow same-sex couples to marry while some do not permit marriage but recognize domestic partnerships or civil unions and still others do not grant legal recognition to same-sex relationships at all. In some states the rights conferred by a civil union or a domestic partnership approximate the state-law rights of marriage. In other states, civil unions and domestic partnerships may confer a lesser set of rights. LGBT people must familiarize themselves with the laws of the state where they live to properly assess their family status. Understanding the relevant law is the first task for lesbian and gay family members.

Yet even when one has properly assessed one's family status under home-state law, the state-law based structure of American family law generates further complexity for LGBT-parent families. Whatever the legal status of a family in its home state, there is no guarantee that other states will recognize and respect that legal status. The marriage of a same-sex couple that is proper in New

York or Massachusetts will not be recognized as a marriage in New Jersey (which does not currently permit same-sex couples to marry), though it may be treated as though it was a civil union. Perhaps more importantly, the relationship will not be recognized *at all* in Virginia or Ohio (O.R.C. § 3101.01, 2004; VA Code Ann. § 20–45.3, 2004). None of the rights and obligations of marriage would be afforded to the couple in these states. Thus, if one member of the couple were hospitalized while traveling in Virginia, the other might be denied the right to visit or to make medical decisions—rights that would routinely be extended to a different-sex spouse.

Recognition of legal parentage may be subject to similar interstate variation. For example, suppose P (parent) and C (child) live in state A and that the law in state A recognizes a legal parent–child relationship between P and C. Now suppose that there is a neighboring state, B, where the law is different so that as a general matter, state B would not recognize a person in P's position as a parent of C. If P and C move from state A to state B, is P still a legal parent? Does P's legal status as a parent evaporate when the state line is crossed? This question of parental status is not an academic one. Parental status is of immense practical importance. Will state B allow P to authorize medical care for C, as a parent is undoubtedly able to do? Can P visit C in a hospital? Can P enroll C in school? If P died, would C inherit as a child of P? These questions cannot always be answered generally. LGBT parents confront a world rife with legal uncertainty.

As was noted above, there is little direct federal family law. Instead, generally speaking, the federal government will recognize family relationships that are properly established under the relevant state's law. Thus, if the parent–child relationship between P and C is recognized by state A it will generally be recognized by the federal government (Crockin & Jones, 2010). This recognition provides the child with access to federal programs based on the parent/child relationship, such as social security survivor benefits or veteran's benefits.

The notable exception to the rule that family law is generally state law is the federal Defense of Marriage Act (DOMA). DOMA has two main provisions. One purports to regulate the interstate recognition of marriage, explicitly allowing states to deny recognition to out-of-state marriages between same-sex couples (28 U.S.C. § 1738C, 1996). The second provision, more important to the discussion here, prohibits the federal government from recognizing lawful state marriages between people of the same sex (1 U.S.C.A. § 7). This means that while a same-sex couple can be lawfully married in Massachusetts, the federal government is prohibited from recognizing the couple as married. The practical effect of this is important. Federal benefits ordinarily available to a couple—Social Security benefits or exclusion from federal estate tax, for example—are not available if the married couple is a same-sex couple. The validity of this provision of DOMA is also being litigated in several lawsuits (see, e.g., Gill v. Office of Personnel Management, 2010). The Obama Administration has concluded that DOMA is unconstitutional and is no longer defending the statute. Nonetheless it may take several years before the validity of the provision is resolved (Cooper, 2011).

The next section of this chapter examines general family law principles that apply in all states. It will also consider constitutional law—which is to say those family law principles found to be rooted in the United States Constitution. Because the Constitution is binding in all states, principles of constitutional law necessarily apply to all states. It is only because the principles introduced here are stated relatively abstractly that generalizations can be offered. The specifics of family law vary significantly state to state. Thus, the outcomes of particular cases may vary by state.

The Importance of Legal Parenthood

"Parent" is a word with many meanings. In common speech it is often coupled with different modifiers. Thus, there can be stepparents and social parents, natural parents and adoptive parents, and so on. The critical category for law is, unsurprisingly, that of *legal parent*. A legal parent is a person who the law recognizes as a parent of the child in question. People who function as social parents may or may not be legal parents, just as legal parents may or may not be social parents.

It is difficult to overstate the importance of being a legal parent. Legal parents are assigned a wide array of both rights and obligations with regard to a child. As long as the actions of a legal parent do not directly endanger the child, neither the state nor other individuals (who are not themselves parents) can interfere with them. Legal parents have great latitude within their families and can invoke powerful protections to prevent outside interference (Polikoff, 2009).

Throughout the USA, as in many countries throughout the world, the legal rights of those recognized as parents are far superior to the legal rights of those who are not legal parents. Legal parents have the right to make important decisions for their children as to education, upbringing, religion, and health care. Legal parents can decide who their children see and spend time with and can exclude nonparents from their children's lives. At the same time, legal parents have obligations to care for, protect, and support their children and can be subject to prosecution where they fail to fulfill their obligations (Polikoff, 2009).

The Supreme Court has recognized that the rights of a legal parent are constitutionally protected (Troxel v. Granville, 2000). In Troxel, a trial court ordered visitation between two children and their paternal grandparents over the objections of the children's mother. (The children's father was deceased.) The trial judge did so because he found that visiting the grandparents would be beneficial to the children. The United States Supreme Court concluded that the trial court's action violated the constitutionally protected parental rights of the mother. (The mother's status as a legal parent was never in doubt.) The Supreme Court did so even though it might well have been beneficial to the children to visit the grandparents. The choice of who the children were to see properly lay with their mother, and the state (here acting through the trial judge) could not constitutionally interfere with her choice absent some specific circumstances. While those precise circumstances might

remain ill defined, the general import of Troxel is clear: All states are required to recognize and enforce strong parental rights. Absent special circumstances, a legal parent's decisions will stand.

The circumstances under which a legal parent's judgment will be overridden are narrow but have historically been of some concern to LGBT-parent families. A legal parent loses the protections described above where the parent is found to be unfit. In the past, there have been cases where unfitness has been premised on a parent's identification as lesbian or gay. In some instances, proof that a parent was a lesbian or a gay man constituted proof that the parent was per se unfit (N.K.M. v. L.E.M., 1980). These cases arose where a heterosexual relationship that had produced children dissolved and one of the parties subsequently identified himself or herself as gay or lesbian. The heterosexual parent would invoke the sexuality of the parent newly identified as LGBT as a basis for disqualifying that parent from receiving custody (Joslin & Minter, 2011).

In more recent years, this approach has been rejected in favor of a nexus test focused on the relationship between parental conduct and harm to the child (Shapiro, 1996). Use of the nexus test is now nearly universal. Only actual conduct which is shown to cause harm to the child may be a basis for a finding of unfitness (Joslin & Minter, 2011). This test requires an individualized analysis based on the specific facts of each case. In the hands of a fair judge, it places lesbian and gay parents on an equal footing with all other parents with regard to unfitness inquiries. Findings of parental unfitness are relatively rare and the overwhelming majority of lesbian and gay people who have obtained legal recognition as parents will be fit parents.

To summarize, the only person who can directly challenge a fit legal parent's decisions in court is another fit legal parent. Where two fit legal parents disagree over the custody/control of a child or children, a court will determine the outcome in a conventional custody case. In such a case, the best interests of the child become the court's guiding principle. But if a fit legal parent has a disagreement with a person who is *not* a legal parent, the fit legal parent has an immense and typically insurmountable advantage. It is the fit legal parent's right to determine the outcome, and courts will be loath to interfere. Where they do interfere, they will grant the fit legal parent's decision great, typically dispositive, deference.

In contrast to the earlier era where many cases arose upon dissolution of heterosexual relationships and subsequent identification as lesbian or gay, modern LGBT family law is distinguished by a series of cases where two people—most often lesbians but increasingly gay men as well—raising a child together separate and disagree over the continuing care and custody of the child. A review of the active cases on the websites of the organizations cited above reveals that there are now more intra-lesbian cases than there are cases involving a lesbian parent and a heterosexual parent. Of course these cases may come to court as ordinary custody cases where two legal parents compete, but in the most troubling cases, the dynamic is quite different. One woman argues that she alone is a legal parent. She asserts that her former partner, who may have functioned as a parent for any number of years, is not a legal parent. If this argument succeeds, the end is virtually certain—the nonlegal parent's relationship with the child (and the child's relationship with her) has no protection (Alison D. v Virginia M., 1991). The legal mother alone is entitled to decide with whom the child spends time. If she prefers that the child not see her former partner, the child will not see her. These cases graphically illustrate the power of the legal parent and the necessity of attention to legal status in family formation. These problematic outcomes are best avoided if LGBT people forming families take steps to ensure recognition of legal parentage in both parties.[2] The following section examines the law governing the methods by which LGBT people bring children into their relationships.

Bringing Children into a Family

Broadly speaking there are two alternative paths to legal parenthood: One can become a parent to an already existing child via adoption or one can participate in the creation of a new child via the process of conception/birth. Each path has its own complications and potentials, particularly for LGBT prospective parents. In the first two of the following sections, these options will be examined in more detail. Because the original formation of a family sometimes only involves recognition of one legal parent, legal devices for securing rights for additional legal parents will then be considered.

Adoption

Generally speaking adoption is a process by which a child acquires a new parent or set of parents who take the place of an earlier parent or set of parents.[3] While adoptions can be (and often are) arranged in advance of the birth of a child, there is always some period of time after the birth of the child during which the birth parent(s) can revoke their consent to the adoption. This period varies from place to place and may be quite short, but it is important to recognize that it exists.

There is no general right to adopt. Thus, prospective parents must apply to the state for approval to adopt. The process for assessing prospective parents is typically delegated to either a state or private agency, but the legal process for the adoption and the requirements for adoptive parents are essentially similar in the public and private systems in any given state. The approval process may be quite time-consuming, intensive,

---

[2]Litigation of these cases can be destructive for the lesbian and gay communities as well as for the individuals involved. This is the motivation for the recent pamphlet "Protecting Families"—a coproduction of GLAD and NCLR. http://www.glad.org/uploads/docs/publications/protecting-families-standards-for-lgbt-families.pdf.

[3]The important exception to this generalization is second-parent or stepparent adoption, which is discussed below. Absent adoption, a stepparent is typically not a legal parent. To the extent the stepparent has any legal parental rights, they depend on the legal relationship with a preexisting legal parent and terminate if the relationship with the legal parent terminates.

and expensive. It usually includes a home study as well as criminal background checks. Home studies are generally an evaluation of the fitness of the prospective parent(s) to raise a child or children and may or may not include an actual visit to the home. Prospective LGBT parents may face a variety of special concerns, particularly with respect to laws restricting access to adoption. Restrictive access to adoption is discussed further below.

Once an adoption is properly completed, adoptive parents are full legal parents. Thus, they have the full range of parental rights regarding custody and control of their children as well as the full set of parental obligations. A dispute over custody of a child between two adoptive parents or between an adoptive parent and a natural legal parent should be handled as any dispute between two recognized legal parents of the child would be. In most instances this means that a court will attempt to determine the best interests of the child and that the two parents stand on an equal footing at the beginning of this inquiry.

Adoption is generally said to be irrevocable, though parental rights can be terminated due to unfitness. It is extremely difficult to challenge a completed adoption.[4] It is important, however, for prospective parents to be forthright and honest during the evaluative process involved in adoption. Fraud (which is deliberately misstating facts) and/or concealment of significant facts about past conduct or about one's qualifications as an adoptive parent may undermine the validity of an adoption. While candid disclosure of some matters (a criminal record or a history of mental illness, for instance) may make the path to adoption more difficult, it ensures that once completed the adoption will stand. Careful attention to disclosure

requirements may be especially important to prospective LGBT parents who find themselves in a hostile legal environment as allegations of fraud could provide a basis for a hostile court to invalidate an adoption. Consultation with experienced legal counsel is strongly advised.

As noted above, state restrictions on who may adopt vary. Some of the restrictions are of particular importance to prospective LGBT parents. Perhaps most notably, until 2010 Florida barred lesbian and gay people from adopting. This explicit restriction was unique to Florida and was enacted as a result of the Anita Bryant campaign of the late 1970s. At the same time, Florida did not bar lesbian and gay people from acting as foster parents. Martin Gill was a committed foster parent for two boys over the course of several years. In time he sought to adopt the boys to establish a permanent relationship with them. Strong testimony was offered to demonstrate that it was in the interests of these children to be adopted by Gill and also that lesbian and gay people make suitable parents. As a result the Florida appellate court struck down the ban on lesbian and gay adoption (Florida Department of Children and Families v. In re Matter of Adoption of X.X.G. and N.R.G, 2010). No further appeal was taken (Joslin & Minter, 2011). Thus, at this time, no state explicitly bars lesbian and gay people from adopting because they identify as lesbian or gay (Joslin & Minter, 2011).

The course of the Gill case is noteworthy in part because of Gill's progression from foster parent to adoptive parent. Some states may be more accommodating of LGBT people who wish to be foster parents. It is not uncommon for foster parents to seek to adopt the children they foster where the placement has proved enduring and successful. Indeed, many would say this is a desirable outcome. Once a parent/child bond has developed between an LGBT person and a foster child, courts and agencies may be more willing to recognize the importance of an adoption to ensure stability and permanence to that relationship, as was the case in Gill.

All states permit adoption by unmarried individuals who are otherwise qualified to adopt. With the demise of the Florida ban, single LGBT

---

[4]A recent case from the North Carolina Supreme Court, Bozeman v. Jarrell, is a disturbing exception to this rule (Boseman v. Jarrell, 2010). In this case the NC Supreme Court voided a second-parent adoption years after it was completed. In addition, the court appears to have voided all other second-parent adoptions completed in North Carolina. While the case is an extreme outlier, it is also a sobering reminder that on rare occasions adoptions *can* be challenged long after the fact.

people are generally eligible to adopt in all states.

The prospect for same-sex couples seeking to adopt jointly is more complicated. A number of states now limit joint adoptions to married couples only. For instance, in Louisiana, an adoption can be completed by a single person or by a married couple (LA. CHILD. CODE ANN. art., 1221, 2004). However, two people who are not married to each other cannot adopt jointly. Since Louisiana does not permit or recognize marriage between two people of the same sex, lesbian and gay couples cannot adopt jointly in Louisiana.

This combination of laws is not unusual. The states that restrict joint adoptions to married couples uniformly deny access to marriage for same-sex couples. Thus, the requirement that joint adopters be married effectively excludes same-sex couples from joint adoption in those states. This is hardly coincidence. The majority of the married-couple-only restrictions were enacted after the struggle over access to marriage for same-sex couples intensified in the early 2000s. They generally followed state enactment of restrictions, either constitutional or statutory, on access to marriage and were promoted by the same coalitions of conservative political and religious actors. Efforts by these same political coalitions to directly restrict access to adoption for all lesbian and gay individuals were unsuccessful and restrictions on joint adoptions were substituted instead. Thus, in states like Louisiana the law establishes a seemingly peculiar rule that a single lesbian or gay man can adopt even though a lesbian or gay couple cannot.

In most states where joint adoption is not possible, one member of the same-sex couple would still be eligible to adopt, as nonmarital cohabitation is not a bar to adoption.[5] While this may be an important avenue to parenthood for a same-sex couple, it is at best an imperfect solution. The end result is a family where one member of the couple has status as a legal parent and the other does not. As is discussed elsewhere in this chapter, this can have very serious consequences. The nonlegal parent will be at a severe disadvantage in the event that the relationship between the adults dissolves or the legal parent dies. Further, benefits and obligations that ordinarily run between parent and child may not be recognized or imposed. Thus, it is possible that a child will not receive social security if the nonlegal parent dies or is injured. The nonlegal parent may not be able to make medical decisions for the child in the event of an emergency or to visit the child in a hospital. Further, a child may have difficulty establishing an entitlement to financial support from a nonlegal parent.

Lawyers may be able to prepare documents which will ameliorate some of the legal disadvantages experienced by the nonlegal parent and should be consulted, but these documents may not be honored in all states, and the powers granted by them may be revoked in the event the legal parent wishes to do so. Other possible avenues by which a nonlegal parent may gain legal protection are discussed below.

Couples seeking to adopt may wish to consider relocating to a more hospitable state. Most states require residence for a period of time (the precise time varies but is often around six months) before a couple can invoke that state's adoption laws.

Transgender people may face unique challenges during adoption. While no state specifically addresses the eligibility of transgender people as adoptive parents, doubtless individual agencies and judges would consider this a significant factor (Joslin & Minter, 2011). Similarly, many judges and agencies would view the failure to disclose transgender status as a meaningful omission. Thus, careful consultation with a lawyer is essential.

Many LGBT people consider international adoptions (Joslin & Minter, 2011). As is true with the states, different countries have different rules about who is permitted to adopt. Some permit single people but not unmarried couples. Many do not permit LGBT people to adopt. Issues about the extent to which full disclosure is required or advisable are not uncommon. Individualized legal advice is strongly recommended as international adoption adds additional layers of complexity to

---

[5]Utah is an exception to this. Nonmarital cohabitation does preclude eligibility to adopt there.

the adoption process. Lack of candor during the adoption process may be a basis on which the adoption itself can be undermined.

The Portability of Adoption

Given the confusing array of state laws governing adoption, it is valuable to note that once an adoption is properly concluded in one state, all other states must recognize the adoption. Thus, if a second-parent adoption is completed in Pennsylvania, Nebraska must recognize that adoption, even though Nebraska itself does not permit second-parent adoptions (Russell v. Bridgens, 2002).

This result is required by the Full Faith and Credit Clause of the United States Constitution. That Clause obliges the states to give full effect to a valid court judgment from another state (USCA CONST Art. IV § 1). Thus, Nebraska must recognize all out-of-state judgments of adoption and treat such adoptions just as it would its own adoptions. This means that adoptions are portable and can be effective as one travels from state to state. (It is prudent to carry some proof of adoption as one travels state to state.) The same cannot be said for marriages.[6]

Birth Certificates

When an adoption is completed it is common for a court to order that a new birth certificate be prepared for the child. The new birth certificate will list the legally recognized parents of the child, post-adoption. Thus, in the case of a second-parent adoption, the name of the second parent will be added. The original birth certificate is then typically sealed.

A certified copy of the post-adoption birth certificate can be produced by adoptive parents to demonstrate their status as legal parents. The birth certificate allows parents to register a child for school or enroll a child for health insurance. It is also required to obtain a passport.

Some states that do not permit two parents of the same sex to adopt jointly have resisted issuing new birth certificates for children after a second-parent adoption is completed in the couple's home state. For example, Louisiana declined to issue a new birth certificate to two gay men who had adopted a child born in Louisiana. The men had completed an adoption in New York State and thus were both legal parents. The men sued in federal court. Louisiana lost the early rounds of this litigation but prevailed in the most recent court decision from the United States Court of Appeal for the Fifth Circuit (Adar v. Smith, 2011). Thus, as things stand now Louisiana does not have to issue a birth certificate with the two men's names on it. This decision does not have any impact on the validity of the adoption but does create practical difficulties for the family.

Assisted Reproduction

The alternative to adoption for LGBT-parent families is some form of assisted reproduction. Assisted reproductive technology (ART) offers an array of options. The law has been slow to respond to rapidly developing technology, and legal responses vary widely state to state and country to country. It is therefore difficult to make any general statements about ART and parentage. Further, as the ART industry has developed, ART transactions often touch on multiple states if not multiple countries (Chapter 5). Since the different entities often have different laws, this further complicates the legal picture.

Given the nature of human reproduction, the needs of women are generally different from the needs of men. Single women and lesbian couples need a source of sperm while single men and gay male couples need both an egg and a woman to gestate and give birth to the child. Thus,

---

[6]It is widely agreed that marriages, which do not result in court judgments, need not receive Full Faith and Credit. Whether a state recognizes a marriage concluded in another state is a matter of comity. While the general practice is that states do recognize each other's marriages, marriages between people of the same gender are often treated as exceptions to this rule. A significant number of states have statutes or constitutional provisions mandating this result.

lesbians and gay men generally use different ART techniques and so encounter different legal issues. The following section considers these distinct issues.

ART for Lesbians

Lesbians have used assisted insemination (AI) to become pregnant for many years. As a general matter, when a woman gives birth to a child, she is automatically recognized as a legal parent of that child (Jacobs, 2006).[7] Whether she is a lesbian has no bearing on this question. The two main legal questions presented by assisted insemination are the potential parental rights of the man who provides the sperm and the legal status of a nonpregnant lesbian partner. These are considered in turn.

First, regarding legal issues around the rights of the sperm provider, lesbians using third-party sperm have several options. They can use sperm from a man they know, they can use sperm from a man who can be identified in the future, or they can use sperm from an anonymous provider. The decision as to the source of sperm is one that involves both legal and nonlegal factors. Thus, one may choose a known provider so that one's child can have a relationship with that person during childhood. Alternatively, one might choose a donor who can be identified when the child reaches adulthood so that the child can locate the person at that time. There is a great deal of current discussion about the potential social or psychological value of these options, but there are important legal ramifications that should be considered as well.

This is an area where the law varies significantly state to state. In some states a man who provides sperm for the insemination of a woman who is not his wife will not be recognized as a legal parent of any resulting child. In other states, his status will depend on whether there is an agreement regarding parental status in place or on whether or not the insemination was conducted by a medical professional. In still other states the man will have the status of a legal parent no matter what agreement is in place.[8] The first task should be to determine the relevant law. Establishing relevant law often requires consultation with a lawyer or a local LGBT rights organization. It is crucial that the information obtained be both current and reliable. It is not enough to rely on an agreement between the donor and the recipient.

If the law states that a provider is not a legal parent, then a lesbian may freely choose a known or an identifiable provider without concern that he will acquire parental rights. But if a provider is considered to be a legal father then use of a known provider means that the provider will be a legal parent of the child. Use of an anonymous provider ensures that no man will step forward to claim the legal rights of a parent and the rights of the unknown man can generally be terminated by proper legal proceedings. It may also be possible for a known provider to give up his legal rights post-birth, but the provider may change his mind and elect not to give up his rights. Further, some judges may refuse to allow him to give up his rights if it creates a single-parent family. Thus, using a known provider in those jurisdictions where a sperm provider is deemed to be a legal parent requires extremely careful consideration, preferably including input from a legal professional. In those states where the legal status of the provider depends on an agreement between the parties, care must be taken to ensure the agreement is properly crafted and expresses the clear understanding of all those involved. In most states, however, while agreements between the parties may be useful to clarify the intent of the parties, they will not have legal effect.

---

[7]There are limited exceptions in some states for women who are acting as surrogates (Johnson v. Calvert, 1993). These are not of considered here. Surrogacy is discussed below.

[8]These variations occur *only* when using assisted reproduction—which is to say, where conception occurs without intercourse. If a lesbian becomes pregnant via intercourse, the man who provides the sperm will almost assuredly be recognized as the legal father of the child. This is true even if there is an explicit agreement that he will not be a legal parent. It is critical that women considering family formation via this path recognize this consequence.

Second, regarding legal issues around status of the nonpregnant lesbian partner, the woman who gives birth automatically gains recognition as a legal parent. Generally speaking, the same is not the case for her lesbian partner. In some states a second-parent adoption may secure the rights of the partner. Over time she may also qualify as a de facto parent. Each of these possibilities is discussed below in the section on adding parents.

In states allowing access to marriage for same-sex couples and/or with robust domestic partnership or civil union statutes, the lesbian spouse/partner may gain legal recognition as a parent by virtue of her legal relationship (marriage/domestic partnership/civil union) with the woman who gives birth. This is an extension of a broadly recognized legal principle that the spouse of a married woman who gives birth is deemed to be a legal parent of the child. Thus, where a married woman gives birth in Massachusetts her spouse—male or female—is recognized as a legal parent as well.

The problem is that her legal status may only be recognized by states that recognize the relationship between the adult parties. Thus, states which do not recognize the Massachusetts marriage will not recognize her parental status and, as DOMA presently prevents the federal government from recognizing the marriage, it may not recognize parental status either (Polikoff, 2009). In other words, parental status gained in this fashion is not fully portable. Due to this serious limitation, it is generally advisable to take further steps to secure the legal rights of the woman who did not give birth. This generally means completing a second-parent adoption.

ART for Gay Men

Gay men who are considering ART generally use some form of surrogacy. In surrogacy a woman agrees to become pregnant and give birth without intending to be a parent to the child. Instead, she acts for another individual or individuals who are planning to be the parent or parents of the child. Those individuals are often called the "intended parents." The surrogate may be the source of the ovum (in which case the practice is called "traditional surrogacy") or the ovum may be obtained from a third party (Joslin & Minter, 2011). If the pregnant woman is genetically unrelated to the fetus she carries, this is called gestational surrogacy.

There are additional divisions among types of surrogates. Some women (such as close relatives or friends of the men intending to be parents) serve as surrogates without compensation. More commonly, surrogates are compensated.

As with most other aspects of family law, the law governing surrogacy varies a great deal state to state. In some states (California is one) surrogacy is relatively well accepted and the legal course of action is well understood, but in many states surrogacy is either illegal or of questionable status. Because of the complexity of the legal issues involved, surrogacy should never be pursued without consultation with a lawyer who has some expertise in the matter.

In some states (New Jersey, for example) a judge may conclude that any woman who gives birth is a legal parent, whether she is genetically related to the child or not. While this does not necessarily mean that surrogacy is barred in those states, it does mean that the surrogate has to confirm her intention to relinquish parental rights *after* the birth of the child. This gives her an opportunity to change her mind. For many intended parents, the prospect that the surrogate might reconsider creates difficult uncertainty, though in reality the instances in which a surrogate changes her mind appear to be quite rare.

In any surrogacy arrangement, an extensive written agreement is common. A written agreement is an expression of the understandings of the surrogate and the intended parents as to the expectations of all the parties. Even though the agreement may not be legally enforceable, it may be useful to draft an agreement to clarify the expectations. In general, the surrogate must retain the right to control her own medical care and the option to terminate or not terminate her pregnancy.

Adding Parents

Lesbian and gay male couples who form families may find that the initial steps of family formation leave them with only one legal parent. It might be the woman who gives birth or a man who provides the sperm in surrogacy. It may be that only one member of the couple could complete a foreign adoption. However it occurs, the situation in which there is only one legal parent should be addressed since, as is discussed above, it creates a serious power imbalance within the couple.

The most certain way to secure rights for the second parent is through a second-parent adoption. They are not available in all locations. In the absence of a second-parent adoption, a person may qualify as a de facto parent. In addition, parties may enter into various forms of parenting agreements. These agreements in general will be revocable at the will of the legal parent and so do not provide a great deal of protection for the non-legal parent. To supplement an agreement legal documentation may be prepared, but this may not increase the security of the nonlegal parent.

Second-Parent Adoptions

Second-parent adoptions are a critical legal tool in the formation of LGBT-parent families. They are to be distinguished from traditional adoptions. As is noted above, in adoption the general case is that a new parent or parents take the place of the original parent or parents. On many occasions, however, LGBT couples wish to add an additional parent while maintaining the status of the original parent. Second-parent adoptions make this possible. Second-parent adoptions are modeled on stepparent adoptions, which are widely available in proper cases. In the absence of an adoption, stepparents are not legal parents. Second-parent adoptions are not, however, available in all states.[9]

Second-parent adoptions allow the creation of LGBT-parent families with two recognized legal parents. For example, if one member of a lesbian couple gives birth to a child, she will be recognized as a parent by the operation of law.[10] She and her partner may wish to secure recognition for the partner as a second legal parent of the child. While the partner may be able to adopt the child, an ordinary adoption would require the termination of the first woman's parental rights. Thus, at the end of the day the child would still only have one legal parent, albeit a different legal parent. A second-parent adoption allows the addition of the second woman as a parent without the first woman losing legal status. Once the adoption is completed, the parental status of both women is fully secured.

While the situation just described may be the most common instance where a second-parent adoption is concluded, there are a number of other circumstances where they are useful. If only one member of an LGBT couple completes an overseas adoption (to comply with the laws of the other country), the second person may complete a second-parent adoption upon return to their home state. Similarly, one member of an LGBT couple may complete an adoption in a state where joint adoptions by unmarried couples are not permitted. Here, too, the other member of the couple may be able to complete a second-parent adoption in the couple's home state. Or one member of a gay male couple may claim legal parentage by virtue of his genetic connection to a child born to a surrogate. As with adoption generally, once a second-parent adoption is properly completed, all other states must recognize and respect it.

When a second-parent adoption is completed, the rights of the original parent are necessarily diminished. Before the adoption, the original parent is the sole legal parent. As such, she or

---

[9]It is difficult to compile a definitive list of the states where second-parent adoptions are permitted, but the Websites noted in footnote 1 are generally kept up to date. In some jurisdictions there are no authoritative precedents or statutes, so the matter may be left to the discretion of individual judges. This means that some judges are sympathetic and supportive and will approve second-parent adoptions while others will not. Overall, second-parent adoptions can be concluded in most major cities even where there is no authoritative legal ruling allowing them, provided one can find a supportive judge. Typically local lawyers are knowledgeable about judicial selection. It is clear that some states do not permit second-parent adoptions. (See the discussion of the North Carolina case above.)

---

[10]Often she is referred to as a natural parent, but the critical thing here is the operation of law, not nature. The law generally recognizes a woman who gives birth as the mother of a child. The important exception here is surrogacy, which is discussed above.

he stands largely unrivaled when it comes to decision making for the child. In agreeing to a second-parent adoption, the original parent agrees to the recognition of a second-parent who is coequal. No longer is the first parent's position unrivaled. While there are many substantial reasons why a second-parent adoption is desirable, it is nevertheless important that the original parent, in granting consent to the second-parent adoption, is agreeing to share control of and responsibility for the child. While a second-parent adoption can only be completed with the consent of the original parent, once it is given the consent is irrevocable.

In this regard, second-parent adoptions are quite different from less formal arrangements where a legal parent allows another person to co-parent a child. While in some states the other person may acquire some legal status (see the discussion of de facto parentage, below), in general the person who has not completed an adoption is vulnerable. The legal parent is generally entitled to change her or his mind and terminate the relationship between the co-parent and the child. Drafting a co-parenting agreement may be a helpful tool in delineating the expectations and understandings of the parties, but it will typically not be given legal force.

While many children are raised by single parents or in two-parent families, some children have more than two social parents. One situation where this may arise is where two parents separate and continue to share custody of the child although they live apart. If one or both of those parents repartner, the child may have three or four social parents. Additionally, some children may be part of intact family groups with more than two social parents.

De Facto Parenthood

By now it should be clear that, absent legal action, it is quite possible for a family to consist of one legal parent, one nonlegal parent, and a child or children. This might be the case where only one member of a same-sex couple is permitted to adopt a child or where a woman establishes parental rights by giving birth while no provisions of state law confer similar legal rights on her partner. As has been explained, the nonlegal parent is vulnerable in this situation. There are a regrettably large number of instances where the adult members of couples in this situation have separated and the legal mother has attempted to gain advantage by virtue of being the sole legal parent of the child. Unfortunately this has often been a successful tactic.

In response to these cases a doctrine of de facto parentage was developed. De facto parentage, in its strongest form, grants legal recognition as a parent to a person who has acted like a parent for a substantial period of time. This doctrine exists in a variety of forms in a minority of states. There are no fixed definitions for what it means to act like a parent or for the required period of time, but the test is generally fairly stringent.

De facto parentage is only established after the fact. In all of the cases litigated it was determined after a couple separates. While it provides a potential avenue for a person to continue his/her relationship with a child and may provide full parental rights, it does not give the person parental status *during* the relationship. It is also not clear whether this status is in any way portable, although if a person is determined by litigation to have been a de facto parent in the past, that judgment is very likely binding on other states (Joslin & Minter, 2011).

Establishing status as a de facto parent can be long, contested, and expensive. The court will examine the nature and duration of the relationship between the adult and the child, the extent to which the relationship was encouraged by the legal parent, and a variety of other factors. LGBT legal advocacy groups have worked long and hard to establish and fortify the de facto parent doctrine and where it is well established claiming de facto status may be somewhat more routinized (Joslin & Minter, 2011). But even in the best of the jurisdictions, entering the dispute with status as a legal parent is preferable.

Separating with Children

Law is most important at two points in the life of most LGBT-parent families. First, law matters at the time the family is formed. Second, law matters when the family dissolves, particularly if the adults in the family separate.[11]

It is often difficult for separating couples who have been raising children to reach agreement about the children, yet it is frequently better for all involved to reach agreement rather than choose the path of litigation. This advice is particularly true for LGBT-parent families. Courts are not always hospitable forums for these families. While judges may be receptive to some arguments offered by individual LGBT litigants, some judges are most likely to be receptive to those that will, in the long run, injure LGBT communities. If litigation is necessary, then care should be taken that the arguments raised do not undermine the status of LGBT-parent families generally.[12]

At the time of separation the most critical question for families with children will be whether the people separating are legal parents. If they are, then the case will be handled as a conventional custody dispute. The court will in the end approve a plan for the division of decision-making authority with regard to the child as well as a plan for the child's residence. The plan will be drawn up based on an analysis of the best interests of the child.

If one of the parties is not a legal parent, she or he could be at a substantial disadvantage if her former partner chooses to argue that she should not have any legal rights. Leading LGBT legal organizations have prepared a statement of principles outlining approaches to custody matters that allow the parties to vigorously air their disagreement without harming the communities to which they belong. Consideration of the broader effects of specific arguments that may be offered is warranted.[13]

For example, in 1991 the New York State Court of Appeals decided a case involving lesbian co-parents who were separating Alison v. Virginia, (1991). Though Alison D had acted as a social parent to the child, Virginia M argued that she was not entitled to recognition as a legal parent. The Court of Appeals agreed with Virginia M, and Alison D was found to have no right to maintain contact with the child. Beyond the effect on the parties in this case, the precedent has stood for 20 years and to this day, New York State does not recognize de facto parents. This lack of recognition has undermined the ability of lesbians and gay men to create stable families.

If both the separating parties are legal parents then there is a strong presumption that the child will continue to have contact with both parents and that both parents will continue to be involved with the children, both as decision makers and as sources of financial support. Thus, discussion will focus on allocation of decision-making authority (sometimes called legal custody) and on residential provisions (sometimes called physical custody).

In general, day-to-day decision-making authority is assumed to reside with whomever the child is living with at the time. This allocation of authority is premised on the assumption that day-to-day decisions are small ones. Typically, there is an expectation that major decisions (about elective medical procedures, religion, and education, for example) are expected to be made jointly between the parents even if the parents do not spend equal amounts of time with the child.

Different states may have different starting presumptions for the allocation of residential time with the child. Factors such as the age of the children and the physical proximity of the parents' residences will be important.

As with litigation generally, most custody cases do not go to trial. The vast majority of them

---

[11]If the adults do not separate, the relationship will eventually end with the death of one or both of the adults/parents. This, too, raises legal questions, but they are beyond the scope of this chapter.

[12]Those considering litigation should carefully consider the points raised in *Protecting Families*, a joint production of GLAD and NCLR that can be obtained at http://www.glad.org/protecting-families.

---

[13]See note 12.

settle as a result of negotiations between the parties. While the outlines of settlements are no doubt influenced by the governing law, they also reflect the parties' ability to work with each other and reach agreement about what is best for the children involved. Even where the parties separate, they will need to continue to work together as co-parents for the life of the children.

Conclusion

Lesbians and gay men have been creating families with children for several decades, but legal protection of those families is at best imperfect and uneven. While some states recognize relationships between adults as well as those between adults and children, other states refuse recognition. Some legal protections may travel with a family as it moves state to state while others may not. Federal recognition of LGBT families is similarly complicated as parent/child relationships may be recognized while adult/adult relationships cannot be recognized because of DOMA. Thus, in addition to the challenges any family with children confronts, LGBT-parent families confront complex legal questions in many different contexts.

The trend over the last several years is encouraging. More states grant at least some formal recognition to relationships between adults of the same gender. Restrictions on adoption aimed at lesbians and gay men have been rejected by courts and voters. But there is no prospect that all states will progress at the same pace. LGBT families residing in hostile states will likely endure many more years of legal invisibility. The patchwork of laws will remain and thus, for the foreseeable future, LGBT-parent families will need to be aware of potential legal problems that may arise so that these problems can be addressed.

References

Adar v. Smith, 639 F.3d 146 (5th Cir. 2011).

Alison D. v. Virginia M., 572 N.E.2d 27 (Court of Appeals of New York, 1991).

Boseman v. Jarrell, 704 S.E.2d 494 (Supreme Court of North Carolina 2010).

Cooper, H. (2011, July 20). Obama to back repeal of law restricting marriage. *The New York Times.* Retrieved from http://www.nytimes.com/2011/07/20/us/politics/20obama.html?_r=1&scp=3&sq=obama%20doma%20cooper&st=cse

Crockin, S., & Jones, H. (2010). *Legal conceptions: The evolving law and policy of assisted reproductive technologies.* Baltimore, MD: Johns Hopkins University Press.

Florida Department of Children and Families v. In re Matter of Adoption of X.X.G. and N.R.G., 45 So.3d 79, (District Court of Appeal of Florida 2010).

Full Faith and Credit Act, USCA CONST Art. IV § 1.

Gill v. Office of Personnel Management, 699 F.Supp.2d 374 (2010).

Goldberg, A. E. (2010). *Lesbian and gay parents and their children: Research on the family life cycle.* Washington, DC: American Psychological Association.

Herek, G. M. (2006). Legal recognition of same-sex relationships in the United States: A social science perspective. *American Psychologist, 61,* 607–621. doi:10.1037/0003-066X.61.6.607.

Jacobs, M. (2006). Procreation through ART: Why the adoption process should not apply. *Capital University Law Review, 35,* 399–411.

Johnson v. Calvert, 851 P.2d 776, (Supreme Court of California 1993).

Joslin, C. G., & Minter, S. P. (2011). *Lesbian, gay, bisexual and transgender family law.* Egan, MN: West.

LA. CHILD. CODE ANN. art. 1221 (2004).

N.K.M. v. L.E.M., 606 S.W.2d 169 (Missouri Court of Appeals, Western District, 1980).

O.R.C. § 3101.01. (2004).

Polikoff, N. (1990). This child does have two mothers: Redefining parenthood to meet the needs of children in lesbian-mother and other nontraditional families. *Georgetown Law Journal, 78,* 459–575.

Polikoff, N. (2009). A mother should not have to adopt her own child: Parentage law for children of lesbian couples in the twenty-first century. *Stanford Journal of Civil Rights & Civil Liberties, 5,* 201–270.

Protecting Families: Standards for LGBT Families. Retrieved from http://www.glad.org/protecting-families

Russell v. Bridgens, 647 N.W.2d 56 (Supreme Court of Nebraska 2002).

Shapiro, J. (1996). How the law fails lesbian and gay parents and their children. *Indiana Law Journal, 721,* 623–671.

Troxel v. Granville, 530 U.S. 57 (Supreme Court of the United States 2000).

VA Code Ann. § 20–45.3 (2004).

Part IV

Methodology: Research Strategies

JuliAnna Z. Smith, Aline G. Sayer, and Abbie E. Goldberg

One of the most central pursuits of family theory and research is to better understand and explore the dynamics of interpersonal family relationships. Understanding these relationships is furthered by collecting information on multiple family members (Jenkins et al., 2009). However, by their very nature, family members' experiences are interdependent, and this interdependence complicates the question of how to analyze data from multiple family members (Atkins, 2005; Bolger & Shrout, 2007; Jenkins et al., 2009; Sayer & Klute, 2005). Indeed, data interdependence precludes the use of many statistical methods that assume the errors are independent, such as ordinary least squares (OLS) regression or standard analysis of variance (ANOVA). Several statistical methods that take into account the dependency in family members' outcomes are available to researchers and have become the standard in family research journals. Many of the most commonly used approaches, however, require one to distinguish family members on the basis of some characteristic meaningful to the analyses (Sayer & Klute, 2005). For example, in parent/child dyads one can easily distinguish dyad members on the basis of whether they are the parent or child (Papp, Pendry, & Adam, 2009). In research on heterosexual couples, partners are most commonly distinguished on the basis of gender (Atkins, Klann, Marín, Lo, & Hahlweg, 2010; Claxton, O'Rourke, Smith, & DeLongis, 2012; Papp, Goeke-Morey, & Cummings, 2007; Perry-Jenkins, Smith, Goldberg, & Logan, 2011; Raudenbush, Brennan, & Barnett, 1995). Such approaches to distinguishing partners on the basis of gender, however, are clearly not useful to researchers of same-sex couples. In some cases same-sex partners may be distinguished on the basis of some other characteristic, such as biological versus nonbiological parent (Goldberg & Perry-Jenkins, 2007; Goldberg & Sayer, 2006), where that distinction is relevant to the analyses. In other cases, however, no such meaningful distinctions can be made—for example, in many analyses of lesbian/gay nonparent couples or lesbian/gay adoptive parents, wherein neither partner is the biological parent. In these instances, alternate statistical methods must be employed.

This chapter discusses the challenges faced by researchers analyzing data from multiple family members. It focuses on couples, as well as

J.Z. Smith, M.A. (✉)
Department of Psychology, Center for Research on Families, University of Massachusetts, 135 Hicks Way, 622 Tobin Hall, Amherst, MA 01003, USA
e-mail: juliannzsmith@mac.com; julianns@acad.umass.edu

A.G. Sayer, Ph.D.
Department of Psychology, Center for Research on Families, University of Massachusetts, 616 Tobin Hall, 135 Hicks Way, Amherst, MA 01003, USA
e-mail: sayer@psych.umass.edu

A.E. Goldberg, Ph.D.
Department of Psychology, Clark University, 950 Main Street, Worcester, MA 01610, USA
e-mail: agoldberg@clarku.edu

A.E. Goldberg and K.R. Allen (eds.), *LGBT-Parent Families: Innovations in Research and Implications for Practice*, DOI 10.1007/978-1-4614-4556-2_20, © Springer Science+Business Media New York 2013

advances in research methods using multilevel modeling (MLM). MLM, which is a fairly straightforward extension of the more familiar OLS multiple regression, provides one of the more versatile and accessible approaches available to model couple and family data (Sayer & Klute, 2005). We begin by discussing the role of multilevel modeling in family research, in general, and in analyzing dyadic (or paired) data, more specifically. Next, we consider some of the common difficulties encountered by LGBT researchers examining family data. We then describe the basic multilevel models available to researchers analyzing (a) cross-sectional and (b) longitudinal dyadic data. Next, we address the application of these models to analyses of multiple informant data, when multiple family members provide reports of the same outcome. In addition, we present some considerations that researchers using these statistical methods should take into account.

Multilevel Modeling in Family Research

The use of MLM has become common in family journals (e.g., Brincks, Feaster, & Mitrani, 2010; Kretschmer & Pike, 2010; Soliz, Thorson, & Rittenour, 2009), particularly in research on heterosexual couples (e.g., Atkins et al., 2010; Papp et al., 2007; Perry-Jenkins et al., 2011). Notably, its adoption by researchers who study LGBT couples and families has been somewhat slower. In part, this is because the area of LGBT couples and families is relatively new, and much of the research has been qualitative and exploratory as opposed to quantitative (see Goldberg, 2010, for a review). In addition, studies that do use quantitative methods often rely on fairly small sample sizes of LGBT couples and families (e.g., Goldberg & Sayer, 2006; Patterson, Sutfin, & Fulcher, 2004), thereby decreasing power and the ability to detect effects. Small sample sizes may lead researchers to use other methods in preference to maximum likelihood methods such as multilevel modeling which perform best with large samples (Raudenbush, 2008). Finally,

there are often additional complications when analyzing same-sex couples whose members are not clearly distinguishable from one another on the basis of some central characteristic such as gender. Such couples or dyads are termed "indistinguishable" or "exchangeable" and require methods designed to take this indistinguishability into account. Treating dyad members as indistinguishable requires the use of MLM approaches that may be less familiar to many family researchers.

Several excellent recent papers address the use of structural equation modeling (SEM) strategies to analyze data from indistinguishable dyads (Olsen & Kenny, 2006; Woody & Sadler, 2005). For applied family researchers, however, multilevel modeling provides a more straightforward way to analyze data collected on multiple family members. A fairly large and growing body of work discusses the application of MLM to heterosexual couples using models for distinguishable dyads (Bolger & Shrout, 2007; Raudenbush et al., 1995; Sayer & Klute, 2005). Much less is available on its application to indistinguishable couples (Kenny, Kashy, & Cook, 2006). In particular, there is a need to bring together recent advances in several areas: (a) the analyses of indistinguishable dyads, (b) advances in longitudinal analyses (Kashy, Donnellan, Burt, & McGue, 2008), and (c) the analyses of mixed samples, such as analyses including lesbian, gay male, and heterosexual couples (West, Popp, & Kenny, 2008). Consequently, this chapter focuses on multilevel modeling approaches to analyzing dyadic data when couple members can be considered indistinguishable. While these approaches are valuable for the study of same-sex couples, they are also useful in the study of twins, friends, roommates, and other types of relationships where members cannot be distinguished from each other on some meaningful characteristic (Kenny et al., 2006). For this reason, the information presented in this chapter may be useful and relevant to family scholars more generally.

Family theorists from a wide range of perspectives including family systems theory, life course theory, social exchange theory, symbolic interaction theory, conflict theory, and social ecological theory have long been interested in the relationships between family members and how those relationships affect family members. For example, family systems theory views individuals as part, not only of a family, but also of multiple, mutually influencing family subsystems (Cox & Paley, 1997). Individuals' experiences and their dyadic relationships with other family members affect not only those directly involved but other individuals and relationships within the family system as well. Life course theory examines changes in the intertwined lives of family members over the life span (Bengtson & Allen, 1993). Finally, ecological theory posits the importance of understanding the family as a central social context that influences all of the individuals within it (Bronfenbrenner, 1988). Research examining data from multiple family members allows researchers to start to tease apart these complex family relationships. For example, Georgiades, Boyle, Jenkins, Sanford, and Lipman (2008) examined multiple family members' reports of family functioning ($N=26,614$ individuals in 11,023 families). Using MLM enabled them to distinguish shared perceptions of family functioning from unique individual perceptions.

In addition, collecting information from more than one individual per family allows for the examination of the association between family members' scores (Bolger & Shrout, 2007). Multilevel modeling provides a means of better understanding the relationship between separate reports of the same outcomes, while accounting for the correlation between family members' outcomes. In addition, it provides a means of disentangling the variability in the outcome. The variance in the outcome is due to two sources: within-family variability and between-family variability. MLM methods provide a means for separating the variability in the outcome into these two sources, as well as appropriately testing both family-level and individual-level predictors of that variability. It is not surprising, therefore, that MLM has become widely used in family research. The nature of family research has subsequently led to adaptations of MLM approaches to suit the specialized needs of this field, most notably in the area of modeling couple

data (or dyadic data more generally; e.g., Barnett, Marshall, Raudenbush, & Brennan, 1993; Raudenbush et al., 1995).

Key Issues in Analyzing Data from LGBT Couples and Families

The Issue of Dependence

It is important to clarify why special statistical methods may be required when analyzing data from multiple family members. An assumption underlying conventional statistical methods such as OLS regression and standard ANOVAs is that the residuals (errors) are independent. This assumption is untenable in the case of dyadic or family data. Partners who are in a relationship are likely to have outcomes that are similar, and this similarity or dependency must be taken into account when performing statistical analyses. Failure to take into account dependence in the outcome scores results in inaccurate estimates of the standard errors, leading to both Type I and Type II errors (Griffin & Gonzalez, 1995; Kenny & Judd, 1986; Kashy & Kenny, 2000; Kenny et al., 2006). In addition, failure to account for dependency in the outcome can also lead to incorrect estimates of effect sizes (West et al., 2008).

There are a number of reasons why family members' outcomes may be associated (Kenny et al., 2006). For example, partners may have chosen each other at least partly on the basis of shared interests in community involvement (mate selection). Alternately, a small family income may affect the financial confidence of all of the members of a particular family (shared context). Similarly, family members who live together are likely to be affected by each other's moods (mutual influence). Statistical methods such as paired sample t-tests and repeated measures ANOVA do adjust the estimates for the dependency in the outcome and can be used to answer many basic research questions. For example, a researcher may investigate if lesbian mothers and their teen daughters have mean differences in the level of conflict they report in their relationship. Addressing more complex questions requires the application of methods that allow for the estimation of both the average effect for the entire group and the variability of each dyad around the dyad average. In addition, MLM enables the examination of the effects of both individual- (e.g., age or stress level) and family-level (e.g., number of children or family income) variables (Kenny et al., 2006; Sayer & Klute, 2005). In other words, instead of treating the dependence between family members' reports as a nuisance to be adjusted for, MLM enables researchers to treat this dependence as interesting in its own right and to explore predictors of it.

The Issue of Distinguishability

When studying same-sex couples, researchers are often faced with an additional methodological difficulty. For example, most analyses of heterosexual couples within family studies distinguish between the two members of the couple on the basis of gender (Atkins et al., 2010; Claxton et al., 2012; Papp et al., 2007; Perry-Jenkins et al., 2011; Raudenbush et al., 1995). In research on same-sex couples, distinguishing partners by gender is obviously not an option. In some instances same-sex partners should be distinguished on the basis of some other characteristic, as that distinction is important for the analyses conducted. For example, in Abbie Goldberg's work on lesbian couples who used alternative insemination to become parents ($N = 29$–34 couples), she distinguished between the biological mothers and the nonbiological mothers and found differential predictors of relationship quality and mental health across the transition to parenthood (Goldberg & Sayer, 2006; Goldberg & Smith, 2008a). Other distinguishing features that may be relevant to analyses might be work status (e.g., working/not working, in single-earner couples), primary/secondary child caregiver status, or diseased/not diseased (O'Rourke et al., 2010).

It is important that the distinction between dyad members is justified by the research questions being asked and the analyses being conducted and is thereby meaningful in a substantive sense. As it is always possible to find some a distinguishing feature, however arbitrary, it is important to carefully evaluate whether the distinguishing feature is in fact relevant. There are, for example, times when distinguishing heterosexual couples based on gender may not be relevant to the analyses being conducted (Atkins, 2005; Kenny et al., 2006). The use of a particular distinguishing feature should be supported by the theoretical frameworks guiding the research, prior research findings suggesting that this is a meaningful distinction for the analyses being conducted, and by empirical investigation of the data being examined (Kenny et al., 2006). Kenny and Ledermann (2010) contend that distinguishability must be supported empirically. In other words, if dyad members are to be treated as distinguishable in the analyses, additional analyses should be conducted to give empirical support for this decision. Kenny et al. (2006) suggest that an Omnibus Test of Distinguishability be conducted using structural equation modeling, to examine the covariances between all variables in a model, for every model presented in the analyses, in order to show that the data support distinguishing dyad members.

There are also methods that can be used within the context of multilevel modeling to empirically support the use of a particular feature to distinguish between dyad members. Consider, for example, the analyses of mental health in lesbian inseminating couples, where partners were distinguished by whether or not they were the biological mother of the child (Goldberg & Smith, 2008a). The MLM approach for distinguishable dyads provides separate parameter estimates for the two partners based on the distinguishing feature (in our example, biological mother or nonbiological mother). Researchers can test whether these estimates are statistically significantly different from each other, by fitting a second model, in which these two separate parameter estimates are constrained to be equal. Model comparison tests are then used to determine which model is a better fit to the data. If there is no significant decrement in model fit, then there is not enough of a difference in the partners' estimates to justify the estimation of two separate parameters. If there is a significant decrement, this supports the decision to treat partners as being meaningfully distinguished on the basis of the selected distinguishing feature (i.e., in this case, biological versus nonbiological mother).

It is possible that researchers will find that only some parameter estimates differ. Those parameters that are not found to be significantly different can then be constrained to be equal, creating a more parsimonious model. Such an approach was used in Goldberg and Smith's (2008a) examination of changes in the anxiety of lesbian inseminating couples over time ($N = 34$ couples). Their analyses revealed that while the effect of some factors such as neuroticism did not significantly differ for biological and nonbiological lesbian mothers, other factors did have a differential effect on biological and nonbiological mothers. For example, work hours and proportional contribution to housework were related to higher levels of anxiety only for biological mothers, while high infant distress and low instrumental social support were related to greater increases in anxiety only in nonbiological mothers. Such differential findings strongly supported the decision to distinguish partners on the basis of whether or not they were the biological mother.

MLM Approaches to Analyzing Data from Indistinguishable Dyads

In many cases in LGBT couple research, a salient, distinguishing feature will not be available for researchers. Having a distinguishing feature simplifies analyses as it allows the researcher to assign each member to a group based on that distinction and then examine these separate groups in the analyses. As a result, some researchers may be tempted to deal with the lack of a distinguishing feature on which to assign dyad members to groups by randomly assigning members to one of two groups (e.g., partner A and partner B) and then treating them as if they were distinguishable or by using an arbitrary characteristic to distinguish them (see Kenny et al., 2006). The problem with such an approach is that it can lead to erroneous findings. The assignment to a group is purely arbitrary and, yet, findings will differ depending on how the individuals are assigned.

For example, when examining couple data, one of the first questions a researcher may want to consider is "How correlated are partners' scores?" Once the researcher has distinguished between the two partners and assigned them to separate groups, the researcher can simply examine the correlation between the two partners' scores. Unfortunately, however, the estimate of this correlation will differ depending on the way in which partners were assigned to groups (see Kenny et al., 2006, for a more detailed discussion of this issue).

It is important to arrive at an accurate estimate of this correlation between partners' scores. This estimate is the interclass correlation coefficient (ICC), and it provides crucial information about the extent to which family members' scores are associated (and, thereby, the degree of dependence in their reports). As mentioned above, in the case of distinguishable dyads, the correlation between partners' scores can be easily assessed using a Pearson's product moment correlation. While it is more difficult to obtain an accurate estimate of the ICC in the case of indistinguishable dyads, there are two basic methods. Kenny et al. (2006) describe how ANOVA can be used to correctly estimate this correlation, but the ICC is more commonly and more easily estimated using multilevel modeling.

Cross-Sectional Model for Indistinguishable Dyads

Multilevel modeling provides a relatively simple extension of OLS regression, which takes into account the nesting of data within families or couples. In this statistical approach, the variance in the outcome is partitioned into the variance that occurs *within* couples (how partners differ from each other) and the variance that occurs *between* couples (how couples differ from each other). Predictors, both those that vary by couples (such as number of children and length of relationship) and those that vary by partner (such as age or mental health status), can then be added to explain this variance. In the model for the cross-sectional analysis of dyadic data, the

	FAMID	MEMBER	FAMSUP	A1AGE	P1AGE	A1EDUC	P1EDUC	A1PINC	P1PINC
1	1	1	3.10	43	43	5	5	$9.50	2.10
2	1	2	1.45	43	43	5	5	$2.10	9.50
3	2	1	3.50	40	53	5	6	$9.00	14.00
4	2	2	1.95	53	40	6	5	$14.00	9.00
5	3	1	2.85	36	37	5	6	$4.50	9.50
6	3	2	3.50	37	36	6	5	$9.50	4.50
7	4	1	1.85	38	41	4	2	$6.60	3.85
8	4	2	3.55	41	38	2	4	$3.85	6.60

Fig. 20.1 Example of a Level-1 (within couples) data file for the analysis of cross-sectional dyadic data

multilevel model generally used to examine individuals who are nested within groups (such as students within classrooms, workers within organizations, or patients within hospitals) is adapted in very specific ways to deal with the small number of cases or individuals in each dyad. For example, one common area of adaptation is in the specification of the error structure (i.e., using compound symmetry), which is the way in which the dependence of the outcome scores is modeled.

The MLM approach to indistinguishable dyads is actually a simpler model than the one most commonly used for distinguishable dyads (Kenny et al., 2006). Several studies of same-sex couples have used this approach (e.g., Goldberg & Smith, 2008b, 2009b; Kurdek, 1998). For example, Lawrence Kurdek (2003) used this approach to analyze differences between gay and lesbian cohabiting partners' relationship beliefs, conflict resolution strategies, and level of perceived social support variables in a sample of 80 gay male and 53 lesbian couples.

The most basic model is an unconditional model, with no predictors at either level; this is often referred to as a random intercept model (Raudenbush & Bryk, 2002). This model provides estimates for the grand mean of the outcome across all couples as well as estimates for the two sources of variability: within couples and between couples. We calculate the ICC from these two estimates of variability. The ICC provides two central pieces of information: (a) the extent of the dependence within couples on the outcome and (b) the proportion of variance that

lies *between* couples versus the proportion that lies *within* couples. Any ICC larger than a few percentage points indicates a degree of dependence in the data that cannot be overlooked and justifies the use of MLM.

It is easiest to understand multilevel models if one looks at the levels separately. In the cross-sectional model for dyads, Level 1 provides the *within*-couple model, in which individual responses are nested within couples, while Level 2 provides the *between*-couples model. (Examining the structure of the data for the two levels, as required by the software program HLM, can help one better understand the distinction between these levels; see Figs. 20.1 and 20.2; Raudenbush, Bryk, & Congdon, 2004.) In (20.1) of the unconditional model, the intercept, β_{0j}, represents the average outcome score for each couple, and r_{ij} represents the deviation of each member of the couple from the couple average. This intercept is treated as randomly varying; that is, it is allowed to take on different values for each couple. The intercepts that are estimated for each couple are treated as an outcome variable at Level 2. The intercept in the Level-2 equation, (20.2), γ_{00}, provides an estimate of the average outcome score across couples and u_{0j} represents the deviation of each couple from the overall average across all couples.

Level 1 (*within* couples):

$$Y_{ij} = \beta_{0j} + r_{ij}, \tag{20.1}$$

Level 2 (*between* couples):

$$\beta_{0j} = \gamma_{00} + u_{0j}, \tag{20.2}$$

	FAMILYID	lesbian	PrivAdop	PubAdopt	IntAdopt
1	1	1	1	0	0
2	2	1	1	0	0
3	3	1	0	0	1
4	4	1	1	0	0
5	5	1	1	0	0
6	6	1	0	1	0
7	7	1	0	0	1
8	8	1	1	0	0

Fig. 20.2   Example of a Level-2 (between couples) data file for the analysis of cross-sectional dyadic data

where Y_{ij} represents the outcome score of partner i in dyad j, where $i = 1, 2$ for the two members of the dyad. In addition to the above "fixed effect" estimates (e.g., the γ_{00}'s), estimates of the variance of the "random effects" both within and between couples are provided (e.g., the variance of the r_{ij}'s and the u_{0j}'s), as well as the covariance between partners. Predictors can then be added to the model, with those that vary within couples (e.g., partners' ages) added at Level 1:

$$Y_{ij} = \beta_{0j} + \beta_{1j}(\text{Age})_{ij} + r_{ij}, \qquad (20.3)$$

and those that vary between couples (e.g., duration of time in a relationship together) added at Level 2:

$$\beta_{0j} = \gamma_{00} + \gamma_{01}(\text{Duration}) + u_{0j}. \qquad (20.4)$$

We can add a variable at Level 2 that provides us with a way to tease out important group differences in the couple averages, such as the type of couple. For example, in Abbie Goldberg's research on lesbian, gay male, and heterosexual adoptive couples, this multilevel modeling approach is used to provide estimates of means for each group (on reports of love, conflict, and ambivalence), as well as to test for differences in these means (Goldberg, Smith, & Kashy, 2010).

To examine group means, a dichotomous variable is created that indicates the type of couple (e.g., gay male or heterosexual), which is then entered at Level 2. The intercept provides the mean level of the outcome for the reference group (lesbian, in this case), while the coefficient for the predictor (e.g., gay male) indicates the difference between that group and the reference group.

Considering Partner Effects

Personal relationship theory, which examines the predictors, processes, and outcomes of close relationships, has shown the importance of considering the role of partner characteristics in dyadic research (Kenny & Cook, 1999). It may not be immediately evident how such a model can be used to examine partner effects — that is, the association between one partner's predictor with the other partner's outcome score. It is helpful to think of these associations within the context of the Actor–Partner Interdependence Model (APIM; Campbell & Kashy, 2002; Cook & Kenny, 2005). Using this approach, one simultaneously considers the respondent's value on a predictor such as age as well as the respondent's partner's value in relationship to the outcome. For example, Fergus, Lewis, Darbes, and Kral (2009) found that in examining the HIV risk of gay men ($N = 59$ couples), it was important to consider not only individuals' own integration into the gay community but also their partners' integration. In the MLM approach, both of these predictors are entered into the model at Level 1 (Kenny et al., 2006).

Level 1 (within couples):

$$Y_{ij} = \beta_{0j} + \beta_{1j}(\text{Actor Race})_{ij} \\ + \beta_{2j}(\text{Partner Race}) \; ij + r_{ij}, \quad (20.5)$$

Level 2 (between couples):

$$\beta_{0j} = \gamma_{00} + u_{0j} \\ \beta_{1j} = \gamma_{10} + u_{1j} \quad (20.6) \\ \beta_{2j} = \gamma_{20} + u_{2j}.$$

The APIM model goes further, however, suggesting that it is necessary not only to consider both actor and partner characteristics as main effects but also to consider the interaction between them. This models the specific pairing of the two individuals in the couple. For example, the effect of parents' disciplinary style on the child's behavior may vary as a function of their partners' disciplinary style. In such a case, it would be important to test an interaction between actors' disciplinary style and partners' disciplinary style. Whenever the theoretical framework guiding the analyses and past research suggest the potential importance of such an interaction, and sample size permits its inclusion, it is crucial that the interaction term be included (Cook & Kenny, 2005).

Recent work in personal relationship theory has extended the APIM approach to specifically address the role of gender and sexual orientation (particularly in the area of partner preferences; West et al., 2008). West et al. (2008) argue for the need to include lesbian and gay male couples in research on the effects of partner gender. In addition, they contend that both actor gender and partner gender should be considered in analyses that examine data from both heterosexual (distinguishable) and same-sex (indistinguishable) couples.

While they applaud the increasing work that includes all three of the above types of couples (e.g., Bailey, Kim, Hills, & Linsenmeier, 1997; Kurdek, 1997; Kurdek & Schmitt, 1986a, 1986b; Regan, Medina, & Joshi, 2001), they express regret that the analyses performed are too often limited to looking at differences among the three groups and do not include analyses that consider the effect of partner gender in conjunction with the actor's gender. They propose what they term a "factorial method" that considers respondent gender, partner gender, and "dyad gender" (i.e., the difference between same-gendered and different-gendered respondents, where dyad gender is the interaction between actor and partner gender). Examining group differences between lesbian, gay, and heterosexual couples without taking into account the gender differences within heterosexual couples may lead to an inadequate understanding of the data, as it conflates the scores for men and women within heterosexual couples. West and colleagues provide an example in which findings from a group difference approach (i.e., looking only at differences between lesbian, gay male, and heterosexual couples) showed that lesbian and gay male couples placed less importance on the social value of a partner (e.g., appeal to friends, similar social class background, financial worth) than heterosexual couples ($N = 784$ lesbian, 969 gay male, and 4,292 heterosexual couples). When within-dyad gender differences are taken into account, however, the results showed that it was not that lesbians and gay men placed less emphasis on the social value of a partner than heterosexuals, but that heterosexual *women* placed much more emphasis on the social value of a partner than gay men and heterosexual men, with lesbians placing slightly more emphasis on social value than gay men.

Examining Change Over Time in Indistinguishable Dyads

To get a better grasp of longitudinal multilevel models for dyadic data, it is useful to understand how change is modeled in a basic (non-dyadic) multilevel model. The cross-sectional approach to dyads addressed individuals nested within dyads, modeling individuals at Level 1 and couples at Level 2. When examining change over time, we are looking at multiple time points nested within each individual. Level 1 models change within individuals, while Level 2 models differences in change between individuals. There are essentially two MLM approaches to modeling change over time within dyads: (a) a 2-level model in which trajectories of change for both dyad members are modeled at Level 1, while between-dyad differences in change are modeled at Level 2 (Raudenbush et al., 1995), and (b) a 3-level model in which change over time within each individual is modeled at Level 1, individuals within dyads at Level 2, and between-dyad differences at Level 3 (Atkins, 2005; Christensen, Atkins, Yi, Baucom, & George, 2006; Kurdek, 1998, 2008; Simpson, Atkins, Gattis, & Christensen, 2008).

While conceptually, the 3-level approach might appear to make perfect sense, there is a statistical problem in terms of the random effects. That is, while it is a 3-level model in terms of the data structure, it is only a 2-level model in terms of the within-level variation. Consequently, most articles on dyadic multilevel modeling recommend the 2-level approach (Bolger & Shrout, 2007; Raudenbush et al., 1995; Sayer & Klute, 2005). Even proponents of the 3-level model admit to a reduction in power and related changes in findings when using this model in comparison to the 2-level model most commonly used for distinguishable dyads (Atkins, 2005). Recently, Deborah Kashy has developed an extension of the 2-level multilevel model generally used to examine change in distinguishable dyads, which can be applied in the case of indistinguishable dyads (Kashy et al., 2008). While Kashy's initial work was on twin research, more recent work has extended the use of this model to lesbian and gay male parents (Goldberg et al., 2010; Goldberg & Smith, 2009a, 2011). For example, in a study of lesbian, gay male, and heterosexual adoptive parents, this approach was used to examine preadoptive factors on relationship quality (love, conflict, and ambivalence) across the transition to adoptive parenthood (Goldberg et al., 2010; $N=44$ lesbian,

30 gay male, and 51 heterosexual couples). Parents who reported higher levels of depression, greater use of avoidant coping, lower levels of relationship maintenance behaviors, and less satisfaction with their adoption agencies before adoption reported lower relationship quality at the time of the adoption. The effect of avoidant coping on relationship quality varied by gender. The use of a longitudinal model enabled them to examine change in relationship quality across this transition as well: Parents who reported higher levels of depression, greater use of confrontative coping, and higher levels of relationship maintenance behaviors prior to the adoption reported greater declines in relationship quality.

The longitudinal model for indistinguishable dyads is very similar to the distinguishable dyad model in which trajectories for both dyad members are modeled at Level 1, with separate intercepts and slopes modeled for each member of the dyad (Raudenbush et al., 1995). The two partners' intercepts are allowed to covary, as are their rates of change (slopes). Due to the inability to distinguish between dyad members, however, parameter estimates for the average intercept and average slope (the fixed effects) are pooled across partners as well as dyads (Kashy et al., 2008). In addition, drawing from approaches to modeling indistinguishable dyads in structural equation modeling (Olsen & Kenny, 2006; Woody & Sadler, 2005), this approach constrains the estimates of variance to be equal for partners. Similar to the distinguishable model, two (redundant) dummy variables, $P1$ and $P2$, are used to systematically differentiate between the two partners. In other words, if the outcome score is from partner 1, $P1=1$, and otherwise $P1=0$, and if the outcome score is from partner 2, $P2=1$, and otherwise $P2=0$. At Level 1 of the model (in which there are no predictors aside from Time), an intercept and slope for time for each partner is modeled:

Level 1 (within couples):

$$Y_{ijk} = \beta_{01j}(P1) + \beta_{11j}(P1 \times \text{Time})_{1jk} \\ + \beta_{02j}(P2) + \beta_{12j}(P2 \times \text{Time})_{2jk} \quad (20.7) \\ + r_{ijk},$$

where Y_{ijk} represents the outcome score of partner i in dyad j at time k, and $i = 1, 2$ for the two members of the dyad.

In this model, intercepts and slopes can vary both within and between dyads. The inability to distinguish between dyad members would make it meaningless to have separate parameter estimates for member 1 and member 2; therefore the parameter estimates for the fixed effects are aggregated across dyad members. In the Level-1 equation (20.7), β_{01j} and β_{02j} represent the intercepts, for partner 1 and 2 in couple j, and estimate the level of depressive or anxious symptoms at the time of the adoption. Likewise, β_{11j} and β_{12j} represent the slopes for the two partners. These slopes estimate the change in the outcome over time. Unlike the distinguishable model, however, the intercepts and slopes are then pooled into only two Level-2 equations.

Level 2 (between couples):

$$\beta_{0ij} = \gamma_{00} + u_{0ij}$$
$$\beta_{1ij} = \gamma_{10} + u_{1ij}. \tag{20.8}$$

As these two equations show, the intercepts are pooled not only between but also *within* dyads (i.e., across both i and j) to estimate the fixed effect, γ_{00}, which is the average intercept (or the average level of the outcome when Time=0), and similarly, the slopes for time are pooled both between and within dyads to estimate the average slope, γ_{10} (or the average rate of change in the outcome across all partners).

The variance components are also pooled both between and *within* dyads. At Level 2, the variance in the intercept, Var(u_{0ij}), represents the variability in the outcome at the time of the adoptive placement, and the variance in the slopes, Var(u_{1ij}), represents the variability in how depressive or anxious symptoms change over time. The third variance component, Var(r_{ijk}), is the variance of the Level-1 residuals (or the difference between the observed values of the outcome and the predicted values from the fitted trajectories). The variance of the Level-1 residuals is constrained to be equal for both partners and across all time points. In addition to the variances, several

covariances commonly estimated in dyadic growth models are also included in this model. For example, the covariance between the two slopes estimating change for each person uniquely shows the degree of similarity in partners' patterns of change.[1]

Considerations When Modeling Change Over Time

When modeling change, the reliability of the change trajectories will be greatly improved with a greater number of assessment points (Raudenbush & Bryk, 2002; Willett, 1989). In addition, the use of more assessment points allows researchers to examine more complex patterns of change. For example, research on heterosexual-parent couples has shown relationship quality and many mental health outcomes such as depression to follow curvilinear trajectories particularly across the transition to parenthood (Perry-Jenkins, Goldberg, Pierce, & Sayer, 2007). Such patterns cannot be captured with only three time points.

While more time points are preferable, it is possible to fit the change models to examine change between two time points. Goldberg and Smith (2009a) used this approach to examine changes in perceived parenting skill in lesbian, gay male, and heterosexual adoptive couples after the adoption of their first child. Examination of change between only two time points is essentially a difference score. While not ideal, the use of multilevel modeling to generate difference scores provides better estimates of change than observed difference scores, as it provides a correction for

---

[1] In addition to the variances, Kashy et al.'s (2008) model for analyzing longitudinal data from indistinguishable dyads provides estimates for several covariances. Dyadic growth models often include three covariances. First, the covariance between the intercepts estimates the degree of similarity in partners' outcome scores when Time=0. Second, the covariance between the slopes estimates the degree of similarity in partners' patterns of change. Third, a time-specific covariance assesses the similarity in the two partners' outcome scores at each time point after controlling for all of the predictors in the model.

Two additional covariances are estimated using Kashy et al.'s (2008) approach. An intrapersonal covariance between the intercept and slope can be estimated to examine, for example, if having higher depressive symptoms at

measurement error. For an example in the distinguishable case, see Goldberg and Sayer's (2006) examination of change in relationship quality in 29 lesbian inseminating couples across the transition to parenthood.

Additional data preparation is necessary to estimate change between two time points. With only two time points at Level 1, there would be too few degrees of freedom to estimate two fixed effects (an intercept and rate of change) and the residual or error around the fitted regression line, unless additional information on the outcome was available and introduced into the modeling procedure. This additional information can be provided, however, by dividing the outcome measure into two parallel scales with comparable variance and reliability, allowing for the estimation of error (Raudenbush et al., 1995; Sayer & Klute, 2005).[2] In addition, the use of parallel scales provides a limited measurement component to the multilevel model and consequently a somewhat more accurate measure of both error and latent change scores. Future research, however, is needed to examine the reliability of the estimates for change from such models.

---

the time of adoption is related to greater increases in depressive symptoms over time. An interpersonal covariance between the intercept and slope can also be estimated to examine, for example, if partners of individuals with high initial stress experience greater increases in stress over time. As some software such as SPSS does not allow for estimation of these covariances, these are not always included in the models (Goldberg & Smith, 2009a, 2011; Goldberg et al., 2010). As these covariance estimates are less important, and less likely to affect findings, the use of models without them may well be adequate for most research. In fact, identical patterns of results have been found with and without the covariance constraints in the existing published literature (Goldberg & Smith, 2009a, 2011; Goldberg et al., 2010).

Note that the software program HLM does not allow for either variances or covariances to be constrained.

[2]Parallel scales are generally created based on the items variance. First, the variances of all of the items in the scale are determined. The items are then assigned to each of the two scales on the basis of their variance. In other words, the item with the most variance would be assigned to scale A. The item with the second highest variance would go in scale B. The item with the third highest variance would also go in scale B. The items with the next highest variance would go in scale A, as would the next, and so forth.

Multiple Informants

In family research, one often attains multiple reports of the same outcomes. For example, a researcher examining the behavior of children of lesbian mothers may have both mothers report on the child's behavior. While structural equation modeling provides the best available method of handling data from multiple reporters, multilevel modeling may also be used to examine these data. By using reports from both parents, researchers can introduce a limited measurement component to the model. While this is a new area for LGBT research, it is a growing area in family research. A particularly interesting study was conducted by Georgiades et al. (2008), who used MLM to examine reports of family functioning gathered from multiple family members ($N=26,614$ individuals in 11,023 families). While using reports from multiple members of the family provided a better measure of family functioning, the use of MLM enabled the researchers to distinguish shared perceptions of family functioning from unique individual perceptions, as well as to examine predictors of these perceptions.

Dyadic models such as those presented in this paper can also be employed to examine reports from multiple informants. In the simplest application, MLM can provide a composite score across multiple reporters, as well as provide a measure of the degree of association between dyad members' reports. This approach was used by Meteyer and Perry-Jenkins (2010) to examine change in fathers' involvement in child care across the transition to parenthood in a sample of 98 heterosexual couples. The authors used a multilevel model with a single intercept and slope at Level 1 for each couple. This provided a composite estimate of the level of father involvement and the rate of change in involvement, based on both fathers' and mothers' reports of father involvement.

As an example, predictors of gay fathers' reports of their child's school involvement—an area that has received no scholarly attention—could be modeled using the indistinguishable models presented earlier in this chapter. In the dyadic, cross-sectional model, the composite score for the dyad (dyad average) would be represented by the Level-1 intercept. MLM estimates the covariance between the fathers' scores, indicating the strength of the relationship between fathers' reports. Recall that in the MLM models, variance in the reports is partitioned into two sources: that which lies *between* dyads and that which lies *within* dyads. Researchers gain a better understanding of how much is within the dyads and hence between the two individuals who are reporting. Finally, couple-level predictors (e.g., relationship length, family income, number of children) of this composite could be entered at Level 2. Predictors of individual reports could be introduced at Level 1 (i.e., within couples).

With distinguishable dyads, the two-intercept model makes it easy to examine differential predictors of the two respondents' reports. For example, in the case of parent and child reports of child well-being, the model would include separate estimates for child reports and parent reports at Level 1. Predictors, such as family income, would be entered at Level 2. This model provides separate parameter estimates for the effect of income on parents' and children's reports. It is then possible to test whether these estimates are statistically different by constraining the two estimates to be the same and conducting model comparison tests (as discussed early in the section on distinguishability). This approach was used by Kuo and colleagues (Kuo, Mohler, Raudenbush, & Earls, 2000) to examine the relationship between demographic risk factors and reports of children's exposure to violence (*N*=1,880 children and 1,776 parents). The researchers also used the traditional method of conducting analyses separately on fathers' and children's reports and found the results for individual parameter estimates to be very similar. However, it is only possible to statistically test for the differences between informants using the MLM approach, as the two reports must be modeled simultaneously.

Conducting similar analyses is not feasible using the indistinguishable model, as that model does not provide separate parameter estimates of the effects of a couple-level (Level 2) predictor on the two partners' reports (as the two partners are not distinguished). The APIM model could, however, be used to examine differential effects of characteristics that vary for individuals. For example, one could examine the effects of individuals' own characteristics and their partners' characteristics on individuals' reports.

An alternate approach for distinguishable dyads is to examine discrepancies between the reports of the two dyad members (Lyons, Zarit, Sayer, & Whitlach, 2002). Coley and Morris (2002) use this approach to examine discrepancies in mothers' and fathers' reports of father involvement in 228 low-income families. Specifically, reports of the outcome are regressed onto dummy indicators for the mother (−0.5) and father (0.5).

$$Y_{ij} = \beta_{0j} + \beta_{1j}(\text{indicator}) + r_{ij}. \quad (20.9)$$

In this model, the intercept represents the *average* of the two parents' reports of father involvement, and the slope represents the *discrepancy* between the two reports, as there is exactly 1.0 unit between indicators. Predictors for the average and the discrepancy can then be added at Level 2. Coley and Morris (2002) found that parental conflict, fathers' nonresidence, and fathers' age, as well as mothers' education and employment, predicted larger discrepancies between fathers' and mothers' reports. Use of the discrepancy approach, however, requires the ability to differentiate between dyad members.

Examining reports from multiple informants is just one of the areas in which there have been recent advances in MLM approaches to dyadic data analysis. Other areas include the dyadic analysis of diary data (Bolger & Shrout, 2007), issues in interpreting cross-level interactions in dyadic models (West et al., 2008), and the use of simulations to conduct accurate power analyses for complex MLM (and SEM) models such as those for dyads (Muthén & Muthén, 2002).

Limitations of Dyadic Multilevel Modeling

Limitations Due to Small Number Per Family

While multilevel modeling provides a useful method for examining family data, it also has important limitations. Most importantly, MLM is a large sample statistical approach; it is at its best when examining a large number of groups (like families) with a large number of individuals per group. Having too few groups or too few individuals per group (as with dyads) presents a power issue as there is not enough information to reliably detect effects and can lead to a lack of precision in certain parameter estimates (Maas & Hox, 2005; Raudenbush, 2008).

Number of Families Required

Given the limited number of individuals in families and dyads, a large number of groups (at least 100) are required to obtain accurate estimates of the fixed effects, such as the intercept, rate of change and the predictors, as well as their standard errors (Raudenbush, 2008). While there are alternative estimation procedures that provide more accurate estimates when there are a small number of groups at highest level (Level 2 for the models presented here) with many people per group, these cannot address the problem of the small number of individuals per dyad.

While having a sample of at least 100 dyads will provide accurate parameter estimates of the fixed effects and their standard errors, other parameter estimates lack precision due to the small number of individuals per dyad: specifically the estimates of the Level-2 variance components may be inaccurate (e.g., the amount of variability between dyads; Raudenbush, 2008). Consequently, researchers should not rely on statistical tests regarding the amount of variability when deciding whether or not to enter predictors into their model. In addition, the MLM estimates of individual scores for each dyad (the estimated Bayesian coefficients) are unreliable. This is of greatest concern with cross-sectional models, as well-fitting longitudinal models with assessments across multiple time points allow for more accurate estimation.

Noncontinuous Outcomes

Another important limitation to having a small number of individuals per family or dyad is that these models should only be applied to the analysis of continuous outcomes (Raudenbush, 2008). When examining outcomes that are not continuously distributed, such as categorical or count data, MLM cannot provide accurate estimates when there are only a few number of individuals per group, even if there are a large number of these small groups. When there are a large number of dyads, SEM would be the preferred approach to analyzing dichotomous or count data (or any other outcome which requires a link function to transform the outcome into a normal distribution). Unfortunately, there are no published studies comparing the reliability of estimates provided using different approaches (e.g., MLM, cluster-adjusted standard errors, SEM) to dealing with the dependence of dyadic data in the face of small sample sizes. Consequently, it is unclear which approaches should be recommended to researchers confronting these problems.

The Same Number of Individuals Per Family

A limitation specific to dyadic (or triadic) MLM models is the need to have the same number of individuals in each family. While the basic organizational, cross-sectional model can be used to examine reports from a variable number of family members, such as families with different numbers of siblings, dyadic models are more restricted. Dyadic models are designed to examine pairs of individuals. This limitation means that you can only analyze data in which there are two reporters from each family (although the data from some of the second reporters can be missing). Consequently, the dyadic model precludes the analysis of data from both coupled and single parents. For example, the longitudinal model for indistinguishable dyads could not be used to examine a sample of lesbian parents that included both single and coupled lesbian mothers. While the dyadic models for indistinguishable dyads can easily handle couple data, they cannot accommodate a combination of coupled and single parents. Note that examining outcomes from both single and coupled parents is distinct from examining data from couples and having missing data from some partners. While multilevel modeling can accommodate missing data on the outcome, it assumes that these data are missing at random (MAR).

Future Directions

While there have been many important recent advances in the use of MLM (and SEM) for the analysis of dyadic data, particularly in the indistinguishable case, much more work is needed. To better understand the strengths and limitations of these models, studies are needed to examine the extent to which estimates may be affected by the small number of members per dyad. Currently, the smallest within-group size examined in the published literature contained 5 individuals per group, while dyads only have 2 individuals per group (Maas & Hox, 2005). While MLM has become the norm for dyadic data analysis, some researchers contend that the lack of precision in the estimates of the standard errors is sufficient to call the entire approach into question; these researchers tend to prefer the use of SEM approaches to dyadic data. In the absence of additional studies in this area, researchers may best be guided by the guidelines that Raudenbush (2008) presents in his chapter, "Many Small Groups." Raudenbush clearly articulates when MLM approaches to examining small groups such as families and dyads are appropriate (i.e., a large number of groups, continuous outcomes, focus on fixed effects), and where specific applications are inappropriate (i.e., small number of groups, dichotomous or count outcomes, a focus on Level-2 random effects, estimated Bayesian coefficients for individuals).

Given that a great deal of research on LGBT parents and families is conducted on samples with fewer than 100 families, MLM modeling (and SEM) will not provide an appropriate method to address the questions of many researchers. There is great need for a clear articulation of the most appropriate methods for dealing with the dependent data in small samples. While Raudenbush (2008) clearly explains the limitations of MLM approaches to examining small groups such as families and dyads, he fails to indicate appropriate alternative approaches where MLM is not appropriate. While there are good recent papers introducing multilevel modeling approaches to dyadic data (e.g., Atkins, 2005; Kashy et al., 2008; Sayer & Klute, 2005), as well as general recommendations for researchers gathering dyadic data (Ackerman, Donnellan, & Kashy, 2011), there is a need for a paper on the state-of-the-art practices for examining such data in small samples.

While there are still many areas requiring further development in the application of multilevel modeling to the examination of family data, the most important need in the area of LGBT research is the need to make existing methods more available to researchers. To use MLM approaches to dyadic data analysis, researchers must learn both the basics of MLM and the ins and outs of dyadic models. While multilevel modeling is increasingly being taught in departments such as family studies, human development, and psychology, training is still unavailable to students in many programs. Most researchers who study LGBT couples, parents, and families will need to seek out training beyond the courses they were offered in their graduate program. There are training workshops in MLM available across the country (see Appendix A for current programs offering dyadic workshops using MLM). Only a small number of these, however, specifically address approaches for dyads in which members are indistinguishable (most notably David Kenny's workshop). There are however many useful resources available on the web (see Appendix B).

If researchers who study LGBT couples, parents, and families are unable to employ the statistical methods appropriate for their data and research questions, it hinders the development of the field. Researchers who are unfamiliar with the appropriate statistical methods to analyze their data are unable to publish, particularly in the leading journals in fields such as family studies, psychology, and others. In addition, they are often unable to capitalize on the richness of their datasets. Currently, the greatest need in this area is to provide statistical training in methods such as multilevel modeling to junior and senior researchers and to facilitate collaborations between LGBT researchers who lack this training and both established and emerging methodologists in the field of dyadic data analysis.

Appendix A. Organizations Providing Workshops on Multilevel (and Other) Modeling Approaches to Dyadic Data Analysis

Data Analysis Training Institute of Connecticut (DATIC; U of Connecticut) http://datic.uconn.edu/

Center for Research on Families (U of Mass) http://www.umass.edu/family/methodology

ICPSR Summer Program in Quantitative Methods of Social Research (U of Michigan) http://www.icpsr.umich.edu/icpsrweb/content/sumprog/about.html

Note: Many of the foremost scholars in the field of dyadic data analysis have offered workshops through the above or other institutions (e.g., David Kenny, Deborah Kashy, Nial Bolger, Jean-Philippe Laurenceau, and Aline Sayer).

Appendix B. Online Resources for Dyadic Data Analysis

Overview of Dyadic Data Analysis http://www.davidakenny.net/dyad.htm

Materials and Syntax to Accompany Kenny et al. (2006), Dyadic Data Analysis http://www.davidakenny.net/kkc/kkc.htm

Introductory Materials on Dyadic Data Analysis http://www.umass.edu/family/methodology/ncfr.htm

Videos Introducing Dyadic Analysis and Explaining Dyadic Modelling Approaches by Bolger and Laurenceau http://methodology.psu.edu/training/mcsi10media

Mulilevel Listserv http://www.nursing.manchester.ac.uk/learning/staff/mcampbell/multilevel.html

References

Ackerman, R. A., Donnellan, M., & Kashy, D. A. (2011). Working with dyadic data in studies of emerging adulthood: Specific recommendations, general advice, and practical tips. In F. D. Fincham & M. Cui (Eds.), *Romantic relationships in emerging adulthood* (pp. 67–97). New York, NY: Cambridge University Press.

Atkins, D. (2005). Using multilevel models to analyze couple and family treatment data: Basic and advanced issues. *Journal of Family Psychology, 19*, 86–97. doi:10.1037/0893-3200.19.1.98

Atkins, D. C., Klann, N., Marín, R. A., Lo, T. Y., & Hahlweg, K. (2010). Outcomes of couples with infidelity in a community-based sample of couple therapy. *Journal of Family Psychology, 24*, 212–216. doi:10.1037/a0018789

Bailey, J., Kim, P. Y., Hills, A., & Linsenmeier, J. W. (1997). Butch, femme, or straight acting? Partner preferences of gay men and lesbians. *Journal of Personality and Social Psychology, 73*, 960–973. doi:10.1037/0022-3514.73.5.960

Barnett, R. C., Marshall, N. L., Raudenbush, S. W., & Brennan, R. T. (1993). Gender and the relationship between job experiences and psychological distress: A study of dual-earner couples. *Journal of Personality and Social Psychology, 64*, 794–806. doi:10.1037/0022-3514.64.5.794

Bengtson, V. L., & Allen, K. R. (1993). The life course perspective applied to families over time. In P. G. Boss, W. J. Doherty, R. LaRossa, W. R. Schumm, S. & K. Steinmetz (Eds.), *Sourcebook of family theories and methods: A contextual approach* (pp. 469–504). New York, NY: Plenum Press.

Bolger, N., & Shrout, P. E. (2007). Accounting for statistical dependency in longitudinal data on dyads. In T. D. Little, J. A. Bovaird, & N. A. Card (Eds.), *Modeling contextual effects in longitudinal studies* (pp. 285–298). Mahwah, NJ: Lawrence Erlbaum Associates.

Brincks, A. M., Feaster, D. J., & Mitrani, V. B. (2010). A multilevel mediation model of stress and coping for women with HIV and their families. *Family Process, 49*, 517–529. doi:10.1111/j.1545-5300.2010.01337.x

Bronfenbrenner, U. (1988). Interacting systems in human development. In N. Bolger, A. Caspi, G. Downey, & M. Moorehouse (Eds.), *Persons in context: Developmental processes* (pp. 25–49). New York, NY: Cambridge University Press.

Campbell, L. J., & Kashy, D. A. (2002). Estimating actor, partner, and interaction effects for dyadic data using PROC MIXED and HLM5: A user-friendly guide.

Personal Relationships, 9, 327–342. doi:10.1111/1475-6811.00023

Christensen, A., Atkins, D. C., Yi, J., Baucom, D. H., & George, W. H. (2006). Couple and individual adjustment for 2 years following a randomized clinical trial comparing traditional versus integrative behavioral couple therapy. *Journal of Consulting and Clinical Psychology, 74,* 1180–1191. doi:10.1037/0022-006X.74.6.1180

Claxton, A., O'Rourke, N., Smith, J. Z., & DeLongis, A. (2012). Personality traits and marital satisfaction within enduring relationships: An intra-couple concurrence and discrepancy approach. *Journal of Social and Personal Relationships, 29,* 375–396.

Coley, R., & Morris, J. (2002). Comparing father and mother reports of father involvement among low-income minority families. *Journal of Marriage and Family, 64,* 982–997. doi:10.1111/j.1741-3737.2002.00982.x

Cook, W. L., & Kenny, D. A. (2005). The actor-partner interdependence model: A model of directional effects in developmental studies. *International Journal of Behavioral Development, 29,* 101–109. doi:10.1080/01650250444000405

Cox, M. J., & Paley, B. (1997). Families as systems. *Annual Review of Psychology, 48,* 243–267. doi:10.1146/annurev.psych.48.1.243

Fergus, S., Lewis, M. A., Darbes, L. A., & Kral, A. H. (2009). Social support moderates the relationship between gay community integration and sexual risk behavior among gay male couples. *Health Education & Behavior, 36,* 846–859. doi:10.1177/1090198108319891

Georgiades, K., Boyle, M. H., Jenkins, J. M., Sanford, M., & Lipman, E. (2008). A multilevel analysis of whole family functioning using the McMaster family assessment device. *Journal of Family Psychology, 22,* 344–354. doi:10.1037/0893-3200.22.3.344

Goldberg, A. E. (2010). *Lesbian and gay parents and their children: Research on the family life cycle.* Washington, DC: American Psychological Association

Goldberg, A. E., & Perry-Jenkins, M. (2007). The division of labor and perceptions of parental roles: Lesbian couples across the transition to parenthood. *Journal of Social and Personal Relationships, 24,* 297–318. doi:10.1177/0265407507075415

Goldberg, A. E., & Sayer, A. G. (2006). Lesbian couples' relationship quality across the transition to parenthood. *Journal of Marriage and Family, 68,* 87–100. doi:10.1111/j.1741-3737.2006.00235.x

Goldberg, A. E., & Smith, J. Z. (2008a). The social context of lesbian mothers' anxiety during early parenthood. *Parenting: Science & Practice, 8,* 213–239. doi:10.1080/15295190802204801

Goldberg, A. E., & Smith, J. Z. (2008b). Social support and well-being in lesbian and heterosexual preadoptive couples. *Family Relations, 57,* 281–291. doi:10.1111/j.1741-3729.2008.00500.x

Goldberg, A. E., & Smith, J. Z. (2009a). Perceived parenting skill across the transition to adoptive parenthood: A study of lesbian, gay and heterosexual couples.

Journal of Family Psychology, 23, 861–870. doi:10.1037/a0017009

Goldberg, A. E., & Smith, J. Z. (2009b). Predicting non-African American lesbian and heterosexual preadoptive couples' openness to adopting an African American child. *Family Relations, 58,* 346–360. doi:10.1111/j.1741-3729.2009.00557.x

Goldberg, A. E., & Smith, J. Z. (2011). Stigma, support and mental health: Lesbian and gay male couples across the transition parenthood. *Journal of Counseling Psychology, 58,* 139–150. doi:10.1037/a0021684

Goldberg, A. E., Smith, J. Z., & Kashy, D. (2010). Preadoptive factors predicting lesbian, gay and heterosexual couples relationship quality across the transition parenthood. *Journal of Family Psychology, 24,* 221–232. doi:10.1037/a0019615

Griffin, D., & Gonzalez, R. (1995). Correlational analysis of dyad-level data in the exchangeable case. *Psychological Bulletin, 118,* 430–439. doi:10.1037/0033-2909.118.3.430

Jenkins, J. M., Cheung, C., Frampton, K., Rasbash, J., Boyle, M. H., & Georgiades, K. (2009). The use of multilevel modeling for the investigation of family process. *European Journal of Developmental Science, 3,* 131–149.

Kashy, D. A., Donnellan, M. B., Burt, S. A., & McGue, M. (2008). Growth curve models for indistinguishable dyads using multilevel modeling and structural equation modeling: The case of adolescent twins' conflict with their mothers. *Developmental Psychology, 44,* 316–329. doi:10.1037/0012-1649.44.2.316

Kashy, D. A., & Kenny, D. A. (2000). The analysis of data from dyads and groups. In H. Reis & C. M. Judd (Eds.), *Handbook of research methods in social psychology* (pp. 451–477). New York, NY: Cambridge University Press

Kenny, D. A., & Cook, W. (1999). Partner effects in relationship research: Conceptual issues, analytic difficulties, and illustrations. *Personal Relationships, 6,* 433–448. doi:10.1111/j.1475-6811.1999.tb00202.x

Kenny, D. A., & Judd, C. M. (1986). Consequences of violating the independence assumption in analysis of variance. *Psychological Bulletin, 99,* 422–431. doi:10.1037/0033-2909.99.3.422

Kenny, D., Kashy, D., & Cook, W. (2006). *Dyadic data analysis.* New York, NY: Guilford Press

Kenny, D. A., & Ledermann, T. (2010). Detecting, measuring, and testing dyadic patterns in the actor–partner interdependence model. *Journal of Family Psychology, 24,* 359–366. doi:10.1037/a0019651

Kretschmer, T., & Pike, A. (2010). Associations between adolescent siblings' relationship quality and similarity and differences in values. *Journal of Family Psychology, 24,* 411–418. doi:10.1037/a0020060

Kuo, M., Mohler, B., Raudenbush, S. L., & Earls, F. J. (2000). Assessing exposure to violence using multiple informants: Application of hierarchical linear model. *Journal of Child Psychology and Psychiatry, 41,* 1049–1056. doi:10.1111/1469-7610.00692

Kurdek, L. A. (1997). The link between facets of neuroticism and dimensions of relationship commitment:

Evidence from gay, lesbian, and heterosexual couples. *Journal of Family Psychology, 11,* 503–514. doi:10.1037/0893-3200.11.4.503

Kurdek, L. A. (1998). Relationship outcomes and their predictors: Longitudinal evidence from heterosexual married, gay cohabiting, and lesbian cohabiting couples. *Journal of Marriage and the Family, 60,* 553–568. doi:10.2307/353528

Kurdek, L. A. (2003). Differences between gay and lesbian cohabiting couples. *Journal of Social and Personal Relationships, 20,* 411–436. doi:10.1177/02654075030204001

Kurdek, L. A. (2008). Change in relationship quality for partners from lesbian, gay male, and heterosexual couples. *Journal of Family Psychology, 22,* 701–711. doi:10.1037/0893-3200.22.5.701

Kurdek, L. A., & Schmitt, J. P. (1986a). Interaction of sex role self-concept with relationship quality and relationship beliefs in married, heterosexual cohabiting, gay, and lesbian couples. *Journal of Personality and Social Psychology, 51,* 365–370. doi:10.1037/0022-3514.51.2.365

Kurdek, L. A., & Schmitt, J. P. (1986b). Relationship quality of partners in heterosexual married, heterosexual cohabitating, and gay and lesbian relationships. *Journal of Personality and Social Psychology, 51,* 711–720. doi:10.1037/0022-3514.51.4.711

Lyons, K. S., Zarit, S. H., Sayer, A. G., & Whitlach, C. J. (2002). Caregiving as a dyadic process: Perspectives from caregiver and receiver. *Journal of Gerontology: Psychological Sciences, 57B,* 195–204.

Maas, C. J. M., & Hox, J. J. (2005). Sufficient sample size for multilevel modeling. *Methodology, 1,* 86–92. doi:10.1027/1614-2241.1.3.86

Meteyer, K., & Perry-Jenkins, M. (2010). Father involvement among working-class, dual-earner couples. *Fathering: A Journal of Theory, Research, & Practice about Men as Fathers, 8,* 379–403.

Muthén, L. K., & Muthén, B. O. (2002). How to use a Monte Carlo study to decide on sample size and determine power. *Structural Equation Modeling, 9,* 599–620. doi:10.1207/S15328007SEM0904_8

O'Rourke, N., Kupferschmidt, A. L., Claxton, A., Smith, J. Z., Chappell, N., & Beattie, B. L. (2010). Psychological resilience predicts depressive symptoms among spouses of persons with Alzheimer disease over time. *Aging and Mental Health, 14,* 984–993. doi:10.1080/13607863.2010.501063

Olsen, J. A., & Kenny, D. A. (2006). Structural equation modeling with interchangeable dyads. *Psychological Methods, 11,* 127–141. doi:10.1037/1082-989X.11.2.127

Papp, L. M., Goeke-Morey, M. C., & Cummings, E. (2007). Linkages between spouses' psychological distress and marital conflict in the home. *Journal of Family Psychology, 21,* 533–537. doi:10.1037/0893-3200.21.3.533

Papp, L. M., Pendry, P., & Adam, E. K. (2009). Mother-adolescent physiological synchrony in naturalistic settings: Within-family cortisol associations and moderators. *Journal of Family Psychology, 23,* 882–894. doi:10.1037/a0017147

Patterson, C. J., Sutfin, E. L., & Fulcher, M. (2004). Division of labor among lesbian and heterosexual parenting couples: Correlates of specialized versus shared patterns. *Journal of Adult Development, 11,* 179–189. doi:10.1023/B:JADE.0000035626.90331.47

Perry-Jenkins, M., Goldberg, A. E., Pierce, C. P., & Sayer, A. G. (2007). Shift work, role overload, and the transition to parenthood. *Journal of Marriage & Family, 69,* 123–138. doi:10.1111/j.1741-3737.2006.00349.x

Perry-Jenkins, M., Smith, J. Z., Goldberg, A., & Logan, J. N. (2011). Working-class jobs and new parents' mental health. *Journal of Marriage and Family, 73,* 1117–1132. doi:10.1111/j.1741-3737.2011.00871.x

Raudenbush, S. W. (2008). Many small groups. In J. de Leeuw, E. Meijer, J. de Leeuw, & E. Meijer (Eds.), *Handbook of multilevel analysis* (pp. 207–236). New York, NY: Springer. doi:10.1007/978-0-387-73186-5_5

Raudenbush, S. W., Brennan, R., & Barnett, R. (1995). A multivariate hierarchical model for studying psychological change within married couples. *Journal of Family Psychology, 9,* 161–174. doi:10.1037/0893-3200.9.2.161

Raudenbush, S. W., & Bryk, A. S. (2002). *Hierarchical linear models: Applications and data analysis methods.* Thousand Oaks, CA: Sage.

Raudenbush, S., Bryk, A., & Congdon, R. (2004). *HLM6: Hierarchical linear and nonlinear modeling.* Chicago, IL: Scientific Software International.

Regan, P. C., Medina, R., & Joshi, A. (2001). Partner preferences among homosexual men and women: What is desirable in a sex partner is not necessarily desirable in a romantic partner. *Social Behavior and Personality, 29,* 625–633. doi:10.2224/sbp.2001.29.7.625

Sayer, A. G., & Klute, M. M. (2005). Analyzing couples and families: Multilevel methods. In V. L. Bengtson, A. Acock, K. R. Allen, P. Dilworth-Anderson, & D. M. Klein (Eds.), *Sourcebook of family theory and research* (pp. 289–313). Thousand Oaks, CA: Sage.

Simpson, L. E., Atkins, D. C., Gattis, K. S., & Christensen, A. (2008). Low-level relationship aggression and couple therapy outcomes. *Journal of Family Psychology, 22,* 102–111. doi:10.1037/0893-3200.22.1.102

Soliz, J., Thorson, A. R., & Rittenour, C. E. (2009). Communicative correlates of satisfaction, family identity, and group salience in multiracial/ethnic families. *Journal of Marriage and Family, 71,* 819–832. doi:10.1111/j.1741-3737.2009.00637.x

West, T. V., Popp, D., & Kenny, D. A. (2008). A guide for the estimation of gender and sexual orientation effects in dyadic data: An actor-partner interdependence model approach. *Personality & Social Psychology Bulletin, 34,* 321–336. doi:10.1177/0146167207311199

Willett, J. B. (1989). Some results on reliability for the longitudinal measurement of change: Implications for the design of studies of individual growth. *Educational and Psychological Measurement, 49,* 587–602. doi:10.1177/001316448904900309

Woody, E., & Sadler, P. (2005). Structural equation models for interchangeable dyads: Being the same makes a difference. *Psychological Methods, 10,* 139–158. doi:10.1037/1082-989X.10.2.139

Qualitative Research on LGBT-Parent Families

Jacqui Gabb

Qualitative analyses of lesbian, gay, bisexual, and transgender (LGBT)-parent families tend to reside in and develop out of sexuality studies, being peripheral to mainstream agendas in family studies. Contemporary family studies can be characterized as a dynamic interdisciplinary engagement with shifting trends in the patterning of family and intimate networks of care (Williams, 2004), which create and consolidate wide-ranging relationships (Budgeon & Roseneil, 2004; Jamieson, Morgan, Crow, & Allan, 2006). In sociology, research methodologies are predominantly qualitative, focusing on how families are made and remade through "family practices" (Morgan, 1996), largely oriented around the connections between parent and child. In psychology, there remains a tendency to measure and assess family functioning and the impact of changing circumstances on children's well-being and development.

In many ways, studies of LGBT-parent families follow a similar conceptual trajectory; however, there is perhaps slightly more attention paid to narratives of planned conception (Nordqvist, 2011) and the negotiation and *meanings* of parenthood and kin-ties in lesbian father-free families (Almack, 2008; Clarke, 2006; Goldberg & Allen, 2007). In this work, the sameness and difference of (predominantly lesbian) same-sex parent families are afforded particular attention, as well as how these impact on children's emotional well-being and personal development (Clarke, 2002; Golombok, 2000; Hicks, 2005; Stacey & Biblarz, 2001).

Notwithstanding the richness of this interdisciplinary work, across both fields of study, their conceptual separateness has arguably perpetuated gaps in knowledge. We actually know very little about the ordinary experiences of *sexuality practices* in families per se, while the *sexual identities* of LGBT parents are afforded an excess of significance, determining parenthood through queer sexuality. As such, there is a schism between sexuality studies and studies of family life. In this chapter I pull together these two fields of study, demonstrating how a qualitative mixed methods (QMM) approach, defined below, can shed new light on everyday practices of "family sexuality" (Gabb, 2001a), enabling us to better understand the multidimensional identities of LGBT parents and the negotiated absence–presence of sexuality in queer family living.

I use the terms "family sexuality" and "family intimacy" to demonstrate the intersections of and distinctions between these terms and to simultaneously locate intimacy and sexuality in the context of everyday family relationships. My circumspection in how I use and define these terms stems from the (past and present) need to tread carefully around issues of sexuality in the context of parent–child relationships and LGBT-parent

J. Gabb (✉)
Department of Social Policy and Criminology,
The Open University, Walton Hall, Milton Keynes,
7 6AA, UK
e-mail: J.A.Gabb@open.ac.uk

A.E. Goldberg and K.R. Allen (eds.), *LGBT-Parent Families: Innovations in Research and Implications for Practice*, DOI 10.1007/978-1-4614-4556-2_21, © Springer Science+Business Media New York 2013

families in particular. Sexuality and children remain antithetical in the popular imagination (Jackson, 1982); intergenerational sexuality of any description is taboo both within and outside of the academy (Kinkaid, 1998). As a consequence, and with only a few notable exceptions (including Fineman, 1995; Gabb, 2004b; Malone & Cleary, 2002; Smith, 1992), social science research tends to "desex" families. I aim to resituate sexuality as part of family life. I deploy "family" or "families" as interactional units that are created and maintained through sets of relationship practices. This focus on everyday practice facilitates insight on the ways that partner and parenting dynamics are materialized in LGBT-parent families.

The conceptual thread that runs throughout this chapter is, therefore, my desire to nudge forward debate on how we can make sense of sexuality in the context of LGBT-parent families. The primary focus of the chapter is, however, methodological. I will demonstrate the usefulness of qualitative research in the study of LGBT-parent families. In particular, I evince the benefits of using a QMM approach to advance understandings of everyday family living, showing how it can help us to unpack the conundrum of LGBT parents' (sexual–parental) identities.

Although "mixed methods" is most commonly associated with the combination of quantitative and qualitative data (see Creswell & Plano Clark, 2007), the term qualitative mixed methods (QMM) refers to research that deploys multiple qualitative methods. Research in this vein, my own work included, does not seek to cross-check data from different methods, to either prove the validity of findings from one method to another or to build up a definitive case to address a particular hypothesis. Instead, the rich data that are generated through a QMM approach are used to gain insight into multidimensional experience. The approach acknowledges the *contingency of experience* and seeks to retain and examine this through the methodological and analytical techniques that are adopted.

To illustrate the effectiveness of a QMM approach and the kinds of multidimensional insights that can be generated, I draw on data from

two empirical research projects. Research on LGBT-parent families is dominated by studies on lesbian motherhood (Biblarz & Savci, 2010), and likewise my focus here remains limited to lesbian mother households. The first study focuses on families and intimacy (Gabb, 2008).[1] Data were collected from heterosexual and lesbian parents and their children: mothers ($n=9$), fathers ($n=5$), and children ($n=10$). The second study examined lesbian parenthood and sexuality.[2] Data were collected from lesbian mothers ($n=18$) and children ($n=13$). All participants lived in the North of England, UK. The sampling scale of QMM research is inevitably small; however, where the approach pays dividends is in drilling down through the multidimensional layers of practices, meanings, biography, and emotional attachments, to reveal the *fabric* of family processes. As I will demonstrate in this chapter, a QMM approach is therefore primarily useful when deployed to gain insight into the decision-making processes which inform family relationships and ordinary practices of sexuality and intimacy.

A QMMs Approach

In QMM research there are rich analytical rewards offered through creativity in research design. The methods that I detail here include emotion maps, diaries, participant observation, semi-structured and psychosocial (biographical narrative) interviews, photo elicitation, and discussion of vignettes. This is by no means an exhaustive list of techniques used in QMM research, and the

---

[1] *Behind Closed Doors* was an ESRC-funded project (RES-000-22-0854), completed in 2004–2005.

[2] *Perverting Motherhood? Sexuality and Lesbian Motherhood* was ESRC-funded doctoral research completed in 1999–2000.

Both studies focused recruitment strategies on parents who were not engaged in lesbian community activity. The content and scope of these projects were discussed in full with parents and children, using age-appropriate description. Children's age and maturity are important factors in making sense of family practices. I have therefore included the age of children when citing extracts from their data (for example, Reece, 10). Pseudonyms are used for all participants.

range of methods successfully deployed in studies of childhood and children's lives is particularly wide and dynamic (Clark & Moss, 2001; Mauthner, 1997). The primary benefit of the QMM approach is that different methods generate distinctive kinds of data, adding novel dimensions and distinctive perspectives that can be drawn together to enrich understandings of the phenomenon being investigated.

Emotion Maps

This method, which I pioneered in the *Behind Closed Doors* study, adds depth to our understandings of the materiality of personal relationships. Emotion maps locate interactions in the context of the family home, facilitating analysis on the boundaries of family intimacy and sexuality. The method was developed from the household portrait technique introduced by Andrea Doucet (2001) in her study of gendered roles and responsibilities among heterosexual couples. In principle, the emotion map method is a form of sticker chart. The researcher is taken on a guided tour of the family home, an opportunity which can also allow children to talk through how they perceive different "territories" around the household. After this tour either the researcher or a family member sketches out a floor plan. This sketch is then reproduced using *Microsoft Draw* (or a similar word processing package). Several days later a large format (A3, 420×297 mm) copy of the floor plan is given out to each participant along with a set of colored emoticon stickers that denote happiness, sadness, anger, and love/affection. Family members (broadly defined) are individually assigned a color. Participants then place these different colored emoticon stickers on their copy of the household floor plan to indicate where an interaction occurs and between whom—that is to say, to spatially locate relational encounters. The merits of the emotion map method are that it is fun to complete and not reliant on language skills. It serves to flatten out intergenerational competencies among parents and children, and because children are familiar with sticker charts they tend to be extremely adept in completing this method. Later on in this chapter I will provide an illustration of this technique and the kinds of data that can be generated.

Diaries

Diary data add a temporal dimension to QMM research, generating information on everydayness and routine family processes (Laurenceau & Bolger, 2005). They are also useful in the analysis of family lives because they can elucidate the personal meanings of relating practices. For example, in my studies they highlighted the "affective currencies" (Gabb, 2008, p. 141) that operate within a family. That is to say, how families use symbolic phrases, such as "hugs and kisses" and "I love you" as affective shorthand to stand in for more complex emotion work and/or ambivalent feelings. They can facilitate research in that they introduce the research topic to participants at a pace and pitch that feels comfortable to them and provide background information which enables the researcher to tailor subsequent interview questions around the individual family situation. In the *Behind Closed Doors* project, diaries were completed over a 1–2 week period. Most parents committed considerable time and thought to the completion of their diaries. Children were invited to complete them if they wanted to, although they were often perceived as a form of homework by older children, especially adolescents, and as such participation rates were low among this age group. Participants were all requested to use diaries to produce an account of everyday family interactions and as a space to think through their family practices and where appropriate their parental/partner roles.

Observations

Observation data add another layer to the participatory materials from diaries and emotion maps, giving a glimpse of everyday practices of intimacy and drawing attention to the *performances of family* which participants chose to render public. These data on the texture of intimate family life and the mediation of lived experience bring to the fore where and how the absence–presence of sexuality becomes enacted, which opens up space for an interrogation of what determines the parameters of "family displays" (Finch, 2007).

Interviews

Notwithstanding the insights afforded through methodological creativity, interviews remain the method of choice in qualitative research (Silverman, 1996). Interviews enable participants to give their version of interpersonal relationships. Psychosocial biographical narrative or free association (open) interviews situate experiences of intimacy and sexuality across the life course, within the participants' own terms of reference, through events which they define as significant. Semi-structured interviews can be used to pick up particular (thematic) threads which feature in these biographical accounts, enabling more targeted research questions.

Vignettes and Photo Elicitation

Discussion of third-party vignettes and photographs facilitates examination of participants' perceptions and beliefs, at the social level (Schoenberg & Ravdal, 2000). These techniques enable the researcher to approach highly sensitive topics that might otherwise be deemed too risky if tackled through personal experience. In my research, using vignettes and photo methods has enabled me to talk directly about the management of boundaries around children and sexuality and adult–child intimacy more widely. For example, an image taken from a parenting handbook depicting a man sharing a bath with a child facilitated conversation on how men, as fathers, negotiate issues of nudity and bodily contact. This opened up wider discussion on "family rules" and the normative judgments that are invoked to manage perceptions of risk associated with different practices of intimacy.

QMM data, such as those described above, produce a multilayered, richly textured account of *where, when, how,* and *why* family intimacy is experienced, adding in-depth knowledge on everyday practices of LGBT parenthood. Recent developments in mixed methods studies evince an eclectic approach (Bryman, 2006), with researchers adopting "complex methodological hybridity and elasticity" (Green & Preston, 2005, p. 171). This creativity in research design is requiring researchers to develop equally dynamic analytical strategies. There are various ways to bring together data generated through QMM research. In the *Behind Closed Doors* project the intensity and complexity of data inclined me toward an "integrative" approach (Mason, 2006). This analytical strategy aims to increase subject knowledge while simultaneously retaining the paradigmatic nature of each method (Moran-Ellis et al., 2006). Through case study analysis the relational threads of a story can be traced; cross-sectional analysis brings social–personal connections to the fore (Gabb, 2008, p. 63). The integration of QMM data has enabled me to connect these different dimensions, to interrogate the fabric of everyday family intimacy. The use of critical discourse analysis has enabled me to focus attention on the patterning of language and how meaning-making can be read through the written and spoken word (Wetherall, Taylor, & Yates, 2001). Looking at language as a social practice has shown how wider power relations are embedded (and contested) in everyday talk and descriptions of family living. In the following sections I will now illustrate some of the kinds of data that are generated by using different qualitative methods before moving on to consider how these data can be combined in ways that represent the vitality of lived lives.

Listening to Children: The Value of Participatory Methods

Research on children's lives in many ways exemplifies the benefits of creativity in research design and a QMM approach. European scholars in the field of qualitative studies of childhood have presented a compelling argument that we need to listen to children when writing about subjects that involve them (James & Prout, 1990).

We can no longer rely on adults' reported accounts of children's lives if we want to fully understand how young people experience changes in family relationships (Smart & Neale, 1999). Similar arguments have been made about the incompleteness of LGBT-parent family research when intergenerational perspectives are omitted (Gabb, 2008; Perlesz et al., 2006). It is therefore surprising that in queer families' research, children's perspectives are often excluded (Dunne, 1998; Weeks, Heaphy, & Donovan, 2001). Some psychological accounts of lesbian and gay families do involve interviews with children (Goldberg, 2010; Patterson, 1992; Tasker & Golombok, 1997), and anthologies of children's experiences are produced by the "community press" (Saffron, 1996), but most sociological and ethnographic qualitative research on LGBT-parent families relies on second-hand accounts of childhood experience (Barrett & Tasker, 2001), often focusing on routes into planned parenthood (Almack, 2008; Nordqvist, 2011).

In my studies, listening to children enabled me to piece together an *intergenerational* perspective that located young people as an integral part of family life. Research with children does not require highly specialized skills (Harden, Scott, Backett-Milburn, & Jackson, 2000); however it does require a creative methodological imagination. I deployed a "mosaic approach" (Clark & Moss, 2001), utilizing participatory methods that engaged children's interest, at an age-appropriate pitch, facilitating talk on the subject of study (Gabb, 2009). Task-centered activities have proven to be particularly effective (Morrow, 1998) in part because visual participatory methods avoid the need for eye contact and so reduce imbalances of power (Mauthner, 1997). Visual methods decrease the significance of age-related competencies which normally divide parents and children (Gabb, 2008); for similar reasons they are also useful for working with both adults and children whose first language is not English or whose language skills may be limited. Qualitative researchers who use "draw and talk" techniques suggest that this approach can help to structure children's descriptions of emotionally charged events and add depth of insight

on complex phenomenon and/or abstract ideas such as family relationships, which may be otherwise hard to verbalize (Clark & Moss, 2001; Gabb, 2005a; Mauthner, 1997).

The youngest children that I have interviewed were 6-years-old, and even at this young age, by using participatory methods they were able to meaningfully contribute to the research projects. Individual informed consent from all children must always be obtained. For me this was achieved by talking each child through the research, in a way that was age-appropriate and comprehensible. This consent was subject to ongoing negotiation throughout the duration of the fieldwork, following ethical procedures that have been developed for research with children (Gabb, 2010). Younger children, up to adolescence, are often keen to speak about their families, and this includes an openness to talk about the impact of their mothers' sexual orientation on their lives and how they experience and perceive different relationships. Asking these children to describe their families can yield unexpected rewards and generate immensely rich data. Their accounts illustrate the power of family discourses and how these structure young people's perception and experience of relationships.

Children were largely adamant that their families are indistinguishable from any other.

Reece (10):	Erm…. [we're] just like a normal family really but with two women in it instead of a woman and a man really.
Interviewer:	Can you think of any differences between you and other kids?
Reece:	Only that I'm vegetarian and my friends aren't!
Interviewer:	Would you think of your family as a "lesbian family"?
Harriet (15):	(Laughs) Well I'm not a lesbian! No really it's just a family and a person in it happens to be a lesbian: "Wow big deal!" kind of thing.

Many children used the word "normal" to describe their families, because to them same-sex parent families were simply part of everyday life. Some children did, however, appear to perceive their families as different in some ways.

What constituted this difference was typically unclear although explanations tended to focus on difficulties in *fitting* the non-birth mother into traditional understandings of family. That is to say, the presence of the "other mother" represented an identifiable source of family difference which required explanation, and it was this which made children susceptible to being teased.

In all interviews with children, I did not directly ask them about similarities and differences between heterosexual-parent and lesbian-parent families. I used the words and concepts familiar to them, only asking about their mother(s)' lesbian sexuality if they ventured onto this subject. By taking my cue from them, and only referring to lesbianism at their instigation, I ensured as far as possible that I did not create anxieties where none previously existed. Asking young children to talk about such sensitive issues would have been hard to approach head-on. Instead, sitting down with these children, usually on the floor in their bedrooms, and unpacking my bag full of drawing paper and sets of pencils and colored crayons, eased the awkwardness of the situation because the power imbalance was lessened and the occasion was oriented around an activity that was familiar to them.

I usually started by asking children if they could draw me a picture of their family. This could include anyone and the drawings could and did often take on many forms. Some children's pictures were figurative; one child drew vehicles, because he "couldn't draw people" (see Gabb, 2005a). Schools and playgroups often focus teaching on stories and pictures of home and family life because these feature centrally children's worlds; the subject was therefore familiar to young children. Drawing pictures enabled children to focus on something that captured their imagination while facilitating conversation on my chosen topic. Thus, we both got something out of the encounter. Once I had made a copy of the pictures, the originals were all returned to the children, as promised.

Close analysis of children's pictures alongside their interview data can provide significant insight into their perceptions and experiences of LGBT-parent families. It is sometimes, however,

children's silences that speak volumes. A qualitative approach that advances critical discourse analysis is able to incorporate pauses, diversions, and associations as part of children's data, paying careful attention to what is said and unsaid and the way that descriptions are articulated. For example, in my study of lesbian parenthood, one child (James) did not explicitly identify Jill ("other mother") as the source of difference, but his *train of thought* suggests this may be the case.

Interviewer:	Are you going to draw Jill [other mother] in this picture? (see Fig. 21.1)
James (7):	I'm not really sure about that [Interviewer: Why aren't you sure?] I don't know
Interviewer:	Is your family the same as all your friends' families?
James:	A bit different [Interviewer: In what ways different?] I don't know, just a bit different
Interviewer:	So can you think of any things that make your family different?
James:	I can try and draw Jill, but she's just dyed her hair.

While "draw and talk" techniques may be highly successful in research with young children (aged 6–12 years old), with teenagers, research encounters are typically most successful when they are framed as gentle conversations. In my research, young people from this age group often welcomed the opportunity of getting their viewpoint heard. For example, Jeffrey spoke quite eloquently about the politics of sexuality, using the space of the interview to "have his say." He was keen to question the distinction between the homo/heterosexual divide and expressed dissatisfaction with the categorization process of sexual identity-based politics.

Jeffrey (19):	I don't know why anybody makes a big deal about anything. I mean Gay Pride, why are you proud to be gay. It's nothing to be proud or ashamed of. It just is and if everybody thought like that then there would be no bigotry in the

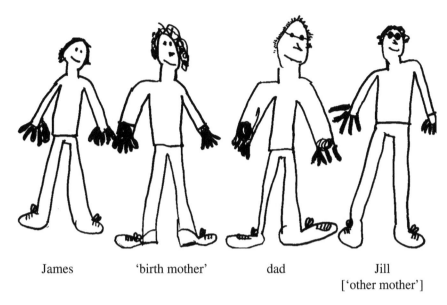

James   'birth mother'   dad   Jill
                                              ['other mother']

Fig. 21.1   James (aged 7). "My family"

world. It's not "oh you're a lesbian we'll treat you different."
It's not. Or "we're lesbians so
we have to treat you the same"
it's just you're you. So what,
who cares! It just doesn't make
a difference, or at least it
shouldn't. Nobody's different
anymore. There's a broad spectrum and we're sitting here cat-
egorizing people.

From the evidence of my data, it would appear
that Jeffrey is most perceptive; the differentiation
between homo- and heterosexual families may be
ultimately more discursive than experiential. That
is to say, research and writing may be foregrounding sexuality differences in ways that obscure the
similarities between all kinds of families.
Children's data may be opaque and sometimes
even contradictory, but a child-centered approach
to LGBT-parent family studies holds great promise because it adds an intergenerational dimension to the picture. Taking account of children
refocuses the analytical lens onto lived experience rather than sexual identity politics; it requires
that we begin to look at families "from the ground
up," demonstrating the value of family practices
above and beyond categories of family and fam-

ily function (Dunn & Deater-Deckard, 2001;
Morrow, 1998). From the child's point of view,
all parents, kin, and even significant friendships
may constitute family (Allen & Demo, 1995).
The shift in emphasis—from adult to children,
discursive to experiential—reorients our thinking, and calls into question the merit of reifying
different kinds of family through sexuality
descriptors (Gabb, 2005a). As Judith Stacey
(2002) points out:

> Why would we want to designate a family type
> according to the sexual identity of one or more of
> its members? ... The more one attempts to arrive at
> a coherent, defensible sorting principle, the more
> evident it becomes that the category "gay and les-
> bian family" signals nothing so much as the conse-
> quential   social   factor   of   widespread,
> institutionalized homophobia. (p. 396)

Highlighting lesbian parents' *sexuality difference* simply reaffirms an imaginary heteronormative model against which we are measured and to
which we remain deferent. It may be, as Stacey
goes on to argue, that a more productive way to
proceed would be to acknowledge that the monolithic cultural regime that governs our intimate
bonds is in fact collapsing. "Gay and lesbian
families simply brave intensified versions of
widespread contemporary challenges" (Stacey,

2002, p. 404). Data from children add credence to this assertion, querying the significance afforded to parents' sexuality. This does not contest the particularities that may comprise same-sex family forms, nor does it occlude the queering of parental categories that takes place in LGBT-parent families (Gabb, 2005a). What it does do is to shift the emphasis away from sexuality as *the* defining criterion of these particularities.

Balancing Sexual–Maternal Identities: Combining Interview and Visual Data

Lesbianism and motherhood are not antithetical. Discourses on homosexuality may suggest that sexuality is to be found at the juncture of our subjectivity, making us who and what we are (Weeks, 1995, p. 235), but lesbianism especially has never been *just* an identity or wholly typified by (homo)sexual activity and same-sex desire. Empirical research contests the ontological basis of this kind of demarcation (Gabb, 2005a; Stacey, 2002). What a QMM approach can effectively demonstrate are the particularities of experience and understandings of sexuality and maternity *in context*, and it provides the methodological tools to interrogate the slippery boundaries *between* these two factors. Combining data from methods that interrogate the materiality of sexuality practices and identity formations adds rich insight to existing knowledge on parents' strategies to manage sexual and maternal identities (Malone & Cleary, 2002; Rust, 2001). Findings from my research demonstrate how parents' parental–sexual selves are not experienced as mutually exclusive; they are experienced through sets of circumstances with sexuality and parental responsibility being negotiated around the absence–presence of children (Gabb, 2005b). In the *Perverting Motherhood?* project, this was articulated in open and often quite explicit terms:

Michelle: Obviously […] you don't shag in front of your kids, anyone will tell you that hopefully, but we're quite openly affectionate in front of Rob [son, aged 7].

Janis: [Bedrooms] become baby-feeding spaces actually (laughs)! Well that's

what happened. Oh yeh, that's definitely true. […] So in a way the bedroom has always kind of been a cross between sort of where you go to sleep and where you go and do 'it' or whatever, or have a cuddle. […] If she [daughter] was a problem it was because she woke up every night until she was three and a half, and not just once (laughs). […] Which doesn't leave a lot of time to think about the bedroom as a place for sex (laughs) let's face it!

Data such as these substantiate the truism that "having a child changes your life," but this does not set maternal and familial identities beyond sexuality. Instead, it illustrates intersections between sexual–maternal feelings and expressions of intimacy (Gabb, 2004b, p. 409) and the need for linguistic management of these shifting identities (Gabb, 2005a). Data generated through semi-structured interviews, talking to mothers about the significance of their sexuality on everyday family life, produced on one level broadly conflicting accounts. Whether lesbian sexuality was manifestly *on display* fell into two camps: "It's everywhere!" (Michelle) and "It's not really noticeable!" (Matilda). Notwithstanding mothers' polarized assertions, when QMM data were combined together, there was far more commonality of experience than was presented in interviews. Observations detailed the underlying presence of lesbian sexuality. "Subtle signifiers of lesbian identity" (Valentine, 1996, p. 150), such as lesbian iconography and media aimed at the queer market, were visible in all homes, here and there, if you knew where to look and what to look for. However, more often than not it was the abundance of pictures of women and the absence of male equivalents that provided the most "telling signs." Iconic images of favorite celebrities, snapshots of family and friends, and pictures of women predominately adorned the walls and shelves of rooms. Research may have shown that many lesbian parents go to elaborate lengths to include men and male role models in their family networks (for example, Clarke, 2006; Goldberg & Allen, 2007), but in my studies' observational data indicate that this does not necessarily translate into ambient surroundings. Lesbian-parent homes were not essentially feminized, but images, keepsakes, and decorations were predominantly associated with women, and there was a notable lack of paraphernalia that could be linked with men and masculinity. Observations of this kind, documented in field notes, add another layer to interview data on how maternal and sexual identities are experienced, adding depth of insight on the impact of the absence of male presence in lesbian households. This information may have easily slipped beneath my analytical radar if I had relied on interview data only.

Visual data shed yet further light on the opaqueness of LGBT-parent family living. In the *Perverting Motherhood?* Project, I asked parents and children to take pictures that represented their "lesbian families." Anonymity was assured and I guaranteed that none of these images would be used in publication; for this reason I am reliant here on descriptive detail. The photos that were produced were extremely interesting not just because of what they depicted but also because they illustrated how difficult it was for parents and children to represent lesbian parenthood. In some cases, after their interviews, families who did not take photographs described conceptual images—pictures they would have taken had the pressures of simply *being* a family not taken up all of their available time. One parent presented an existing "family album" as a substitute, using this to talk through what and who constituted family.

The images that were produced, and likewise the discussion over why pictures were not taken, illustrated the uncertainty about what constitutes lesbian-parent family life. Images of people reinforced ideas of "the couple," valorizing normative ideals of the dyadic two-parent family model. Other images were either concerned with household chores or with showing loving relationships—closeness and embodied intimacy that was captured in family embraces. Images were also interesting, in part, because of what they did not show. Sexuality was notably absent and the "family displays" (Finch, 2007) that were depicted said more about normative ideals of family rather than advance understandings of the particularities of lesbian-parent family living (Gabb, 2011b).

As such, perhaps the most insightful depiction was of a bathroom shelf which included three toothbrushes in a pot, two adult, colored blue and green, and the third a child's toothbrush depicting a superhero. Simply stated, this signified the "lesbian family," ordinary, like any other, concerned with mundane everyday life.

Taking Account of Biographical Data and Psychosocial Dimensions

In the *Behind Closed Doors* project, I used this rich methodological palette alongside biographical narrative (free association) interviews, with the aim of adding another layer of understanding focused on the emotional–social biographical factors that combine to shape LGBT-parent experience. To demonstrate the depth of insight that can be achieved through this psychosocial method and its combination with other data, I will primarily draw on one case study. This case study data also serve to illustrate the ways that a QMM approach can begin to build up multidimensional understandings of a phenomenon, in this instance a person's family story. Claire is a 43-year-old lesbian single parent. She has three sons aged 21, 19, and 17 who were conceived in a previous heterosexual relationship. She is in full-time employment in a professional job and lives in a comfortable semi-detached suburban home. She is in a LAT (living apart together) relationship with Jade (aged 48) who lives nearby.

Developed from the biographical narrative integrative method (BNIM) (Wengraf, 2001) and free association narrative interview (FANI) (Hollway & Jefferson, 2000), the "open" interview enabled me to examine the interplay between the psychic and the social, located in the cultural context and biography of the individual (Roseneil, 2006, p. 851). The legitimacy and limitations of this approach remain hotly contested (Layton, 2008), being primarily focused around the authority that researchers have to make sense of and interpret participants' psychic reality, transposing methodological and analytic techniques which originate in clinical settings onto academic empirical research data. It does nevertheless usefully reorient the analytical lens onto the connections between past and present experience, foregrounding relationality and emotions in studies of family living. The psychosocial approach is based on the *Gestalt* principle, suggesting that through the framing and telling of stories the speaker produces a *biographical narrative* (Wengraf, 2001, p. 113) that reveals the *significance* of experiences and/or events. Psychosocial interviews are wholly nondirective, with the researcher asking a single open question at the start of the interview and thereafter the interview narrative is participant-directed, framed in their own terms of reference.

Participants were asked: "Tell me about significant emotional events in your life." This question, at first glance, may not appear to be particularly relevant to research on LGBT-parent family lives, but in my description of Claire's account I will show how posing an open question of this kind can reap unforeseen analytical rewards. It enables participants to orient the interview around events and encounters that are meaningful to them, producing sometimes unexpected data. For example, in my project on family relationships I had presumed that becoming and being a mother would feature centrally in women's lives. In their psychosocial interviews, however, many women focused on other emotionally significant events in their lives. A couple of mothers did not raise the subject of motherhood at all. For others, in line with findings on motherhood more generally, maternal experience and becoming a mother remained a source of great ambivalence and was surrounded with many mixed emotions, including happiness, depression, and distress. Individuals stitched connections between different life events and in so doing shed light on some of the underlying factors that shape personal decision making.

The nature of biographical narrative interviews means that in the following section I have needed to paraphrase much of Claire's data, dipping in and out of extracts to illustrate the analytical point being made or provoke new insight. This is because this method typically produces a long unbroken monologue, which is not structured around tightly framed questions and answers. The

kind of descriptive writing that I will therefore use is in some ways akin to a detailed pen portrait, this is to say, fragmentary notes which when combined together begin to sketch out an outline picture of an individual and her "story." Claire's interview describes a life steeped in change, peppered with moments of emotional–physical disruption and continuity. She recalls paternal death, difficult stepfamily relations, failing to achieve at school, unplanned pregnancy, marriage, domestic violence, divorce, remarriage, and coming out. The narrative that she recounts appears well rehearsed and neatly packaged. It is told in "fast forward," moving from one event to another, in quick succession. She talks about how her personal needs and those of her family and the couple relationship are often hard to balance.

Claire is evidently struggling to incorporate Jade within her family life. Trying to make sense of why this separation exists, she distinguishes her own family from that of the ideal (heterosexual) norm, based on parent–child relationships that are grounded in birth origin. Whereas the children cited earlier in this chapter seemed inclined to accept diversity in family composition, Claire sets up an imaginary ideal as something that her situation can only ever imitate: "it's not a day-to-day family existence as a whole family unit." Her lesbian-parent family is "a recreation" and not a "*family* family." She appears to be unable to trust that adult couple relationships may last and that things may work out for the best:

Claire: Probably during a car drive somewhere, we've had little discussions and it's been touched upon, "Why doesn't Jade move in?" and, and things like that. And I said because I preferred the separation […] I think the boys are probably happier. They would have accepted it, but I know that they, they feel more comfortable that this is their home […] we were a nice little family unit for a couple of years while the children…. [were young]. It, it was a nice time for all of us. There was no bad feeling anywhere it was just nice, comfortable, content, but it couldn't last, it really couldn't.

Claire can be seen here to be moving back and forth, imagining and justifying her decisions, working hard to make the right decision. After reading these kinds of data there is a temptation to fall back on psychoanalytically determined interpretations: to join up the experiential dots and make sense of Claire's experience for her. I contend that this delimits the potential of psychosocial interviews (Gabb, 2010). One of the key strengths of this kind of method is to illustrate the connections that are made *by the narrator/interviewee*, between different life events. To overwrite these individually crafted associations disregards the fabric of the accounts that are presented. Going back to the data again and again, often in the context of research group analysis, requires that we keep looking at what is there while holding at bay the analytical compulsion to tie up loose ends. Taking as an example the extract from Claire (above), it is possible to see how different facets of her experience come to bear in dynamic and contested ways that resist clear-cut interpretation.

Reading and rereading this extract, I am still unclear what the "it" is which Claire is referring to in her last sentence. It is probable that "it" has various meanings here. *It* could be referring to the contained family unit that she shared with her children while they were growing up, before they started to work and live away from home. *It* could be that she is talking more hypothetically, about how introducing her partner into their household might not be a long-lasting arrangement and therefore *it* is not an option that she wants to risk. Alternatively, in the broader context of the whole interview, *it* may be happiness. The flux and lack of surety which characterize her biographical narrative have shown that things do not last—adult relationships, family cohesion, and the closeness of mother–child relationships—all things change and lack constancy. Goodbyes are commonplace. The point I am trying to make here is that there is no need to close down meanings through tightly defined interpretations. It is highly plausible that the extract, as with Claire's family story, has multiple meanings which shift over time and in accordance with different sets of circumstance. Retaining this dynamic perspective is a crucial part of the QMM approach, something that I will return to later on.

The Spatial–Temporal Patterning of Intimacy: Emotion Maps and Diaries

In the *Behind Closed Doors* project, I tried to develop methods that generated data on *how* intimacy and family sexuality are experienced in *different contexts* around the home, and to extend the methodological toolkit to include techniques that engage with the abstract realm of our emotions, feelings, and connections with others. To facilitate insight on the deeply personal and often strictly guarded aspects of families' private lives, I used two simultaneous participatory methods—diaries and emotion maps. Claire was a diligent diarist and she indicated that she thoroughly enjoyed this method. Her diary facilitated self-reflection, enabling her to think through the day's events and the significance of different interactions.

Claire: Day 6 [date]. [Jade] is not responding very well to my needs. She's also struggling with flightiness and hormonal imbalance due to the menopause and I am actually quite relieved to see her go. I want to be by myself […] I went to make a cup of tea and have come to my room to write this down, read and then sleep alone.

Diary data such as these provide insight not only on everyday events but also on personal thought processes, describing how decisions are reached and the emotional impact of events on the diarist. For Claire, being a mother is a crucial part of her identity and her lifestyle. Jade has no investment in either "the boys" or this area of Claire's biography. The only solution that seems to work for them is to carve out an emotional–spatial–temporal separation between these different parts of their lives. Diaries produced by participants were steeped in temporal referents—clock time, age and generation, personal time, family time, precious time for the self, and the time needed to maintain and manage relationships. Emotion maps data on the boundaries of family intimacy added a *spatial* dimension to these understandings of LGBT-parent family living.

Emotion map data and the conversation generated through these graphic materials chart the emotional geographies of the family home.

Rooms and intimate space were described as having multiple uses that change over time, as children grow up. Considerable mobility was evident in the uses of space, which countermanded the otherwise static environment of demarcated rooms. Some mothers talked about "bed hopping" as they moved in and out of the "marital" bed to provide comfort and/or company for children. Others identified certain spaces, such as the kitchen, as both a "hot spot" for family tension and a site for family togetherness. Combined diary and emotion data illustrated how furtive embraces and brief moments of intimacy were fitted into the spatial and temporal cracks of family living.

In studying the "boundaries of intimacy" (Jamieson, 2005, p. 189) in LGBT-parent families, one of the most potent sites to investigate is the parents' bedroom, and yet not surprisingly it remains one of the hardest spaces to effectively research. The bedroom is traditionally afforded great symbolic resonance. It is a *cultural sign* of sexuality that personifies "the sexual family" (Fineman, 1995). As the site of parental sex it marks the child's separation from the mother and signifies the hierarchical difference between parent and child. In psychoanalytic terms, the "maternal bed" is a sign of sexual activity and adult intimacy, a space where children are supplanted in the mother's affections by the father The double bed thus signifies the real and cultural difference between generationally defined adult (sexual) relations and parent/child (nurturing) relationships (Hollway, 1997).

Participatory methods, such as the emotion map, begin to open up such private space for qualitative investigation. The interview data which this method generates elicit rich insight on how different kinds of relations are kept separate and how ordinary family intimacy is policed. They add to understandings on the factors which inform decision making on who gets entry into certain spaces and how permissions are granted and by whom. This advances knowledge on how and why "rules" are set up to separate self and other (Gabb, 2011a), with the policing of relations often being informed by social understandings of risk and gender:

Claire: Probably keep the intimacy within the family rather than a family friend or an uncle.

Claire was keen to establish clear boundaries around codes of conduct, "just in case." The in/significance of gender in lesbian-parent families is much debated (Gabb, 2001b, 2004b). In parents' accounts of family relationships and the boundaries of intimacy, it was never far from view and often shaped opinions and practice. Talking about the intimate behavior depicted on her emotion map (Fig. 21.2), Claire seeks to categorically disassociate denoted interactions from any inference of sex, including those between her and her partner. In her account she therefore shuts down all possibilities for misinterpretation, but in so doing she also removes sexuality from the lesbian-parent family equation and from family intimacy more widely.

Interviewer: Right, so on the bed in your room, erm there's kind of stickers at one end and stickers at the other end. Is that significant?

Claire: Yeah, well that was because she [Jade, partner] stayed over one night and this is because erm I've got a hug but it wasn't sort of, of a, a sexual nature or anything like that … it's changed, it does change over the years. No this doesn't surprise me. This is, is fairly usual. But things have changed and I think that's the noticeable thing for me is that Jake often comes into my bedroom and has a chat. They'll always knock at the door and they'll always come in and, and have a chat and that doesn't happen so much now. Probably because they're older.

The approach adds rich insight into parents' management of family sexuality practices, enabling us to trace the spatial–temporal patterning of intimate behavior in LGBT-parent households. In the above quote Claire alludes to earlier relationship incarnations, when sexual activity between her and Jade was more frequent. As time has passed, this dimension of the relationship has cooled down, something that is commented upon as unsurprising. She identifies the children's freedom to come into her bedroom "on demand" as a

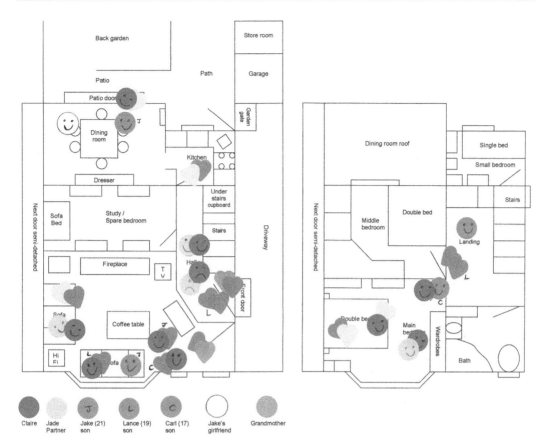

Fig. 21.2 Claire's emotion map

factor that has delimited sex when they were younger. It is plausible that this practice and the "open door" policy that existed during this time have had a lasting impact on her experience of adult-sexual relationships. Her bed (the maternal bedroom) now remains associated with being a family space rather than a site of adult-sexual intimacy.

Mapping Categories of Behavior: Inhabiting Class

In qualitative analysis of the patterning of family intimacy at home, it is important to remain attentive to the ways that affective practices are shaped by sets of circumstances and "choices" that are not always of parents' own making. Separate spaces and personal privacy at home are luxuries

that not every family can afford (Phoenix & Woollett, 1991). Widening the scope of the academic research lens to incorporate socioeconomic diversity is crucial in opening up understandings of LGBT-parent families. Family studies research on heterosexual motherhood has clearly demonstrated the impact of financial factors and cultural resources on the pragmatics of parenting (Gillies, 2006; Vincent & Ball, 2006). Social circumstance affects the ways that women mother, and these maternal practices are then duly mapped onto categories of mothering (Phoenix & Woollett, 1991). This stigmatizing process reinforces ideas of good and bad parenting, wherein the working class parent can never fully attain the status of respectability because she does not have access to the financial resources and cultural capital that are needed to achieve this (Skeggs, 1997). In LGBT-parent family research, however, issues of class and the material impact of socioeconomic status on the practices and identities of queer parents remain under-researched (Biblarz & Savci, 2010) and samples selected remain predominantly middle class (Almack, 2008; Dunne, 1998; Nordqvist, 2011). This is in part a consequence of the costs involved in pursuing assisted conception through official routes. Even in the UK, where the National Health Service subsidizes fertility treatment, significant sums of money are involved for each insemination attempt. Other reasons for the sample composition are likely to be informed by the demographic profile of those who participate in organized parenting activities and by the personal biography of the researcher (Gabb, 2004a).

Some qualitative studies of lesbian and gay parenting are beginning to examine the ways that class simultaneously reproduces and ruptures understandings and experiences of sexuality (Taylor, 2009). Such analysis adds another much needed perspective in the otherwise partial LGBT-parent family narrative, usefully accounting for the ways that class positioning, educational advantage, and cultural capital shape perceptions and experiences of parenthood. In my own research I have ensured that the sample comprises socioeconomic diversity so that the picture painted is not steeped in privilege, thereby furthering the marginalization of traditionally stigmatized families. Notwithstanding the richness of data which this sampling provides, I can nevertheless find little correlation between socioeconomic factors and discernible differences in the patterning of intimate behavior (Gabb, 2009). The decision-making processes around risk and family sexuality practices and the boundaries that are set up around intimacy do not appear to readily map onto differences in cultural resources or class status. Instead findings seem to indicate that it is emotional–social biographical experience combined with wider sets of sociocultural meanings which variously shape patterns of behavior, contributing to where boundaries are set up around understandings of "appropriate" codes of sexuality conduct.

Managing Public–Private Space: Vignettes and Photo Elicitation

While there are undoubtedly specificities in circumstance and experience that can be teased out, what I want to focus on here are the common methodological challenges that are presented in trying to investigate sensitive and closely guarded aspects of people's personal lives. One strategy that I have found useful in working my way around such barriers is to approach the topic using methods that draw on the third person, asking the participant to respond to an abstract scenario rather than begin from their personal experience. This can be a central feature in the design of the photo interview. Used in this way, the method can produce data on where parents set boundaries around intimacy and the codes of conduct that are invoked to legitimize personal–family sexuality management. In the *Behind Closed Doors* project parents were shown six images. One was an illustration that depicted a double bed, occupied by a man and woman, separated by a happy sleeping child in between them, with a cat curled up on the end of the bed. In response Claire says:

Claire: Yeah. Mmm quite typical I think isn't it (laughs) yeah… Sleeping quite happily, yeah nothing wrong with that, I would have thought […] My cat used to sleep on my bed and yeah. I'm probably a little bit relaxed about things like that and a lot of people are more strict, they don't want pets in the bedroom but I'm not like that […] the boys have on occasion, on regular occasions, come into [my] bed, up until, the last time I remember was when [son] was about 13 and he'd had a really bad dream so mmmm…

In the previous section I discussed Claire's desire to set up categorical boundaries around different activities and practices of intimacy. Here, talking in the third person, she becomes less prescriptive. When talking earlier about her sleeping arrangements, she presented a quite defensive response which emphasizes the need to protect children. This tells us something about the impact of societal pressures to conform and parents' role in the management of sexuality and risk, but it does not, however, tell us much about everyday practices of intimacy. By tackling the subject *indirectly* I was able to facilitate Claire to talk about her experience *in comparison*. This generated another layer of information on personal past experience, times when she shared a bed with her teenage son, something that had previously been only inferred.

Methods which use third-party scenarios aim to generate information on people's beliefs and opinions; conversations which then ordinarily move on to include how these beliefs and opinions translate in everyday practice and experience in their own families. In response to another scenario, presented in a vignette, Claire again shifts between third and first person. She reflects on the ways that a scenario relates to issues of boundary setting in lesbian relationships generally, before moving on to describe more personally revealing details concerning her relationship with Jade. The vignette described an intimate (nonsexual) relationship that is developing between a "married" woman and male colleague at work. Participants were then asked what the woman's partner should do:

Claire: Oh this is exactly what's going on with [my friend] at the moment […] I mean same sex relationships are more difficult in that respect because it's difficult for me to have friends, female friends over […] very difficult because there's a, there's a boundary there but for some of them, for others it's fine, if the boundary is set, but for others it isn't and it's difficult for Jade…

Issues of boundaries feature high in Claire's account of her family and different kinds of relationship. These data from discussion of the vignette added another piece of the jigsaw, helping me to begin to understand why boundary setting is so important. Again, Claire is caught between her own needs and those of others, in this instance her partner, Jade; these data generated through third person narratives would be difficult to access through other means. They add a crucial dimension to understandings of both the participant (as an individual) and some of the factors that combine to shape LGBT-parent family living. Combined together with findings from other methods, a dynamic and highly illuminating picture begins to emerge, providing depth of knowledge to understandings of sexuality management and how parents balance sexual–parental identities in everyday practices of intimacy.

Concluding Thoughts

In this chapter I have demonstrated how a QMM approach can provide rich multilayered accounts. To conclude, I want to caution against trying to piece together these layers of data to either reconstruct holistic portraits of individual participants or to make grand claims about trends in the patterning of intimate behavior and sexuality conduct. In my analysis of Claire's data I have tried to demonstrate the benefits of retaining the frayed ends and incongruities that weave in and out across her data, resisting the temptation to produce a finished case study portrait from the composite pieces of data that are available. QMM research does produce comprehensive findings on LGBT-parent family relationships, but I propose that we need to find ways to retain and reflect the *complexity of relational experience* and, in so doing, to challenge the sanitization of queer family lives that characterizes so many studies in this area. I want to tease open the contained picture which edits out sections that make for uncomfortable reading (Gabb, 2004a), looking across the constellation of multiple methods in the dataset to create multifaceted pictures of phenomenon (Moran-Ellis et al., 2006, p. 54).

I concede that on a sheer practical level the amount of data collected through a QMM approach, per participant, per family, does require the researcher to edit, synthesize, and paraphrase these complex and capacious data. This process does not, however, lead us inexorably toward the narrativization of experience. We should be mindful of any individual and/or external impetus to neaten the research picture: "life experience is messy, we may do well, in our portrayals of that experience, to hold onto some of that messiness in our writings" (Daly, 2007, pp. 259–260). This desire to retain messiness calls into question epistemological certainties, a theme that has been taken up in recent work on the relationship between research and meaning-making (Law & Urry, 2004). It has been argued that social phenomena can be captured only fleetingly in momentary stability because the research process aims to open space for the indefinite. Method, therefore, should be slow and uncertain: a risky and troubling process (Law, 2004).

Undoing the certainties created through methods has great salience in making sense of everyday family relationships (Gabb, 2009). Thematic analysis of different threads *across* the dataset can freeze the frame and conjure up a series of analytical snapshots of LGBT-parent families, but it is attentiveness to the subtle interplay of threads which crisscross the breadth and depth of data which evinces the *contingency* of lived lives. Meanings are produced through relational connections which shift as we twist the analytical kaleidoscope (McCarthy Ribbens, Holland, & Gillies, 2003, p. 19) and which shift again as different dimensions are brought into view. This dynamic mode of analysis is not designed to trace trends in family formation and networks of kin; this task is better suited to micro–macro, qualitative–quantitative analyses. Instead I suggest that a QMM approach is best suited to the examination of the materiality of LGBT-parent family lives, a messy process that inevitably produces loose ends. Leaving in methodological and emotional uncertainties is not analytical sloppiness rather it reflects the ephemera and flux of LGBT relationships across the life course.

References

Allen, K. R., & Demo, D. H. (1995). The families of lesbian and gay men: A new frontier in family research. *Journal of Marriage and the Family, 57*, 111–127. doi:10.2307/353821

Almack, K. (2008). Display work: Lesbian parent couples and their families of origin negotiating new kin relationships. *Sociology, 42*, 1183–1199. doi:10.1177/0038038508096940

Barrett, H., & Tasker, F. (2001). Growing up with a gay parent: Views of 101 gay fathers on their sons' and daughters' experiences. *Educational and Child Psychology, 18*, 62–77.

Biblarz, T. J., & Savci, E. (2010). Lesbian, gay, bisexual, and transgender families. *Journal of Marriage and Family, 72*, 480–497. doi:10.1111/j.1741-3737.2010.00714.x

Bryman, A. (2006). Editorial. *Qualitative Research, 6*, 5–7. doi:10.1177/1468794106058865

Budgeon, S., & Roseneil, S. (2004). Editors' introduction: Beyond the conventional family. *Current Sociology, 52*, 127–134. doi:10.1177/0011392104041797

Clark, A., & Moss, P. (2001). *Listening to young children: The mosaic approach*. Trowbridge, Wiltshire UK: National Children's Bureau.

Clarke, V. (2002). Sameness and difference in research on lesbian parenting. *Journal of Community & Applied Social Psychology, 12*, 210–222. doi:10.1002/casp.673

Clarke, V. (2006). "Gay men, gay men and more gay men": Traditional, liberal and critical perspectives on male role models in lesbian families. *Lesbian and Gay Psychology Review, 7*(1), 19–35.

Creswell, J. W., & Plano Clark, V. L. (2007). *Designing & conducting mixed methods research*. Thousand Oaks, CA: Sage.

Daly, K. J. (2007). *Qualitative methods for family studies and human development*. Thousand Oaks, CA: Sage.

Doucet, A. (2001). "You see the need perhaps more clearly than I have": Exploring gendered processes of domestic responsibility. *Journal of Family Issues, 22*, 328–348. doi:10.1177/019251301022003004

Dunn, J., & Deater-Deckard, K. (2001). *Children's views of their changing families*. York, UK: Joseph Rowntree Foundation.

Dunne, G. A. (1998). *Opting into motherhood: Blurring the boundaries and redefining the meaning of parenthood*. London: London School of Economics (No. 6).

Finch, J. (2007). Displaying families. *Sociology, 41*, 65–81. doi:10.1177/0038038507072284

Fineman, M. A. (1995). *The neutered mother, the sexual family, and other twentieth century tragedies*. New York: Routledge.

Gabb, J. (2001a). Desirous subjects and parental identities: Toward a radical theory on (lesbian) family sexuality. *Sexualities, 4*, 333–352. doi:10.1177/1363460010040030004

Gabb, J. (2001b). Querying the discourses of love: An analysis of contemporary patterns of love and the stratification of intimacy. *European Journal of Women's Studies, 8*, 313–328. doi:10.1177/135050680100800304

Gabb, J. (2004a). Critical differentials: Querying the contrarieties between research on lesbian parent families. *Sexualities, 7*, 171–187. doi:10.1177/1363460704042162

Gabb, J. (2004b). 'I could eat my baby to bits'; passion and desire in lesbian mother-children love. *Gender, Place, Culture, 11*, 399–415. doi:10.1080/0966369042000258703

Gabb, J. (2005a). Lesbian m/otherhood: Strategies of familial-linguistic management in lesbian parent families. *Sociology, 39,* 585–603. doi:10.1177/0038038505056025

Gabb, J. (2005b). Locating lesbian parent families. *Gender, Place, Culture, 12,* 419–432. doi:10.1080/09663690500356768

Gabb, J. (2008). *Researching intimacy in families.* Basingstoke, UK: Palgrave Macmillan. doi:10.1057/9780230227668

Gabb, J. (2009). Researching family relationships: A qualitative mixed methods approach. *Methodological Innovations Online, 4*(2), 37–52.

Gabb, J. (2010). Home truths: Ethical issues in family research. *Qualitative Research, 10,* 461–478. doi:10.1177/1468794110366807

Gabb, J. (2011a). Family lives and relational living: Taking account of otherness. *Sociological Research Online, 16*(4).

Gabb, J. (2011b). Troubling displays: The affect of gender, sexuality and class. In E. Dermott & J. Seymour (Eds.), *Displaying families* (pp. 38–60). Palgrave Macmillan: Basingstoke, UK.

Gillies, V. (2006). *Marginalised mothers. Exploring working class experiences of parenting.* London: Routledge.

Goldberg, A. E. (2010). *Lesbian and gay parents and their children: Research on the family life cycle.* Washington, DC: American Psychological Association. doi:10.1037/12055-000

Goldberg, A. E., & Allen, K. R. (2007). Lesbian mothers' ideas and intentions about male involvement across the transition to parenthood. *Journal of Marriage and Family, 69,* 352–365. doi:10.1111/j.1741-3737.2007.00370.x

Golombok, S. (2000). *Parenting - what really counts?* London: Routledge.

Green, A., & Preston, J. (2005). Editorial: Speaking in tongues - diversity in mixed methods research. *International Journal of Social Research Methodology, 8,* 167–171. doi:10.1080/13645570500154626

Harden, J., Scott, S., Backett-Milburn, K., & Jackson, S. (2000). Can't talk, won't talk?: Methodological issues in researching children. *Sociological Research Online, 5*(2). doi:10.5153/sro.486.

Hicks, S. (2005). Is gay parenting bad for kids? Responding to the 'very idea of difference' in research on lesbian and gay parents. *Sexualities, 8,* 153–168. doi:10.1177/1363460705050852

Hollway, W. (1997). The maternal bed. In W. Holloway & B. Featherstone (Eds.), *Mothering and ambivalence* (pp. 54–79). London: Routledge. doi:10.4324/9780203284018

Hollway, W., & Jefferson, T. (2000). *Doing qualitative research differently: Free association, narrative and the interview method.* Thousand Oaks, CA: Sage.

Jackson, S. (1982). *Childhood and sexuality.* Oxford, UK: Basil Blackwell.

James, A., & Prout, A. (Eds.). (1990). *Constructing and reconstructing childhood: Contemporary issues in the sociological study of childhood.* London: Falmer Press.

Jamieson, L. (2005). Boundaries of intimacy. In L. McKie & S. Cunningham-Burley (Eds.), *Families in society: Boundaries and relationships* (pp. 189–206). Bristol, UK: The Policy Press.

Jamieson, L., Morgan, D., Crow, G., & Allan, G. (2006). Friends, neighbours and distant partners: Extending or decentring family relationships? *Sociological Research Online, 11*(3). doi:10.5153/sro.1421

Kinkaid, J. (1998). *Erotic innocence.* Durham, N. C.: Duke University Press.

Laurenceau, J.-P., & Bolger, N. (2005). Using diary methods to study marital and family processes. *Journal of Family Psychology, 19,* 86–97. doi:10.1037/0893-3200.19.1.86

Law, J. (2004). *After method. Mess in social science research.* London: Routledge.

Law, J., & Urry, J. (2004). Enacting the social. *Economy and Society, 33,* 390–410. doi:10.1080/0308514042000225716

Layton, L. (2008). Editor's introduction to special issue on British psycho(−)social studies. *Psychoanalysis, Culture and Society, 13,* 339–340. doi:10.1057/pcs.2008.34

Malone, K., & Cleary, R. (2002). (de)sexing the family. Theorizing the social science of lesbian families. *Feminist Theory, 3,* 271–293. doi:10.1177/146470002762492006

Mason, J. (2006). Mixing methods in a qualitatively-driven way. *Qualitative Research, 6,* 9–25. doi:10.1177/1468794106058866

Mauthner, M. (1997). Methodological aspects of collecting data from children: Lessons from three research projects. *Children & Society, 11,* 16–28. doi:10.1111/j.1099-0860.1997.tb00003.x

McCarthy Ribbens, J., Holland, J., & Gillies, V. (2003). Multiple perspectives on the family lives of young people: Methodological and theoretical issues in case study research. *International Journal of Social Research Methodology, 6,* 1–23. doi:10.1080/13645570305052

Moran-Ellis, J., Alexander, V. D., Cronin, A., Dickinson, M., Fielding, J., Sleney, J., et al. (2006). Triangulation and integration: Processes, claims and implications. *Qualitative Research, 6,* 45–59. doi:10.1177/1468794106058870

Morgan, D. H. J. (1996). *Family connections: An introduction to family studies.* Cambridge: Cambridge, Polity Press.

Morrow, V. (1998). *Understanding families: Children's perspectives.* London: National Children's Bureau.

Nordqvist, P. (2011). Out of sight, out of mind. Family resemblances in lesbian donor conception. *Sociology, 44,* 1128–1144. doi:10.1177/0038038510381616

Patterson, C. (1992). Children of lesbian and gay parents. *Child Development, 63,* 1025–1042. doi:10.2307/1131517

Perlesz, A., Brown, R., Lindsay, J., McNair, R., De Vaus, D., & Pitts, M. (2006). Family in transition: Parents, children and grandparents in lesbian families give meaning to 'doing family'. *Journal of Family Therapy, 28,* 175–199. doi:10.1111/j.1467-6427.2006.00345.x

Phoenix, A., & Woollett, A. (1991). Motherhood: Meanings, practices, and ideologies. In A. Phoenix, A. Woollett, & E. Lloyd (Eds.), *Motherhood. Meanings, practices, and ideologies* (pp. 13–27). London: Sage.

Roseneil, S. (2006). The ambivalences of angel's 'arrangement': A psychosocial lens on the contemporary condition of personal life. *The Sociological Review, 54*, 847–869. doi:10.1111/j.1467-954X.2006.00674.x

Rust, P. C. R. (2001). Too many and not enough: The meanings of bisexual identities. *Journal of Bisexuality, 1*, 33–68.

Saffron, L. (1996). *What about the children? Sons and daughters of lesbians and gay men speak about their lives*. London: Cassell.

Schoenberg, N. E., & Ravdal, H. (2000). Using vignettes in awareness and attitudinal research. *International Journal of Social Research Methodology, 3*, 63–75. doi:10.1080/136455700294932

Silverman, D. (1996, July). *Telling it like it is: The interview in the interview society*. Paper presented to the International Sociology Association, University of Essex, UK.

Skeggs, B. (1997). *Formations of class and gender. Becoming respectable*. London: Sage.

Smart, C., & Neale, B. (1999). *Family fragments?* Cambridge: Polity Press.

Smith, A. M. (1992). Resisting the erasure of lesbian sexuality: A challenge for queer activism. In K. Plummer (Ed.), *Modern homosexualities. Fragments of lesbian and gay experience* (pp. 200–216). London: Routledge.

Stacey, J. (2002). Gay and lesbian families are here; all our families are queer; let's get used to it! In C. L. Williams & A. Stein (Eds.), *Sexuality and gender* (pp. 395–407). Cambridge, MA: Blackwell.

Stacey, J., & Biblarz, T. J. (2001). (How) does sexual orientation of parents matter? *American Sociological Review, 66*, 159–183. doi:10.2307/2657413

Tasker, F. L., & Golombok, S. (1997). *Growing up in a lesbian family. Effects on child development*. New York: Guilford.

Taylor, Y. (2009). *Lesbian and gay parenting: Securing social and educational capital*. Basingstoke, Palgrave Macmillan.

Valentine, G. (1996). (Re)negotiating the "heterosexual street". Lesbian productions of space. In N. Duncan (Ed.), *Body space. Destabilizing geographies of gender and sexuality* (pp. 146–155). London: Routledge.

Vincent, C., & Ball, S. J. (2006). *Childcare, choice and class practices*. London: Taylor & Francis.

Weeks, J. (1995). The body and sexuality. In The Polity Press (Ed.), *The Polity reader in gender studies* (pp. 235–239). Cambridge, UK: Polity Press. doi:10.4324/9780203167168

Weeks, J., Heaphy, B., & Donovan, C. (2001). *Same sex intimacies: Families of choice and other life experiments*. New York: Routledge.

Wengraf, T. (2001). *Qualitative research interviewing: Biographic narrative and semi-structured method*. London: Sage.

Wetherall, M., Taylor, S., & Yates, S. (2001). *Discourse theory and practice*. London: Sage.

Williams, F. (2004). *Rethinking families; Moral tales of parenting and step-parenting*. London, Calouste Gulbenkian Foundation.

22

Stephen T. Russell and Joel A. Muraco

The Use of Representative Data Sets to Study LGBT-Parent Families: Challenges, Advantages, and Opportunities

New understandings of LGBT-parent families have emerged in the last decade through the analysis of several important national or population-based data sources. Until recently, heterosexism in the social, health, and behavioral sciences rendered LGBT-parent families invisible in large-scale surveys of family life: There simply were no attempts to identify LGBT-parent families in studies of families and children. It was not until the 1990s that scholars, along with the general public, began to recognize LGBT-parent families as a legitimate family form that was not going to go away. The growing research literature on LGBT-parent families during the 1990s (see Goldberg, 2010) prompted the designers of large-scale family surveys to begin to consider non-heterosexual family forms. Thus, new possibilities emerged with, for example, the U.S. Census (Simmons & O'Connell, 2003) and the National Longitudinal Survey of Adolescent Health

(Add Health: e.g., Wainright, Russell, & Patterson, 2004), which began to include the possibility for respondents to identify same-sex partners in families and households.[1]

With the growing visibility of LGBT people, we may anticipate that a growing number of large-scale data sets in the USA and around the world will be extended to include attention to LGBT-parent families. These studies offer the potential to greatly advance our understandings of contemporary families. In this chapter we consider the use of large-scale secondary data sources (many of which are population-based and nationally or regionally representative) for the study of LGBT-parent families. We include a detailed list of large-scale secondary data sources in the Appendix at the end of this chapter. We also discuss the advantages and opportunities that such data sets offer, as well as the challenges that define working with secondary data on such an understudied and marginalized population.

In this chapter we consider several types of data sets that hold potential for the study of LGBT-parent families. First are population-based, representative surveys that may be local,

S.T. Russell, Ph.D. (✉) • J.A. Muraco, B.S.
Norton School of Family and Consumer Sciences,
University of Arizona, PO Box 210078,
650 N. Park Ave, Tucson, AZ 85721-0078, USA
e-mail: strussell@arizona.edu;
muraco@email.arizona.edu

---

[1] We use "LGBT-parent families" to be consistent with the nomenclature of this book, acknowledging the complexities of individual personal LGBT identities and experiences. As we describe in more detail later in this chapter, the data sets to which we refer often include measures of same-sex partnerships in households, and thus the personal sexual identities of household members are often unknown.

A.E. Goldberg and K.R. Allen (eds.), *LGBT-Parent Families: Innovations in Research and Implications for Practice*, DOI 10.1007/978-1-4614-4556-2_22, © Springer Science+Business Media New York 2013

regional, or national in scope, and typically are designed as samples that allow generalizations to the larger populations that they represent. Examples include the U.S. Census, which includes information on same-sex couple householders, or the Add Health study, which includes questions about young adult sexual identity and orientation as well as marital or family status. A second group of studies are large-scale cohort studies: The 1,970 British Cohort Study (BCS) and the 1958 National Child Development Study (NCDS) are unique in that the design of both studies includes a complete population (rather than a "sample" per se) at a given point in time (all births in 1 week, followed across childhood and into adulthood). Both studies ask respondents in adulthood about their marital (or marriage-like) relationships and household composition, including information about gender and how study members are related to other householders. Results from these studies are generalizable to similar age cohorts. A third group of studies are large scale but are not representative of or generalizable to a broader population. Nonrepresentative local, regional, or multisite samples that provide sufficient numbers of LGBT-parent families for study may not be specifically generalizable to a broader population, but may illuminate important associations or processes that characterize LGBT-parent family life. An example is the US National Longitudinal Lesbian Family Study (NLLFS). The Appendix includes examples of each of these types of data sets.

It is important to understand the potential of these data sources within the context of the body of existing research on LGBT-parent families. Historically, research on LGBT-parent families developed from and was grounded in a particular set of methodological approaches and disciplines. Early questions about child adjustment (with particular attention to sexual orientation, gender identity, and psychological adjustment) in LGBT-parent families emerged from the fields of psychology, child development, and family studies, fields that were already attuned to diverse family forms (Patterson, 1992). Further, studies based on small samples of distinct populations that are not population based were typical in those fields: Early studies were based largely on community

or regional samples (Patterson, 2006). These studies focused on child adjustment and the well-being of mothers, not only because these constructs were central in these fields but also because scholars were responding to fears that lesbians were mentally unwell and would therefore negatively influence their children (Goldberg, 2010). Over time, LGBT-parent research extended to include parenting, family processes, and the well-being of LGBT parents (Goldberg, 2010). As this body of work grew it attracted the attention of other fields of study relevant to families and children, including demography, sociology, economics, and health. Thus, beginning a decade ago a number of studies in these fields were among the first to provide a vantage point for understanding LGBT-parent families that was population based and generalizable to regions or countries and that allowed comparisons with heterosexual-parent families (see Biblarz & Savci, 2010, for a review).

Today there are a number of large-scale data sets available that afford the possibility of studying LGBT-parent families—but most have rarely or never been used for this purpose. Some nationally representative studies of families and households in the USA have begun to include questions about the LGBT identity status of adult householders, many of whom have children: The Survey of Income and Program Participation (SIPP); the Panel Study of Income Dynamics (PSID); and the U.S. Census. Other large-scale studies began as population-based, longitudinal studies of children: As the study members have grown up and been followed into adulthood, some have become LGBT parents themselves. For instance, it is possible with the Add Health study to follow those who reported same-sex attractions or relationships in adolescence into adulthood, affording the opportunity to study their coupling and parenting in adulthood. The prospective birth cohort studies such as the NCDS and the BCS make it possible to identify same-sex couple and parent households when cohort members are adults, but we know of few published studies that have capitalized on this opportunity. While the NCDS has been used, for example, to examine how family composition differences influence child well-being, published comparisons only include two-parent heterosexual families with single mother households (e.g., Joshi et al., 1999). Unpublished analyses of the BCS and NCDS have examined the associations between relationship type (same-sex cohabitating, opposite-sex cohabitating, and marriage) and relationship stability. Results indicate that same-sex cohabitators have higher rates of relationship dissolution than do opposite-sex cohabitating and married couples, with male same-sex couples having slightly higher dissolution rates than female same-sex couples (Strohm, 2011).

In this chapter we review findings based on some of these existing data sources while identifying challenges as well as advantages of using population-based representative data sets to study LGBT-parent families. Given the growing number of large-scale representative studies that now allow for the study of LGBT-parent families, we identify a number of areas of research that are largely understudied, but from which much could be learned in the coming years.

Challenges in Using Secondary Data to Study LGBT-Parent Families

There are a number of challenges in any research based on analyses of existing secondary data sources, some of which are further complicated in studies of LGBT-parent families. We consider challenges associated with conceptual breadth as well as measurement inclusion in existing studies. The use of secondary data is relatively new among researchers of LGBT-parent families, in part because relevant measures have only recently been included in secondary data sources, and also in part due to the origins of the study of LGBT-parent families in disciplines where secondary data analysis was less common. Thus, we also briefly review other basic challenges and suggest strategies to address these challenges.

Conceptual Challenges

At the most basic level, scholars who use secondary data sets must negotiate the discrepancies between their research question/s and available data (Hofferth, 2005; Russell & Matthews, 2011). Unless the researcher was directly involved with the data collection process, it is unlikely that full information will be available to address their precise questions. However, they may find that sufficient data exist to partially address their questions, or to allow an adjustment of the question based on available data. Most data sets that are focused on broad populations have been developed by economists and sociologists who may not be concerned with many of the constructs important to family studies scholars and psychologists (Russell & Matthews, 2011). Thus, the researcher undoubtedly will be required to be flexible with the conceptual design and creative in posing research questions that can be addressed with available data. At a fundamental level this is a conceptual problem, but one that typically plays out as problems with measurement (what is measured and how).

The most obvious example of this conceptual (and measurement) challenge is that most of what is known from nationally representative studies is based on families in same-sex couple households rather than couples or individuals who specifically identify themselves as lesbian, gay, bisexual, or transgender (measurement strategies to identify LGBT-parent families are presented with each data set in the Appendix). For example, the U.S. Census includes the option that a primary householder may report an "unmarried partner." There are no known examples of a single item question to ascertain LGBT-parent family status; rather, researchers must combine multiple questions to identify households with children in which the parent(s) are same-sex partners, householders, or engage in same-sex sexual practices or behaviors. Measures of self-identification as LGBT on large-scale surveys continue to be relatively rare; however, participant gender and the gender of their partner/s may be available (Gates & Romero, 2009). Of the 16 data sets included in the Appendix, only 7 include measures of self-reported sexual identity of parenting-aged adults: Add Health, the Behavioral Risk Factor Surveillance System (BRFSS; which varies by state), the National Health and Social Life Survey (NHSLS), the National Survey of Family Growth (NSFG), the California Health Interview Survey

(CHIS), the California Quality of Life Survey (CQLS), and the NLLFS.

Another conceptual challenge for using secondary data sources to study LGBT-parent families is that many of the important constructs in this field are LGBT specific and are unavailable in population-based studies. Thus, important questions specific to LGBT-parent families may be missing. For example: How and why do LGBT couples decide to have children? How do same-sex couples manage historically gendered parenting roles (Goldberg, 2010)? What is the impact of LGBT-specific minority stress (the experiences of stigma, prejudice, or discrimination due to LGBT status; Meyer, 2003) on parenting options, processes, and family life (Dudley et al., 2005)? These questions have been addressed using samples of LGBT-parent families, but not population-based samples. Given the low prevalence of LGBT people in the general population and pragmatic concerns for the cost of each item on large-scale survey (combined with pervasive heterosexism in science and sexual prejudice in the general public), it is unlikely that questions specific to LGBT populations will be included in population-based surveys. For example, one published study used the National Survey of Midlife Development in the United States (MIDUS) to show that discrimination partly explained compromised mental health among LGB adults (Mays & Cochran, 2001); however, the measure was a single item that included discrimination based on race, ethnicity, gender, age, religion, physical appearance, sexual orientation, or other reasons. Thus, although general minority stress was assessed in this population-based survey through questions about discrimination, the specific nature of the discrimination (as due to LGBT status versus some other personal characteristic) was unmeasured.

Overall, most of the research literature on LGBT-parent families concerns constructs that are generalizable to all populations: child adjustment, parent relationship quality, and parenting practices. Yet for questions about LGBT-specific dimensions of social or family life (e.g., LGBT-specific discrimination; method for becoming parents and related decision making), secondary data sources may simply not be suitable unless purposefully constructed to investigate such areas (e.g., the NLLFS). There is one important exception involving methodological innovation to study LGBT individual and families. Strohm, Seltzer, Cochran, and Mays (2009) used the CHIS sample to identify LGB participants who were then recontacted for participation in the CQLS. They selected all participants of the CHIS who reported their sexual identity as gay, lesbian, or bisexual, or as having had same-sex sexual activity and who agreed to participate in future surveys on the CHIS (Strohm et al., 2009). The CQLS included questions specific to LGBT individuals and families. Through this innovative strategy these researchers were able to identify a population-based sample of LGBT adults for in-depth study.

Measuring LGBT-Parent Families

In terms of measurement, there are a number of challenges specific to the availability of measures in secondary data sources. Research based on any one data source must be interpreted in light of other studies, yet there is variability across studies in the specific measures that can be used to identify LGBT-parent families. For example, several federally initiated surveys such as the BRFSS surveys are administered by states, and while some states have begun to include measures that would allow the study of LGBT individuals and thus LGBT-parents and families, the measures are not consistent across states.

Within the BRFSS, for example, Massachusetts is unusual because it includes measures since 2000 (some that differ across the years) for same-sex sexual behavior as well as sexual identity (whether one identifies as lesbian, gay, or bisexual); beginning in 2007, a measure for transgender identity was included (Behavioral Risk Factor Surveillance System, 2011). No one, to our knowledge, has used these data to examine LGBT-parent families. Other states have included either no measures or only a single measure of sexual identity or same-sex sexual behavior. Such variation limits comparisons to other states, and to studies published from other data sources, and thus limits conclusions regarding generalizability. Further, the inability to make valid comparisons prevents the study of how state characteristics—such as state laws, policies, and practices—affect LGBT-parent families.

There are also a number of measurement challenges particularly relevant for longitudinal studies of LGBT-parent families. Sometimes the measures used in prospective studies change over the span of the study (measures for young children will not be identical to those for adolescents and adults; Russell & Matthews, 2011). For repeated cross-sectional studies there are challenges when measures are changed. For example, the U.S. Census maintains that, as a result of flaws in the way they classified same-sex households in 1990,[2] the data from 1990 to 2000 cannot be compared (Smith & Gates, 2001). In addition to data errors that result from classifications, some argue that there has been notable change over only a few decades in sexual self-identity labels: Some individuals or couples may prefer, for example, the term "queer" to "gay" or "lesbian." The existing variability in measures across studies may only be compounded by changes over time in the ways that LGBT parents self-label and disclose their identities and family statuses to researchers.

There are well-known debates about the appropriate measurement of the multiple and distinct dimensions of sexual identity, orientation, and behavior (see Chandra, Mosher, Copen, & Sionean, 2011 for a review), as well as a growing body of research that points to fluidity or change in same-sex identities across adolescence and adulthood (Ott, Corliss, Wypij, Rosario, & Austin, 2010; Udry & Chantala, 2005). Family composition, as well, may change over time. Longitudinal studies will inevitably include participants who report change in the constructs that scholars hope to study, including LGBT identities, same-sex sexualities, and family composi-

tion. For example, "living apart together" or nonresidential partnerships are gaining visibility in Western countries (Strohm et al., 2009). As more studies add measures that allow for the study of LGBT family life, scholars will have to navigate differences between studies in available measures, potential differences in available measures across time within the same study, or changes over time in who qualifies as an LGBT-parent family. To our knowledge, no known study attempts such a complex undertaking regarding LGBT-parent families; however, demographers have utilized multiple data sources to examine characteristics of the gay and lesbian population. For example, Black, Gates, Sanders and Taylor (2000) used data from the General Social Survey (GSS), NHSLS, and the U.S. Census to examine geographical distribution, veteran status, family structure of the household, education, earnings, and wealth of the gay and lesbian population.

To address these challenges it is crucial at a most basic level to carefully sort out the opportunities and limitations of the match between one's research question and the data available through secondary sources. For example, one could use the National Health Interview Survey (NHIS) to examine same-sex couple household access to health care (the NHIS collects respondents' gender and the gender of others in the household and their relationship to the respondent). However, if one's theory of health-care access and utilization relies on arguments about homophobic discrimination in the health-care setting, the absence of data for householders' sexual identities is crucial. Clarity will help formulate a strong case for a study's rationale and ultimately for persuading reviewers that the opportunity the data afford outweighs any limitations. In the example above, it may be an important first step for the field to simply document differences in health-care access and utilization based on householder couple status. The researcher must be flexible and creative in matching the research question to available data (Russell & Matthews, 2011). In addition to the need for conceptual and analytic flexibility and creativity with regard to measurement, we turn to several other basic challenges and suggestions for addressing them.

---

[2]In the 1990 U.S. Census, when the responding householder identified two persons of the same sex as being spouses, or legally married, the Census Bureau administratively changed the reported gender of the spouse in most cases. Thus, same-sex couple households were undercounted, and reported as heterosexual married couple households.

Basic Challenges to Consider

There are several challenges that are basic to all research with secondary data sets. Becoming familiar with a large and complex existing data set is time consuming and researchers often overlook the "costs" of learning. One must understand a study's design, data structure, and distinct methodological characteristics that may influence analyses (Hofferth, 2005). Studies often employ complex sampling designs which require specialized statistical analytic techniques: Researchers may need to learn methods for adjusting for complex sample designs (e.g., nested samples or cluster designs), or methods for the use of weighted data responses (Russell & Matthews, 2011). There is a common perception that using existing data simply circumvents a data collection phase of research; however, recoding existing variables into useful constructs is time consuming (after 20 years of experience, the first author has found it necessary to estimate the time it will take, and multiple by four!). At the same time there are often opportunities for learning: Many large-scale studies have user groups or conferences designed to allow researchers to network with one another.[3] These networks offer possibilities for collaboration or the sharing of strategies for analysis, as well as for learning about others' questions and research efforts. Although when working with publicly available data there is a possibility of having one's idea "scooped" or taken, tested, and published before one is able to do so oneself, participating in scholarly networks of study users can keep one abreast of developments by other scholars in the field.

Finally, a unique challenge is potential professional costs. In many fields and at many institutions, original data collection may be more highly valued, partly because of the higher costs and thus larger extramural grants required to collect data. As institutions place greater demand on researchers to receive external funding it is important to acknowledge that grants for secondary data analyses tend to require less overall time and staff.

Advantages of Secondary Data for Studies of LGBT-Parent Families

Having discussed some of the challenges, we now describe the potential advantages of using large-scale or population-based secondary data sets for the study of LGBT-parent families. Important advantages include generalizability to broad populations, large sample sizes (including sufficient numbers of underrepresented populations and power for statistical analyses), and the ability to conduct comparative analyses with populations of heterosexual-parent families. Some data sources allow for additional advantages: They may be longitudinal, include data from multiple reporters, allow insights about multiple contexts and processes of development, or allow cross-historical or cross-national comparisons (Russell & Matthews, 2011). An obvious practical advantage is low cost and ease of access (Hofferth, 2005) compared to the labor-intensive work of sample selection and data collection to begin a new study of LGBT-parent families.

First, the possibility for making generalizations to broader populations of LGBT-parent families is a crucial advantage that can advance this field of study. For example, the 2000 U.S. Census counted 594,391 same-sex couples (Simmons & O'Connell, 2003); of those same-sex couples, about a quarter reported a child under the age of 18 living in their household (Gates & Ost, 2004). Never before had there been a true census of LGBT-parent families (or more accurately, households headed by parenting same-sex couples): For the first time researchers

---

[3]For example, Add Health offers a reference list with over 3,800 publications, presentations, unpublished manuscripts, and dissertations that use Add Health data. Add Health is not alone, with MIDUS, NCDS, and others offering similar databases. Add Health also offers user seminars, conferences, and meetings that take place at various times and locations throughout the year. Beginning in 2010, The National Conference on Health Statistics began offering hands-on and education sessions on the full range of data systems they offer including the NHIS and NSFG.

asserted that they had "identified same-sex couples in every state and virtually every county in the United States" (Sears, Gates, & Rubenstein, 2005, p. 1) and provided population estimates of the proportion of households headed by same-sex couples who are parenting in every state (the proportion of same-sex couples out of all households ranged from 27% to 80%). Notably, the same statistics have also been challenged because, with data only available for relationships among adult householders and thus on couples, it dramatically undercounts the total number of single LGBT people, and single LGBT-parent families in the USA. Yet these results have been groundbreaking for establishing the presence of these families for policy makers and planners. The results have also been instrumental in challenging stereotypes about LGBT-parent families—for example, that they are White, affluent, coastal, and urban. Indeed, these data have established that although same-sex couples without children are more likely to reside in California and Vermont, same-sex couples with children are more likely to reside in rural states (Mississippi, South Dakota, Alaska, South Carolina, and Louisiana; Gates & Ost, 2004). Yet California is where gay and lesbian adoptive and foster families are most likely to live (Gates, Badgett, Macomber, & Chambers, 2007). Further, African-American same-sex couples are more likely to include children compared to their White counterparts (Bennett & Gates, 2004; Black, Sanders, & Taylor, 2007; Carpenter & Gates, 2008).

Second, large sample sizes are beneficial because they allow for both the study of small and often marginalized subpopulations and statistical power for complex analyses (Russell & Matthews, 2011). Obviously, LGBT people and LGBT-parent families are present in all large-scale studies: The question is whether data are obtained to acknowledge them or whether they are invisible. Given their very small proportion within the total population, only huge studies will yield sufficient numbers of LGBT-parent families to allow for statistical analyses. For example, over 20,000 adolescents were included in the in-home portion of the Add Health study collected in 1994–1995; over 17,000 of their parents completed surveys. Wainright et al. (2004) were among the first investigators to use these data to investigate the well-being of adolescents growing up in same-sex parent households. They investigated psychosocial adjustment, school outcomes, and romantic relationships for 44 adolescents determined to be parented by same-sex couples based on parent reports of their gender and the gender of their partner (all were mothers; there were too few two-father families for inclusion in the study). Compared to a matched group of adolescents from heterosexual-parent families, no differences were found in adolescent adjustment (Wainright et al., 2004).

This study was the first of its kind based on a nationally representative sample to allow comparisons across family types, yet even with over 17,000 responding parents in that study only 44 adolescents parented by female same-sex couples were identified. It is important to note that these low numbers may also be explained by heteronormative assumptions in the design of the household measures in the original waves of the Add Health study that (a) did not ask the sexual orientation/identity of responding parents, (b) gave preference to female parents on the parent survey, and (c) precluded the possibility for adolescents to indicate on the adolescent-reported household roster that an adult living in the household could be the same-sex partner of a parent.

Add Health data have since been utilized for a number of studies examining children of mothers in same-sex couples. Wainright and Patterson (2006) found that regardless of family type, adolescents whose mothers described closer relationships with their children reported less delinquent behavior and substance use. Further, Wainright and Patterson (2008) found that regardless of family type, adolescents whose mothers described closer relationships with their children reported higher quality peer relations and more friends in school. These findings support the assertion that the quality of the parent–adolescent relationship better predicts adolescent outcomes than family type (Wainright & Patterson, 2006, 2008). Future studies should examine whether such findings remain true for children of male same-sex couples.

An additional benefit of very large samples is the possibility to study differences among LGBT-parent families based on race, ethnicity, age, and gender. Granted, perhaps the only data set large enough to make this possible is the U.S. Census. Gates and Romero (2009) report that African-American and Latina women in same-sex couples are more than twice as likely to be raising children as their White counterparts, and African-American and Latino men in such relationships are more than four times as likely to be raising children compared to their White counterparts (see also Bennett & Gates, 2004; Black et al., 2007; Carpenter & Gates, 2008). These findings are groundbreaking in identifying far more racial and ethnic diversity in LGBT-parent families than has been represented in the existing literature, because this literature has been largely derived from community-based samples of LGBT-identified parents of whom, until recently, consisted of primarily White lesbian mothers. As a result, these findings from the Census caution against generalizing from the existing literature to "all" LGBT-parent families.[4]

Another advantage to the use of population-based data sources is that some utilize longitudinal designs (Russell & Matthews, 2011). Some, like the GSS and the NHIS, collect data longitudinally by collecting representative data across time (but do not follow the same participants prospectively from year to year); few if any published studies based on these data have examined LGBT-parent families. Other data sets, such as Add Health, the NCDS and the BCS allow for the study of individuals across time so that hypotheses concerning human development and change can be explored. The members of the Add Health and both the NCDS and BCS cohorts are now adults or young adults, many of whom are becoming parents. These data sets offer unique opportunities to study characteristics from the early life course (childhood and adolescence) that may be associated with the well-being of LGBT adults and their children, or the adult lives of children

who were parented in same-sex households; again, we are aware of no studies that have taken this approach.

Other benefits of large-scale survey studies include reports from multiple reporters (children and parents), which allows for more than one perspective on family life. Finally, another potential advantage is the ability to conduct cross-historical or cross-national comparisons (Russell & Matthews, 2011). For example, a component of the GSS, the International Social Survey Program, was specifically developed to allow for cross-cultural comparisons between the USA, Australia, Great Britain, and West Germany. Such surveys may allow for future comparisons of LGBT-parent families across multiple countries.

Opportunities and Conclusions

There is a rich tradition of population-based survey research in the social and behavioral sciences that has provided a baseline for scientific and public understanding of the social and economic health and development of families, yet for generations, LGBT people and families have been invisible. Developments in recent decades have begun to change that. More large-scale surveys now include possibilities to identify, study, and understand LGBT-parent families. These developments come at the same time that many have begun to demand equal rights for LGBT people and families. Simultaneously, scholars are demanding both inclusion of LGBT people and families in research, as well as equal scientific rigor in the ways that LGBT families are studied. Large-scale representative studies are one path for building scientific understanding of LGBT-parent families. The Appendix includes descriptions of relevant data sources, some of which to our knowledge have never been used for the study of LGBT-parent families.

In addition to the challenges and opportunities we have discussed, we note some areas in the study of LGBT-parent families that have been particularly underexamined and for which the use of secondary data sources may provide important new possibilities. Gay fathers have

---

[4]We note that while this work advances understandings of the racial and gender diversity among LGBT-parent families, we still know little about social class differences.

been underrepresented in existing studies of LGBT-parent families. In 1990, 1 in 5 female same-sex couples were raising children compared to 1 in 20 male same-sex couples (Gates & Ost, 2004). By 2000, 1 in 3 female same-sex couples were raising children and 1 in 5 male same-sex couples were raising children (Gates & Ost, 2004). No data source is comparable to the NLLFS (Gartrell et al., 1996) for the study of male same-sex couples raising children. Although it is not population based and thus is not representative of all lesbian-parent families, it is a large sample that includes a birth mother and a co-mother with at least one child from whom data have been collected five times (before the child was born, and then when the child was 2, 5, 10, and 17). Results find, for example, that the development of psychological well-being in children of lesbian mothers over a 7-year period from childhood through adolescence is the same for those with known and unknown donors (Bos & Gartrell, 2010); no similar information exists about the children of gay fathers. As the number of LGBT-parent families (including both female and male same-sex couples raising children) continues to increase, more attention to gay-male parenting is warranted.

Further, there are few, if any, studies based on population-representative data sources that examine bisexual- or transgender-parent families (further, there are few existing studies of bisexual or transgender persons and family life in general; examples are discussed in other chapters of this book). Large-scale population-based data sets are a strategic place to look to find samples large enough for studies of bisexual and transgender people and families. Of the sources included in the Appendix, the BRFSS (select states), BCS, and the NCDS include measures that allow identification of transgender people. Even these sources are largely untapped: They could afford unprecedented opportunities for scholarship. Lastly, little is known about LGBT-parent families and socioeconomic status; much of the existing research focuses on middle-class LGBT-parent families. Population-based data sets such as the NHSLS, the GSS, the U.S. Census, and the ACS

allow for studies of same-sex headed households and their socioeconomic status.

In conclusion, we have identified challenges as well as opportunities for scholars who may pursue the study of LGBT-parent families through analysis of secondary data sources or large-scale surveys. There are many new possibilities for the study of LGBT-parent families (and even more possibilities to study LGBT individuals). To date, findings from such studies have been groundbreaking. Not only have they demonstrated, for example, that child and family well-being does not differ in LGBT-parent and heterosexual-parent families (Wainright & Patterson, 2006, 2008; Wainright et al., 2004); they have dispelled myths about who LGBT-parents are and where they live (Gates & Ost, 2004; Gates & Romero, 2009), and have shown simply—yet radically—that LGBT-parent families are everywhere (Simmons & O'Connell, 2003). There are remarkable possibilities waiting in these data sources—opportunities to propel the field of LGBT-parent families—and thus our understanding of all contemporary families—forward.

Acknowledgments The authors acknowledge support for this research from the Fitch Nesbitt Endowment of the Norton School of Family and Consumer Sciences, the Frances McClelland Institute for Children, Youth, and Families.

Appendix: Secondary Data Opportunities

American Community Survey (ACS, 2010)
Population: Representative of U.S. population.
Measure for LGBT-parent family: Combination of gender of participant, gender of others living in household, and type of relationship between participant and others living in household.
Parent Data: Demographic, financial, housing, and economic data.
Child Data: Assesses if children are in the home and their ages.
Parenting Data: Not applicable.

Description: Started in 2000, the yearly ACS mimics the decennial Population and Housing Census (commonly referred to as the U.S. Census), but rather than show the number of people who live in the USA the ACS shows how people live, with the goal of proportioning of funds for services.

Behavioral Risk Factor Surveillance System (BRFSS, 2010)

Population: Representative at state level.

Measure: Varies by state: sexual orientation; transgender status.

Parent Data: Demographic, health behaviors, and contextual factors (varies by state).

Child Data: If children live in household and demographics (varies by state).

Parenting Data: Assesses care giving to individuals (including children) with health problems, long-term illnesses, or disabilities, and the following vary by state: childhood asthma prevalence, childhood immunization, and child Human Papilloma Virus.

Description: The BRFSS is a state-based system of health surveys that tracks health conditions and risk behaviors in the USA on a monthly basis by telephone in all 50 states, the District of Columbia, Puerto Rico, the U.S. Virgin Islands, and Guam; approximately 350,000 adults are included annually.

British Cohort Study (BCS)

Population: All infants ($N = 17,200$) born during a 1 week period in England, Scotland, Wales, and Northern Ireland in April 1970.

Measure: Combination of sex of respondent, marital status, sex of individuals living in household, and relationship between household members, and sex change status.

Parent Data: Demographics, physical health, mental health, drug and alcohol use, attitudes and beliefs, and economic development.

Child Data: Demographic.

Parenting Data: How often children see the other parent if parents are divorced, type of relationship child has with each member of the household.

Description: Six follow-up surveys, and plan for 2012; Initial survey data from midwives and information from clinical records; data have

also been collected from parents, teachers, school health services, and participants in subsequent waves. One wave included daily diary reports.

Relevant Reference: Strohm (2011).

California Health Interview Survey: Adult (CHIS, 2011)

Population: Representative of the state of California.

Measure: Gender of sexual partners, sexual orientation, and type of partnership assessed.

Parent Data: Demographic and health topics are primarily assessed. Topics cover health conditions, health behaviors, general health, disabilities, sexual health, women's health, mental health, and health insurance.

Child Data: Demographics and health insurance.

Parenting Data: Not applicable.

Description: The CHIS is a random-dial telephone survey conducted every 2 years. Each round more than 50,000 California residents, including adults, teenagers, and children, are surveyed. The sample is extensive enough to be statistically representative of California's diverse population.

Relevant Reference: Carpenter & Gates (2008).

California Quality of Life Survey (Cal-QOS)

Population: Gay, lesbian, and bisexual individuals in the state of California.

Measure: Data collected from the CHIS was used which assessed gender of sexual partners, sexual orientation, and type of partnership.

Parent Data: Demographic and health topics are primarily assessed. Topics cover health conditions, health behaviors, general health, disabilities, sexual health, women's health, mental health, and health insurance.

Child Data: Demographics and health insurance.

Parenting Data: Not applicable.

Description: The Cal-QOS was a follow-up survey to the CHIS. Participants who reported a gay, lesbian, or bisexual identity or same-sex sexual activity and who agreed to participate in future surveys on the CHIS were reinterviewed. Additionally, as a heterosexual comparison group, a random sample of remaining 18–70 year olds was also reinterviewed. Of those contacted, 56% were successfully reinterviewed 6–18 months after they were contacted.

Relevant Reference: Strohm et al. (2009).

General Social Survey (GSS, 2010)

Population: Representative of U.S. population.

Measure: Sexual behavior can be assessed in older data (1972–1988); same-sex relationships can be addressed in newer data (1988–present).

Parent Data: Demographics, attitudes, and behaviors.

Child Data: Demographic.

Parenting Data: Extensive data on parenting attitudes and behaviors.

Description: The GSS is unique in its aim to "take the pulse of America" through data on opinions and beliefs, and the ability to conduct comparisons with other nations. Sample sizes range from 1,500 to 3,000 each year.

Relevant References: Black et al. (2000, 2007); Strohm et al., (2009).

The National Survey of Midlife Development in the United States (MIDUS)

Population: Over 7,000 Americans aged 25–74.

Measure: Sexual orientation assessed via a single item measure.

Parent Data: Primarily concerned with physical and mental health, including medical history, history or risk behaviors, work history, and demographics.

Child Data: Demographic.

Parenting Data: General feelings about relationship with children and how children affected their work situation.

Description: MIDUS began in 1994 with the intention of investigating the role of behavioral psychological and social factors in understanding age-related differences in physical and mental health. Data collection for the second wave began in 2004 and was completed in 2009. The second wave provides follow-up data on the psychosocial, sociodemographic, health, daily diary data collected at the first wave as well as new data including cognitive assessments, biomarker assessments (subsample), and neuroscience assessments (subsample).

Relevant Reference: Mays and Cochran (2001).

National Child Development Study (NCDS)

Population: All infants ($N = 17,500$) born during a 1 week period in England, Scotland, and Wales in March 1958.

Measure: Combination of sex of respondent, marital status, sex of individuals living in household, and relationship between household members; sex change status.

Parent Data: Demographic, physical health, mental health, drug and alcohol use, attitudes and beliefs, and economic development.

Child Data: Demographic.

Parenting Data: How often children see the other parent if parents are divorced, type of relationship child has with each member of the household.

Description: The NCDS included an interview and medical assessment of mothers during the week of birth and eight follow-up surveys regarding physical, educational, social, and economic development across the life span. Like the BCS early waves included multiple informants and school and medical records. In subsequent waves data when cohort members were adults, data were collected from partners and children.

Relevant Reference: Strohm (2011).

National Health and Social Life Survey (NHSLS, 2010)

Population: Approximately 2,500 adults, aged 18–44, from two middle-sized metropolitan areas.

Measure: Combination of gender of participant and gender of others they have cohabitated with longer than 1 month (cohabitation defined by sexual relationship), attraction, and identification.

Parent Data: Demographic, sexual practices, sexual histories, pregnancies, drug and alcohol use, physical health, attitudes.

Child Data: Demographic.

Parenting Data: Not applicable.

Description: The aim of NHSLS is to investigate social organization of sexual behavior, including identifying a full range of sexual behaviors and examining patterns associated with specific types of partnerships and attitudes.

Relevant References: Black et al. (2000, 2007)

National Health Interview Survey (NHIS, 2010)

Population: Representative of U.S. population.

Measure: Combination of gender of participant, gender of others living in household, and type of relationship between participant and others living in household.

Parent Data: Demographic, health conditions, insurance, access to health care and utilization, and health behaviors.

Child Data: Child health status and limitations.

Parenting Data: Child access to health care and utilization.

Description: The purpose of the NHIS is to monitor the health of the U.S. population; approximately 36,000 households are included annually.

National Longitudinal Study of Adolescent Health (Add Health, 2010)

Population: Representative of U.S. population.

Measure: Sexual behaviors, romantic attractions, and orientation assessed (most recent wave).

Parent Data: Demographic, social, economic, psychological, and physical well-being, contextual data on the family, neighborhood, community, school, friendships, peer groups, and romantic relationships.

Child Data: Demographics and health.

Parenting Data: Parent–child relationship, general feelings about being parent.

Description: Add Health began with a representative sample of over 12,000 adolescents in grades 7–12 and has since followed them into young adulthood. The most recent wave of data was collected in 2008 with an in-home interview of the now 24–32-year-old participants and includes biological data. Add Health offers data on respondent's social, economic, psychological, and physical well-being with contextual data on the family, neighborhood, community, school, friendships, peer groups, and romantic relationships.

Relevant References: Wainright and Patterson (2006, 2008), Wainright et al. (2004).

National Survey of Family Growth (NSFG, 2011)

Population: Prior to 2002, the sample was representative of women 15–44 living in the USA. Starting with the sixth wave in 2002, the population became representative of all people 15–44 living in the USA.

Measure: Sexual behavior, sexual attraction, and sexual identity are assessed.

Parent Data: Demographics and health.

Child Data: Demographics.

Parenting Data: Family life, marriage and divorce, infertility, use of contraception.

Description: Began in 1973, NSFG only surveyed women. During this period, five waves of data were collected. Starting with the sixth wave, in 2002, men were included. A seventh wave of data was collected in 2010.

Relevant Reference: Chandra et al. (2011).

Survey of Income and Program Participation (2010)

Population: Representative of U.S. population.

Measure: Combination of gender of participant, gender of others living in household, and type of relationship between participant and others living in household.

Parent Data: Demographics, poverty, income, employment, work experience, program participation, transfer income, asset income, and health coverage.

Child Data: Within topic module children's well-being is assessed.

Parenting Data: Within topic module child care, family activities, rules governing TV viewing, and quality of the neighborhood are assessed.

Description: SIPP provides detailed information on respondent's income and program participation, principal determinants of income and program participation, detailed information on various forms of income, and data on taxes, assets, liabilities, and participation in government transfer programs.

United States Census (2010)

Population: Representative of U.S. population.

Measure: Combination of gender of participant, gender of others living in household, and type of relationship between participant and others living in household.

Parent Data: Demographics.

Child Data: Demographics.

Parenting Data: Not applicable.

Description: The U.S. Population and Housing Census is collected every 10 years while the Economic Census and Census of Governments are conducted every 5 years. The Population and Housing Census offers the most comprehensive estimates of the number of LGBT-families living in the country.

Relevant References: Bennett and Gates (2004), Black et al. (2000), Gates and Ost (2004), Gates and Romero (2009), Gates et al. (2007), Sears et al. (2005), Simmons and O'Connell (2003), and Smith and Gates (2001).

U.S. National Longitudinal Lesbian Family Study (NLLFS, 2010)

Population: Recruitment occurred in Boston, Washington, DC, and San Francisco.

Measure: Self-identified as lesbian.

Parent Data: Demographics, parental relationships, social supports, pregnancy motivations and preferences, stigmatization, and coping.

Child Data: Peer and school contexts, socialization, externalizing problem behavior, and well-being.

Parenting Data: Family dynamics, parent–child relationship.

Description: The NLLFS follows a cohort of nearly 70 planned lesbian families with the goal of examining the social, psychological, and emotional development of the children, and the dynamics of planned lesbian families.

Relevant References: Bos & Gartrell (2010), Gartrell et al. (1996).

Welfare, Children, & Families: A Three-City Study (WCF, 2010)

Population: Low income families in Boston, Chicago, and San Antonio.

Measure: Combination of gender of participant, gender of others living in household, and type of relationship between participant and others living in household.

Parent Data: Demographics, self-esteem/self-concept, family routines, home environment, welfare participation, health and disability, illegal activities, and domestic violence.

Child Data: Behavior checklist, schooling, delinquency, and ages and stages (younger children).

Parenting Data: Parenting styles, farther involvement, parent–child relationships (older children), and parental monitoring.

Description: The WCF assesses the well-being of low income children and families in the Boston, Chicago, and San Antonio areas.

References

American Community Survey. (2010). Retrieved from http://www.census.gov/acs/www/

Behavioral Risk Factor Surveillance System. (2010). *About the BRFSS.* Retrieved from http://www.cdc.gov/brfss/

Behavioral Risk Factor Surveillance System. (2011). *State-added question database.* Retrieved from https://www.ark.org/adh_brfss_questions/results.aspx

Bennett, L., & Gates, G. J. (2004). The cost of marriage inequality to children and their same-sex parents. *Report.* Washington, DC: Human Rights Campaign Foundation. Retrieved from http://www.hrc.org/costkids/pdf

Biblarz, T. J., & Savci, E. (2010). Lesbian, gay, bisexual, and transgender families. *Journal of Marriage and Family, 72,* 480–497. doi:10.1111/j.1741-3737.2010.00714.x

Black, D., Gates, G. J., Sanders, S., & Taylor, L. (2000). Demographics of the gay and lesbian population in the United States: Evidence from available systematic data sources. *Demography, 37,* 139–154. doi:10.2307/2648117

Black, D. A., Sanders, S. G., & Taylor, L. J. (2007). The economics of lesbian and gay families. *Journal of Economic Perspectives, 21*(2), 53–70.

Bos, H. M. W., & Gartrell, N. K. (2010). Adolescents of the US National Longitudinal Lesbian Family Study: The impact of having a known or an unknown donor on the stability of psychological adjustment. *Human Reproduction, 26,* 630–637. doi:10.1093/humrep/deq359

California Health Interview Survey. (2011). Retrieved from http://www.chis.ucla.edu/about.html

Carpenter, C., & Gates, G. (2008). Gay and lesbian partnerships: Evidence from California. *Demography, 45,* 573–590. doi:10.1353/dem.0.0014

Chandra, A., Mosher, W. D., Copen, C., & Sionean, C. (2011). Sexual behavior, sexual attraction, and sexual identity in the United States: Data from the 2006–2008 National Survey of Family Growth. *National Health Statistics Reports, 36.* Retrieved from http://www.cdc.gov/nchs/data/nhsr/nhsr036.pdf

Dudley, M. J., Rostosky, S. S., Riggle, E. D. B., Duhigg, J., Brodnicki, C., & Couch, R. (2005). Same-sex couples' experiences with homonegativity. *Journal of GLBT Family Studies, 1,* 68–93. doi:10.1300/J461v01n04_04

Gartrell, N., Hamilton, J., Banks, A., Mosbacher, D., Reed, N., Sparks, C. H., & Bishop, H. (1996). The national lesbian family study: 1. Interviews with prospective mothers. *American Journal of Orthopsychiatry, 66,* 272–281. doi:10.1037/h0080178

Gates, G. J., Badgett, M. V. L., Macomber, J. E., & Chambers, K. (2007). *Adoption and foster care by gay and lesbian parents in the United States.* Los Angeles, CA: The Williams Project on Sexual Orientation Law and Public Policy, UCLA School of Law. Retrieved from http://escholarship.org/uc/item/2v4528cx

Gates, G. J., & Ost, J. (2004). *The gay and lesbian atlas.* Washington, DC: Urban Institute

Gates, G. J., & Romero, A. (2009). Parenting by gay men and lesbians: Beyond the current research. In E. Peters & C. M. Kamp Dush (Eds.), *Marriage and family: Perspectives and complexities* (pp. 227–246). New York, NY: Columbia University Press

General Social Survey. (2010). *About GSS.* Retrieved from http://www.norc.org/GSS+Website/About+GSS/

Goldberg, A. E. (2010). *Lesbian and gay parents and their children: Research on the family life cycle.* Washington, DC: American Psychological Association.

Hofferth, S. L. (2005). Secondary data analysis in family research. *Journal of Marriage and Family, 67,* 891–907. doi:10.1111/j.1741-3737.2005.00182.x

Joshi, H., Cooksey, E. C., Wiggins, R. D., McCulloch, A., Verropoulou, G., & Clarke, L. (1999). Diverse family living situations and child development: A multilevel analysis comparing longitudinal evidence from Britain and the United States. *International Journal of Law, Policy and the Family, 13,* 292–314. doi:10.1093/lawfam/13.3.292

Mays, V. M., & Cochran, S. D. (2001). Mental health correlates of perceived discrimination among lesbian, gay, and bisexual adults in the United States. *American Journal of Public Health, 91,* 1869–1876.

Meyer, I. H. (2003). Prejudice, social stress, and mental health in lesbian, gay, and bisexual populations: Conceptual issues and research evidence. *Psychological Bulletin, 129,* 674–697. doi:10.1037/0033-2909.129.5.674

National Health and Social Life Survey. (2010). *Abstract.* Retrieved from http://popcenter.uchicago.edu/data/nhsls.shtml

National Health Interview Study. (2010). *About the National Health Interview Survey.* Retrieved from http://www.cdc.gov/nchs/nhis/about_nhis.htm

National Longitudinal Lesbian Family Study. (2010). *About.* Retrieved from http://www.nllfs.org/about/

National Longitudinal Study of Adolescent Health. (2010). *About Add Health.* Retrieved from http://www.cpc.unc.edu/projects/addhealth/about

National Survey of Family Growth. (2011). Retrieved from http://www.cdc.gov/nchs/nsfg.htm

Ott, M. Q., Corliss, H. L., Wypij, D., Rosario, M., & Austin, S. B. (2010). Stability and change in self-reported sexual orientation identity in young people: Application of mobility metrics. *Archives of Sexual Behavior, 40,* 519–532. doi:10.1007/s10508-010-9691-3

Patterson, C. J. (1992). Children of lesbian and gay parents. *Child Development, 63,* 1025–1042.

Patterson, C. J. (2006). Children of lesbian and gay parents. *Current Directions in Psychological Science, 15,* 241–244. doi:10.1111/j.1467-8721.2006.00444.x

Russell, S. T., & Matthews, E. (2011). Using secondary data to study adolescence and adolescent development. In K. Trzesniewki, M. B. Donnellan, & R. E. Lucas (Eds.), *Obtaining and analyzing secondary data: Methods and illustrations* (pp. 163–176). Washington, DC: American Psychological Association.

Sears, R. B., Gates, G., & Rubenstein, W. B. (2005). *Same-sex couples and same-sex couples raising children in the United States: Data from Census 2000.* Los Angeles, CA: The Williams Project on Sexual Orientation Law and Public Policy, UCLA School of Law. Retrieved from http://www.law.ucla.edu/Williamsinstitute/publications/USReport.pdf

Simmons, T., & O'Connell, M. (2003). Married-couple and unmarried-couple households: 2000, *Census 2000 Special Reports.* Washington, DC: U.S. Census Bureau

Smith, D. M., & Gates, G. J. (2001). Gay and lesbian families in the United States: Same-sex unmarried partner households. *A Human Rights Campaign Report.* Washington, DC. Retrieved from http://www.urban.org/url.cfm?ID=1000494

Strohm, C. Q. (2011). *The stability of same-sex cohabitation, different-sex cohabitation, and marriage* (Report No. PWP-CCPR-2010-013). Retrieved from California Center for Population Research Website: http://papers.ccpr.ucla.edu/papers/

Strohm, C. Q., Seltzer, J. A., Cochran, S. D., & Mays, V. M. (2009). "Living apart together" relationships in the United States. *Demographic Research, 21,* 177–214. doi:10.4054/DemRes.2009.21.7.

Survey of Income and Program Participation. (2010). *Introduction to SIPP.* Retrieved from http://www.census.gov/sipp/intro.html

Udry, J. R., & Chantala, K. (2005). Risk factors differ according to same-sex and opposite-sex interest. *Journal of Biosocial Science, 37,* 481–497. doi:10.1017/S0021932004006765

United States Census. (2010). Retrieved from http://2010.census.gov/2010census/index.php

Wainright, J. L., & Patterson, C. J. (2006). Delinquency, victimization, and drug, tobacco, and alcohol use among adolescents with female same-sex parents. *Journal of Family Psychology, 20,* 526–530. doi:10.1037/0893-3200.20.3.526

Wainright, J. L., & Patterson, C. (2008). Peer relations among adolescents with female same-sex parents. *Developmental Psychology, 44,* 117–126. doi:10.1037/0012-1649.44.1.117

Wainright, J. L., Russell, S. T., & Patterson, C. (2004). Psychosocial adjustment, school outcomes, and romantic attractions of adolescents with same-sex parents. *Child Development, 75,* 1886–1898. doi:10.1111/j1467-8624.2004.00823.x

Welfare, Children, & Families: A Three City Study (2010). *Home.* Retrieved from http://web.jhu.edu/threecitystudy/index.html

Part V
Conclusion

Abbie E. Goldberg and Katherine R. Allen

Thirty years ago, the publication of a book like *LGBT-Parent Families: Innovations in Research and Implications for Practice* would not have been conceivable. The fact that such a book now exists, and with such compelling contributions, is an indication of how far the field has progressed. Beginning with the pioneering and innovative scholarship of Larry Kurdek on same-sex couples; Jerry Bigner and Frederick Bozett on gay fathers; Martha Kirkpatrick, Susan Golombok, and Charlotte Patterson on lesbian mothers; and other key scholars, the scholarship on LGBT families has become increasingly prolific and more complex.

Building upon the foundations of this earlier work on LGBT couples and families, as well as the shifting social norms that have allowed new access into hard-to-find populations, scholars have begun to imagine—and explore in depth—the intricacies and diversity inherent in LGBT-parent families. Increasing research attention, for example, is now being paid to LGBT-parent families of color, as well as the role of social class and gender in LGBT-parent

families' experiences. Research has exploded into understudied and truly innovative topics, such as the experiences of youth with LGBT parents who also identify as LGBT, the experiences of LGBT grandparents, and the experiences of LGBT-parent families living in non-Western cultures. Research and practice associated with these topics, and many others, form the basis of this book. In what follows, we revisit the question that guided our vision for each chapter—What do we, and what do we not, know regarding the field of LGBT-parent families?—in the context of the major themes that emerge throughout the volume. We conclude with our assessment of the future of research, theory, and praxis on LGBT parenting, addressing, as well, the value of interdisciplinary and intergenerational collaboration in LGBT family scholarship.

Major Substantive Issues in LGBT-Parent Research: What Have We Learned?

The overview chapters in this volume addressed the major research areas that have been generated over the past three decades. These chapters use a comparative and historical lens to trace the evolution of each of these research areas. Notably, these chapters focus largely on lesbian-mother families, given the relative paucity of work on gay fathering. Chapters 1 and 2 on lesbian-mother families formed post-heterosexual divorce and intentional lesbian-mother families, respectively,

A.E. Goldberg, Ph.D.(✉)
Department of Psychology, Clark University,
950 Main Street, Worcester, MA 01610, USA
e-mail: agoldberg@clarku.edu

K.R. Allen, Ph.D.
Department of Human Development,
Virginia Polytechnic Institute & State University,
401C Wallace Hall (0416), Blacksburg, VA 24061, USA
e-mail: kallen@vt.edu

A.E. Goldberg and K.R. Allen (eds.), *LGBT-Parent Families: Innovations in Research and Implications for Practice*, DOI 10.1007/978-1-4614-4556-2_23, © Springer Science+Business Media New York 2013

most sharply illuminate a major shift in the field: Whereas early research was largely conducted on lesbian mothers postdivorce, the current wave of studies has focused on two-mother families formed after the women come out. Yet, it is important to emphasize that studies of lesbian mothers parenting post-heterosexual divorce—as well as lesbian mother step-families—are still a key part of the landscape of LGBT-parent families, insomuch as some women will inevitably continue to come out and form same-sex relationships post-heterosexual divorce. A question for future research is how the experiences of contemporary women differ from past cohorts of lesbians parenting post-heterosexual divorce. Another question is whether it will be less relevant and meaningful to focus on "coming out" as a discrete and one-time transition. Sexual orientation can be fairly fluid across the life course, particularly for certain subgroups of women (Diamond, 2008). Given new research into fluidity in sexual identities over the life course (Diamond, 2008), and the diverse ways in which women form partnerships and parent with other women, regardless of previous relationship history (Moore, 2011), it is increasingly important to incorporate an understanding of and attention to sexual fluidity in research on lesbian and gay parenting.

As Bos describes in Chapter 2, lesbian-mother families formed through alternative insemination, although a relatively "new" family form, have been the focus of considerable research in the past two decades. This focus is appropriate and warranted, given advancements in reproductive technology (see Chapter 5 as well), and the increased social acceptance of lesbian motherhood. It is notable that, despite being a relatively new area of research, lesbian-mother families formed through insemination are already being studied in several different cultural contexts, and several cross-national comparative studies have been initiated. Yet, as Bos points out, the groups being studied continue to be middle-class to upper-middle-class, White lesbians. In part, this sampling issue may reflect that fewer working-class and racial minority lesbians pursue insemination, as compared to other routes (e.g., adoption, conceiving via heterosexual sex), as emphasized in Chapter 4 by Mezey on deciding to become

parents or remain childfree and in Chapter 9 by Moore and Brainer on race and ethnicity in the lives of sexual minority parents and their children. Indeed, Moore and Brainer point out that middle-class and upper-middle-class White lesbians who support an egalitarian feminism are the most likely to be able to afford insemination; working-class and racial/ethnic minority women, correspondingly, often pursue other methods. Thus, new research should not aim to simply include more racial and social class diversity in studies of lesbians who pursue insemination, but, rather, should look within groups (e.g., working-class lesbians; Black lesbians; Latina lesbians) to see what parenting routes are most common.

Chapter 3 on adoptive families reveals how an even newer research area has taken shape. As a research area still in its infancy, research questions abound regarding lesbian and gay adoptive family formation and experiences. Indeed, lesbian and gay adoptive families are uniquely distinguished by the fact that neither parent is biologically related to her/his child; parents may be of a different race (and potentially culture) than their child; birth parents may be symbolically and/or physically present in the child's (and adoptive parents') lives. Of great interest is how family members navigate these diverse issues as they develop. How do they define themselves, develop over time, and nourish their relationships in a broader context that defines families as heterosexual and biologically related?

Further, reflective of its status as a relatively new research area, most of the research on lesbian and gay adoptive families is on lesbian mothers. Gay adoptive fathers are beginning to be studied, although, like lesbian mothers, the samples that have been investigated to date tend to be middle-class and upper-middle-class and White. Yet, U.S. Census data reveal that gay adoptive mothers and fathers are much more racially diverse than existing research has captured: 61% of male same-sex couples with adopted children and 77% of female same-sex couples are racial minorities (Gates, Badgett, Macomber, & Chambers, 2007). Scholars need to become more attentive to this diversity to better understand the multiplicative stresses and strengths that characterize these families.

Themes in Understudied Research Areas: What Are We Learning?

The understudied topic chapters provide insights into "new" research areas and raise a number of exciting questions for future work. Several themes are evident across these chapters, demonstrating the progress that scholars have made in advancing knowledge about LGBT-parent families. Making such inroads into new territory is a long-awaited desire that is now being fulfilled. Over the past several decades, for example, scholars have championed the need to implement the theory of intersectionality into actual research (Crenshaw, 1991; Lorde, 1984); emphasized the need for empirical research to augment personal narratives of parenting experiences (Pollack & Vaughn, 1987); and called for scholars to clarify and elaborate how to define LGBT identities within families (i.e., to get beyond the lesbian and gay family nomenclature) (Allen & Demo, 1995). Many of these early hopes are being fulfilled with answers to the complex dilemmas and questions that inaugurated the field. We now turn to overarching themes in how the understudied topics in this volume are expanding the knowledge in LGBT-parent family research.

Intersectionality

Nearly all of the authors in this volume address the issue of samples restricted to White, middle-class and upper-middle-class lesbians and gay men. But in this book, there are new inroads into expanding knowledge into unchartered territory, in the form of investigations that link sexual orientation diversity with gender, race, class, place, nationality, and other axes of stratification, oppression, and privilege.

In Chapters 9 and 14, the examination of Western non-White lesbians reveals the limitations of concepts such as "same-sex parenting." Indeed, as these chapters point out, much more expansion is needed beyond the Western world (e.g., to indigenous cultures, non-White cultures), so that individualistic conceptualizations of gender and sexual orientation in the construction of family relationships are critiqued and thus expanded. In many non-Western cultures, it is clear that same-sex sexual behavior is not synonymous with a homosexual or bisexual orientation; a woman may marry another woman, have sexual relations with her, pass on inheritance rights to the children she bears, but not be defined as a lesbian. Hicks, in Chapter 10, also critiques the reified concepts of gender role and identity that have informed much of the recent theory and research regarding LGBT parenting, thus demonstrating the relevance of a social constructionist perspective on the fluidity of the categories of gender and sexual orientation. The challenge for researchers is not to be constrained by Western notions of homosexuality, coupling, and parenthood, and to expand the depth and breadth of inquiry beyond these constructs, when studying issues related to "same-sex parenting" in non-Western cultures.

Many authors also emphasize the need for more critical attention and insight into the multiple contexts that shape LGBT people's lives. For example, one's immediate community context, and the broader legal context (e.g., at the state and federal level) may powerfully influence the experiences of LGBT-parent family members, as Oswald and Holman (Chapter 13) point out. Likewise, one's experience at work can be instrumental in shaping one's experience at home and vice versa; indeed, the workplace is an understudied context in the lives of LGBT people and parents, as King, Huffman, and Peddie (Chapter 15) describe. The chapters in this volume also bring together scholarship that demonstrates the intersectionality of rural, working-class LGBT-parent families, whose experiences are often not captured in current research, and yet, like many lesbian and gay men of color, are often engaged in parenting (e.g., Moore & Brainer; Oswald & Holman).

Intergenerational Relationships in Families

All of the chapters that address understudied topics provide some new insight into intergenerational relationships in families that extend a narrow way of viewing family beyond the nuclear family model. Beginning with the way that families are formed, Mezey in Chapter 4 highlights the class-inscribed nature of lesbian women's decision making about parenthood. Further, her research raises intriguing questions about the need to differentiate between motivation to parent and motivation to be pregnant, and the multiplicative forces and contexts that may influence decision making about both pregnancy and parenting.

Along the lines of the nuances of parenting motivations and decision making, Berkowitz (Chapter 5) advances current scholarship by focusing on gay fathers who decide to have biological children. Granted, surrogacy is the province of highly educated and economically well off, primarily White men, given the often prohibitive cost; but, the phenomenon raises new questions about the nature of nuclear families, and the relative importance of gender versus biology in creating a family.

Chapter 11 on second-generation LGBT persons, Chapter 8 on parents and children in polyamorous parent families, and Chapter 12 on LGBT grandparenting further illustrate the importance of attending to intergenerational relationships within LGBT-parent families. As Kuvalanka reveals, the meaning and experience of being LGBT changes from generation to generation; therefore, adolescents or young adults who identify as LGBT may not necessarily feel as though their LGBT parent(s) fully understand or can relate to their experience. Indeed, one question this chapter raises is the reality that each new generation brings new meanings to defining LGBT identity. Do "labels" have the same meaning for the current generation? Do they "matter" in the same way that they have for previous generations (Russell, Clarke, & Clary, 2009)? Likewise, Pallotta-Chiarolli and colleagues demonstrate the sensitivity that polyamorous parents must have when considering their children's relationships to individuals and institutions outside the immediate social environment. Of interest is the degree to which parents' and children's concerns intersect or overlap—for example, do parents and children share similar types of concerns about privacy and protecting their families? Do children "take their cue" from their parents in terms of their attitudes and practices related to

disclosure of their families? Finally, Chapter 12 on LGBT grandparenting highlights how a family member's identification as LGBT may affect family members of different generations in different ways: that is, one's child and one's grandchild will likely respond to and experience one's lesbianism in different ways. Much more research is needed that examines these intergenerational relationships, and of course, greater attention needs to be paid to the experiences and familial roles of gay grandfathers, as well as bisexual and transgender grandparents.

Making Bisexual and Transgender-Parent Families Visible

One of the most important contributions of this volume is the current assessment of research and theory about bisexuality and transgender parenting, thus, as Biblarz and Savci (2010) note, loosening the B and T from L and G. The invisibility of the "B" and the "T" in LGBT is taken on by Ross and Dobinson (Chapter 6) and Downing (Chapter 7), respectively. These authors highlight the limitations of the LGBT umbrella to capture the full range of experiences of bisexual and trans parents, and the need for future research to more explicitly and systematically study these populations—especially given the practical and theoretical utility of examining these groups. Ross and Dobinson, for example, point out that bisexual parenting challenges scholars to think more carefully about the research methods used to obtain and define samples (e.g., members of same-sex couples may be lesbian or bisexual; members of heterosexual couples may be heterosexual or bisexual). Downing, on the other hand, shows how transgender parenting has challenged the field not just substantively but also theoretically, in terms of the social construction of gender and sexual orientation. Both, together, point to the emergence of new conceptualizations about identity: for example, Ross introduces the notion of trans bisexual people, thereby complicating static notions of gender identity, gender, and sexual orientation—complexities which need to be addressed in depth in future research.

Research Methods: What Have We Learned?

With increased interest in LGBT families, many methodological questions have arisen, leading to possibilities and challenges in how studies are framed and in the quality of data that are collected. Several chapters in this volume address methodological innovations and new strategies for studying LGBT-parent families.

As Gabb (Chapter 21) demonstrates, the richness of in-depth, small-scale samples are demonstrated in what can be learned through the complex data collection methods allowed by qualitative research paradigms. These "deep" accounts and insights are only possible when using the creative kinds of approaches that Gabb describes, and are still so necessary when investigating understudied populations or not yet understood populations. Indeed, it is no coincidence that many of the chapters about understudied research rely heavily on data collected through qualitative methods; gaining insight into little explored phenomena such as the experiences of LGBT children with LGBT parents, or the experiences of transgender-parent families, requires methods that allow for flexibility, nuance, and depth.

Yet at the same time, new quantitative methods are also emerging that hold exciting promise for capturing the complexity in LGBT-parent families. For example, Smith, Sayer, and Goldberg (Chapter 20) outline a range of exciting and innovative approaches to handling various statistical issues that arise in studying LGBT couples and families. And yet, the continued challenge facing the field is that these methods are often not taught in graduate programs, and workshops that teach statistical methods such as multilevel modeling are expensive and still not widely available. More widespread training and knowledge of these methods is necessary, in that it will help to eliminate or decrease the "file drawer problem" whereby studies that use less-than-ideal methods to analyze data from same-sex couples and families are rejected or simply not submitted to top- and middle-tier journals in the field.

A different methodological challenge was raised by Russell and Muraco. They emphasize that large-scale population-based data sets can be mined to answer questions related to same-sex couples and parenting; yet, measures of sexual orientation are inconsistent across surveys and often do not capture all dimensions of sexuality (e.g., attraction, behavior, identity), thus limiting the ability to answer questions of interest. At the same time, the bigger challenge is perhaps not the limitations of these data sets but the reality that these data sets have not, as of yet, been sufficiently utilized to analyze data relevant to same-sex couples and families. Perhaps scholars who study LGBT couples and families but who lack familiarity with these data sets can partner with scholars who have expertise in working with these data sets. Such collaborations have the capacity to be mutually fulfilling and productive.

Applications: What Have We Learned?

The implications and applications of research on LGBT-parent families matter. The series of cutting edge clinical and applied chapters in this volume address the role of therapists and educators in the lives of today's LGBT-parent families. These chapters (namely, Chapters 16, 17, and 18) highlight key issues for researchers to attend to in their work, which are salient in the lives of LGBT-parent families. For example, Chapter 16 highlights the new "normativity" of family building for sexual minorities, which may change the focus of therapy from "can we become parents?" to "when, with whom, and how will we become parents?" Chapter 17 raises the issue that there may be more than two "parents" in LGBT-parent families, a reality that may need to be negotiated and renegotiated in the clinical context at various points during the parenting life cycle. The clinical issues that are raised in these chapters bring light to the new opportunities and challenges posed in this "brave new world" of LGBT family building (Stacey, 1990).

The applied chapters also offer a number of practical "tools" to assist LGBT-parent families and their advocates in navigating the varied settings in which they live their lives. For example, as Byard and Kosciw point out, schools play an important role in the lives of LGBT family members, and there are increasingly a large number of resources to help schools create inclusive environments for families, as well as resources for LGBT family members wishing to advocate for their families. Likewise, Shapiro provides knowledge and resources that can assist LGBT-parent families in navigating the ever-complex legal climate. As evident in Telingator's and Lev and Sennott's case studies, it is important for practitioners who work with LGBT-parent families to allow children to define their complex families from their own frame of reference, a perspective that might differ from their primary set of parents.

Conclusion

The research on LGBT-parent families is diverse in terms of approach and method. Although we, and many of the volume's contributors, have pointed to the need to gain more representative samples, we do not wish to send the message that we regard this as the hallmark of success or the most important goal for future research. Rather, we should embrace a diversity of approaches and types of knowledge, valuing, and not ghettoizing, qualitative research and small samples. We take the approach that both qualitative and quantitative approaches are important, and that both small and large samples are valuable. Different methods capture different levels and types of family complexity, and yield different insights.

As this volume has documented, the field of LGBT-parent families has grown significantly over the past several decades. What does the future hold, then? What new questions are on the horizon? Do we continue to build on, even replicate, the foundation of studies that we have built; or do we begin to ask new questions, going into uncharted territories, and exploring the "messiness" of families' lives?

Indeed, there are many messy, but altogether exciting and innovative, questions that scholars can, and perhaps should, be asking and addressing, at this point in time. For example, there are new data showing that when intentional lesbian mother families split up, children often report feeling closer to, and often reside with, their biological mother (Gartrell, Bos, Peyser,

Deck, & Rodas, 2011). Certainly, the uneven legal terrain for biological versus social mothers has implications for these dynamics. But, perhaps scholars should also be probing how societal notions about biology play into these post-dissolution dynamics. How and why do children prefer the biological mother over the social mother, in some cases? Similarly, studies could more closely probe and investigate parents' reasons for seeking biological parenthood. Do some women want to be pregnant because they understand it will allow them greater "power" in a situation where the couple breaks up?

Another interesting and somewhat related question is the degree to which, and the ways in which, gender identity may influence decision making about pregnancy. For example, to what extent do masculine or butch-identified sexual minority women shy away from becoming pregnant because it is dissonant with their gender identity; and, under what conditions do they pursue pregnancy? Additionally, how might pregnancy change or alter a butch-identified woman's sense of gender identity and identity in general? Indeed, Epstein (2002) argued that butch-identified lesbian mothers in general—and those who are pregnant in particular—reconfigure what it means to be butch and broaden the range, depth, and meaning of the butch experience.

These and other interesting and provocative questions may be avoided, however, because of concerns about how the pursuit of such questions, and the data that are obtained, might be viewed by both "insiders" (other scholars who study LGBT-parent families) and "outsiders" (i.e., antigay politicians and researchers). That is, "pro-gay family" scholars and activists may be concerned about how the telling of such stories may be used to discriminate against LGBT-parent families, and the "antigay family" camp may indeed use controversial data to argue against LGBT rights. But our perspective is that we cannot avoid wading into these deeper waters—otherwise, we come to a polarized standstill whereby the field cannot move forward with telling the more complicated and nuanced stories with our data, thus demonstrating the inherent complexity of people's lives. In turn, many of the benefits of studying people, where they are—benefits that include adding to the body of empirical science and improving policy and education—are lost.

Finally, a pressing and related question that remains, and which should continue to dominate scholars' thinking as they pursue their research in this area, is: Who are we doing this research *for*? Some scholars likely believe that scholarship on LGBT-parent families should be driven by a desire or goal to improve marginalized peoples' lives. But, is there no room for basic research in this area—research that is not "activist" in nature but which is aimed to explore, for example, whether theories of human development or family processes can be applied to, and hold up in, LGBT-parent families? We argue for an inclusive approach, whereby diverse approaches and goals are respected, emphasizing a healthy science that is tempered by a concern for the outcomes of real people's lives.

Indeed, it is notable that many of the chapters share a common theme of highlighting what the understudied population under investigation wants us to know about them. By asking understudied and marginalized populations such as these what they want scholars, practitioners, policymakers, and the lay public to know about them, researchers communicate a respect and curiosity for the group's experiences, as well as possibly generating more meaningful and innovative data. For example, what does it really mean to be a daughter of working-class lesbian parents in a school where most of the other children have more affluent parents? That is, in what ways does being from a lesbian-parent family, alongside of social class disadvantages and other forms of discrimination, "disadvantage" a child's experience and position with her peers? We encourage researchers to continue to ask their participants what they believe are the most relevant issues in their lives, and what is important for scholars, policymakers, and the lay public to know about them.

We can imagine a future where these competing discourses can actually live side by side. We can imagine scientific collaborations among and between people who embody these diverse discourses, who can, together, produce richer

knowledge that helps us to understand what is actually going on in people's lives. We can imagine application of this research to a wide range of settings, including educational, therapeutic, and policy arenas. As we look ahead to the future, we are excited by the innovations and possibilities that are emerging, and we welcome both new and seasoned scholars to help define the path that lies before us.

References

Allen, K. R., & Demo, D. H. (1995). The families of lesbian and gay men: A new frontier in family research. *Journal of Marriage and the Family, 57*, 111–127. doi:10.2307/353821

Biblarz, T. J., & Savci, E. (2010). Lesbian, gay, bisexual, and transgender families. *Journal of Marriage and Family, 72*, 480–497. doi:10.1111/j.1741-3737. 2010.00714.x

Crenshaw, K. (1991). Mapping the margins: Intersectionality, identity politics, and violence against women of color. *Stanford Law Review, 43*, 1241–1299. doi:10.2307/1229039

Diamond, L. (2008). *Sexual fluidity: Understanding women's love and desire*. Cambridge, MA: Harvard University Press.

Epstein, R. (2002). Butches with babies: Reconfiguring gender and motherhood. *Journal of Lesbian Studies, 6*, 41–57. doi:10.1300/J155v06n02_06

Gartrell, N., Bos, H., Peyser, H., Deck, A., & Rodas, C. (2011). Family characteristics, custody arrangements, and adolescent psychological well-being after lesbian mothers break up. *Family Relations, 60*, 572–585. doi:10.1111/j.1741-3729.2011.00667.x

Gates, G., Badgett, M. V. L., Macomber, J. E., & Chambers, K. (2007). *Adoption and foster care by gay and lesbian parents in the United States*. Washington, DC: The Urban Institute.

Lorde, A. (1984). Age, race, class, and sex: Women redefining difference. In A. Lorde (Ed.), *Sister outsider: Essays and speeches* (pp. 114–123). Freedom, CA: The Crossing Press.

Moore, M. (2011). *Invisible families: Gay identities, relationships, and motherhood among Black women*. Berkeley, CA: University of California Press.

Pollack, S., & Vaughn, J. (Eds.). (1987). *Politics of the heart: A lesbian parenting anthology*. Ithaca, NY: Firebrand Books.

Russell, S. T., Clarke, T. J., & Clary, J. (2009). Are teens "post-gay"? Contemporary adolescents' sexual identity labels. *Journal of Youth and Adolescence, 38*, 884–890. doi:10.1007/s10964-008-9388-2

Stacey, J. (1990). *Brave new families: Stories of domestic upheaval in late twentieth century America*. New York: Basic Books.

Index

A

Actor–partner interdependence model, 313
Adolescents, 7, 8, 25–27, 30, 32, 33, 47, 49, 50, 108,
        111, 120, 127, 163, 218, 243, 255, 261–273,
        327, 343, 347, 349, 354, 362
Adoption, 11, 21, 39, 60, 71, 93, 109, 135, 150, 182, 197,
        211, 227, 242, 263, 291, 308, 360
Adoptive families, 39–42, 46–52, 360
Advocacy, 100, 137, 168, 214, 254, 275–289, 302
Africa, 142, 210, 211, 217–221
African-American LGBT families, 211
Aging, 80, 177, 178, 184, 187, 188, 304
Alternative insemination, 138, 154, 310, 360
American Indian Two-Spirit parents, 138
ART. *See* Assisted reproductive technology (ART)
Asian/Pacific Islander LGBT families, 134, 136–137
Assisted reproductive technology (ART), 73, 219, 298

B

Bias, 26, 27, 32, 44, 68, 145, 241, 245, 246, 261,
        275–279, 282, 284, 288
Biographical narrative interviews, 326, 334
Biological mothers, 27, 28, 215, 216, 245, 310,
        311, 364
Biological relatedness, 27, 71, 76, 83
Biphobia, 96
Bisexual, 7, 22, 44, 60, 87, 105, 117, 133, 149, 163, 177,
        193, 209, 225, 241, 261, 275, 325, 345, 361
Bisexuality, 88, 89, 91–93, 96–98, 101, 117, 124, 149,
        184, 362
Border dwellers, 120

C

Case studies, 113, 143, 213, 220, 328, 333, 339
Child
    adjustment, 344, 346
    custody, 6, 89, 90, 98, 109, 123, 292
    welfare, 44, 51, 88, 98, 246
Childfree, 59–69, 360
Childless, 59–69, 360

Childrearing

Childrearing, 33, 79, 138, 140, 144, 150, 241, 256
Children, 3, 21, 39, 59, 71, 93, 105, 117, 133, 149, 163,
        177, 193, 209–221, 227, 241, 261–273, 275,
        291, 310, 325, 343, 360
Chunde T women, 143
Citizenship, 67, 136, 137, 142, 145, 146, 197, 202, 242
Clinical practice, 137, 142
Clinical work, 241–257, 261–273
Clinicians, 4, 14, 72, 81, 83, 111, 187, 242, 256, 257,
        261, 262, 267, 271
Cohort studies, 344
Collaborative parenting, 125
Coming out, 4, 7–9, 12, 14–16, 21, 33, 47, 62, 63, 71, 88,
        96, 97, 105, 107–109, 113, 122, 163, 164,
        167–169, 172, 173, 178, 179, 184–189, 194,
        242–244, 248–250, 252, 253, 255, 261, 266,
        267, 270–272, 334, 360
Communication privacy management (CPM), 121
Community climate, 196–197, 201, 203, 204, 279
Community programs and social services, 123
Comparative analysis, 348
Co-parent, 9, 23, 48, 83, 110, 135, 153, 216, 245, 291,
        302–304
Coworkers, 50, 202, 225, 229–231
CPM. *See* Communication privacy
        management (CPM)
Cross-cultural, 6, 209, 211, 212, 249, 350
Culture, 62, 92, 117, 119, 126–129, 139–142, 144, 153,
        165, 169, 171, 179, 180, 183, 185, 187, 188,
        209–211, 214, 216, 218–220, 228, 229, 243,
        244, 246, 251, 273, 359–361

D

Datasets, 321, 339, 340
Decision-making, 27–28, 59, 60, 64, 66–69, 71, 184,
        252, 267, 271, 279, 280, 303, 326, 338
De facto parent, 300–303
De facto parentage, 302
Dependency, in data, 309–312, 319
Developmental outcomes, 5, 6, 16
Diaries, 154, 326, 327, 335–337

Lightning Source UK Ltd.
Milton Keynes UK
UKHW052022230220
359168UK00009B/469